REOPERATIVE ABDOMINAL SURGERY

REOPERATIVE ABDOMINAL SURGERY

EDITED BY

Solly Mizrahi, MD, FACS
Professor of Surgery and Transplantation
Chairman, Department of Surgery A
Soroka Medical Center
Faculty of Health Sciences
Ben-Gurion University of the Negev
Beer Sheva
Israel

Hiram C. Polk Jr., MD
Professor of Surgery Emeritus
Department of Surgery
University of Louisville
Louisville, Kentucky
USA

Petachia Reissman, MD, FACS
Associate Professor of Surgery
Chairman, Department of Surgery
Shaare – Zedek Medical Center
The Hebrew University School of Medicine
Jerusalem
Israel

JP medical publishers

London • Philadelphia • Panama City • New Delhi

Published by JP Medical Ltd, 83 Victoria Street, London, SW1H 0HW, UK
Tel: +44 (0)20 3170 8910 Fax: +44 (0)20 3008 6180
Email: info@jpmedpub.com Web: www.jpmedpub.com

ISBN: 978-1-907816-55-0

British Library Cataloguing in Publication Data
A catalogue record for this book is available from the British Library

Library of Congress Cataloging in Publication Data
A catalog record for this book is available from the Library of Congress

Publisher: Geoff Greenwood
Development Editors: Gavin Smith
Design: Designers Collective Ltd

Typeset, indexed, printed and bound in India.

Preface

Our decision to produce a comprehensive textbook on reoperative abdominal surgery was driven by the limited availability of literature devoted to the postoperative considerations and clinical decisions required of the surgeon when rescuing deteriorating patients. Moreover, the truncated training times for resident and trainee surgeons today make a book like this one more valuable than ever before.

In assembling a team of authors to prepare chapters we invited experienced surgeons with the ability to communicate clearly and provide the best possible surgical advice. We are delighted by the various qualities - judgment, wisdom and maturity – that all our authors have brought to the content. Anatomic and technical experience is evident in every chapter, as is the emphasis on the importance of involving patients, their families, and the entire surgical team in the management process.

No textbook can hope to cover every possible clinical eventuality. So we acknowledge that this book cannot provide guidance on every possible reoperative problem associated with the abdomen that will ever be encountered. However, we firmly believe that *Reoperative Abdominal Surgery* achieves our original goals of providing solid, reliable advice to all surgeons involved in this area of care and of ensuring the safety of their patients.

Solly Mizrahi
Hiram C. Polk, Jr.
Petachia Reissman

Contents

Preface v

Contributors ix

Dedications xiii

Chapter 1
Orientation to reoperative surgery with an emphasis on communication and safety 1
Hiram C. Polk, Jr.

Chapter 2
The ethical legal implications of reoperative surgery 3
Rosalind Cordini, Beth Hendrickson McMasters

Chapter 3
The broad view of reoperative surgery 9
Thilo Hackert, Markus W. Büchler

Chapter 4
Anesthetic considerations 19
Stuart Bertsch, Rainer Lenhardt, Ozan Akca

Chapter 5
Reoperative surgery for abdominal wall infection and intra-abdominal abscess 29
Donald E. Fry

Chapter 6
The modern approach to the open abdomen and abdominal compartment syndrome 37
William P. Schecter, Asher Hirshberg

Chapter 7
Laparoscopic reoperative surgery after open and laparoscopic abdominal operations 47
Petachia Reissman, Yair Edden

Chapter 8
Resuscitation and intervention for postoperative hemorrhage after abdominal surgery 59
Ronald V. Maier, Scott C. Brakenridge

Chapter 9
Reoperative surgery in trauma 71
Joyce I. Kaufman, Howard M. Lieberman, Mauricio Lynn

Chapter 10
Urgent reoperative vascular surgery 83
Jessica L. Secor, K. Craig Kent

Chapter 11
Postoperative intestinal anastomotic leak and enterocutaneous fistula 91
Solly Mizrahi

Chapter 12
Reoperation for open and laparoscopic groin hernia 95
Shahzad M. Ali, David R. Farley

Chapter 13
Repair of the recurrent ventral hernia 101
Alla Zemlyak, Paul D. Colavita, B. Todd Heniford

Chapter 14
Reoperative bariatric surgery 109
Yaniv Cozacov, Raul Rosenthal

Chapter 15
Reoperations for pancreatic surgery complications 121
Mitsugi Shimoda, Keiichi Kubota

Chapter 16
Reoperative liver surgery 129
Myron E. Schwartz, Parissa Tabrizian, Sasan Roayaie

Chapter 17
Reoperations for complications of biliary tract surgery 137
Kristina V. Spate, Michael H. Bahr, Gary C. Vitale

Chapter 18
Reoperations after abdominal organ transplants 149
Christoph E. Broelsch, G. Felix Broelsch

Chapter 19
Reoperative surgery for chronic inflammatory bowel disease 159
Fabrizio Michelassi, Léon Maggiori

Chapter 20
Reoperative management of acute and chronic small and large bowel stoma complications 171
Susan Galandiuk

Chapter 21
Surgical management of *Clostridium difficile* colitis 177
P. Ronan O'Connell, Olivier Gié

Chapter 22
Reoperative abdominal surgery for chronic vascular events 185
Peter Lamont

Chapter 23
Surgery for recurrent small bowel obstruction 193
Herbert R. Freund

Chapter 24
The surgical approach to acute and chronic complications of radiation injury and chemotherapy 197
Sandra L. Wong, Khaled S. Hafez

Chapter 25
The approach to reoperations in the geriatric population 205
Paul J. Speicher, Sandhya A. Lagoo-Deenadayalan

Index 211

Contributors

Ozan Akca, MD, FCCM
Associate Professor of Anesthesiology and Perioperative Medicine
Department of Anesthesiology and Perioperative Medicine
University of Louisville
Louisville, Kentucky
USA

Shahzad M. Ali, MD
General Surgery Resident (PGY 2)
Division of Gastrointestinal and General Surgery
Mayo Clinic
Rochester, Minnesota
USA

Michael H. Bahr, MD
Assistant Professor of Surgery
Department of Surgery
University of Louisville
Louisville, Kentucky
USA

Stuart Bertsch, MD
Chief Resident
Department of Anesthesiology and Perioperative Medicine
University of Louisville
Louisville, Kentucky
USA

Scott C. Brakenridge, MD, MSCS
Assistant Professor of Surgery and Anesthesiology
Division of Acute Care Surgery
Department of Surgery
University of Florida Health Science Center
Gainesville, Florida
USA

Christoph E. Broelsch, MD, PhD
Professor Emeritus of Surgery
Duesseldorf
Germany

G. Felix Broelsch, MD
Resident, Department of Plastic, Hand and Reconstructive Surgery
Hannover Medical School
Hannover
Germany

Markus W. Büchler, MD
Professor and Chairman
Department of Surgery
University of Heidelberg
Heidelberg
Germany

Paul D. Colavita, MD
General Surgery Resident
Department of General Surgery
Carolinas Medical Center
Charlotte, North Carolina
USA

Rosalind Cordini, RN, MSN, JD
Attorney
Healthcare Service Team
Wyatt, Tarrant & Combs, LLP
Louisville, Kentucky
USA

Yaniv Cozacov, MD
Clinical Research Fellow, Surgery
Metabolic and Bariatric Institute, Section of Minimally Invasive Surgery
Cleveland Clinic Florida
Weston, Florida
USA

Yair Edden, MD
Colorectal Surgeon
Residency Program Director
Department of General Surgery
Shaare Zedek Medical Center
The Hebrew University School of Medicine
Jerusalem
Israel

David R. Farley, MD
Professor of Surgery
Department of Surgery
Mayo Clinic
Rochester, Minnesota
USA

Herbert R. Freund, MD
Professor of Surgery (Emeritus) and Chief Of Surgery (Emeritus)
Hadassah-Hebrew University Medical Center
Jerusalem
Israel

Donald E. Fry, MD
Adjunct Professor of Surgery
Department of Surgery
Northwestern University Feinberg School of Medicine
Chicago, Illinois
Emeritus Professor of Surgery
Department of Surgery
University of New Mexico School of Medicine
Albuquerque, New Mexico
USA

Susan Galandiuk, MD, FACS, FASCRS
Professor of Surgery
Director, Price Institute of Surgical Research
Department of Surgery
University of Louisville School of Medicine
Louisville, Kentucky
USA

Olivier Gié, MD
Department of Visceral Surgery
CHUV – Lausanne
Switzerland

Thilo Hackert, MD
Consultant Surgeon
Department of Surgery
University of Heidelberg
Heidelberg
Germany

Khaled S. Hafez, MD
Associate Professor of Urology
Department of Urology
University of Michigan
Ann Arbor, Michigan
USA

B. Todd Heniford, MD
Professor of Surgery
Chief, Division of Gastrointestinal and Minimally Invasive Surgery
Department of General Surgery
Division of Gastrointestinal and Minimally Invasive Surgery
Carolinas Medical Center
Charlotte, North Carolina
USA

Asher Hirshberg, MD, FACS
Director, Emergency Vascular Surgery
Department of Surgery
Kings County Hospital Center
Brooklyn, New York
USA

Joyce I. Kaufman, MD
Trauma Surgery and Surgical Critical Care Fellow
Jackson Memorial Hospital Ryder Trauma Center
Miami, Florida
USA

K. Craig Kent, MD
A. R. Curreri Professor and Chairman, Department of Surgery
University of Wisconsin School of Medicine and Public Health
Madison, Wisconsin
USA

Keiichi Kubota, MD, PhD
Professor of General Surgery and Hepato-Biliary-Pancreas Surgery
Second Department of Surgery
Dokkyo Medical University
Mibu, Tochigi
Japan

Sandhya A. Lagoo-Deenadayalan, MD, PhD
Associate Professor
Senior Fellow, Center for Aging
Division of General and Advanced GI Surgery
Department of Surgery
Duke University Medical Center
Durham, North Carolina
USA

Peter Lamont, MD, FRCS, FEBVS, FFSTEd
Consultant Vascular Surgeon
Department of Vascular Surgery
Bristol Royal Infirmary
University Hospitals Bristol
Bristol
UK

Howard M. Lieberman, MD, MS
Assistant Professor of Surgery
University of Miami Miller School of Medicine
DeWitt Daughtry Family Department of Surgery
Division of Trauma Surgery and Critical Care
Miami, Florida
USA

Rainer Lenhardt, MD, MBA
Associate Professor of Anesthesiology and Critical Care
Department of Anesthesiology and Perioperative Medicine
University of Louisville
Louisville, Kentucky
USA

Mauricio Lynn, MD
Professor of Surgery
University of Miami Miller School of Medicine
DeWitt Daughtry Family Department of Surgery
Division of Trauma Surgery and Critical Care
Miami, Florida
USA

Léon Maggiori, MD
Assistant Professor of Surgery
Department of Colorectal Surgery
Pôle des Maladies de l'Appareil Digestif (PMAD)
Beaujon Hospital, Assistance publique-Hôpitaux de Paris (AP-HP)
University Denis Diderot (Paris VII)
Clichy, France

Ronald V. Maier, MD
Professor of Surgery
Division of Trauma, Burn and Critical Care
Department of Surgery
University of Washington
Seattle, Washington
USA

Beth Hendrickson McMasters, BSN, JD
Managing Partner
McMasters Keith Butler, Inc.
Louisville, Kentucky
USA

Fabrizio Michelassi, MD
Lewis Atterbury Stimson Professor of Surgery
Chairman, Department of Surgery
Surgeon-in-Chief
Department of Surgery
New York-Presbyterian Weill Cornell Medical Center
New York, New York
USA

Solly Mizrahi, MD, FACS
Professor of Surgery and Transplantation
Chairman, Department of Surgery A
Soroka Medical Center
Faculty of Health Sciences
Ben-Gurion University of the Negev
Beer sheva
Israel

P. Ronan O'Connell, MD, FRCSI, FRCS(Glas)
Professor of Surgery
School of Medicine and Medical Sciences
University College Dublin
Centre for Colorectal Disease
St Vincent's University Hospital
Dublin
Ireland

Hiram C. Polk, Jr., MD
Professor of Surgery Emeritus
Department of Surgery
University of Louisville
Louisville, Kentucky
USA

Petachia Reissman, MD, FACS
Associate Professor of Surgery
Chairman, Department of Surgery
Shaare – Zedek Medical Center
The Hebrew University School of Medicine
Jerusalem
Israel

Sasan Roayaie, MD
Chief, Hepatobiliary Surgery
Hofstra-North Shore-LIJ School of Medicine
Lenox Hill Hospital
New York, New York
USA

Raul Rosenthal, MD, FASMBS, FACS
Professor of Surgery and Chairman, Department of General Surgery
Director of Minimally Invasive Surgery and The Bariatric and Metabolic Institute
Director, General Surgery Residency Program
Director, Fellowship in MIS and Bariatric Surgery
Cleveland Clinic Florida
Weston, Florida
USA

William P. Schecter, MD
Professor of Clinical Surgery Emeritus
Department of Surgery
University of California, San Francisco
San Francisco General Hospital
San Francisco, CA
USA

Myron E. Schwartz, MD, FACS
Professor of Surgery
Mount Sinai Liver Cancer Program
Icahn School of Medicine at Mount Sinai
New York, New York
USA

Jessica L. Secor, MD
Vascular Surgery Resident
Division of Vascular Surgery
University of Wisconsin
Wisconsin
USA

Mitsugi Shimoda, MD, PhD
Associate Professor of Hepato-Biliary-Pancreas Surgery
Second Department of Surgery
Dokkyo Medical University
Mibu, Tochigi
Japan

Kristina V. Spate, MD
Department of Surgery
University of Louisville
Louisville, Kentucky
USA

Paul J. Speicher, MD
Research Fellow
Department of Surgery
Duke University Medical Center
Durham, North Carolina
USA

Parissa Tabrizian, MD
Fellow, Mount Sinai Liver Cancer Program
Icahn School of Medicine at Mount Sinai
New York, New York
USA

Gary C. Vitale, MD
Professor of Surgery
Department of Surgery
University of Louisville
Louisville, Kentucky
USA

Sandra L. Wong, MD, MS
Associate Professor of Surgery
Department of Surgery
University of Michigan
Ann Arbor, Michigan
USA

Alla Zemlyak, MD
Attending Physician
Union Surgical Associates
Carolinas Medical Center –Union
Monroe, North Carolina
USA

Dedications

To my late mentors in surgery, Dr Beni Shtamler and Dr Ida Lunski, for their inspiration, surgical education and training. To my students and residents in surgery who always keep me challenged. In blessed memory of my late parents, Cesar and Allegra Mizrahi, who encouraged and supported me throughout my professional lifetime.

SM

To the large number of 'good doctors' I have helped to train, in appreciation of their numerous and diverse contributions to medicine, surgery and the health of the public as a whole. Reoperative surgery is seldom 'pretty' but it is an ongoing and essential component of good patient care.

HCP

To my wife Aviva and my four children, Einav, Tom, Nitzan and Noa, without whose endless understanding and support of my everlasting work, this project, like many others, would not have been possible. Thanks to my teachers and mentors, as well as my residents, to whom I owe my ongoing learning of the art of surgery.

PR

Chapter 1 Orientation to reoperative surgery with an emphasis on communication and safety

Hiram C. Polk, Jr.

Reoperative surgery requires an entirely different approach from any other kind of surgical care. The implication that the first or prior effort had failed or that the disease recurred is the essence of the problem and creates another sequence of pain, anxiety, and recovery that must be directly addressed. There are always multiple parties with an interest in the reasons for failure, the prospects of lasting recovery, and other therapeutic options. When the surgeon proposing reoperation differs from the earlier operator, there will always be the wish that younger/older, wiser or more or less aggressive, better facilities, or other aspects of the change of characters on the surgical team will lead to a better outcome. When any surgeon faces reoperation on his own patient, the psychological milieu is different in that there should always be a sense of fault or constructive self-blame, even when no error has been made:

- Could I have used different techniques?
- Better timing?
- More overall support, such as nutrition or anesthetics?
- Different antibiotics and shorter or longer use?
- An endless list of questions about materials, strategies, and devices:
- Minimal versus maximal access?
- Absorbable or nonabsorbable sutures?
- Staged operations as opposed to a single coup?
- Alimentary diversion or not?
- More or less utilization of image-dependent adjunctive therapy?
- Had I done something differently, would the outcome have been better?

Before proceeding, I rightly should recognize some specific efforts of now senior and respected protégés in keeping me focused upon the goals of surgical education; the patient is best served by the curative and innovative surgeon who is also totally honest! Gaar, Mitchell, Fry, Bland, Edwards, Evers, Voyles, and McMasters: these former residents' books and articles on reoperation and surgical infection have hugely influenced this 2013 version of Reoperative Surgery.

Given a reoperation by the same surgeon, a conscious initial assessment, including formal or informal consultation with colleagues, must be made and plans for alternate strategies and techniques set forth with the patient and immediate family. What will lead to a more satisfactory outcome this time? In all cases, the approach to the operation should be undertaken with specific but often different goals, assured that preoperative total patient preparation and optimum imaging will have been done. The most certain predictor of failure is 'let's see what we find and go from there.'

Again assuming the same surgeon or team is going to do the reoperative procedure, expectations must be finite and carefully laid out for the patient and family. Although preoperative consultation is given, intraoperative consultation may be even more important; a peer in the field should always be available – even if by telephone – to discuss unanticipated discoveries or diseases.

It is a psychologically easier scenario when reoperation is undertaken by a different surgeon; it is never too early to remind the reader–surgeon that many professional liability lawsuits are spawned by overt or even subtle inferences that the first operation was less than ideally done. A personal conversation between the two surgeons is not always done but is most desirable.

Senior surgeons always savor judgment and wisdom, and younger ones are fascinated by new technologies and devices. In the last decade's obsession with quality and outcomes (has it not always been so?), a study of major abdominal operations done by fully trained surgeons in a Midwestern state showed that among sequenced age groups of surgeons, only recent (<5 years of experience) graduate surgeons had a higher than expected operative mortality rate (Billeter et al. 2012, Galandiuk et al. 2004, Prystowsky et al. 2002). Regardless of the situation, two heads are often better than one! In that same vein, the surgeon's evening preceding a reoperation should dwell on details of the case ahead: think and rethink! Reoperative surgery is seldom pretty and virtually never easy.

A good example for many of these principles is the re-repair of ventral or incisional hernia; increasingly, it is agreed that nearly half such operations fail and fail again. This scenario is familiar to all general surgeons. Often in North America the predisposing cause is overt abdominal obesity. Pleas for weight reduction are seldom heeded, but the optimistic second surgeon is easily seduced. When the hernia is very large or 'massive,' pneumoperitoneum preoperatively in the doctor's office is an advantageous maneuver, virtually always overlooked and historically ignored. If the patient is obese, excision of the omentum as a battering ram to a new repair as well as the previous one is useful and regularly forgotten. Tension is the producer of failure and one of the advantages of component release as a technique is its de facto requirement for wide dissection (Kanaan et al. 2011). Although the sundry, innumerable meshes, or combinations thereof are regularly placed by their seriously conflicted surgeon advocates, combinations of the technically demanding component release bridged with permanent mesh are increasingly the fashion among the most experienced abdominal surgeons. Again communication failure sets the stage for disappointment; 'do not lift anything over 4 kg (10 lbs) until the 100th days after operation' is the most important pre- and postoperative admonition, to be repeated at every follow-up visit!

If there is any nontechnical common thread to the requirement for reoperation, it is the failure to understand and, to the extent possible, eliminate predisposing causes. Here, an alimentary fistula is a highly representative case. While the litany is known to all, distal obstruction and foreign bodies, such as mesh, and cancer lead the list. All the prescribed medications in the world will not close a fistula due to any of the unholy trinity – all of which must be systematically corrected or eliminated at reoperation.

Safety issues apply to all operations, but reoperation is the ideal scenario in which to practice the surgical time-out (Altpeter et al. 2007). Preoperative description of the plan and goals should be followed by the postoperative 'huddle' - what did we achieve and what are the necessary adjuncts to postoperative care? Drains and other devices must be appreciated for what they are: early for blood, late for intestinal discharge, and removal accordingly but always with the consent of the senior surgeon.

The postoperative report to the family and the next day to the patient must emphasize essential aspects of the reoperation:

1. We found no cancer

   Or

   We found some recurrent cancer, removed it, and believe we can slow the progress of the disease to some degree with further therapy
2. We found a blockage and were able to remove it

   Or

   Bypass it, which often works as well
3. We found a tack or suture of the mesh underneath and corrected it

   Or

   We removed all of the mesh and used your own tissue for repair

Surgeon, patient, team, family need to enter the reoperative arena with understanding, trust, and tempered optimism. Finally, if at all possible, reoperation should be undertaken as the first case of an uncrowded day. So be it.

REFERENCES

Altpeter T, Luckhardt K, Lewis JN, et al. Expanded surgical time out: a key to real-time data collection and quality improvement. J Am Coll Surg 2007; 204:527–532. PubMed PMID: 17382210.

Billeter AT, Polk HC Jr, Hohmann SF, et al. Mortality after elective colon resection: the search for outcomes that define quality in surgical practice. J Am Coll Surg 2012; 214:436–443; discussion 443–444. PubMed PMID: 22397975.

Galandiuk S, Rao MK, Heine MF, Scherm MJ, Polk HC. Mutual reporting of process and outcomes enhances quality outcomes for colon and rectal resections. Surgery 2004; 136:833–841. PubMed PMID: 15467669.

Kanaan Z, Hicks N, Weller C, et al. Abdominal wall component release is a sensible choice for patients requiring complicated closure of abdominal defects. Langenbecks Arch Surg 2011; 396:1263–1270. PubMed PMID: 21870175.

Prystowsky JB, Bordage G, Feinglass JM. Patients outcomes for segmental colon resection according to surgeon's training, certification, and experience. Surgery 2002; 132:663–670.

FURTHER READING

Bland KI, Sarr RG, eds. The practice of general surgery. Philadelphia, PA: WB Saunders, 2002.

Edwards MJ, Heniford BT, Klar EA, Doak KW, Miller FN. Pentoxifylline inhibits interleukin-2 induced toxicity in C57BL/6 mice but preserves antitumor efficacy. J Clin Invest 1992; 90:637–641.

Evers BM, Cryer HM, Miller FB. Pelvic fracture hemorrhage. Priorities in management. Arch Surg 1989; 124:422–424. PubMed PMID: 2930351.

Fry DE, ed. Reoperative surgery of the abdomen. New York: Marcel Dekker, 1986.

Gaar EE, ed. E-General Surgery Review [Kindle version]. Louisville, KY: Earl Gaar, 2102. Available from: http://www.amazon.com/General-Surgery-Review-Earl-Gaar-ebook/dp/B00B6FH4VG (accessed 31 Mar 2014).

Garrison RN. The Association for Academic Surgery: what a concept! J Surg Res 1992; 52:287–292. PubMed PMID: 1593865.

McMasters KM, Vauthey JN, eds. Hepatocellular carcinoma: targeted therapy and multidisciplinary care. New York: Springer, 2011.

Townsend C, Beauchamp RD, Evers BM, Mattox KL, eds. Sabiston textbook of surgery, 19th edn. New York: Saunders, 2012.

Voyles CR, Petro AB, Meena AL, Haick AJ, Koury AM. A practical approach to laparoscopic cholecystectomy. Am J Surg 1991; 161:365–370. PubMed PMID: 1825759.

Voyles CR, Richardson JD, Bland KI, et al. Emergency abdominal wall reconstruction with polypropylene mesh: short-term benefits versus long-term complications. Ann Surg 1981; 194:219–223. PubMed PMID: 6455099; PubMed Central PMCID: PMC1345243.

Chapter 2 The ethical legal implications of reoperative surgery

Rosalind Cordini, Beth Hendrickson McMasters

INTRODUCTION

Reoperative abdominal surgery is not an unexpected phenomenon, occurring in both the immediate post operative period and remote from the primary surgery. Acute reoperative surgery generally results from infection, bleeding, or failed procedures, whereas remote occurrence tends to result from late procedure failure, scar tissue development, or other complications. Regardless of when the reoperation occurs, the surgeon is faced with making a clinical judgment as to the best course of action for the patient, as few definitive studies may exist to provide a roadmap for the surgeon and the anticipated anatomy and potential complications may be different than those experienced in an initial operation. Where complications, morbidity, and mortality occur in the medical setting, the stage is set for malpractice claims. Not only must a physician concern himself with a simple negligence claim, he must also consider whether the patient will pursue an informed consent claim.

To illustrate the importance of the necessary clinical judgment, consider Fry and Osler (1991), who noted that care and caution must be exercised when selecting the site for incision in a second abdominal wall surgery due to the potential that adhesions may have developed and attached to the underlying bowel where a previous incision exists, increasing the potential for complications. The authors surmise that a separate incision might be the best course of action to prevent or reduce the risk of complications in a patient undergoing reoperative abdominal wall surgery. They further suggest that the surgeon must have a comprehensive understanding of abdominal wall blood supply so as to avoid serious morbidity associated with a poorly planned site. In a medical malpractice claim, the surgeon is held to the standard of whether his actions were those of a reasonable physician acting under the same or similar circumstances. Assuming Fry and Osler's conclusions are, in fact, the medical standard of care, a surgeon who operates outside of these parameters risks not only being sued under a medical malpractice theory, but potentially found liable for his actions, even where his incision site for a primary procedure may have been appropriate.

Fry and Osler further state that a reoperation of the abdominal wall is associated with an increased risk of complications including dehiscence, infection, or ventral herniation. Infection, potentially the most serious of these problems, can range from a simple wound infection to necrotizing fasciitis. Armed with this knowledge, a surgeon who fails to disclose this known cluster of risks to a patient undergoing abdominal wall reoperative surgery places himself at risk of liability in an informed consent suit, in addition to those pursued for alleged negligence related to either the first operation or performance of the second operation.

As the above example illustrates, complication rates from reoperative surgery vary significantly and are dependent on a host of factors such as the type of surgical procedure to be performed, the previous procedure performed, patient-related risk factors, and surgical skill and experience. Consider for example, the following: Generally, 10–25% of patients who have bariatric surgery undergo such a surgery for either complications arising from initial surgery or for further weight control. It is also known that patients with morbid obesity have a mortality risk of up to 12 times that of the general population. And, in approximately 11% of these bariatric reoperations, serious morbidity will occur (Behrns et al 1993). In ileal pouch reoperative surgery, one study examined the complication rates, finding that two thirds of patients undergoing such a reoperative surgery experienced excellent clinical outcomes but one third did not, and up to one in five patients experienced a loss of their reservoir altogether (Galandiuk et al 1990). This is information most patients would consider critical to their decision making as to whether to undergo additional surgery, and it is incumbent upon the surgeon to stress the risks and potential benefits in obtaining informed consent.

In addition to procedure-specific complication rates, the surgeon must determine whether laparoscopy is available and advisable as a technique. When utilized, consideration must be given as to whether there has been a previous laparotomy, the surgeon's level of experience, the peritoneal access technique to be used, and patient-related factors such as the type and number of previous abdominal operations, the location of previous incision(s), and the likelihood of existing adhesions (Arnell 2006). Indeed, pneumoperitoneum access during laparoscopy can account for significant morbidity. In one report, 40% of bowel injuries occurring during laparoscopy were attributed to the establishment of the pneumoperitoneum – 60% of which occurred in patients who had undergone previous abdominal surgery (Arnell 2006). Finally, as a special consideration, where there has been a complication or other reason for reoperative surgery, the surgeon must disclose to the patient whether there are options for remediation/repair outside the scope of his expertise and should consider consultation with a subspecialist, where appropriate. The surgeon must be honest with himself and the patient regarding what options are available, what procedure best addresses the reoperative need, and whether the surgeon is in the best position to offer that option to the patient. A common theme in lawsuits filed after surgical complication (whether from primary or reoperative care) is that the surgeon was not trained, or was minimally trained in the particular procedure performed or that the surgeon simply did not perform the procedure correctly. The eye on the complication becomes more critical when the surgeon has operative failure a second time.

Thus, certain particularized elements of risk exist and are known at the outset when a decision is made to proceed with reoperative abdominal surgery. The decision to proceed with such a procedure is under the sound discretion of the competent surgeon in conjunction with the patient following a thorough discussion of the risks, benefits, and alternatives to the proposed procedure. This of course, is wholly aligned with the long-standing principles of medical ethics.

MEDICAL ETHICS

> **I WILL FOLLOW that method of treatment which according to my ability and judgment, I consider for the benefit of my patient and abstain from whatever is harmful or mischievous. . . .WITH PURITY, HOLINESS AND BENEFICENCE I will pass my life and practice my art. Except for the prudent correction of an imminent danger, I will neither treat any patient nor carry out any research on any human being without the valid informed consent of the subject or the appropriate legal protector thereof . . .**
>
> ***—The Hippocratic Oath***
> ***Harvard Classics Volume 38***

The Hippocratic Oath has long provided physicians with an ethical framework to guide medical practice; however, the advancement of both technology and medical knowledge has resulted in ever increasing moral and ethical dilemmas for today's physicians. Beauchamp's model of ethical and moral principles incorporates the four generally accepted principles of medical ethics: autonomy, justice, beneficence, and nonmaleficence, providing a meaningful ethical framework in today's climate (Beauchamp & Childress 2008).

Autonomy is the principle of self-governance, viewed my many as an irrefutable value, the crux of which is the ability to be one's own person. In the medical ethical arena, autonomy permits a greater equilibrium in the doctor–patient relationship and power structure. It embodies a respect for the patient's wishes and a facilitation of a patient's input into the medical decision-making process. Autonomy requires the physician to not only consult with the patient regarding their care and treatment, but also to obtain their agreement to any proposed treatment prior to performing the procedure. The principle of justice is equated to 'fairness' and the conscious effort not to permit ones prejudices to directly influence their professional work by prejudicing their assessment of a patient's needs or restricting or delaying their access to care. Beneficence is the concept of doing that which benefits one's patients and nonmaleficence involves the avoidance of harm. Thus, a natural conflict arises between upholding each of these principles, as a procedure that is intended to promote the well-being of a patient may carry significant risks and potential harm to the same patient. These principles must, therefore, be considered together. Each proposed action upon a patient requires a careful cost-benefit balancing, the aim of which is to produce a net benefit over harm to the patient. These principles are likewise intertwined with the principle of autonomy. By informing the patient of what the net benefits and risks are to a procedure, a patient is able to deliberate on the options, and participate fully in the decision to proceed.

LEGAL CONSIDERATIONS: INFORMED CONSENT

Background

In the context of reoperative surgery, the aforementioned ethical principles align with the legal doctrine of informed consent. The doctrine of informed consent as pertains to physician–patient relationships reaches far back into the English Common Law. As early as 1767, physicians were charged with the tort of battery if they performed a procedure on a patient without having secured their consent. In an early United States case, Justice Cardoza stated, 'every human being of adult years and sound mind has a right to determine what shall be done with his own body; and a surgeon who performs an operation without his patient's consent commits an assault, for which he is liable in damages (Schloendorff v. Society of New York Hospital, 211 NY 125, 129-30;1914).' Today, informed consent actions are based in negligence rather than battery and in each of the 50 United States, the requirements are expressed by either case law or statute.

INFORMED CONSENT: REQUIREMENTS

The informed consent process is much more than the obtaining of a patient's signature on a consent form. Rather, informed consent is the process of communication between the physician and patient, which results in the patient's authorization to proceed with a proposed procedure or their decision to refuse the proposed procedure. In discussing a proposed procedure with a patient, a physician should discuss the nature of the proposed procedure, the risks and benefits of the proposed procedure, alternatives to the proposed procedure, risks and benefits of the alternative procedures, and the risks and benefits of choosing not to undergo any procedure. Heightened requirements exist for certain populations, including those participating in human subjects research. Physicians participating in clinical research are encouraged to familiarize themselves with these heightened requirements. As the purpose of informed consent is to enable the patient to make an informed decision, this communications process should provide the patient with the opportunity to ask questions to better understand both his illness and the proposed treatment or procedure. This communications process has long been an ethical obligation of the physician, and today, it is also the legal duty of the physician to engage in this process prior to proceeding with any proposed treatment. Obtaining informed consent is not properly delegated to nurses or nonclinical staff. The communication requires knowledge regarding the patient and the procedure possessed by the surgeon.

Unlike a standard malpractice claim where the patient alleges that the doctor negligently performed a given procedure, the crux of an informed consent action is the patient's allegation that the physician never told him that there was the possibility of the occurrence of a resulting injury or harm and had he known, he would not have undergone the procedure. The patient must prove he experienced a complication of the procedure, and had he known about the specific complication he experienced, he would have opted not to undergo the proposed procedure. In other words, the patient has the burden of showing that the physician's failure to disclose a given risk resulted in the patient having a procedure he would have otherwise refused, resulting in the ultimate harm or injury suffered.

INFORMED CONSENT DISCLOSURE STANDARD

The question often asked, is how much information is adequate when a physician sets out to disclose the risks involved in a given procedure. States are divided in the standards they set forth in this regard (**Table 2.1**). The most widely applied approach is the 'Professional Standard' or the standard of the 'reasonable physician.' States utilizing this approach require a physician to disclose the amount of information, or particularized risks, as would a reasonably prudent physician with the same background, training, and experience in the same or similar situation. This approach is the same standard

Table 2.1 State-specific informed consent standards (July 2012)

State	Reasonable physician	Materiality standard	Case name or statute
Alabama	x		Giles v. Brookwood Health Services, Inc., 5 So. 3d 533, 554 (Ala. 2008)
Alaska		x	Alaska Stat. Ann. § 09.55.556 (West)
Arizona	x		Shetter v. Rochelle, 2 Ariz. App. 358, 370, 409 P.2d 74, 86 (1965) modified, 2 Ariz. App. 607, 411 P.2d 45 (1966)
Arkansas	x		Ark. Code Ann. § 16-114-206 (West)
California		x	Cobbs v. Grant, 8 Cal. 3d 229, 245, 502 P.2d 1, 11 (1972)
Colorado	x		Gorab v. Zook, 943 P.2d 423, 427 (Colo. 1997)
Connecticut		x	Duffy v. Flagg, 279 Conn. 682, 691-92, 905 A.2d 15, 20 (2006)
Delaware	x		Del. Code Ann. tit. 18, § 6852 (West)
Florida	x		Fla. Stat. Ann. § 766.103 (West)
Georgia		x	Ga. Code Ann. § 31-9-6.1 (West)
Hawaii		x	Carr v. Strode, 904 P.2d 489, 500 (Haw. 1995)
Idaho	x		2012 Idaho Laws Ch. 302 (S.B. 1294), 2012 Idaho Laws Ch. 302 (S.B. 1294)
Illinois	x		Lisowski v. MacNeal Mem'l Hosp. Ass'n, 381 Ill. App. 3d 275, 290, 885 N.E.2d 1120, 1136 (2008)
Indiana	x		Spar v. Cha, 907 N.E.2d 974, 984 (Ind. 2009)
Iowa		x	Kennis v. Mercy Hosp. Med. Ctr., 491 N.W.2d 161, 166 (Iowa 1992)
Kansas	x		Rojas v. Barker, 40 Kan. App. 2d 758, 763, 195 P.3d 785, 789 (2008)
Kentucky	x	x	Ky. Rev. Stat. Ann. § 304.40-320 (West)
Louisiana		x	Hondroulis v. Schuhmacher, 553 So. 2d 398, 411-12 (La. 1988)
Maine	x		Me. Rev. Stat. tit. 24, § 2905
Maryland		x	McQuitty v. Spangler, 410 Md. 1, 18-19, 976 A.2d 1020, 1030 (2009)
Massachusetts		x	Roukounakis v. Messer, 63 Mass. App. Ct. 482, 485, 826 N.E.2d 777, 780 (2005)
Michigan	x		Roberts v. Young, 369 Mich. 133, 140, 119 N.W.2d 627, 630 (1963)
Minnesota	x		K.A.C. v. Benson, 527 N.W.2d 553, 561 (Minn. 1995)
Mississippi		x	Latham v. Hayes, 495 So. 2d 453 (Miss. 1986)
Missouri	x		Wilkerson v. Mid-Am. Cardiology, 908 S.W.2d 691, 696 (Mo. Ct. App. 1995)
Montana	x		Llera v. Wisner, 171 Mont. 254, 262, 557 P.2d 805, 810 (1976)
Nebraska	x		Neb. Rev. Stat. § 44-2816
Nevada	x		Smith v. Cotter, 107 Nev. 267, 272, 810 P.2d 1204, 1207 (1991)
New Hampshire	x		Folger v. Corbett, 118 N.H. 737, 738, 394 A.2d 63, 63-64 (1978)
New Jersey		x	Largey v. Rothman, 110 N.J. 204, 215, 540 A.2d 504, 510 (1988)
New Mexico		x	Gerety v. Demers, 92 N.M. 396, 410, 589 P.2d 180, 194 (1978)
New York	x		N.Y. Pub. Health Law § 2805-d (McKinney)
North Carolina	x		N.C. Gen. Stat. Ann. § 90-21.13 (West)
North Dakota		x	Long v. Jaszczak, 2004 ND 194, 688 N.W.2d 173, 178
Ohio		x	Nickell v. Gonzalez, 17 Ohio St. 3d 136, 139, 477 N.E.2d 1145, 1148-49 (1985)
Oklahoma		x	Parris v. Limes, 2012 OK 18, 277 P.3d 1259, 1263, reh'g denied (May 14, 2012)
Oregon	x		Or. Rev. Stat. Ann. § 677.097 (West)
Pennsylvania	x		40 Pa. Stat. Ann. § 1303.504 (West)
Rhode Island		x	Lauro v. Knowles, 785 A.2d 1140, 1141-42 (R.I. 2001)
South Carolina	x		Melton v. Medtronic, Inc., 389 S.C. 641, 656, 698 S.E.2d 886, 894 (Ct. App. 2010)
South Dakota		x	Wheeldon v. Madison, 374 N.W.2d 367, 374 (S.D. 1985)
Tennessee	x		Tenn. Code Ann. § 29-26-118 (West)
Texas		x	Vaughan v. Nielson, 274 S.W.3d 732, 737 (Tex. App. 2008)
Utah		x	Utah Code Ann. § 78B-3-406 (West)

Continued

State	Reasonable physician	Materiality standard	Case name or statute
Vermont	x		Vt. Stat. Ann. tit. 12, § 1909 (West)
Virginia	x		Tashman v. Gibbs, 263 Va. 65, 73, 556 S.E.2d 772, 777 (2002)
Washington		x	Wash. Rev. Code Ann. § 7.70.050 (West)
West Virginia		x	Cross v. Trapp, 170 W. Va. 459, 468, 294 S.E.2d 446, 455 (1982)
Wisconsin		x	Johnson by Adler v. Kokemoor, 199 Wis. 2d 615, 631, 545 N.W.2d 495, 501 (1996)
Wyoming	x	x	Willis v. Bender, 596 F.3d 1244, 1254 (10th Cir. 2010)

Compiled by Billy Hopkins, summer law clerk, Wyatt, Tarrant & Combs LLP, Louisville, KY, USA (2013)

applied in other medical malpractice actions and requires that a physician expert testify at trial on behalf of the defendant physician as to the appropriateness of the scope of his disclosure. States may expand upon this standard. In Oregon, for example, the physician has a statutory duty to ask the patient if they would like additional information, and if so, must provide the patient with a description of the proposed procedure in substantial detail.

Several states apply what is termed the 'materiality standard' or the reasonable patient standard, another objective standard. These states define appropriate disclosure as including that which a reasonable patient in the same or similar situation would need to know to make an informed and appropriate decision regarding a proposed procedure. In other words, the information deemed 'material' to an informed decision must be provided. Information that is 'material' is that information that a person in the patient's position would be likely to attach significance to in deciding whether or not to undergo the proposed surgery. In these states, no medical expert is required to define the scope of this disclosure, but rather, the jury, who is considered a reasonable group of people, defines the scope of this material disclosure in objective terms. Again, states may vary in their precise standards. For example, in Pennsylvania, the materiality standard is imposed in informed consent actions; however, a physician defendant is permitted to present evidence of the community standard in his defense. Note that both Kentucky and Wyoming standards are hybrids, meaning, they combine the requirements of both the reasonable physician standard and the materiality standard.

Finally, the 'subjective patient standard' is mentioned in various anecdotal reports on informed consent. This standard asks what the particular plaintiff/patient, under his circumstances, would need to know prior to agreeing to proceed with a proposed procedure. This standard would prove very difficult to establish, and the authors were unable to identify a jurisdiction in the United States that applies this standard. Physicians should familiarize with the standard applied in their respective locale to understand the scope of the informed consent duty.

DEFENSES TO AN INFORMED CONSENT CAUSE OF ACTION

There are several scenarios where a defense exists to the physician's duty to obtain informed consent. The best established of these is in an emergency, where any attempt in obtaining informed consent would delay necessary emergency treatment. In such a case, most hospitals require that a physician document in the medical record that informed consent could not be obtained due to the emergency status of the situation. Another viable defense to an informed consent claim is the lack of foreseeability of an injury, or those that are so remote, that they would not give rise to a duty in the physician to advise of its potential. This concept is consistent with both the 'reasonable physician' and 'materiality' standards applied in informed consent actions in the majority of states.

The physician's duty for disclosure may also be successfully defended against in situations where the patient has prior knowledge of the potential risks of a proposed procedure, as in when they have undergone the same procedure previously, or when the potential risks are common knowledge, as in pain after surgery.

Another doctrine that may enable a successful defense against an informed consent claim is what is referred to as the 'therapeutic privilege.' This privilege permits a physician to withhold information from a patient where, in his professional judgment, the physician believes the information would either be too upsetting for the patient to hear, or would in some way interfere with treatment. It seems obvious that reliance on such a privilege ought to be well considered prior to deciding to withhold disclosure of information to a patient, as the patient's right to autonomy is highly regarded. If relied upon, the physician's rationale for withholding certain information must be well documented in the record. This paternalistic approach is one the statutes and case law seek to discourage. Reliance on a single physician's opinion regarding potential harm would provide a weak defense where that physician is also the operating surgeon.

Finally, the best defense in an informed consent action is where the patient has actually been informed of the potential risk and has decided to proceed. A patient's knowledge of these risks is often portrayed by the presence of a written consent form that outlines the risks and benefits of a procedure and includes the patient's signature in acknowledgment thereof and further supported by a written note by the surgeon outlining the consent process. The argument is that the patient knew of the potential risk, and agreed to undergo the operation, despite knowledge of those risks. Notably, Florida's informed consent statute expressly provides for a rebuttable presumption of a valid consent where a signed consent is of record.

Sometimes, a comparative negligence instruction is sought in an effort to share the liability between the patient and physician where a signed consent form exists, yet there is a dispute regarding what was precisely disclosed. As simplistic as this defense seems, it is not always a clean defense. For example, in a recent Kentucky Court of Appeals case, a physician was sued under an informed consent cause of action when his patient suffered postoperative complications after ureteroscopy for removal of a kidney stone. The physician defendant presented a copy of the written operative consent form, signed by the patient, which indicated that the procedure to be performed was ureteroscopy. Despite the presence of the consent form, the Court refused to issue a comparative negligence instruction to the jury because at trial, the plaintiff testified that the only procedure verbally discussed with his wife was shock lithotripsy, the same procedure performed on the patient previously, and neither the physician nor the patient could remember what was precisely discussed in advance of the operation. The Court relied on a Wisconsin case that stated that a contributory negligence instruction may apply in an informed consent case, but only in certain extraordinary circumstances (Oghia v. Hollan, March 16, 2012, Ky. App). Thus, reliance on the signed consent form alone may not provide for the defense a physician presumes it does.

CONCLUSION

Performance of subsequent operations for complications or failure is a reality of every surgical practice. As surgeons are aware, each operative and reoperative procedure carries specific risks – those inherent in the procedure itself, and others compounded by certain patient-related and surgeon-related factors, such as skill and experience. The surgeon must determine the options for treatment and remediation of the complication or failure of the initial procedure; the risks inherent with various options; whether he is the person most suited to providing the continuing surgical care; and provide the patient with sufficient information to decide what is best under the circumstances. The obtaining of a patient's informed consent prior to the performance of an operative procedure is both a moral obligation and the legal duty of a surgeon. Physicians are encouraged to familiarize themselves with the standards applied in an informed consent cause of action in their practicing jurisdiction, as the law and standards vary from state to state, and change from time to time.

Because reoperative surgery often carries higher risk than primary operations, the risk that the surgeon may be sued for complications experienced by the patient also increases. The surgeon must arm himself with a thorough progress note detailing informed consent, but equally as important, the surgeon must give thoughtful attention to his own decision whether to act as the reoperative surgeon for repair of his complication. Only after thorough, honest, meaningful discussion between the physician and his patient, and the implementation of a plan of care that balances the beneficence and nonmaleficence components of the physician's oath in the care and treatment of his patients, should he proceed.

REFERENCES

Arnell, T. Minimally invasive reoperation following laparotomy. Clin Colon Rectal Surg 2006; 19:223–227.

Beauchamp TL, Childress JF. Principles of biomedical ethics. 6th edn. New York: Oxford University Press, 2008.

Behrns, KE, Smith, CD, et al. Reoperative bariatric surgery. Lessons learned to improve patient selection and results. Ann Surg 1993; 218:646–653.

Fry DE, Osler T. Abdominal Wall Considerations and Complications in Reoperative Surgery. Surg Clin North Am 1991 ;71(1):1-11.

Galandiuk S, Scott NA, Dozois RR, et al. Ileal pouch-anal anastomosis. Reoperation for pouch-related complications. Ann Surg 1990; 212:446–454.

Chapter 3 The broad view of reoperative surgery

Thilo Hackert, Markus W. Büchler

BACKGROUND AND HISTORICAL PERSPECTIVE

Reoperative surgery is a complex field within abdominal surgery and remains a clinical challenge in many patients. The interaction between the mechanical irritation induced by surgical manipulation and the pathophysiological changes that can lead to adhesions and cause major technical problems in cases of reoperation have been investigated in numerous historical and current studies. Despite increased understanding of these mechanisms, no established treatment pathway exists to date to avoid the formation of adhesions and thereby facilitate surgical reinterventions. Another aspect of reoperative surgery – is the induction of compromised wound healing with the consequence of abdominal wall defects and the clinical picture of an open abdomen.

From a historical point of view, the problems associated with reoperative surgery can be traced back to the beginning of major abdominal operations in the late 19th and early 20th century. Anecdotal reports of problems with enterocutaneous fistulas after surgical interventions primarily referred to complicated emergencies such as appendicitis or ulcer perforation. In the 1960s, reports on larger patient series tried to systematically address the problem of reoperation and fistulas; however, it should be noted that either of these can always induce the other – a reoperation causing a fistula and vice versa. Directly linked to these problems is another major aspect of reoperative surgery: adhesion formation. Firm adhesions, which are often difficult to understand in origin and etiology, result in reoperations due to passage problems and they increase the risk of accidental enterotomy with postoperative intestinal leakage and the consequent need for another reoperation.

The clinically challenging problem of complications after reoperative surgery has been characterized as 'the hostile' or 'the frozen' abdomen, which linguistically reflects the strenuous and sometimes ineffective surgical efforts required to deal with this unpleasant situation.

ANATOMICAL ISSUES

Access to the abdominal cavity for visceral operations is most frequently via vertical or transverse incisions. Depending on the site and length of the incision, the biomechanical features of the abdominal wall differ to a great extent, resulting in a specific risk of incisional hernia development, which increases in cases of repeated surgical interventions. From the available large series, the overall risk of incisional hernias in abdominal surgery is approximately 10–20% and is not significantly associated with the choice of incision (Seiler et al. 2009, Van't Riet et al. 2002). Although, compared with other incisions, closure of a midline incision seems to be less stable from the biomechanical point of view due to the presence of bradytrophic fascial tissue components only, a similar complication rate, including hernia incidence, has been demonstrated in systematic reviews and meta-analyses (Brown & Goodfellow 2005, Diener et al. 2010). A possible anatomical factor for hernia predisposition in transverse and oblique incisions may be the functional disturbance of the muscle layer by transection of the lateral nerve structures, which results in decreased stability. In the reoperation setting, usually the pre-existing incision is used with the intention of minimizing additional trauma and producing a better cosmetic outcome, although this increases the risk of incisional hernia (O'Dwyer & Courtney 2003, Stumpf et al. 2009).

Besides hernia development as a late complication, difficulty accessing the abdominal cavity is a major issue in reoperative surgery, especially with regard to unintended or accidental enterotomy. Anatomical structures adherent to the abdominal wall include the liver surface, omentum, and stomach as well as the small and large bowel. Anatomically, the omentum serves as a protective layer inside the abdominal wall and, if not removed during a preceding operation, is located immediately below vertical incisions of the upper abdomen. In the right upper quadrant, the surface of the liver is approached first. These vertical incisions therefore seem to provide a relatively safe means of access in revision operations. However, the possibility of accidental transverse colon incision must always be taken into account in these locations. In all other incision sites, the risk of small bowel injury is much higher, which implies that opening of the abdominal cavity must be performed with the utmost caution in order to avoid enterotomy or serosa lesions, which may not be evident initially but may cause delayed intestinal leakage with the need for surgical revision and the risk of long-lasting enterocutaneous fistula development (Ching et al. 2003, Fry and Osler 1991).

Another aspect of adhesion formation relates to the pelvis in female patients. The close proximity of the ovaries and adnexae to neighboring peritoneal and bowel structures causes infertility as a specific complication, especially after recurrent operations in this anatomical region in younger women (Ahmad et al. 2008).

PATHOPHYSIOLOGY OF ADHESION FORMATION

Adhesions may develop after any type of abdominal surgery although this process is highly dependent on individual patient features, the surgical access to the abdominal cavity (open/laparoscopic) and the type of surgery originally performed. Furthermore, intra-abdominal inflammatory complications – such as peritonitis or fistula development – have a strong impact on adhesion formation (Holmdahl et al. 1997).

From the clinical point of view, adhesions should be regarded as a relevant factor for surgical morbidity as they cause obstruction, pain, and infertility in a considerable number of patients (Arung et al. 2011). This results in reoperations, with their associated risks (including reformation of adhesions), and causes hospitalization, with consequent costs for the health care systems (Ellis 1997).

The pathophysiological background of adhesion formation has been extensively investigated in the past, as well as prophylactic approaches for their prevention. As a reaction to surgical trauma, the peritoneum shows a damage control response with both coagulatory and inflammatory aspects. Major cells involved in the latter are leukocytes, macrophages, and mesothelial cells (Arung et al., 2011, Ellis 1997, Reed et al. 2008). Within the first few postoperative hours, inflammatory mediators are liberated, attracting macrophages and polymorphonuclear neutrophil cells to the site of injury. At the end of the first week, this reaction reaches its peak and leads to a regeneration of mesothelial cells on the one hand, but also to a secretion and activation of fibrinogen on the other. This results in a so-called 'fibrin gel matrix', consisting mainly of polymerized fibrin and fibronectin (Ching et al. 2003). In addition to this adhesive process, fibrinolytic proteins (including tissue plasminogen activators) are secreted, mainly by mesothelial cells. This fibrinolytic cascade can therefore be regarded as a control mechanism to restore mesothelial integrity and function, but it may be impaired by an upregulation of plasminogen activator inhibitors in patients with major abdominal operations, with the consequence of extensive adhesion formation. The final and irreversible step in adhesiogenesis is the firm organization of attached surface areas as scar tissue due to persisting fibroblast activity [**Figures 3.1** and **3.2** (Brokelman et al. 2009, Hellebrekers & Kooistra 2011)].

TIME COURSE OF ADHESION FORMATION

The first postoperative week is the crucial time interval for adhesion formation (diZerega 1997). After 7 days, adhesions tend to become more firm, reaching their maximum strength after 14 days. Consequently, reoperations are feasible within the first 7–10 days in an emergency setting. After this period, the conditions for a surgical intervention become measurably worse and the risk of bowel injuries during re-exploration increases significantly. Between weeks 3 and 6, adhesions slowly resolve in most patients and reach a stable state after that time, which may facilitate reoperations. On the basis of clinical experience, most surgeons prefer to wait another 6 weeks before planning any reoperation to let the intra-abdominal conditions improve further.

PROPHYLAXIS OF ADHESION FORMATION

Numerous experimental and clinical studies have dealt with the topic of adhesion prophylaxis (Becker et al. 1996, Brochhausen et al. 2012, Fujii et al. 2009, Kumar et al. 2009, Kosaka et al. 2008, Lalountas et al. 2012, Ouaïssi et al. 2012, Tang et al. 2006, Vrijland et al. 2002, Zeng et al. 2007). This has been investigated not only by general surgeons but also, mainly, from the gynecological point of view as adhesion can be regarded as an important cause of female infertility. However, of all agents used to reduce the inflammatory peritoneal response, only a few have shown reproducible benefits and have been used clinically, despite often encouraging experimental results (Lalountas et al. 2012). Intraoperative measures to prevent adhesions include careful tissue handling, immediate hemostasis, avoidance of bacterial contamination, and the use of starch-free gloves, all of which have been routinely implemented in most departments. Drug therapy for postoperative reduction of the peritoneal inflammatory reaction encompasses both local and systemic agents. The prophylactic systemic use of non-steroidal anti-inflammatory drugs, corticosteroids, histamine antagonists, antioxidants, or calcium channel-blockers has shown benefits in the experimental setting for each of these substances but this has failed to translate to the clinical situation. Furthermore, anticoagulatory and fibrinolytic agents including heparin and warfarin may have an antiadhesive effect

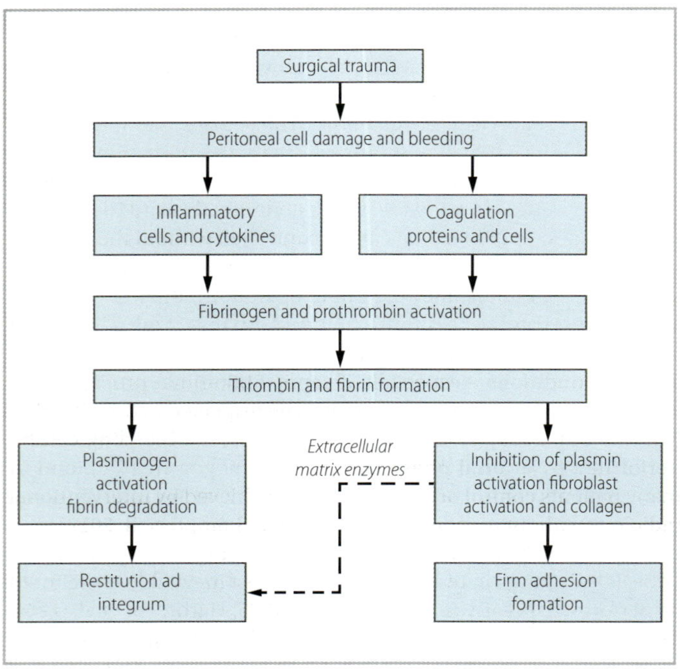

Figure 3.1 Pathogenesis of adhesion formation.

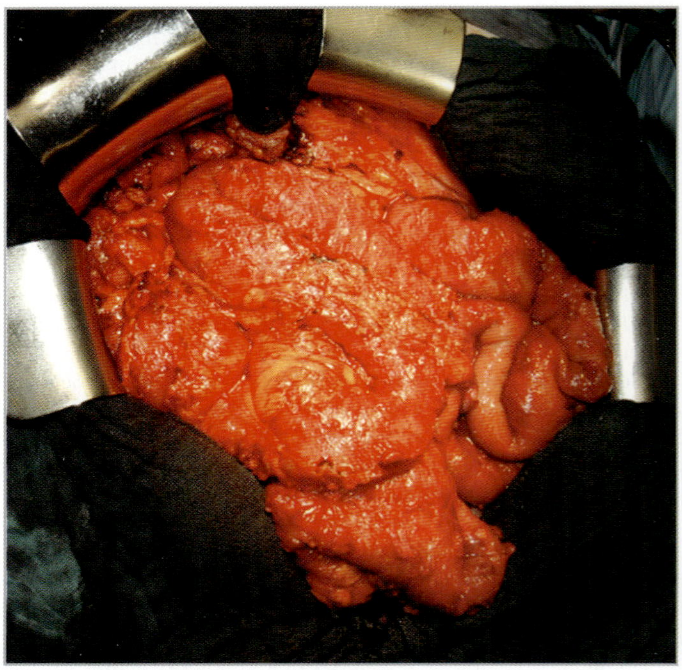

Figure 3.2 Intraoperative sites of severe adhesions after multivisceral resection. Elective reoperation due to tumor recurrence of leiomyosarcoma.

but are not suitable (in an adequate dosage) for this purpose in the clinical situation due to an increased risk of bleeding. With regard to locally applied agents, fibrinolytic enzymes such as streptokinase, plasmin, or rtPA may have a beneficial influence on adhesion formation. To date, these approaches have not been investigated in high-quality randomized trials. In contrast, adhesion prevention by local application of hyaluronic acid/carboxymethyl membranes has been investigated in six randomized controlled trials including >2000 patients in both treatment and control groups (Kumar et al. 2009). A recent meta-analysis of these studies showed evidence of a reduction of the incidence, extent and severity of adhesion formation, although an increased risk of anastomotic leakage may be associated with the application. In contrast, no high-level evidence was found to show that these agents reduce the occurrence of intestinal obstruction and the need for reoperations (Kumar et al. 2009). From these observations, to date, no clear recommendation can be given to use this approach routinely, although certain benefits may be present for individual patients with regard to presumable reoperations in the future.

INDICATIONS FOR REOPERATIVE SURGERY

Patients who require reoperations are mainly operated on in emergency situations, such as bowel perforation, pancreatitis, abdominal compartment syndrome, and abscesses or disorders that cause peritonitis for other reasons. Furthermore, many postoperative complications – especially anastomotic leakage – are frequent indications for reoperative procedures (Ching et al. 2003, Fry & Clevenger 1991, Fry et al. 1980, Polk and Fry 1980).

Regarding bowel perforations, the leading indication is complicated colonic diverticulitis, a very common surgical emergency (Zingg et al. 2010). A two-stage procedure begins with resection of the sigmoid colon, which is usually affected, and completed as a Hartman procedure with a terminal colostomy. This leads to a planned reoperation to restore bowel continuity. Regarding the timing of this second operation, usually a minimum wait of 3 months should be respected, as mentioned below. Other emergency procedures may be required in severe necrotizing pancreatitis, although the frequency of open surgery has dramatically decreased in recent decades as interventional and minimally invasive procedures have progressively replaced the open approach, which was historically associated with planned relaparotomies and often resulted in a laparostoma stage, with the need for a secondary abdominal wall reconstruction (Werner et al. 2005). Other indications include decompression of the abdominal compartment of any origin, second-look laparotomies in bowel ischemia, and emergency packing procedures in uncontrolled bleeding. In these situations, reoperation has to be performed early – usually within 24–72 hours of the first surgical intervention. This implies an adhesion-free situation but may sometimes be associated with difficult closure of the abdominal wall due to retraction of the abdominal fascia and therefore may require augmentation of the abdominal wall by inlay mesh implantation or a very complicated component release procedure to avoid inadequate tension on the suture edges (Mathes et al. 2000).

In contrast to these emergencies, the most common elective surgical indication for relaparotomy is closure of protective enterostomies, for example after low anterior rectal resections. However, in this situation, a circumscript local operation without reopening the main laparotomy is often possible to minimize surgical trauma (Bennis et al. 2012).

TIMING OF REOPERATION

An important aspect of reoperative surgery is the question of timing. If not determined by an emergency situation (e.g. postoperative intestinal leakage or overt sepsis), surgical re-exploration should be performed no earlier than 3 months after the last preceding operations. The rationale for this recommendation is based on the clinical experience that adhesion formation – comparable with superficial wound healing – is a process that follows a more or less uniform time course in patients who are not affected by immunosuppression or compromised healing of any other etiology.

Reoperations that are electively planned (e.g. closure of protective ileostomy or restoration of bowel continuity after Hartmann's procedure) can normally be postponed as long as possible without impairment of the surgical conditions and should seldom be performed before week 13 after the initial operation, although patients sometimes tend to apply psychological pressure on the surgeon due to their strong wish to have their stoma closed (Bennis et al. 2012).

ACUTE REOPERATION

In contrast to elective reoperations, the field of emergency reoperative surgery has specific different aspects that require attention to avoid consecutive complications and additional repeated surgical interventions. An important aspect of emergency reoperations is that the time point of operation cannot be chosen, with the consequence that the surgeon may have to deal with the most difficult conditions regarding adhesions, bleeding, peritonitis, and abdominal wall closure (Büchler et al. 2003, Bunt 1985, Harbrecht et al. 1984, Keller et al. 1983, van Ruler et al. 2007, Wente et al. 2006). This fact naturally means that emergency relaparotomies carry a higher morbidity and mortality risk than elective reoperations. Indications for emergency reoperation include postoperative bleeding, anastomotic or bowel leakage, and burst abdomen. The risk of these complications is highly dependent not only on the preceding operation but also on the individual patient's pre-existing comorbidities (Ching et al. 2003).

Early postoperative bleeding is usually caused by technical failure and occurs within the first 24 hours after the initial operation (Wente et al. 2007). Common reasons for bleeding are dislocations of vessel ligations, either by a clip or suture slipping or by electrocautery failure in the case of small vessel coagulation. In most cases, drains are placed at the sites of resection or anastomoses in abdominal operations, which show early bleeding events. In this situation, immediate surgical revision is preferable as access to the abdominal cavity is easy, and all potential sites of bleeding can be controlled without the need for any time-consuming preoperative imaging. If postoperative bleeding is delayed (>24 hours after the initial operation), the indication for surgical re-exploration should be critically reviewed. The risk of damaging the bowel or anastomoses and of encountering difficult surgical conditions – especially if septic abdominal processes are associated with the bleeding – needs to be respected in this situation (Miura et al. 2009). A diagnostic step to localize bleeding can be performed by arterial phase computed tomography (CT), and in many patients control of bleeding can be achieved by interventional radiology without reopening the abdomen (Stampfl et al. 2012).

In case of bowel leakage, which may occur after difficult adhesiolysis, surgical re-exploration is almost inevitable and should be performed as early as possible (Bunt 1985, Harbrecht et al., 1984, Keller et al., 1983). Bowel leakage can generally be recognized easily by checking the drain fluid, which shows a characteristic quality in terms of fecal colour and often odour and elevated levels of amylase, lipase, and bilirubin. In addition, oral application of colored substances (e.g. diluted methylene blue) can be useful to clarify certain situations. During reoperation, bowel leakage can be closed by direct suture in most patients. In cases of severe peritonitis or a risk of complications of other origin (e.g. preceding radiation of the bowel), an enterostomy at the site of leakage can be a safer option to avoid repeated leakage episodes and can be closed after recovery of the patient within a 3–6-month interval.

Anastomotic leakage is certainly one of the most difficult postoperative surgical complications to handle (Welsch et al. 2011). Depending on the type of leakage, therapeutic options include reoperation, endoscopic, or interventional management. Anastomotic leakage after esophagectomy or gastrectomy is rarely an indication for emergency reoperation. Endoscopic stenting end – if necessary – interventional drainage can often be a sufficient treatment option, especially as revisional surgery may result in cervical esophagostoma and insertion of a jejunal feeding tube and result in delayed and difficult restoration of enteral continuity. Comparable insufficiency of rectal anastomoses can often be treated by diverting ileo- or colostomy and drainage, and operative revision of the anastomosis or Hartmann's procedure can be avoided in most of the patients [**Figure 3.3** (Bennis et al., 2012, Moran & Heald 2001)].

Bile duct anastomosis leakage (e.g. after pancreaticoduodenectomy) does not usually require reoperation unless it occurs very early, within 48 hours of the initial operation. In this situation, a surgical revision of the anastomosis can be performed with promising results. In delayed leakage, interventional therapy by percutaneous transhepatic biliary drainage offers a less invasive alternative with high technical and clinical success rates (Stampfl et al. 2011).

Pancreatic leakage and fistula after pancreaticojejunostomy or gastrostomy should be treated conservatively for as long as possible. Drainage of the pancreatic fluid is essential to avoid intra-abdominal collections and consecutive arrosion complications. Reoperation should only be considered in persisting septic situations or arrosion bleeding that cannot be controlled interventionally (Reid-Lombardo et al. 2007). A remnant pancreatectomy is the therapy of choice in these patients to achieve surgical control and regain stability of the patient. This reoperative approach is associated with a considerable morbidity and mortality but may be the only life-saving option for the patient (Hackert et al. 2011).

Colon or small bowel leaks usually require immediate reoperation and can be successfully treated by revision of the anastomosis, although the accompanying peritonitis increases the risk of releakage, which can be treated by diverting enterostomy as mentioned earlier.

Burst abdomen is another emergency that requires immediate reoperation (Gislason & Viste 1999, van Ramshorst et al. 2010). Risk factors for fascia rupture are extensive wound infections, infectious intra-abdominal complications, obesity, immunosuppression, preceding laparotomies, and existing cachexia. The use of slowly absorbable continuous sutures for abdominal wall closure in elective operations shows the best results with respect to late hernias and can therefore be regarded as the technique of choice to decrease the risk of burst abdomen (Diener et al. 2010). In contrast, the technique for burst abdomen closure has not been standardized with a high level of evidence yet (Van't et al. 2004). The use of continuous or interrupted

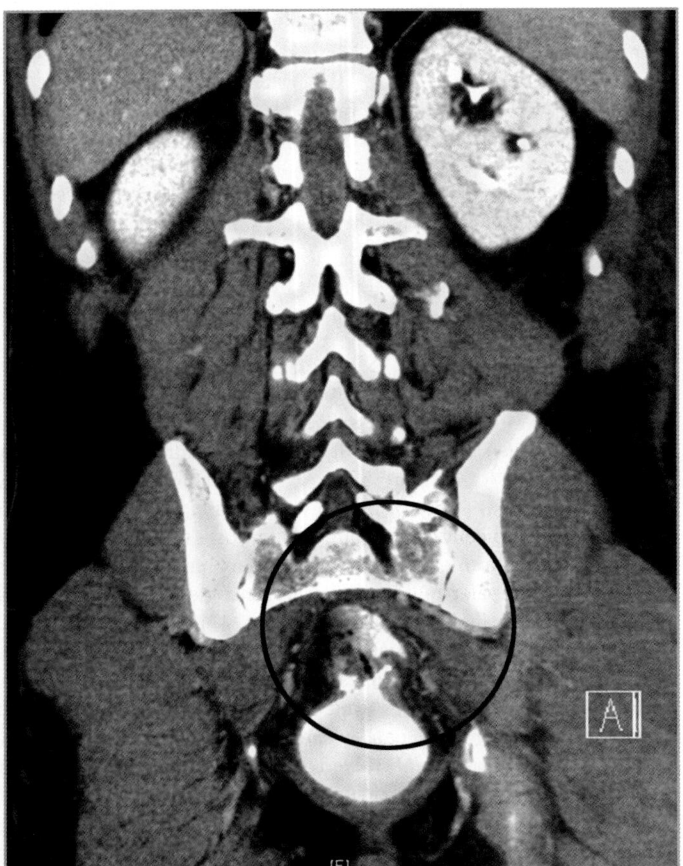

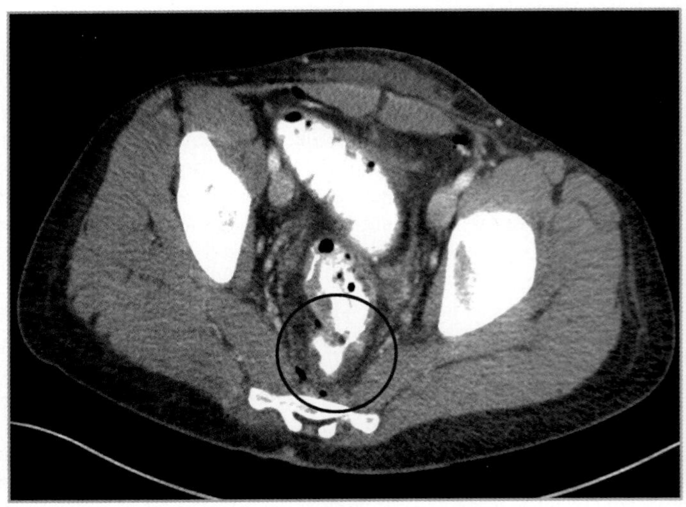

Figure 3.3 Computed tomographic scan showing anastomotic leakage after colectomy with ileorectostomy (black circles). Indication for emergency reoperation with revision of the anastomosis, loop ileostomy, and drainage placement.

sutures can be applied as well as a combination of both techniques, and the suture material can either be resorbable or nonresorbable. The chosen approach is highly dependent on the individual experience of the surgeon; nonresorbable sutures may offer a longer stability in critical patients. The use of a mesh augmentation during reoperation for burst abdomen is also not evidence based. Although this technique may offer more mechanical stability, it remains difficult to evaluate mesh implantation with regard to the risk of infection. As the occurrence of burst abdomen is often associated with infectious complications of the wound or intra-abdominally, the use of nonresorbable meshes seems inadvisable in this situation. However, if no obvious infection is present, mesh implantation can offer advantages in burst abdomen closure without any clear preference for positioning the mesh below (sublay position) or above (onlay position) the rectus muscle layer.

PREOPERATIVE IMAGING

Preoperative imaging before elective reoperation is generally focused on the underlying disease. Specific imaging to evaluate the existence of adhesions, their intensity or localization is not routinely recommended although magnetic resonance imaging (MRI) or a CT scan may be useful for this purpose. Inflammatory changes and scar formation can be visualized especially well using functional MRI, as can stenoses or kinking of bowel segments (Buhmann-Kirchhoff et al. 2008, Kirchhoff et al. 2010). However, the true extent of these changes is not sufficiently reflected by these examinations and they must be carefully exposed by the surgeon during exploration of the abdominal cavity.

If bowel obstruction by postoperative adhesions is the indication for reoperation, conventional or contrast-enhanced abdominal X-ray may provide information on the localization of the obstruction and facilitate exploration. Therefore, this easy-to-perform imaging is routinely performed in most patients, to settle the diagnosis of obstruction and help localize it (Harvey et al. 2005).

If reoperation is performed in patients with a coexisting large incisional hernia, an abdominal CT scan can be useful to evaluate the dimensions of the abdominal wall defect and the volume of bowel or other organs to plan repositioning, mesh implantation if necessary, and avoid intraoperative surprises [**Figure 3.4** (Hadad et al. 2009)].

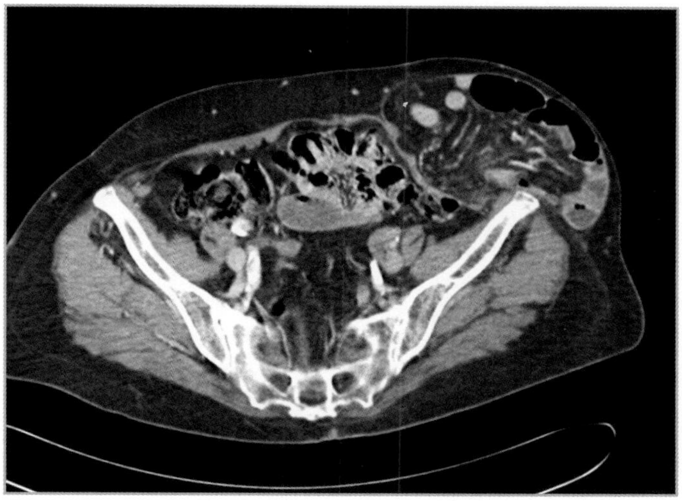

Figure 3.4 Computed tomographic scan showing a large incisional hernia after left pararectal incision. Preoperative imaging for evaluation of the defect size and the exteriorized intestinal volume.

LONG OPERATIONS AND ANTICIPATED HEMORRHAGE

Reoperations that require extensive adhesiolysis are associated with a long operation time and can lead to considerable blood loss due to the large tissue surface that is subjected to surgical manipulation. Although usually only small vessels are involved in adhesive structures, blunt or sharp dissection causes microinjuries with consecutive bleeding. This may accumulate over the long operation time and can additionally be aggravated by a decrease in body temperature due to the nonphysiological heat loss via the large exposed areas. Therefore, special attention has to be paid to these issues and close intraoperative consultation with the anesthesiologist is necessary to avoid any derangements that may result in hemorrhage and consecutive complications (Körner et al. 2012).

If a long operation time is anticipated, with the possibility of associated blood loss, continuous external warming of the patients is recommended, for example by convective air warming or a water-based thermo-wrap system (Qadan et al. 2009). This can be supplemented by warming of the infused fluid components, warm saline solution spilling into the abdominal cavity and an increase in operating-room temperature when required to avoid dangerous hypothermia (Dickinson et al. 2010).

Timely substitution of coagulation components is another important measure to prevent an underestimated and potentially continuing massive blood loss in long-lasting reoperations (Lawson & Murphy 2004, MacLaren 2007). As continuous minor bleeding may trigger a vicious circle resulting in a disseminated coagulation disorder, the application of fresh frozen plasma, selected coagulatory proteins, and platelets may be required and can minimize the need for replacement of packed red blood cells, which are in general less well tolerated by patients and more frequently associated with transfusion reactions or associated lung injury.

PLANNED SECONDARY RECONSTRUCTION

After extensive and long-lasting preparation during reoperative surgery, the problem of bowel edema may occur in some patients despite restrictive intravenous fluid management. Depending on the severity of this condition, it is advisable in some patients to plan a secondary reconstruction not only of bowel or stomach anastomoses, but especially of technically challenging anastomoses such as pancreatico- or hepato-jejunostomies. A planned secondary reconstruction implies the possibility of a safer anastomosis due to less edema within the bowel wall and can usually be performed within 24–48 hours of the initial operation. Temporary drainage of bile and pancreatic ducts before the completion of the operation can be undertaken by percutaneously placed soft catheters that are fixed with purse-string sutures around the duct. Bowel segments can be exteriorized as temporary stomas, and the stomach can be left closed as long as a nasogastric tube or gastrostomy is inserted to avoid dilation.

PATIENT POSITIONING AND THE NEED TO CHANGE POSITIONING DURING AN OPERATION

The positioning of the patient is determined by the planned operation. For visceral surgery, usually a supine position is adequate: sometimes a lithotomy position is required if mobilization of the pelvic organs has to be performed. Alternative positioning is rarely necessary. Positioning in reoperations can be performed in the same manner as the standard positioning used in primary surgery. A change in positioning is required only in exceptional cases. An important issue is to avoid any damage to neural and muscolosceletal structures caused by incorrect positioning. During long-lasting reoperations in the lithotomy position in particular, the legs are at risk of the development of pressure- or weight-induced damage (Zappa & Sugarbaker 2007). The most common injuries that arise as a result are neuropathies of the fibular nerve and compartment syndromes of the lower leg. Therefore, positioning needs to be carefully controlled throughout the operation and a lithotomy position should be used only as long as necessary. The position should be changed to a supine position with straightened legs as soon as possible. If this is not possible, the lower legs need to be released regularly (every 2–3 hours) before continuing the operation to avoid pressure-induced damage. Postoperatively, perfusion, sensation and motor function should be monitored for at least 12 hours (Beraldo & Dodds 2006).

CONDUCT OF THE OPERATION

Infection prophylaxis in reoperative surgery does not differ from the standard routine in primary operations, in terms of perioperative antibiotic application and disinfection or dressing if the abdominal wall is patent at the time of reoperation (Polk 2005). Antibiotic prophylaxis should be given 30 minutes before skin incision and consists of broadly covering penicillin or cephalosporin, combined with metronidazole in cases of planned bowel resection. For hernia surgery alone, cephalosporin prophylaxis is adequate. Application of antibiotics should be repeated every 4 hours during the operation (Enzler et al. 2011, Knebel et al. 2011).

In cases of a pre-existing stoma with planned restoration of bowel continuity, the stoma can be separately dressed and closed at the beginning of the operation, followed by another local disinfection and removal of the first dressing as well as a change of instruments and gloves to guarantee maximum infection prophylaxis.

The choice of incision has to be made taking into account two conflicting aspects. On the one hand, the cosmetic results are best if the pre-existing incision is chosen for relaparatomy. On the other hand, in this approach, a region of the abdominal wall is incised that has already been exposed to incision and healing before, which may lead to an impaired healing process and a mechanical weakness in this areas, predisposing to hernia development. In addition, the extent of adhesions is maximized underneath the prior incision, which may result in very difficult access to the abdominal cavity and an initially unclear anatomical situation in cases of dense adhesions, which in turn increases the risk of accidental enterotomy. Consequently, it may be advisable to choose a different incision (e.g. transverse after median or vice versa) for a reoperation, especially in patients who show a history of two or more preceding laparotomies with concomitant intra-abdominal complications such as peritonitis or abscesses. Access to the abdominal cavity is much easier using a different and new incision and adhesiolysis can often be carried out under better conditions.

Adhesiolysis is probably the most important operative step during reoperations. Careful separation of bowel and organ structures can be carried out by diathermy or sharply under bleeding control (e.g. by bipolar coagulation). Separation of tissue layers can be facilitated by continuous application of saline solution onto the tissue surface by the assisting surgeon. Accidental serosal injuries or enterotomies should be carefully avoided and immediately closed by direct suture or – if a longer segment of the bowel is affected – treated by segmental resection and primary anastomosis to offer the safest conditions for postoperative healing.

At the end of the operation, drain placement is performed to avoid collections, especially after extensive adhesiolysis, as a certain amount of fluid secretion from the tissue surface is inevitable. Generally, soft silicon drainage tubing should be chosen, and drainage of all abdominal quadrants that have been accessed should be considered, resulting in the use of two to four drainage tubes. Drainage removal can be performed after 24–48 hours to avoid drainage-associated ascending abdominal infection (Launay-Savary & Slim 2006).

In the case of a primary infection (abscess, peritonitis, acute pancreatitis), drains for spillage should be used to enable continuous evacuation of the abdominal cavity. Removal of these drains cannot be standardized but is dependent on the quality (clear reflux) of spilling fluid and the clinical situation.

Abdominal wall closure in reoperative surgery is not proven by the evidence from high-quality randomized studies (Diener et al. 2010, Seiler et al. 2009, Van't Riet et al. 2002). If a primary closure is attempted, slowly resorbable running sutures are appropriate and can be augmented by single stitches with slowly- or non-resorbable sutures. There is no evidence that a prophylactic mesh implantation is advisable in this situation. In particular, in reoperations that are associated with stoma closure or bowel resection, a mesh implantation should be avoided, otherwise there will be an increased risk of mesh infection.

Reconstruction of abdominal wall defects which cannot be closed without critical tension can be performed by the use of an inlay mesh [**Figure 3.5** (de Vries Reilingh et al. 2004)]. As this mesh is usually attached to bowel and organ structures, a biologically inert and compatible mesh should be used (e.g. extended polytetrafluoroethylene) to avoid arrosion complications on the

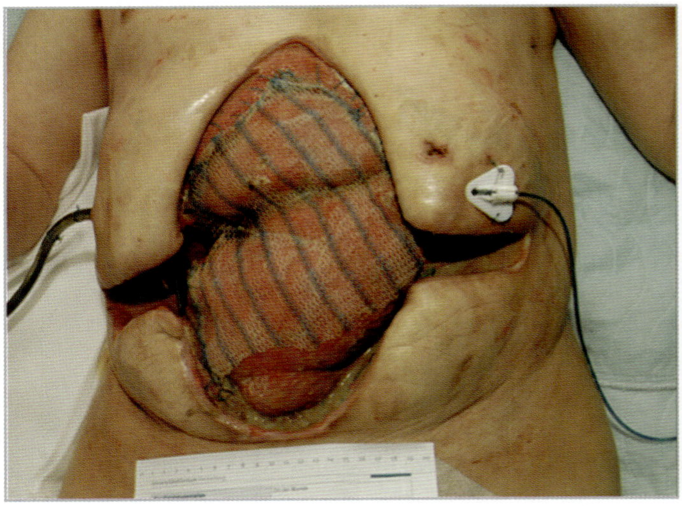

Figure 3.5 Laparostoma closed with inlay mesh. Enteral feeding tube (right side) and drainage (left side) for persisting duodenal leakage after complicated gastric ulcer surgery.

long-term course. Such meshes offer the same mechanical stability as other nonresorbable meshes and cause less irritation of bowel or organ tissue. The complex compartment release procedure requires skill, experience, and patience (Kanaan et al. 2011). For defect reconstruction, in general nonresorbable meshes should be used to avoid later recurrence of the defect and the need for another hernia repair. After mesh reconstruction, subcutaneous placement of a sufficient number of closed-suction drains is necessary to avoid fluid collections and secondary mesh infections.

POSTOPERATIVE PRINCIPLES

Postoperative antibiotic treatment is not generally recommended unless an intra-abdominal infection has been proven during surgery (e.g. abscess or peritonitis). In these patients, antibiotic therapy should be maintained depending on the clinical situation (Knebel et al. 2011). Furthermore, antibiotics use should be extended to adequately cover the septic situation and underlying bacteria. In most patients, this requires the use of carbapenem antibiotics (Mazuski 2007). If complicated bacterial infections (e.g. caused by resistant staphylococccal or enterococcal strains) are proven, standard drugs must be supplemented by suitable substances with regard to the specific sensitivity and resistance.

Nutrition of reoperated patients must be adapted to the intraoperative situation (Warren et al. 2011). Oral food intake can be started early in uncomplicated abdominal situations and safe anastomosis and can be completed within the first postoperative week if bowel motility is present. In cases with high-risk anastomoses or delayed recovery of gastric and bowel function, total parenteral nutrition is preferred, starting at day 3 to avoid a prolonged catabolic state. Concomitant oral feeding can be started as soon as postoperative paralysis resolves and bowel movements are present. A postoperative nasogastric tube may be required, especially in patients who undergo revision surgery for obstruction and who often show a massive dilation of the small or large bowel with a consequent functional impairment that may persist after surgical removal of the obstruction. A supportive stimulation of enteral passage can be performed by careful intravenous application of prokinetics including erythromycin for stomach emptying and metoclopramide for bowel motility (Bonacini et al. 1993, Longo & Vernava 1993).

Wound management is an essential topic in reoperative surgery as the incidence of wound infection is increased in repeated laparotomies as well as the occurrence of wound dehiscence that may eventually lead to a laparostoma as the worst-case scenario (Baharestani & Gabriel 2011, Heller et al. 2006). Uncomplicated infections of the skin and subcutaneous tissue are treated according to the principles of secondary wound healing: in an open manner with regular cleaning and dressing after opening of the infected portion of the wound. In large healing defects, the application of a vacuum-assisted closure system can facilitate the management and accelerate cleaning and healing of the wound which may be secondarily closed after all signs of infection have disappeared (DeFranzo et al. 2008).

Laparostoma care is certainly one of the most difficult and challenging tasks in reoperative surgery (Boele et al. 2009, Eder et al. 2006). From the clinical experience, more than three repeated laparotomies within a short period of time and combined with intra-abdominal infection lead to a fascia dehiscence, which often cannot be directly closed and requires open treatment. Furthermore, intestinal leakage due to insufficiency of anastomoses or accidental enterotomy triggers laparostoma development and prohibits mesh reconstruction due to the presence of infection. In cases of laparostoma occurrence, wound management includes regular cleaning and dressing with saline swabs and foil, which can usually be performed at the bedside with analgesic and sedative medication. Vacuum-assisted wound dressing in laparostoma treatment carries the risk of further suction-associated bowel injury. However, if suction is applied to a laparostoma dressing due to massive secretion, it needs to be downregulated to the lowest level possible, but may be helpful to avoid continuous leakage of the dressing [**Figure 3.6** (Miller et al. 2004)].

A time interval of at least 3 months, preferably 6 months, should be left before any attempts at closure of a laparostoma are considered, otherwise, the risk of recurrent difficult adhesiolysis and consequently bowel injury is considerable (Björck et al. 2011). Exceptions from this time course should only be made in patients who are at risk of severe laparostoma-associated complications, such as uncontrolled extensive fluid and electrolyte loss due to very high jejunal leakage or inadequate wound management.

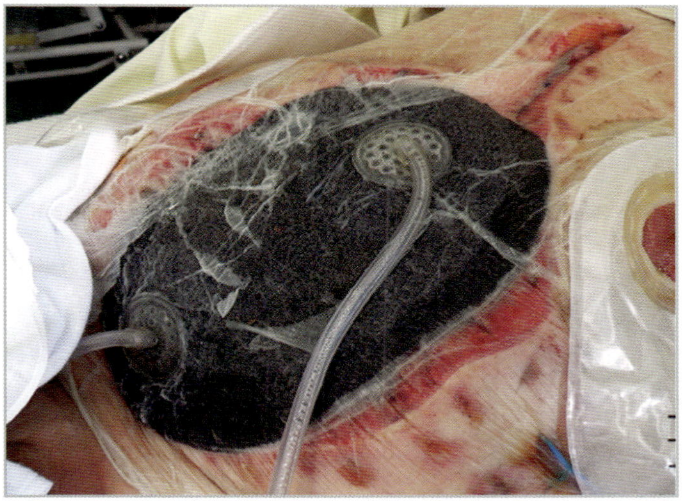

Figure 3.6 Vacuum-assisted laparostoma treatment to achieve a clean wound situation and bridge the interval to secondary abdominal wall reconstruction.

REFERENCES

Ahmad G, Duffy JM, Farquhar C, et al. Barrier agents for adhesion prevention after gynaecological surgery. Cochrane Database Syst Rev. 2012 Feb 15; 2:CD006583.

Arung W, Meurisse M, Detry O. Pathophysiology and prevention of postoperative peritoneal adhesions. World J Gastroenterol 2011; 17:4545–4553. Review.

Baharestani MM, Gabriel A. Use of negative pressure wound therapy in the management of infected abdominal wounds containing mesh: an analysis of outcomes. Int Wound J 2011; 8:118–125.

Becker JM, Dayton MT, Fazio VW, et al. Prevention of postoperative abdominal adhesions by a sodium hyaluronate-based bioresorbable membrane: a prospective, randomized, double-blind multicenter study. J Am Coll Surg 1996; 183:297–306.

Bennis M, Parc Y, Lefevre JH, et al. Morbidity risk factors after low anterior resection with total mesorectal excision and coloanal anastomosis: a retrospective series of 483 patients. Ann Surg 2012; 255:504–510.

Beraldo S, Dodds SR. Lower limb acute compartment syndrome after colorectal surgery in prolonged lithotomy position. Dis Colon Rectum 2006; 49:1772–1780. Review.

Björck M, D'Amours SK, Hamilton AE. Closure of the open abdomen. Am Surg 2011; 77:S58–61.

Boele van Hensbroek P, Wind J, Dijkgraaf MG, Busch OR, Goslings JC. Temporary closure of the open abdomen: a systematic review on delayed primary fascial closure in patients with an open abdomen. World J Surg 2009; 33:199–207.

Bonacini M, Quiason S, Reynolds M, et al. Effect of intravenous erythromycin on postoperative ileus. Am J Gastroenterol 1993; 88:208–211.

Brochhausen C, Schmitt VH, Planck CN, et al. Current strategies and future perspectives for intraperitoneal adhesion prevention [published online ahead of print 2 Feb 2012]. J Brochhausen: J Gastrointest Surg. 2012 Jun; 16(6):1256–74. Review.

Brokelman W, Holmdahl L, Falk P, Klinkenbijl J, Reijnen M. The peritoneal fibrinolytic response to conventional and laparoscopic colonic surgery. J Laparoendosc Adv Surg Tech A 2009; 19:489–493.

Brown SR, Goodfellow PB. Transverse verses midline incisions for abdominal surgery. Brown: Cochrane Database Syst Rev. 2005 Oct 19; (4):CD005199. Review.

Büchler MW, Wagner M, Schmied BM, et al. Changes in morbidity after pancreatic resection: toward the end of completion pancreatectomy. Arch Surg 2003; 138:1310–1314; discussion 1315.

Buhmann-Kirchhoff S, Lang R, Kirchhoff C, et al. Functional cine MR imaging for the detection and mapping of intra-abdominal adhesions: method and surgical correlation. Eur Radiol 2008; 18:1215–1223.

Bunt TJ. Urgent relaparotomy: the high-risk, no-choice operation. Surgery 1985; 98:555–560.

Ching SS, Muralikrishnan VP, Whiteley GS. Relaparotomy: a five-year review of indications and outcome. Int J Clin Pract 2003; 57:333–337.

DeFranzo AJ, Pitzer K, Molnar JA, et al. Vacuum-assisted closure for defects of the abdominal wall. Plast Reconstr Surg 2008; 121:832–839.

de Vries Reilingh TS, van Geldere D, Langenhorst B, et al. Repair of large midline incisional hernias with polypropylene mesh: comparison of three operative techniques. Hernia 2004; 8:56–59.

Dickinson A, Qadan M, Polk HC Jr. Optimizing surgical care: a contemporary assessment of temperature, oxygen, and glucose. Am Surg 2010; 76:571–577.

Diener MK, Voss S, Jensen K, Büchler MW, Seiler CM. Elective midline laparotomy closure: the INLINE systematic review and meta-analysis. Ann Surg 2010; 251:843–856 (Review).

diZerega GS. Biochemical events in peritoneal tissue repair. Eur J Surg Suppl. 1997; (577):10–6. Review.

Eder F, Tautenhahn J, Lippert H. Late complications of open abdomen. Chirurg 2006; 77:602–609.

Ellis H. The clinical significance of adhesions: focus on intestinal obstruction. Eur J Surg Suppl. 1997; (577):5–9. Review.

Enzler MJ, Berbari E, Osmon DR. Antimicrobial prophylaxis in adults. Mayo Clin Proc 2011; 86:686–701. Review.

Fry DE, Clevenger FW. Reoperation for intra-abdominal abscess. Surg Clin North Am 1991; 71:159–174.

Fry DE, Garrison RN, Heitsch RC, Calhoun K, Polk HC Jr. Determinants of death in patients with intra-abdominal abscess. Surgery 1980; 88:517–523.

Fry DE, Osler T. Abdominal wall considerations and complications in reoperative surgery. Surg Clin North Am 1991; 71:1–11.

Fujii S, Shimada H, Ike H, et al. Reduction of postoperative abdominal adhesion and ileus by a bioresorbable membrane. Hepatogastroenterology 2009; 56:725–728.

Gislason H, Viste A. Closure of burst abdomen after major gastrointestinal operations – comparison of different surgical techniques and later development of incisional hernia. Eur J Surg 1999; 165:958–961.

Hadad I, Small W, Dumanian GA. Repair of massive ventral hernias with the separation of parts technique: reversal of the 'lost domain. Am Surg 2009; 75:301–306.

Hackert T, Werner J, Büchler MW. Postoperative pancreatic fistula. Surgeon 2011; 9:211–217. Review.

Harbrecht PJ, Garrison RN, Fry DE. Early urgent relaparotomy. Arch Surg 1984; 119:369–374.

Harvey CJ, Allen S, O'Regan D. Interpretation of the abdominal radiograph: 1. Br J Hosp Med (Lond) 2005; 66:M66–M69. Review

Hellebrekers BW, Kooistra T. Pathogenesis of postoperative adhesion formation. Br J Surg 2011; 98:1503–1516. Review.

Heller L, Levin SL, Butler CE. Management of abdominal wound dehiscence using vacuum assisted closure in patients with compromised healing. Am J Surg 2006; 191:165–172.

Holmdahl L, Risberg B, Beck DE, et al. Adhesions: pathogenesis and prevention-panel discussion and summary. Eur J Surg. 1997 Mar; 163(3):169–174.

Kanaan Z, Bilchuk N, Galandiuk S, et al. Abdominal wall component release is a sensible choice for patients requiring complicated closure of abdominal defects. Langenbeck's archives of surgery/Deutsche Gesellschaft für Chirurgie 2011; 396:1263–1270.

Keller E, Neher M, Schuster HP. Relaparotomy, retrospective analysis and intensive care aspects. Langenbecks Arch Chir 1983; 360:167–177.

Kirchhoff S, Ladurner R, Kirchhoff C, et al. Detection of recurrent hernia and intraabdominal adhesions following incisional hernia repair: a functional cine MRI-study. Abdom Imaging 2010; 35:224–231.

Knebel P, Weigand MA, Büchler MW, Seiler CM. Evidence-based antibiotic prophylaxis in general and visceral surgery. Chirurg 2011; 82:227–234.

Körner CM, Weigand MA, Martin E. Anesthesiology: partner or competitor? [published online ahead of print 15 Feb 2012]. Chirurg. 2012 Apr; 83(4):323–326.

Kosaka H, Yoshimoto T, Yoshimoto T, Fujimoto J, Nakanishi K. Interferon-gamma is a therapeutic target molecule for prevention of postoperative adhesion formation. Nat Med 2008; 14:437–441.

Kumar S, Wong PF, Leaper DJ. Intra-peritoneal prophylactic agents for preventing adhesions and adhesive intestinal obstruction after non-gynaecological abdominal surgery. Cochrane Database Syst Rev. 2009 Jan 21; (1):CD005080.

Lalountas M, Ballas KD, Michalakis A, et al. Postoperative adhesion prevention using a statin-containing cellulose film in an experimental model. Br J Surg 2012; 99:423–429.

Launay-Savary MV, Slim K. Evidence-based analysis of prophylactic abdominal drainage. Ann Chir 2006; 131:302–305. Review.

Lawson JH, Murphy MP. Challenges for providing effective hemostasis in surgery and trauma. Semin Hematol 2004; 41:55–64. Review.

Longo WE, Vernava AM 3rd. Prokinetic agents for lower gastrointestinal motility disorders. Dis Colon Rectum 1993; 36:696–708. Review.

MacLaren R. Key concepts in the management of difficult hemorrhagic cases. Pharmacotherapy 2007; 27:93S–102S.

Mathes SJ, Steinwald PM, Foster RD, Hoffman WY, Anthony JP. Complex abdominal wall reconstruction: a comparison of flap and mesh closure. Ann Surg 2000; 232:586–596.

Mazuski JE. Antimicrobial treatment for intra-abdominal infections. Expert Opin Pharmacother 2007; 8:2933–2945. Review.

Miller PR, Meredith JW, Johnson JC, Chang MC. Prospective evaluation of vacuum-assisted fascial closure after open abdomen: planned ventral hernia rate is substantially reduced. Ann Surg 2004; 239:608–614; discussion 614–616.

Miura F, Asano T, Amano H, et al. Management of postoperative arterial hemorrhage after pancreato-biliary surgery according to the site of bleeding: re-laparotomy or interventional radiology. J Hepatobiliary Pancreat Surg 2009; 16:56–63.

Moran BJ, Heald RJ. Risk factors for and management of anastomotic leakage in rectal surgery. Colorectal Dis 2001; 3:135–137.

Polk HC Jr. Continuing refinements in surgical antibiotic prophylaxis. Arch Surg 2005; 140:1066–1067.

Polk HC Jr, Fry DE. Radical peritoneal debridement for established peritonitis. The results of a prospective randomized clinical trial. Ann Surg 1980; 192:350–355.

O'Dwyer PJ, Courtney CA. Factors involved in abdominal wall closure and subsequent incisional hernia. Surgeon 2003; 1:17–22. Review. Related citations

Qadan M, Gardner SA, Vitale DS, et al. Hypothermia and surgery: immunologic mechanisms for current practice. Ann Surg 2009; 250:134–40.

Ouaïssi M, Gaujoux S, Veyrie N, et al. Post-operative adhesions after digestive surgery: their incidence and prevention: review of the literature [published online ahead of print 20 Jan 2012. J Visc Surg. 2012 Apr; 149(2):e104–114.

Reed KL, Stucchi AF, Leeman SE, Becker JM. Inhibitory effects of a neurokinin-1 receptor antagonist on postoperative peritoneal adhesion formation. Ann N Y Acad Sci 2008; 1144:116–26.

Reid-Lombardo KM, Farnell MB, Crippa S, et al. Pancreatic anastomotic leakage after pancreaticoduodenectomy in 1,507 patients: a report from the Pancreatic Anastomotic Leak Study Group. J Gastrointest Surg 2007; 11:1451–1458; discussion 1459.

Seiler CM, Deckert A, Diener MK, et al. Midline versus transverse incision in major abdominal surgery: a randomized, double-blind equivalence trial (POVATI: ISRCTN60734227). Ann Surg 2009; 249:913–920.

Stampfl U, Hackert T, Radeleff B, et al. Percutaneous management of postoperative bile leaks after upper gastrointestinal surgery. Cardiovasc Intervent Radiol 2011; 34:808–815.

Stampfl U, Hackert T, Sommer CM, et al. Superselective embolization for the management of postpancreatectomy hemorrhage: a single-center experience in 25 patients [published online ahead of print 22 Feb 2012]. J Vasc Interv Radiol. 2012 Apr; 23(4):504–510.

Stumpf M, Conze J, Prescher A, et al. The lateral incisional hernia: anatomical considerations for a standardized retromuscular sublay repair. Hernia 2009; 13:293–297.

Tang CL, Jayne DG, Seow-Choen F, et al. A randomized controlled trial of 0.5% ferric hyaluronate gel (Intergel) in the prevention of adhesions following abdominal surgery. Ann Surg 2006; 243:449–455.

van Ramshorst GH, Eker HH, Harlaar JJ, et al. Therapeutic alternatives for burst abdomen. Surg Technol Int 2010; 19:111–119.

van Ruler O, Lamme B, Gouma DJ, Reitsma JB, Boermeester MA. Variables associated with positive findings at relaparotomy in patients with secondary peritonitis. Crit Care Med 2007; 35:468–476.

van't RM, De Vos Van Steenwijk PJ, Bonjer HJ, Steyerberg EW, Jeekel J. Incisional hernia after repair of wound dehiscence: incidence and risk factors. Am Surg 2004; 70:281–286.

Van't Riet M, Steyerberg EW, Nellensteyn J, Bonjer HJ, Jeekel J. Meta-analysis of techniques for closure of midline abdominal incisions. Br J Surg 2002; 89:1350–1356.

Vrijland WW, Tseng LN, Eijkman HJ, et al. Fewer intraperitoneal adhesions with use of hyaluronic acid-carboxymethylcellulose membrane: a randomized clinical trial. Ann Surg 2002; 235:193–199.

Warren J, Bhalla V, Cresci G. Postoperative diet advancement: surgical dogma vs evidence-based medicine. Nutr Clin Pract 2011; 26:115–125. Review.

Welsch T, von Frankenberg M, Schmidt J, Büchler MW. Diagnosis and definition of anastomotic leakage from the surgeon's perspective. Chirurg 2011; 82:48–55. Review.

Wente MN, Shrikhande SV, Kleeff J, et al. Management of early hemorrhage from pancreatic anastomoses after pancreaticoduodenectomy. Dig Surg 2006; 23:203–208. Epub 2006 July 26.

Wente MN, Veit JA, Bassi C, et al. Postpancreatectomy hemorrhage (PPH): an International Study Group of Pancreatic Surgery (ISGPS) definition. Surgery 2007; 142:20–25. Review.

Werner J, Hartwig W, Hackert T, Büchler MW. Surgery in the treatment of acute pancreatitis – open pancreatic necrosectomy. Scand J Surg 2005; 94:130–4. Review.

Zappa L, Sugarbaker PH. Compartment syndrome of the leg associated with lithotomy position for cytoreductive surgery. J Surg Oncol 2007; 96:619–23.

Zeng Q, Yu Z, You J, Zhang Q. Efficacy and safety of Seprafilm for preventing postoperative abdominal adhesion: systematic review and meta-analysis. World J Surg 2007; 31:2125–2131; discussion 2132. Review.

Zingg U, Pasternak I, Dietrich M, et al. Primary anastomosis vs Hartmann's procedure in patients undergoing emergency left colectomy for perforated diverticulitis. Colorectal Dis 2010; 12:54–60.

Chapter 4 Anesthetic considerations

Stuart Bertsch, Rainer Lenhardt, Ozan Akca

INTRODUCTION

Reoperative surgery presents specific challenges and considerations for the anesthesiologist. In general, patients who undergo reoperations are not as physically fit and optimized as in their initial operation. Moreover, the changed anatomy and various degrees of scarring lead to increased duration of surgery and frequent intraoperative management challenges for both surgeons and anesthesiologists. Thus, higher complication rates may ensue, resulting in increased morbidity for patients undergoing reoperative surgery (Beck 2006). Perioperative management includes minimally invasive techniques, early ambulation, and pain management, all of which have been shown to decrease postoperative recovery times, shorten hospitalizations, and reduce health care costs (Delaney et al. 2003, Kehlet & Dahl 2003, Kehlet & Wilmore 2002). The scope of this chapter focuses on important perioperative anesthetic management techniques to address and reduce complication rates pre-, intra-, and postoperatively.

PREOPERATIVE MANAGEMENT

Cardiovascular assessment

Preoperative cardiovascular assessment of patients for reoperative surgery is one of the main priorities for anesthesiologists. The American College of Cardiology/American Heart Association's (ACC/AHA) recent guidelines on perioperative cardiovascular evaluation and care for noncardiac surgery recommend a focused approach dictated by the patient's background heart disease, physical functional status, and the severity of surgical procedure (Fleisher et al. 2009). Patients requiring emergency surgery should proceed immediately to the operating room regardless of the severity of their heart disease. However, patients with active cardiac conditions often need referral for further cardiac management prior to elective surgery. Active cardiac conditions are defined as unstable angina or myocardial infarction within 30 days prior, new-onset or decompensated heart failure, uncontrolled significant arrhythmia, or severe valvular heart disease. Patients without active cardiac conditions, undergoing low-risk surgery, classified as endoscopic procedures, cataract surgery, breast surgery, may proceed to surgery with no additional workup. Patients without active cardiac conditions and a functional capacity $\geq$ 4 metabolic equivalents (METs) may proceed to surgery with no additional assessment. Finally, patients without any active cardiac conditions but with a functional capacity $<$ 4 METs, who are undergoing intermediate or high-risk surgery need assessment for the presence of risk factors. Major risk factors include a history of ischemic heart disease, heart failure, cerebrovascular disease, diabetes mellitus, and renal insufficiency. Patients without significant risk factors may proceed to surgery, but the presence of three or more risk factors potentially dictates further workup with noninvasive cardiac testing. For all other patients, noninvasive testing ought to be performed prior to surgery, only if a change in perioperative management is expected.

Medical optimization

Beta-blockers and other cardiac medications

Patients' medical comorbidities need to be addressed and optimized preoperatively. Great emphasis is placed on preoperative cardiac risk stratification associated with comorbidities. Patient's medications must be reviewed, and the patient is urged to take all medications important for an optimal perioperative outcome. The mainstay of these medications lies with perioperative beta blockade and statin therapy that should not be discontinued during the perioperative period.

Current ACC/AHA guidelines recommend against the routine preoperative administration of high-dose beta-blockers in low-risk group patients (Fleisher et al. 2009). However, preoperative withdrawal of beta-blockers increases mortality secondary to increased sympathetic stimulation. Therefore, perioperative continuation of beta-blockers is recommended for patients who are already taking them. Starting new treatment with beta-blockers in the perioperative period carries the risk of hypotension and bradycardia, thus decreased cardiac output. Other cardiac medications, such as calcium channel blockers, digoxin, nitrates, and antiarrhythmics, are also recommended to be continued throughout the perioperative period.

Statins

The Dutch Echocardiographic Cardiac Risk Evaluation Applying Stress Echocardiography (DECREASE) III study, which included statin-naïve patients undergoing noncardiac vascular surgery, reported a major reduction in myocardial infarctions (MIs) within 30 days after surgery in patients treated with fluvastatin and a beta-blocker without any difference in adverse outcomes (Schouten et al. 2009). Recent meta-analysis, which included statin-naïve surgical patients, reported a major decrease in MI, atrial fibrillation rates, and reduced length of stay (Chopra et al. 2012). Based on these findings and their pleitropic effects, statins should be continued throughout the perioperative period.

Antibiotic prophylaxis

Anesthesiologists' work hand-in-hand with surgeons, contributing to the prevention of surgical site infections through the administration of perioperative antibiotics. Through the ground-breaking work provided in the 1960s, Polk and Lopez Mayor established the importance of preoperative antibiotics in the reduction of wound infections and sepsis for elective gastrointestinal surgery (Polk & Lopez-Mayor 1969). With administration prior to surgical incision the drug levels in serum and tissue are greater than the minimum inhibitory concentration needed for targeted organisms (Bratzler & Houck 2005). Prior to incision, the proper antibiotics must be verified and administered while also ensuring no interactions with the patient's allergies. Frequently during reoperative surgery, the prolonged operative times require redosing of antibiotics. Bratzler and Houck (2005) recommended redosing the antibiotics two half lives after the first dose to ensure adequate serum levels. As important as the scheduled redosing intraoperatively stands, the discontinuation of antibiotics after surgery remains vital. Multiple studies demonstrated the importance of discontinuation, as it provides no additional benefit in preventing surgical site infection (SSI) after wound closure (ASHP 1999, Dellinger et al. 1994, Kreter & Woods 1992, Mangram et al. 1999, McDonald et al. 1998, Meijer et al. 1990, Page et al. 1993). One study actually exhibited an increased rate of surgical site infections during hospitalization and after hospital discharge when prolonged antibiotics were used (De Chiara et al. 2010). Furthermore, the prolonged use of antibiotics increases the emergence of resistant strains of bacteria (Eggimann & Pittet 2001, Harbarth et al. 2000, Hecker et al. 2003). The Surgical Care Improvement Project (SCIP) highlights these main issues. Each and every day, the proper antibiotics need to be started within one hour of incision and subsequently ceased within 24 hours of the completion of surgery.

Antiplatelet therapy and stents

Patients undergoing noncardiac surgery < 30 days after bare-metal stent implantation or < 6 months after drug-eluting stent implantation may have significantly elevated rates of major cardiac events when compared with patients in whom the interval between stenting and noncardiac surgery is longer (Schouten et al. 2007) (**Figure 4.1**). Similarly, the rate of major cardiac events within the early surgery group is expected to be significantly higher in patients whose antiplatelet therapy discontinued during the preoperative period than in those whose antiplatelet therapy was not stopped (Schouten et al. 2007). A hypercoagulable state develops within 7–10 days after interruption of antiplatelet therapy, rendering the patient vulnerable to thrombosis. In light of existing evidence, a significant consideration to continue antiplatelet therapy is required. Therefore, Fleisher suggests giving ketorolac or aspirin the morning of surgery to the patients whose antiplatelet therapy has been stopped 7–10 days previously (Fleisher 2009). However, no data from randomized trials exist to support this recommendation. It may be reasonable to stop antiplatelet therapy 4–5 days before surgery in patients with an increased risk of bleeding and resume therapy as soon as the bleeding risk becomes negligible, meaning within 1–2 days after surgery. In this way, patients avoid reaching the hypercoagulability time range.

Respiratory assessment, obstructive sleep apnea (OSA), and smoking

Respiratory assessment

No single preoperative assessment tool to consistently diagnose perioperative pulmonary complications exists. Factors along the lines of patients' age, type of surgery, emergency status of surgery, dependent functional status of the patient, low albumin levels, preoperative sepsis, and high American Society of Anesthesiologist (ASA) physical status are reportedly the independent risk predictors of postoperative pulmonary compromise (Gupta et al., Johnson et al. 2007, Qaseem et al. 2006, Smetana 2009) (**Table 4.1**). Because all of these independent risk predictors are very likely to be altered, intensified, and increased in reoperative surgery patients, the rate of pulmonary complications increases. Moreover, chronic obstructive pulmonary disease (COPD) patients with various states of severity need assessment in the preoperative clinic. Inhaled β-2-agonists, anticholinergic drugs, and corticosteroids are recommended to be continued in asthma and COPD patients to help achieve improved peak flow benefit preoperatively (Bapoje et al. 2007).

Obstructive sleep apnea

The ASA recommends the early initiation of continuous positive airway pressure in severe OSA. OSA increases the incidence of postoperative cardiopulmonary complications. The risks of postoperative complications depend on the severity of OSA and the type of surgical procedure to be performed (Gross et al. 2006). Diagnosis often requires polysomnography, which may be difficult to obtain preoperatively due to time constraints, especially with reoperative surgery. Therefore, a presumptive diagnosis of OSA necessitates the help of clinical criteria like snoring, increased body mass index, daytime hypersomnolence, inability to visualize the soft palate, and witnessed apnea episodes during sleep. For this purpose, screening questionnaires, mainly the

Table 4.1 Select independent predictors of respiratory failure from the updated respiratory failure index (Johnson et al. 2007, Smetana 2009)

Risk factors	Odds ratio
ASA class III	2.9
ASA class IV or V	4.9
Orofacial surgery	6.6
Work RVU > 17 (proxy for high-complexity procedures)	4.4
Albumin < 35 g/L (3.5 g/dL)	1.5
Aneurysm surgery	1.6
Age > 65 years	2.1
Smoker	1.1

ASA class III: severe systemic disease; ASA class IV & V: severe disease that is a constant threat to life, or moribund status in which survival is not expected without operation.

ASA, American Society of Anesthesiologists. RVU, Relative Value Units.

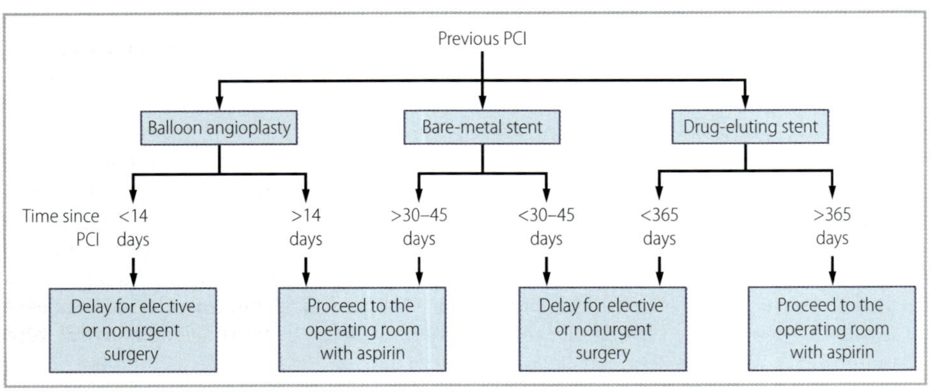

Figure 4.1 Proposed approach to management of patients with prior PCI. Redrawn with permission from Fleisher et al. (2007).

ASA checklist and the STOP-Bang questionnaire, provide guidance for the clinician (Adesanya et al., American Society of Anesthesiologists Task Force on Perioperative Management of patients with obstructive sleep apnea 2014, Gross et al. 2006].

Smoking

According to the Centers for Disease Control and Prevention – although decreasing continually – approximately 1 in 5 Americans are still current smokers despite the increased knowledge of complications and side effects. Many of these individuals undergo surgical procedures within their lifetime providing a prime opportunity to counsel patients on the dangers of tobacco use and its implications within the perioperative period (Shi & Warner). Sorenson highlights the detrimental effects of smoking on wound healing and infection through three main pathways '(1) a temporary reduction in tissue perfusion and oxygenation, (2) impairment of inflammatory cell functions and oxidative bactericidal mechanisms, and (3) attenuation of reparative cell function including synthesis and deposition of collagen' (Sorensen). The vasoconstrictive properties of smoking have been demonstrated through multiple studies, which can potentially lead to a 40% decrease in blood flow to tissue (Black et al. 2001, Emmanuel & Kamm 1999, Jensen et al. 1991, Monfrecola et al. 1998, Morecraft et al. 1994, Sorensen et al. 2009). In addition, the formation of carbon monoxide after smoking further decreases tissue oxygenation as the carbon monoxide binds hemoglobin molecules 200 times more than oxygen and causes a leftward shift of the oxygen-hemoglobin dissociation curve. Through these mechanisms, oxygen delivery to the tissues decreases and local hypoxia may occur (Rietbrock et al. 1992). Like tissue oxygenation, the inflammatory response plays a key role in wound healing and can significantly be impaired by smoking. Smoking compromises neutrophil function thereby decreasing the ability to prevent bacterial contamination, which frequently leads to higher rates of surgical site infections (Sorensen et al. 2005). A recent meta-analysis demonstrated a higher incidence of surgical site infection and wound necrosis in smokers (Sorensen). On the other hand, cessation of smoking leads to reversible changes and allows for improvement of wound healing, better oxygenation, and less respiratory complications. The exact time for when to quit smoking before surgery remains elusive, but the longer time ceased leads to better results. Typically, the effects of poor wound healing may be reversed by quitting 4–6 weeks before surgery, and the effects of carbon monoxide can be minimized by stopping 24 hours prior to incision. The importance of counseling cannot be understated throughout the perioperative period and the impact of anesthesiologists and surgeons in promoting cessation of smoking remain imperative (Mastracci et al., Warner et al. 1984, Warner & Shi).

INTRAOPERATIVE MANAGEMENT

Type of anesthesia

Although the comorbidities and type of surgery dictate certain decisions in managing patient care, anesthesiologists maintain various modalities for the perioperative period. These consist of anything from local to regional anesthesia, including neuraxial techniques and peripheral nerve blocks, as well as monitored anesthesia care with sedation to general anesthesia. Overlapping of different anesthetic types and combinations of regional analgesics to supplement general anesthesia occur frequently.

Debate on the superiority of regional anesthesia to general anesthesia continues to date. Current randomized-controlled trials do not support any difference in mortality between regional and general anesthesia. The largest randomized study to date highlighting this issue, the General Anesthesia Local Anesthesia study group, demonstrated no significant difference among patients receiving local versus general anesthesia for carotid endarterectomy surgery (Lewis et al. 2008). Following that randomized clinical trial, a retrospective review of the American College of Surgeons National Quality Improvement Program (ACS-NSQIP) reported similar results (Schechter et al. 2012). In another report from the ACS-NSQIP focusing on endovascular aortic repair, a lack of difference in mortality among local anesthesia, spinal anesthesia, or general anesthesia emerged (Edwards et al. 2011). Moreover, meta-analyses of regional anesthesia versus general anesthesia for total hip arthroplasty and total knee arthroplasty revealed no difference in mortality (Macfarlane et al. 2009a, 2009b].

Although there may be no difference in mortality, regional and local anesthesia offer other advantages compared with sole general anesthesia. Such advantages may decrease morbidity associated with surgery and the patient's existing medical status. Studies demonstrate a decrease in the rate of surgical site infections when utilizing regional anesthesia compared with general anesthesia (Chang et al. 2010, Tsai et al. 2011). Multiple theories possibly explain this phenomenon. Regional anesthesia impairs the immune system less than general anesthesia (Ciepichal & Kubler 1998), improves tissue oxygenation (Buggy et al. 2002, Ciepichal & Kubler 1998, Treschan et al. 2003) and reduces postoperative pain thus diminishing associated vasoconstriction and further decreased tissue oxygenation (Akca et al. 1999). Many studies and reviews established the significant effect of regional and regional-general combined anesthesia to decrease postoperative pain scores (Catro-Alves et al. 2011, Macfarlane et al. 2009a, 2009b, Parker et al. 2004, Tahiri et al. 2011, Thavaneswaran et al. 2010, Tzovaras et al. 2008). By improving pain control and reducing opioid consumption, regional anesthesia helps diminish the incidence of postoperative nausea and vomiting (PONV) (Chelly et al. 2011, Macfarlane et al. 2009a, 2009b, Tahiri et al. 2011).

Current controversy surrounds cancer recurrence rates and regional anesthesia. Retrospective reviews determined that supplementation of general anesthetics with epidural or paravertebral blocks decreased cancer recurrence and metastasis (Biki et al. 2008, Exadaktylos et al. 2006). However, some observational studies failed to confirm a reduction in recurrence rates (Gottschalk et al. 2010, Ismail et al. 2010, Tsui et al. 2010). Knowledge that opioids reduce the cellular and humoral immune function (Sacerdote et al. 2000) highlights the importance and consideration of offering regional anesthesia to patients undergoing cancer resections despite conflicting results in recurrence and metastasis. Finally, because regional anesthesia decreases complications from pulmonary morbidity, including aspiration, pneumonia, and respiratory failure (Edwards et al. 2011, Neuman et al. 2012, Svircevic et al. 2011], anesthesiologists need to weigh decisions concerning the type of anesthetic carefully, especially in high-risk group patients as in the case of reoperative surgery.

Normothermia

The SCIP considers normothermia a priority in the perioperative period. In maintaining core body temperature through the perioperative period, multiple deleterious effects are easily prevented. These important complications, including increased myocardial morbidity (Frank et al. 1997), surgical site infections (Kurz et al. 1996, Melling et al. 2001), and coagulopathy (Rajagopalan et al. 2008, Schmied et al. 1996, Widman et al. 2002, Winkler et al. 2000), lead to prolonged recovery period and hospitalization, as well as the potential for increased allogenic blood transfusions (Schmied et al. 1996, Widman et al. 2002, Winkler et al. 2000, Kurz et al. 1996, Lenhardt et al. 1997) (**Table 4.2**). Through the vigilance of the anesthesiologist in the operating room, these preventable complications are minimized.

Hypothermia leads to an increased rate of surgical site infections (SSI) through multiple mechanisms. Not only does hypothermia weaken the immune system through impaired leukocyte migration, neutrophil phagocytosis, and by reducing reactive oxygen intermediates, it also causes significant vasoconstriction (Sessler et al. 1988a, 1988b, Wenisch et al. 1996). Decrease in blood flow leads to lower levels of oxygen within the peripheral tissue prompting bacterial growth and eventually surgical site infections (Greif et al. 2000, Sheffield et al.1994a, 1994b, 1996,).

Throughout the perioperative period, hypothermia results in coagulopathy, which leads to transfusion of blood products. When one experiences hypothermia, platelets undergo morphologic changes that decrease the capacity to activate clot formation (Ferrell et al. 1988, Michelson et al. 1994, Rohrer & Natale 1992, Valeri et al. 1992]. Along with the morphologic changes, the prothrombin time and partial thromboplastin time are prolonged when compared with normothermic patients (Bunker & Goldstein 1958, Rohrer & Natale 1992). Lastly, the fibrinolysis pathway becomes altered promoting clot breakdown. Through all of these mechanisms, blood loss possibly

Table 4.2 Major consequences of mild perioperative hypothermia in patients and healthy human volunteers

Potential complications	First author-year	*N*	ΔT_{core} (°C)	Outcomes	*P*
Surgical wound infection	Kurz et al. 1996	200	1.9	Hypothermic patients experienced ~3x more SSI	<0.01
Surgical wound infection	Melling et al. 2001	421	–	Hypothermic patients experienced ~3x more SSI	0.001
Duration of hospitalization	Kurz et al. 1996	200	1.9	Hypothermic patients had ~2.5 days of longer stay in the hospital	<0.01
Duration of hospitalization	Frank et al. 1997	300	1.3	No difference in duration of stay	NS
Blood loss	Schmied et al. 1996	60	1.6	Hypothermic patients had ~0.5 L more blood loss	<0.001
Blood loss	Winkler et al. 2000	150	0.4	Hypothermic patients had ~0.1 L more blood loss	0.002
Blood loss	Widman et al. 2002	46	0.5	Hypothermic patients had ~0.2 L more blood loss	<0.05
Blood loss	Hofer et al. 2005	60	1.8	Hypothermic patients had ~1.0 L more blood loss	0.01
Blood loss	Johansson et al. 1999	50	0.8	No difference in blood loss	NS
Blood loss	Vassiliades et al. 2003	94	0.9	Hypothermic patients had ~0.2 L more blood loss	0.015
Blood loss	Wong et al. 2007	103	-	Hypothermic patients had ~0.2 L more blood loss	0.01
Transfusion requirement	Nesher et al. 2003	60	1.0	Hypothermic patients required ~1.5–2 U more blood transfusion	<0.01
Transfusion requirement	Schmied et al. 1996	60	1.6	Hypothermic patients required ~70 mL more blood transfusion	<0.05
Transfusion requirement	Kurz et al. 1996	200	1.9	Hypothermic patients required ~0.4 U more blood transfusion	0.001
Transfusion requirement	Hofer et al. 2005	60	1.8	Hypothermic patients required ~0.7 L more blood transfusion	0.013
Morbid cardiac events	Frank et al. 1997	300	1.3	Hypothermic patients experienced 6x more cardiac morbid events	<0.05
Myocardial damage – Troponin I	Nesher et al. 2003	60	1.0	Hypothermic patients had ~3x higher troponin I levels	<0.01
Duration of vecuronium	Heier et al. 1991	20	2.0	Vecuronium duration more than doubled in hypothermic patients	<0.001
Duration of atracurium	Leslie et al. 1995	6	3.0	Atracurium duration increased ~50% in hypothermic patients	<0.05
Duration of postanesthetic recovery	Lenhardt et al. 1997	150	1.9	Duration of recovery period was prolonged by ~40 minutes in hypothermic patients	<0.001
Adrenergic activation	Frank et al. 1995	74	1.5	Adrenergic activity increased by ~50% in hypothermic patients	<0.05
Composite complications	Wong et al. 2007	103	-	Composite complications were ~66% higher in hypothermic patients	0.027
Mortality after major trauma	Gentilello et al. 1997	57	-	Mortality was ~6x higher in hypothermic patients	<0.05

N = total number of subjects.

ΔTcore = difference in core temperature between the treatment groups. Results presented as means ±SDs or median [interquartile range] unless otherwise specified.

NS = not significant.

Modified with permission from Dr. Daniel I. Sessler.

increases significantly. Schmied et al. (1996) demonstrated that a 1.6°C decrease in temperature, increased blood loss by 500 mL, and increased the chance of allogeneic blood transfusion. In avoiding hypothermia, clotting mechanisms are preserved, and the risks associated with allogeneic blood transfusions averted.

Perioperative hypothermia increases the risk of cardiac morbidity through increased catecholamine release, systemic vasoconstriction, shivering, and increased blood pressure (Frank et al. 1995, 1997). Hypothermia increases the activation of the sympathetic system, which leads to an increase in cardiac work. This effect is expected to be exaggerated in elderly patients as they have an elevated norepinephrine concentration of three times normothermic levels, leading to cold-induced hypertension (Frank et al. 2000). All of these mechanisms described by Frank et al. were translated to clinical outcomes as a significant reduction in cardiac events, meaning cardiac arrest, myocardial infarction, unstable angina, and electrocardiographic events, existed in normothermic patients (Frank et al. 1997).

Preventing hypothermia to <36°C decreases the risks of SSIs, coagulopathy, prolonged recovery periods, and cardiac morbidity. Despite the existing knowledge and regulations, it is estimated that a third of patients are still hypothermic on arrival to the PACU, significantly prolonging a patient's recovery (Forbes et al. 2008, Hedrick et al. 2007, Lenhardt et al. 1997) (**Figure 4.2**). Simple actions of adjusting the ambient temperature of the operating room, actively warming patients and increasing awareness on the very issue help prevent hypothermia and related complications in the perioperative period.

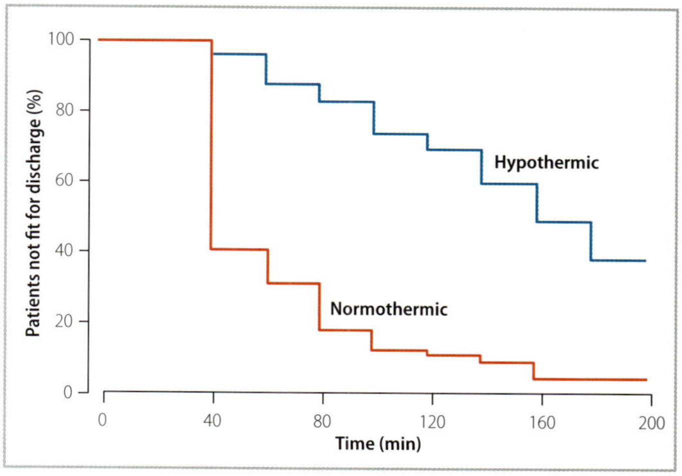

Figure 4.2 Mild intraoperative hypothermia prolongs postoperative recovery. One hundred fifty patients were randomly assigned to normothermia or ≈2.5°C core hypothermia. Fitness for discharge was determined using defined criteria by observers blinded to patient temperature and group assignment. The percentages of patients fit for discharge are plotted against time, using survival curve analysis. Hypothermia significantly delayed discharge by ≈20 minutes (left side of figure). When normothermia (core temperature >36°C) also was required for discharge, the difference between the groups increased to nearly 2 hours (right side of figure). These data indicate that mild hypothermia significantly prolongs postanesthetic recovery. Redrawn with permission from Lenhardt et al. (1997).

Fluid management

The critical role of fluid management is another challenge for perioperative team members. Multiple factors, including type and duration of surgery and anesthesia as well as patient characteristics and types of morbidities, impact the decisions in guiding fluid management. Throughout the perioperative period, fluid therapy helps manage hypotension, impaired tissue oxygenation, and inadequate organ perfusion but may also result in interstitial edema and congestion of the cardiopulmonary system (Arkilic et al. 2003, Bamboat & Bordeianou 2009, Kabon et al. 2005). Currently, there are many controversies regarding the types of fluids, meaning crystalloids versus colloids, and restrictive versus liberal approaches, or a goal directed approach.

The debate on colloid versus crystalloid fluid therapy remains unresolved. Benefits of crystalloid therapy include avoidance of renal impairment, minimal interaction with coagulation, and lack of allergic reactions, whereas colloid therapy possesses volume-expanding properties, minor edema formation, and improved microcirculation (Miller 2010). However, the recent Cochrane Database reviews demonstrated no difference in the treatment of critically ill, trauma, burn, and surgical patients with regards to a reduction in the risk of death, pulmonary edema, or length of hospital stay (Perel & Roberts 2007). Furthermore, no data exist to support the use of a particular colloid in terms of impact on survival (Bunn et al. 2008).

Although the debate regarding fluid type continues, increased controversy surrounds the amount of fluids to be given within the perioperative period as well. Although the goal focuses on reestablishing the effective circulating intravascular volume to ensure tissue oxygenation, (Arkilic et al. 2003, Bamboat & Bordeianou 2009, Kabon et al. 2005) three main strategies currently guide fluid management. Restrictive fluid therapy focuses on limiting fluids to no edema or weight gain, whereas a liberal fluid approach allows for improved perfusion. Each modality carries advantages and disadvantages throughout the perioperative period. A restrictive fluid approach potentially reduces the incidence of anastomic leakage and pulmonary complications (Brandstrup et al. 2003) with the further advantages of earlier resumption of bowel function and motility (Nisanevich et al. 2005). The reverse also exists as liberal fluid therapy impacts poor anastomotic healing (Brandstrup et al. 2003, Lobo et al. 2002, Nisanevich et al. 2005) and may result in delayed return of bowel functions (Brandstrup et al. 2003, Corcoran et al. 2012, Grocott et al. 2005). As technology advances, newer tools focusing on pulse pressure variation and stroke volume variation help individualize fluid management, a term garnered goal-directed therapy. This individualized management typically leads to improved hemodynamics intraoperatively and reduced postoperative complications with the potential to decrease the length of hospital stay (Benes et al. 2010). On average, studies focusing on goal directed therapy typically administered higher rates of colloid therapy and larger amounts of fluid when compared with nongoal directed treatment. When compared with nongoal-directed therapy, the goal-directed therapy patients usually had less pneumonia and renal complications, less time to first bowel movement, and resumption of normal diet earlier (Corcoran et al. 2012). The debate regarding fluid type and administration will continue as newer trials emerge, but as of now, no clear cut answer exists to give the final word in optimal fluid management strategy. Therefore, our recommendation is customizing the amount and type of fluids to each individual patient based on patient's medical background, current cardiovascular functionality, and type and duration of surgery.

Supplemental oxygen – hyperoxia

Oxidative killing function of polymorphonuclear leukocytes is the primary mechanism of defense against surgical pathogens (Allen et al.

1997, Qadan et al.). Tissue oxygenation correlates with oxidative killing and helps predict SSI rates (Govinda et al., Hopf et al. 1997). As a result, some randomized controlled trials have been conducted to assess the benefit of perioperative supplemental oxygen therapy (Belda et al. 2005, Greif et al. 2000, Mayzler et al. 2005, Meyhoff et al. 2009, Myles et al. 2007, Pryor et al. 2004). As discussed in detail by Qadan et al. (2009) results of these trials have been inconsistent due to varying subsets of patients with varying criteria for diagnosing SSI. Therefore, various reports from meta-analyses of the data help perioperative physicians to interpret these conflicting results. Currently, the jury is still out about beneficial effects of hyperoxia. Because supplemental perioperative oxygen ($FiO_2 \leq 0.80$) can be considered harmless, anesthesiologists and surgeons may consider its use intra- and early postoperatively for potential benefits.

Glucose management

The epidemic of diabetes mellitus continues with an estimated 8.3% of the US population being affected (Huang et al. 2009). Diabetes mellitus increases morbidity and mortality through multiple complications, including myocardial ischemia, retinopathy, autonomic and peripheral neuropathy, nephropathy, stroke, and wound infection. Myocardial ischemia, stroke, end-stage renal disease, and wound infections pose the greatest risk of morbidity and mortality for the diabetic patient undergoing elective surgery (Umpierrez et al. 2002). In addition, diabetic neuropathies often cause gastroparesis increasing the risk of aspiration during anesthesia induction. Lastly, diabetes-related cervical joint stiffness renders intubation more difficult.

Long-term improvement of glycemic control reduces and delays the onset of diabetic complications. Hemoglobin A1C values assess the efficacy of treatment better than blood glucose profiles. Instead of assessing long-term glycemic control, patients admitted to the hospital may receive inadequate treatment with blood glucose measurements on admission, which typically prompts an sliding scale insulin (SSI) regimen. However, this treatment seems to be inferior to a more modern, more physiologic approach featuring a long-lasting basal insulin along administered with a short-term prandial (bolus) insulin on a scheduled basis. This basal/bolus insulin (BBI) approach achieves lower glucose levels in hospitalized medical patients without an increase in hypoglycemic events (Umpierrez et al. 2007). When using a BBI regimen for perioperative glycemic control of in-hospital patients, significantly fewer complications ensued compared with the SSI group (9% vs. 26%, respectively) (Umpierrez et al.).

Most all diabetic patients need treatment with insulin during the perioperative period. Although still controversial, physicians are recommended to set a target goal of <7.8 mmol/L (140 mg/dL) in nonintensive care unit patients and between 7.8 and 10.0 mmol/L (140 and 180 mg/dL) in intensive care unit patients (Umpierrez et al.). All diabetic patients who are admitted to the hospital are recommended to receive BBI therapy. Oral antidiabetics should be discontinued. On the day of surgery, diabetic patients may require a near full dose of basal insulin, if glargine or insulin detemir is used. If treated with NPH, half of patients' normal dose is suggested. Avoidance of bolus insulin remains a mainstay while the patient retains an NPO status (Godoy et al. 2012).

Diabetic patients undergoing major surgery, defined as cardiac, vascular, or major abdominal surgery, necessitate administration of insulin via an insulin drip intravenously with hourly blood glucose measurements. Continuation into the immediate postoperative period remains important as well. Once in a steady state, treatment ought to be converted to a subcutaneous BBI regimen. For conversion from intravenous to subcutaneous insulin, a transition protocol should be employed (Ramos et al.).

Many diabetic patients undergo minor surgery in an ambulatory care setting. Basal insulin management must occur as outlined above. However, no evidence exists that perioperative blood glucose control improves outcomes after one-day surgery. Thus, it is not advisable to use a perioperative insulin drip, even if blood glucose values exceed the recommended goal. In the event of an excessively high blood glucose level, deliberation for postponement of elective surgery should be considered. The definition of a cutoff point for cancellation should be in consensus with a hospital policy.

POSTOPERATIVE MANAGEMENT

Management of postoperative pain

Postoperative care encompasses a majority of the time spent during hospitalizations after prolonged operations. One of the main goals of postoperative care includes pain management as improved pain control may shorten the hospital course (Buvanendran et al. 2003, Callesen et al. 1998, Carr & Goudas 1999, Joshi 2005, Kehlet 1997). Optimum postoperative analgesia results in earlier ambulation and rehabilitation postoperatively (Khoo et al. 2007, Tali & Maaroos 2010, Wu et al. 2005). In addition, patient satisfaction greatly improves. Optimal control of pain occurs through the use of multiple analgesics that act on different receptors within the nervous system, a term deemed multimodal analgesia (Kehlet & Dahl 1993). Various neurotransmitters exist and the ability to target each aim to minimize the effects of individual agents (Kehlet & Dahl 1993). In addition to different classes of drug therapy, the anesthesiologist employs regional anesthetic techniques to help reduce pain via neuropathic transmission.

Although the mainstay of postoperative pain control requires opiate therapy, other classes of drugs help reduce opioid consumption and their side effects when utilized. Nonsteroidal anti-inflammatory drugs (NSAIDs) inhibit the synthesis of prostaglandins at periphery, one of the main causes of the heightened pain state. Acetaminophen also inhibits cyclooxygenase and possesses mild if any anti-inflammatory properties. Furthermore, gabapentin and pregabalin target a neuropathic component through GABA and voltage gated calcium channels. Lastly, ketamine acts on multiple pain receptors, the most important being the NMDA receptor. Each of these drugs decreases opioid consumption and improves analgesia by targeting different pain receptors (Aveline et al. 2009, Huang et al. 2008, Remerand et al. 2009, Remy et al. 2005, Sen et al. 2009, Schmid et al. 1999, Sinatra et al. 2005, Subramaniam et al. 2004, Sun et al. 2008, Turan et al. 2004).

Within the opioid-related side effects, preventing PONV, avoiding excessive sedation, and enhancing the return of bowel function without ileus formation are the most common ones concerning the perioperative period. These side effects may prolong hospitalization, prevent early discharge and fast tracking of patients, which all result in increased costs (Oderda et al. 2003).

In addition to the regional anesthetics and targeting various pain receptors, the infiltration of local anesthetic within the wound helps reduce perioperative pain. Side effects from local anesthetic infiltration remain low, and systemic toxicity is extremely rare. Overall, wound infiltration theoretically reduces pain scores, decreases adjuvant analgesics, and delays the time for the first request of analgesics (Joshi et al. 2012).

Management of postoperative nausea and vomiting

Over the past decades, extensive research focused on the prevention and treatment of PONV. Regardless of advances, PONV continues to have an incidence of 30% and even as high as 80% within high-risk patients. Multiple risk indices developed to stratify a patient's likelihood of developing PONV. Apfel's simplified risk score and the score developed by Koivuranta et al. are the most clinically utilized ones (Apfel et al. 1999, Koivuranta et al. 1997). Patient-related risk factors include the female sex, a nonsmoking status, and a history of PONV. Anesthesia-related risk factors are volatile anesthetic use, including nitrous oxide, and opioid consumption. Mainstay therapy with multiple medication attempts to prevent PONV through a risk-based approach. Medications utilized include serotonin antagonists (ondasetron, dolasetron, granisetron), glucocorticoids (dexamethasone), dopamine antagonists (droperidol, metoclopramide), and cholinergic antagonists (scopolamine). Typically, due to their additive effects, the combination of multiple drugs prevent PONV well (Apfel et al. 2004), but occasionally the need for rescue therapy occurs. To effectively treat PONV after failed prevention, a trial of a separate class of medication is warranted. Prolonged operations are common with reoperative surgery, as well as increased amounts of opioid therapy causing higher incidence of PONV (Roberts et al. 2005, Sinclair et al. 1999). Prediction and prevention remain the ideal goal. A combination of multiple drugs is the best method for the management of PONV.

Respiratory management

The American College of Physicians' guidelines recommend deep breathing exercises, incentive spirometry, and selective use of nasogastric tube decompression for those identified as high-risk patients of postoperative pulmonary complications (Qaseem et al. 2006). Noninvasive positive pressure ventilation can be considered for patients who are unable to perform incentive spirometry or deep breathing exercises. OSA patients should be kept in a semirecumbent or recumbent position and monitored with continuous pulse oximetry until the risk of postoperative respiratory depression decreases. Unless a contraindication exists, extubation needs to be planned when the OSA patient is awake and after full reversal of neuromuscular blockade. The ASA also recommends minimizing the perioperative use of narcotics and benzodiazepines in these high-risk patients (Gross et al. 2006).

SUMMARY

Placing emphasis on each aspect of perioperative management, from the initial preoperative evaluation, intraoperative management to postoperative pain management, aspires to improve surgical outcomes through reduced morbidity and mortality. Communication between the surgeons and anesthesiologists about preoperative risks and perioperative management plans is extremely important in reoperative surgery. Vigilance of the anesthesiologist, via meticulous attention to perioperative details, helps improve surgical outcomes and further decrease perioperative morbidity such as surgical site infections, cardiac complications, and fluid overload. The issues highlighted within this chapter are not all inclusive. The importance of perioperative optimization and communication concerning care plans to achieve the best outcomes for patients cannot be emphasized enough and requires daily cooperation among all parties involved with patient care.

REFERENCES

Adesanya AO, Lee W, Greilich NB, Joshi GP. Perioperative management of obstructive sleep apnea. Chest 2011; 138:1489–1498.

Akca O, Melischek M, Scheck T, et al. Postoperative pain and subcutaneous oxygen tension. Lancet 1999; 354:41–42.

Allen DB, Maguire JJ, Mahdavian M, et al. Wound hypoxia and acidosis limit neutrophil bacterial killing mechanisms. Arch Surg 1997; 132:991–996.

American Society of Anesthesiologists Task Force. Practice guidelines for the perioperative management of patients with obstructive sleep apnea: an updated report by the American Society of Anesthesiologists Task Force on perioperative management of patients with obstructive sleep apnea. Anesthesiology 2014; 120:268–286.

Apfel CC, Korttila K, Abdalla M, et al. A factorial trial of six interventions for the prevention of postoperative nausea and vomiting. N Engl J Med 2004; 350:2441–2451.

Apfel CC, Laara E, Koivuranta M, et al. A simplified risk score for predicting postoperative nausea and vomiting: conclusions from cross-validations between two centers. Anesthesiology 1999; 91:693–700.

ASHP Therapeutic Guidelines on Antimicrobial Prophylaxis in Surgery. American Society of Health-System Pharmacists. Am J Health Syst Pharm 1999; 56:1839–1888.

Arkilic CF, Taguchi A, Sharma N, et al. Supplemental perioperative fluid administration increases tissue oxygen pressure. Surgery 2003; 133:49–55.

Aveline C, Gautier JF, Vautier P, et al. Postoperative analgesia and early rehabilitation after total knee replacement: a comparison of continuous low-dose intravenous ketamine versus nefopam. Eur J Pain 2009; 13:613–619.

Bamboat ZM, Bordeianou L. Perioperative fluid management. Clin Colon Rectal Surg 2009; 22:28–33.

Bapoje SR, Whitaker JF, Schulz T, et al. Preoperative evaluation of the patient with pulmonary disease. Chest 2007; 132:1637–1645.

Beck DE. Reoperative surgery: what can we learn from a large randomized prospective trial? Clin Colon Rectal Surg 2006; 19:247–250.

Belda FJ, Aguilera L, Garcia de la Asuncion J, et al. Supplemental perioperative oxygen and the risk of surgical wound infection: a randomized controlled trial. JAMA 2005; 294:2035–2042.

Benes J, Chytra I, Altmann P, et al. Intraoperative fluid optimization using stroke volume variation in high risk surgical patients: results of prospective randomized study. Crit Care 2010; 14:R118.

Biki B, Mascha E, Moriarty DC, et al. Anesthetic technique for radical prostatectomy surgery affects cancer recurrence: a retrospective analysis. Anesthesiology 2008; 109:180–187.

Black CE, Huang N, Neligan PC, et al. Effect of nicotine on vasoconstrictor and vasodilator responses in human skin vasculature. Am J Physiol Regul Integr Comp Physiol 2001; 281:R1097–R1104.

Brandstrup B, Tonnesen H, Beier-Holgersen R, et al. Effects of intravenous fluid restriction on postoperative complications: comparison of two perioperative fluid regimens: a randomized assessor-blinded multicenter trial. Ann Surg 2003; 238:641–648.

Bratzler DW, Houck PM. Antimicrobial prophylaxis for surgery: an advisory statement from the National Surgical Infection Prevention Project. Am J Surg 2005; 189:395–404.

Buggy DJ, Doherty WL, Hart EM, Pallett EJ. Postoperative wound oxygen tension with epidural or intravenous analgesia: a prospective, randomized, single-blind clinical trial. Anesthesiology 2002; 97:952–958.

Bunker JP, Goldstein R. Coagulation during hypothermia in man. Proc Soc Exp Biol Med 1958; 97:199–202.

Bunn F, Trivedi D, Ashraf S. Colloid solutions for fluid resuscitation. Cochrane Database Syst Rev 2008:CD001319.

Buvanendran A, Kroin JS, Tuman KJ, et al. Effects of perioperative administration of a selective cyclooxygenase 2 inhibitor on pain management and recovery of function after knee replacement: a randomized controlled trial. JAMA 2003; 290:2411–2418.

Callesen T, Bech K, Nielsen R, et al. Pain after groin hernia repair. Br J Surg 1998; 85:1412–1414.

Carr DB, Goudas LC. Acute pain. Lancet 1999; 353:2051–2058.

Catro-Alves LJ, De Azevedo VL, De Freitas Braga TF, et al. The effect of neuraxial versus general anesthesia techniques on postoperative quality of recovery and analgesia after abdominal hysterectomy: a prospective, randomized, controlled trial. Anesth Analg 2011; 113:1480–1486.

Chang CC, Lin HC, Lin HW, Lin HC. Anesthetic management and surgical site infections in total hip or knee replacement: a population-based study. Anesthesiology 2010; 113:279–284.

Chelly JE, Ploskanych T, Dai F, Nelson JB. Multimodal analgesic approach incorporating paravertebral blocks for open radical retropubic prostatectomy: a randomized double-blind placebo-controlled study. Can J Anaesth 2011; 58:371–378.

Chopra V, Wesorick DH, Sussman JB, et al. Effect of perioperative statins on death, myocardial infarction, atrial fibrillation, and length of stay: a systematic review and meta-analysis. Arch Surg 2012; 147:181–189.

Ciepichal J, Kubler A. Effect of general and regional anesthesia on some neutrophil functions. Arch Immunol Ther Exp (Warsz) 1998; 46:183–192.

Corcoran T, Rhodes JE, Clarke S, et al. Perioperative fluid management strategies in major surgery: a stratified meta-analysis. Anesth Analg 2012; 114:640–651.

De Chiara S, Chiumello D, Nicolini R, et al. Prolongation of antibiotic prophylaxis after clean and clean-contaminated surgery and surgical site infection. Minerva Anestesiol 2010; 76:413–419.

Delaney CP, Zutshi M, Senagore AJ, et al. Prospective, randomized, controlled trial between a pathway of controlled rehabilitation with early ambulation and diet and traditional postoperative care after laparotomy and intestinal resection. Dis Colon Rectum 2003; 46:851–859.

Dellinger EP, Gross PA, Barrett TL, et al. Quality standard for antimicrobial prophylaxis in surgical procedures. Infectious Diseases Society of America. Clin Infect Dis 1994; 18:422–427.

Edwards MS, Andrews JS, Edwards AF, et al. Results of endovascular aortic aneurysm repair with general, regional, and local/monitored anesthesia care in the American College of Surgeons National Surgical Quality Improvement Program database. J Vasc Surg 2011; 54:1273–1282.

Eggimann P, Pittet D. Infection control in the ICU. Chest 2001; 120:2059–2093.

Emmanuel AV, Kamm MA. Laser Doppler measurement of rectal mucosal blood flow. Gut 1999; 45:64–69.

Exadaktylos AK, Buggy DJ, Moriarty DC, et al. Can anesthetic technique for primary breast cancer surgery affect recurrence or metastasis? Anesthesiology 2006; 105:660–664.

Ferrell JE, Jr, Mitchell KT, Huestis WH. Membrane bilayer balance and platelet shape: morphological and biochemical responses to amphipathic compounds. Biochim Biophys Acta 1988; 939:223–237.

Fleischmann KE, Beckman JA, Buller CE, et al. 2009 ACCF/AHA focused update on perioperative beta blockade. J Am Coll Cardiol 2009; 54:2102–2128.

Fleisher LA. Cardiac risk stratification for noncardiac surgery: update from the American College of Cardiology/American Heart Association 2007 guidelines. Cleve Clin J Med 2009; 76:S9–S15.

Fleisher LA, Beckman JA, Brown KA, et al. ACC/AHA 2007 guidelines on perioperative cardiovascular evaluation and care for noncardiac surgery: executive summary: a report of the American College of Cardiology/American Heart Association Task Force on Practice Guidelines (Writing Committee to Revise the 2002 Guidelines on Perioperative Cardiovascular Evaluation for Noncardiac Surgery) developed in collaboration with the American Society of Echocardiography, American Society of Nuclear Cardiology, Heart Rhythm Society, Society of Cardiovascular Anesthesiologists, Society for Cardiovascular Angiography and Interventions, Society for Vascular Medicine and Biology, and Society for Vascular Surgery. J Am Coll Cardiol 2007; 50:1707–1732.

Fleisher LA, Beckman JA, Brown KA, et al. 2009 ACCF/AHA focused update on perioperative beta blockade incorporated into the ACC/AHA 2007 guidelines on perioperative cardiovascular evaluation and care for noncardiac surgery. J Am Coll Cardiol 2009; 54:e13–e118.

Forbes SS, Stephen WJ, Harper WL, et al. Implementation of evidence-based practices for surgical site infection prophylaxis: results of a pre- and postintervention study. J Am Coll Surg 2008; 207:336–341.

Frank SM, Fleisher LA, Breslow MJ, et al. Perioperative maintenance of normothermia reduces the incidence of morbid cardiac events. A randomized clinical trial. JAMA 1997; 277:1127–1134.

Frank SM, Higgins MS, Breslow MJ, et al. The catecholamine, cortisol, and hemodynamic responses to mild perioperative hypothermia. A randomized clinical trial. Anesthesiology 1995; 82:83–93.

Frank SM, Higgins MS, Fleisher LA, et al. Adrenergic, respiratory, and cardiovascular effects of core cooling in humans. Am J Physiol 1997; 272:R557– R562.

Frank SM, Raja SN, Bulcao C, Goldstein DS. Age-related thermoregulatory differences during core cooling in humans. Am J Physiol Regul Integr Comp Physiol 2000; 279:R349– R354.

Gentilello LM, Jurkovich GJ, Stark MS, et al. Is hypothermia in the victim of major trauma protective or harmful? A randomized, prospective study. Ann Surg 1997; 226:439–447; discussion 447–449.

Godoy DA, Di Napoli M, Biestro A, Lenhardt R. Perioperative glucose control in neurosurgical patients. Anesthesiol Res Pract; 2012:690362.

Gottschalk A, Ford JG, Regelin CC, et al. Association between epidural analgesia and cancer recurrence after colorectal cancer surgery. Anesthesiology 2010; 113:27–34.

Govinda R, Kasuya Y, Bala E, et al. Early postoperative subcutaneous tissue oxygen predicts surgical site infection. Anesth Analg 2010; 111:946–952.

Greif R, Akca O, Horn EP, et al. Supplemental perioperative oxygen to reduce the incidence of surgical-wound infection. N Engl J Med 2000; 342:161–167.

Grocott MP, Mythen MG, Gan TJ. Perioperative fluid management and clinical outcomes in adults. Anesth Analg 2005; 100:1093–1106.

Gross JB, Bachenberg KL, Benumof JL, et al. Practice guidelines for the perioperative management of patients with obstructive sleep apnea: a report by the American Society of Anesthesiologists Task Force on Perioperative Management of patients with obstructive sleep apnea. Anesthesiology 2006; 104:1081–1093; quiz 1117–1118.

Gupta H, Gupta PK, Fang X, et al. Development and validation of a risk calculator predicting postoperative respiratory failure. Chest 2011; 140:1207–1215.

Harbarth S, Samore MH, Lichtenberg D, Carmeli Y. Prolonged antibiotic prophylaxis after cardiovascular surgery and its effect on surgical site infections and antimicrobial resistance. Circulation 2000; 101:2916–2921.

Hecker MT, Aron DC, Patel NP, et al. Unnecessary use of antimicrobials in hospitalized patients: current patterns of misuse with an emphasis on the antianaerobic spectrum of activity. Arch Intern Med 2003; 163:972–978.

Hedrick TL, Heckman JA, Smith RL, et al. Efficacy of protocol implementation on incidence of wound infection in colorectal operations. J Am Coll Surg 2007; 205:432–438.

Heier T, Caldwell JE, Sessler DI, Miller RD. Mild intraoperative hypothermia increases duration of action and spontaneous recovery of vecuronium blockade during nitrous oxide-isoflurane anesthesia in humans. Anesthesiology 1991; 74:815–819.

Hofer CK, Worn M, Tavakoli R, et al. Influence of body core temperature on blood loss and transfusion requirements during off-pump coronary artery bypass grafting: a comparison of 3 warming systems. J Thorac Cardiovasc Surg 2005; 129:838–843.

Hopf HW, Hunt TK, West JM, et al. Wound tissue oxygen tension predicts the risk of wound infection in surgical patients. Arch Surg 1997; 132:997–1004; discussion 1005.

Huang ES, Basu A, O'Grady M, Capretta JC. Projecting the future diabetes population size and related costs for the U.S. Diabetes Care 2009; 32:2225–2229.

Huang YM, Wang CM, Wang CT, et al. Perioperative celecoxib administration for pain management after total knee arthroplasty – a randomized, controlled study. BMC Musculoskelet Disord 2008; 9:77.

Ismail H, Ho KM, Narayan K, Kondalsamy-Chennakesavan S. Effect of neuraxial anaesthesia on tumour progression in cervical cancer patients treated with brachytherapy: a retrospective cohort study. Br J Anaesth 2010; 105:145–149.

Jensen JA, Goodson WH, Hopf HW, Hunt TK. Cigarette smoking decreases tissue oxygen. Arch Surg 1991; 126:1131–1134.

Johansson T, Lisander B, Ivarsson I. Mild hypothermia does not increase blood loss during total hip arthroplasty. Acta Anaesthesiol Scand 1999; 43:1005–1010.

Johnson RG, Arozullah AM, Neumayer L, et al. Multivariable predictors of postoperative respiratory failure after general and vascular surgery: results from the patient safety in surgery study. J Am Coll Surg 2007; 204:1188–1198.

Joshi GP. Multimodal analgesia techniques and postoperative rehabilitation. Anesthesiol Clin North Am 2005; 23:185–202.

Joshi GP, Rawal N, Kehlet H, et al. Evidence-based management of postoperative pain in adults undergoing open inguinal hernia surgery. Br J Surg 2012; 99:168–185.

Kabon B, Akca O, Taguchi A, et al. Supplemental intravenous crystalloid administration does not reduce the risk of surgical wound infection. Anesth Analg 2005; 101:1546–1553.

Kehlet H. Multimodal approach to control postoperative pathophysiology and rehabilitation. Br J Anaesth 1997; 78:606–617.

Kehlet H, Dahl JB. The value of "multimodal" or "balanced analgesia" in postoperative pain treatment. Anesth Analg 1993; 77:1048–1056.

Kehlet H, Dahl JB. Anaesthesia, surgery, and challenges in postoperative recovery. Lancet 2003; 362:1921–1928.

Kehlet H, Wilmore DW. Multimodal strategies to improve surgical outcome. Am J Surg 2002; 183:630–641.

Khoo CK, Vickery CJ, Forsyth N, et al. A prospective randomized controlled trial of multimodal perioperative management protocol in patients undergoing elective colorectal resection for cancer. Ann Surg 2007; 245:867–872.

Koivuranta M, Laara E, Snare L, Alahuhta S. A survey of postoperative nausea and vomiting. Anaesthesia 1997; 52:443–449.

Kreter B, Woods M. Antibiotic prophylaxis for cardiothoracic operations. Meta-analysis of thirty years of clinical trials. J Thorac Cardiovasc Surg 1992; 104:590–599.

Kurz A, Sessler DI, Christensen R, et al. Thermoregulatory vasoconstriction and perianesthetic heat transfer. Acta Anaesthesiol Scand Suppl 1996; 109:30–33.

Kurz A, Sessler DI, Lenhardt R. Perioperative normothermia to reduce the incidence of surgical-wound infection and shorten hospitalization. Study of Wound Infection and Temperature Group. N Engl J Med 1996; 334:1209–1215.

Lenhardt R, Marker E, Goll V, et al. Mild intraoperative hypothermia prolongs postanesthetic recovery. Anesthesiology 1997; 87:1318–1323.

Leslie K, Sessler DI, Bjorksten AR, Moayeri A. Mild hypothermia alters propofol pharmacokinetics and increases the duration of action of atracurium. Anesth Analg 1995; 80:1007–1014.

Lewis SC, Warlow CP, Bodenham AR, et al. General anaesthesia versus local anaesthesia for carotid surgery (GALA): a multicentre, randomised controlled trial. Lancet 2008; 372:2132–2142.

Lobo DN, Bostock KA, Neal KR, et al. Effect of salt and water balance on recovery of gastrointestinal function after elective colonic resection: a randomised controlled trial. Lancet 2002; 359:1812–1818.

Macfarlane AJ, Prasad GA, Chan VW, Brull R. Does regional anaesthesia improve outcome after total hip arthroplasty? A systematic review. Br J Anaesth 2009a,b; 103:335–345.

Macfarlane AJ, Prasad GA, Chan VW, Brull R. Does regional anesthesia improve outcome after total knee arthroplasty? Clin Orthop Relat Res 2009b; 467:2379–2402.

Mangram AJ, Horan TC, Pearson ML, et al. Guideline for prevention of surgical site infection, 1999. Hospital Infection Control Practices Advisory Committee. Infect Control Hosp Epidemiol 1999; 20:250–278; quiz 279–280.

Mastracci TM, Carli F, Finley RJ, et al. Effect of preoperative smoking cessation interventions on postoperative complications. J Am Coll Surg; 2011:1094–1096.

Mayzler O, Weksler N, Domchik S, et al. Does supplemental perioperative oxygen administration reduce the incidence of wound infection in elective colorectal surgery? Minerva Anestesiol 2005; 71:21–25.

McDonald M, Grabsch E, Marshall C, Forbes A. Single-versus multiple-dose antimicrobial prophylaxis for major surgery: a systematic review. Aust N Z J Surg 1998; 68:388–396.

Meijer WS, Schmitz PI, Jeekel J. Meta-analysis of randomized, controlled clinical trials of antibiotic prophylaxis in biliary tract surgery. Br J Surg 1990; 77:283–290.

Melling AC, Ali B, Scott EM, Leaper DJ. Effects of preoperative warming on the incidence of wound infection after clean surgery: a randomised controlled trial. Lancet 2001; 358:876–80.

Meyhoff CS, Wetterslev J, Jorgensen LN, et al. Effect of high perioperative oxygen fraction on surgical site infection and pulmonary complications after abdominal surgery: the PROXI randomized clinical trial. JAMA 2009; 302:1543–1550.

Michelson AD, MacGregor H, Barnard MR, et al. Reversible inhibition of human platelet activation by hypothermia in vivo and in vitro. Thromb Haemost 1994; 71:633–640.

Miller RD, MD Consult LLC. Miller's anesthesia. Philadelphia, PA: Churchill Livingstone/Elsevier, 2010:2 v. ill.

Monfrecola G, Riccio G, Savarese C, et al. The acute effect of smoking on cutaneous microcirculation blood flow in habitual smokers and nonsmokers. Dermatology 1998; 197:115–118.

Morecraft R, Blair WF, Brown TD, Gable RH. Acute effects of smoking on digital artery blood flow in humans. J Hand Surg Am 1994; 19:1–7.

Myles PS, Leslie K, Chan MT, et al. Avoidance of nitrous oxide for patients undergoing major surgery: a randomized controlled trial. Anesthesiology 2007; 107:221–231.

Nesher N, Zisman E, Wolf T, et al. Strict thermoregulation attenuates myocardial injury during coronary artery bypass graft surgery as reflected by reduced levels of cardiac-specific troponin I. Anesth Analg 2003; 96:328–335, table of contents.

Neuman MD, Silber JH, Elkassabany NM, et al. Comparative effectiveness of regional versus general anesthesia for hip fracture surgery in adults. Anesthesiology 2012; 117:72–92.

Nisanevich V, Felsenstein I, Almogy G, et al. Effect of intraoperative fluid management on outcome after intra-abdominal surgery. Anesthesiology 2005; 103:25–32.

Oderda GM, Evans RS, Lloyd J, et al. Cost of opioid-related adverse drug events in surgical patients. J Pain Symptom Manage 2003; 25:276–283.

Page CP, Bohnen JM, Fletcher JR, et al. Antimicrobial prophylaxis for surgical wounds. Guidelines for clinical care. Arch Surg 1993; 128:79–88.

Parker MJ, Handoll HH, Griffiths R. Anaesthesia for hip fracture surgery in adults. Cochrane Database Syst Rev 2004:CD000521.

Perel P, Roberts I. Colloids versus crystalloids for fluid resuscitation in critically ill patients. Cochrane Database Syst Rev 2007:CD000567.

Polk HC, Jr, Lopez-Mayor JF. Postoperative wound infection: a prospective study of determinant factors and prevention. Surgery 1969; 66:97–103.

Pryor KO, Fahey TJ, 3rd, Lien CA, Goldstein PA. Surgical site infection and the routine use of perioperative hyperoxia in a general surgical population: a randomized controlled trial. JAMA 2004; 291:79–87.

Qadan M, Akca O, Mahid SS, et al. Perioperative supplemental oxygen therapy and surgical site infection: a meta-analysis of randomized controlled trials. Arch Surg 2009; 144:359–366; discussion 366–367.

Qadan M, Battista C, Gardner SA, et al. Oxygen and surgical site infection: a study of underlying immunologic mechanisms. Anesthesiology 2010; 113:369–377.

Qaseem A, Snow V, Fitterman N, et al. Risk assessment for and strategies to reduce perioperative pulmonary complications for patients undergoing noncardiothoracic surgery: a guideline from the American College of Physicians. Ann Intern Med 2006; 144:575–580.

Rajagopalan S, Mascha E, Na J, Sessler DI. The effects of mild perioperative hypothermia on blood loss and transfusion requirement. Anesthesiology 2008; 108:71–77.

Ramos P, Childers D, Maynard G, et al. Maintaining glycemic control when transitioning from infusion insulin: a protocol-driven, multidisciplinary approach. J Hosp Med 2010; 5:446–451.

Remerand F, Le Tendre C, Baud A, et al. The early and delayed analgesic effects of ketamine after total hip arthroplasty: a prospective, randomized, controlled, double-blind study. Anesth Analg 2009; 109:1963–1971.

Remy C, Marret E, Bonnet F. Effects of acetaminophen on morphine side-effects and consumption after major surgery: meta-analysis of randomized controlled trials. Br J Anaesth 2005; 94:505–513.

Rietbrock N, Kunkel S, Worner W, Eyer P. Oxygen-dissociation kinetics in the blood of smokers and non-smokers: interaction between oxygen and carbon monoxide at the hemoglobin molecule. Naunyn Schmiedebergs Arch Pharmacol 1992; 345:123–128.

Roberts GW, Bekker TB, Carlsen HH, et al. Postoperative nausea and vomiting are strongly influenced by postoperative opioid use in a dose-related manner. Anesth Analg 2005; 101:1343–1348.

Rohrer MJ, Natale AM. Effect of hypothermia on the coagulation cascade. Crit Care Med 1992; 20:1402–1405.

Sacerdote P, Bianchi M, Gaspani L, et al. The effects of tramadol and morphine on immune responses and pain after surgery in cancer patients. Anesth Analg 2000; 90:1411–1414.

Schechter MA, Shortell CK, Scarborough JE. Regional versus general anesthesia for carotid endarterectomy: the American College of Surgeons National Surgical Quality Improvement Program perspective. Surgery 2012; 152:309–314.

Schmid RL, Sandler AN, Katz J. Use and efficacy of low-dose ketamine in the management of acute postoperative pain: a review of current techniques and outcomes. Pain 1999; 82:111–125.

Schmied H, Kurz A, Sessler DI, et al. Mild hypothermia increases blood loss and transfusion requirements during total hip arthroplasty. Lancet 1996; 347:289–292.

Schouten O, Boersma E, Hoeks SE, et al. Fluvastatin and perioperative events in patients undergoing vascular surgery. N Engl J Med 2009; 361:980–989.

Schouten O, van Domburg RT, Bax JJ, et al. Noncardiac surgery after coronary stenting: early surgery and interruption of antiplatelet therapy are associated with an increase in major adverse cardiac events. J Am Coll Cardiol 2007; 49:122–124.

Sen H, Sizlan A, Yanarates O, et al. A comparison of gabapentin and ketamine in acute and chronic pain after hysterectomy. Anesth Analg 2009; 109:1645–1650.

Sessler DI, Olofsson CI, Rubinstein EH. The thermoregulatory threshold in humans during nitrous oxide-fentanyl anesthesia. Anesthesiology 1988a,b; 69:357–364.

Sessler DI, Olofsson CI, Rubinstein EH, Beebe JJ. The thermoregulatory threshold in humans during halothane anesthesia. Anesthesiology 1988b; 68:836–842.

Sheffield CW, Sessler DI, Hopf HW, et al. Centrally and locally mediated thermoregulatory responses alter subcutaneous oxygen tension. Wound Repair Regen 1996; 4:339–345.

Sheffield CW, Sessler DI, Hunt TK. Mild hypothermia during isoflurane anesthesia decreases resistance to E. coli dermal infection in guinea pigs. Acta Anaesthesiol Scand 1994a; 38:201–205.

Sheffield CW, Sessler DI, Hunt TK, Scheuenstuhl H. Mild hypothermia during halothane-induced anesthesia decreases resistance to Staphylococcus aureus dermal infection in guinea pigs. Wound Repair Regen 1994b; 2:48–56.

Shi Y, Warner DO. Surgery as a teachable moment for smoking cessation. Anesthesiology 2010; 112:102–107.

Sinatra RS, Jahr JS, Reynolds LW, et al. Efficacy and safety of single and repeated administration of 1 gram intravenous acetaminophen injection (paracetamol) for pain management after major orthopedic surgery. Anesthesiology 2005; 102:822–831.

Sinclair DR, Chung F, Mezei G. Can postoperative nausea and vomiting be predicted? Anesthesiology 1999; 91:109–18.

Smetana GW. Postoperative pulmonary complications: an update on risk assessment and reduction. Cleve Clin J Med 2009; 76:S60– S65.

Sorensen LT. Wound healing and infection in surgery: the pathophysiological impact of smoking, smoking cessation, and nicotine replacement therapy: a systematic review. Ann Surg 2012; 255:1069–1079.

Sorensen LT, Hemmingsen U, Kallehave F, et al. Risk factors for tissue and wound complications in gastrointestinal surgery. Ann Surg 2005; 241:654–658.

Sorensen LT, Jorgensen S, Petersen LJ, et al. Acute effects of nicotine and smoking on blood flow, tissue oxygen, and aerobe metabolism of the skin and subcutis. J Surg Res 2009; 152:224–230.

Sorensen LT. Wound healing and infection in surgery. The clinical impact of smoking and smoking cessation: a systematic review and meta-analysis. Arch Surg 2012; 147:373–383.

Subramaniam K, Subramaniam B, Steinbrook RA. Ketamine as adjuvant analgesic to opioids: a quantitative and qualitative systematic review. Anesth Analg 2004; 99:482–495, table of contents.

Sun T, Sacan O, White PF, et al. Perioperative versus postoperative celecoxib on patient outcomes after major plastic surgery procedures. Anesth Analg 2008; 106:950–958, table of contents.

Svircevic V, van Dijk D, Nierich AP, et al. Meta-analysis of thoracic epidural anesthesia versus general anesthesia for cardiac surgery. Anesthesiology 2011; 114:271–282.

Tahiri Y, Tran de QH, Bouteaud J, et al. General anaesthesia versus thoracic paravertebral block for breast surgery: a meta-analysis. J Plast Reconstr Aesthet Surg 2011; 64:1261–1269.

Tali M, Maaroos J. Lower limbs function and pain relationships after unilateral total knee arthroplasty. Int J Rehabil Res 2010; 33:264–267.

Thavaneswaran P, Rudkin GE, Cooter RD, et al. Brief reports: paravertebral block for anesthesia: a systematic review. Anesth Analg 2010; 110:1740–1744.

Tsai PS, Hsu CS, Fan YC, Huang CJ. General anaesthesia is associated with increased risk of surgical site infection after Caesarean delivery compared with neuraxial anaesthesia: a population-based study. Br J Anaesth 2011; 107:757–761.

Tsui BC, Rashiq S, Schopflocher D, et al. Epidural anesthesia and cancer recurrence rates after radical prostatectomy. Can J Anaesth 2010; 57:107–112.

Treschan TA, Taguchi A, Ali SZ, et al. The effects of epidural and general anesthesia on tissue oxygenation. Anesth Analg 2003; 96:1553–1557, table of contents.

Turan A, Karamanlioglu B, Memis D, et al. Analgesic effects of gabapentin after spinal surgery. Anesthesiology 2004; 100:935–938.

Tzovaras G, Fafoulakis F, Pratsas K, et al. Spinal vs general anesthesia for laparoscopic cholecystectomy: interim analysis of a controlled randomized trial. Arch Surg 2008; 143:497–501.

Umpierrez GE, Hellman R, Korytkowski MT, et al. Management of hyperglycemia in hospitalized patients in non-critical care setting: an endocrine society clinical practice guideline. J Clin Endocrinol Metab 2012; 97:16–38.

Umpierrez GE, Isaacs SD, Bazargan N, et al. Hyperglycemia: an independent marker of in-hospital mortality in patients with undiagnosed diabetes. J Clin Endocrinol Metab 2002; 87:978–982.

Umpierrez GE, Smiley D, Jacobs S, et al. Randomized study of basal-bolus insulin therapy in the inpatient management of patients with type 2 diabetes undergoing general surgery (RABBIT 2 surgery). Diabetes Care 2011; 34:256–261.

Umpierrez GE, Smiley D, Zisman A, et al. Randomized study of basal-bolus insulin therapy in the inpatient management of patients with type 2 diabetes (RABBIT 2 trial). Diabetes Care 2007; 30:2181–2186.

Valeri CR, Khabbaz K, Khuri SF, et al. Effect of skin temperature on platelet function in patients undergoing extracorporeal bypass. J Thorac Cardiovasc Surg 1992; 104:108–116.

Vassiliades TA, Jr, Nielsen JL, Lonquist JL. Evaluation of a new temperature management system during off-pump coronary artery bypass. Interact Cardiovasc Thorac Surg 2003; 2:454–457.

Warner DO, Shi Y. Is it dangerous to quit smoking shortly before surgery? Anesthesiology; 2011; 115:1137–1138; author's reply 1138.

Warner MA, Divertie MB, Tinker JH. Preoperative cessation of smoking and pulmonary complications in coronary artery bypass patients. Anesthesiology 1984; 60:380–383.

Wenisch C, Narzt E, Sessler DI, et al. Mild intraoperative hypothermia reduces production of reactive oxygen intermediates by polymorphonuclear leukocytes. Anesth Analg 1996; 82:810–816.

Widman J, Hammarqvist F, Sellden E. Amino acid infusion induces thermogenesis and reduces blood loss during hip arthroplasty under spinal anesthesia. Anesth Analg 2002; 95:1757–1762, table of contents.

Winkler M, Akca O, Birkenberg B, et al. Aggressive warming reduces blood loss during hip arthroplasty. Anesth Analg 2000; 91:978–984.

Wong PF, Kumar S, Bohra A, et al. Randomized clinical trial of perioperative systemic warming in major elective abdominal surgery. Br J Surg 2007; 94:421–426.

Wu CL, Rowlingson AJ, Partin AW, et al. Correlation of postoperative pain to quality of recovery in the immediate postoperative period. Reg Anesth Pain Med 2005; 30:516–522.

Chapter 5 Reoperative surgery for abdominal wall infection and intra-abdominal abscess

Donald E. Fry

The clinical experience of abdominal surgeons in the management of postoperative infections of the abdominal wall and for abscess within the abdominal cavity has progressively declined over recent decades. Forty years ago, there were no laparoscopic procedures such that every abdominal operation had a full incision that was at risk of infection. There were no high-resolution computerized tomography (CT) scans or percutaneous drainage methods, which meant that all suspected intra-abdominal abscesses required a formal reoperation to achieve drainage (Fry et al. 1980). While the progress associated with minimally invasive abdominal surgery and percutaneous radiologic interventions has been considerable, it has created a new generation of surgeons with less experience in the open management of abdominal wall infection and abdominal abscess. The effectiveness of percutaneous drainage has generated an attitude that formal reoperation for abscess and intra-abdominal infection is seldom a necessary event.

Complicated intra-abdominal infection continues to be a morbid and expensive illness to manage. Current evidence indicates that mortality rates remain at 7.5–10% in studies that are inclusive of worldwide participation (Sartelli et al. 2012, 2013). About 12% of patients with complicated intra-abdominal infections require one or more reoperations mostly for continued infection issues. The presentation will identify those clinical circumstances when abdominal reoperation is still necessary and will provide a framework for the open surgical management of these difficult cases.

PATHOGENESIS: POSTOPERATIVE ABDOMINAL WALL/INTRA-ABDOMINAL ABSCESS

Contamination in excess of the capacity of the nonspecific host defenses to eradicate results in intra-abdominal abscess. The primary function of the inflammatory response within the abdominal cavity is the eradication of pathogens, but the second critical function of inflammation is to contain dense collections of pathogenic organisms and prevent wider dissemination within the abdominal cavity or systemically. Thus, while abscess will be treated as a clinical problem in this discussion, it should be understood that it is a positive response of the host to a large pathogenic burden.

The large burden of bacterial pathogens that is required to result in abscess in the abdominal cavity may occur in several clinical scenarios (Fry 1986). When the primary laparotomy encounters a perforated colon or when penetrating injury of the colon or distal small intestine is identified, then abscess within the peritoneal cavity or necrotizing infection of the surgical incision become events of considerable concern. Leaking gastrointestinal suture lines after resections lead to high concentrations of microbial contamination in a vulnerable peritoneal cavity that already is in a state of subacute inflammation from the primary operation. In yet other circumstances, retained clot or inflammatory exudates that attended the original operation may only have relatively modest contamination, but the favorable local environment for microbial proliferation may set the stage for abscess formation. Finally, necrosis of intra-abdominal structures such as the pancreas will result in an intense inflammatory environment that is secondarily contaminated and bacterial abscess is the result. It is a tribute to the efficiency of the peritoneal host defenses that more abscesses are not seen. Specific risk factors, which are present at the time of the reoperation, become predictive of morbidity and mortality rates that are to be expected (**Table 5.1**).

In the scenario of massive contamination, the inflammatory response of the host is robust. Inflammation yields extravasation of extracellular fluid into the inflammatory environment. Plasma proteins are present in abundance. Leukocytes infiltrate the inflammatory milieu in large numbers. Proinflammatory cytokines are released to further enhance the local response. The resultant viscous liquid medium of large bacterial counts, inflammatory fluids and proteins, and dense leukocyte infiltration is pus.

The pus within the abscess obeys the laws of gravity and accumulates within the physiologic drainage basins of the abdominal cavity. Thus, abscesses typically are identified in the subphrenic, the pericolic, and the pelvic spaces. They occur in the lesser sac because of the somewhat restricted and confined space of that area. Abscesses will less frequently occur in artificial dependencies of the subfascial space and as interloop events within the small bowel when prior adhesions create local conditions that prevent suppuration from going to the most dependent location (Fry & Clevenger 1991).

In the surgical incision, a different dynamic occurs with large bacterial contamination. Fomenting infection results in the typical suppuration response, and this infection is ordinarily confined to the potential space that exists between the coapted skin and subcutaneous tissues from wound closure. However, in a small percentage of selected cases, this nascent infection gains access to the perifascial space (**Figure 5.1**). The perifascial space is that potential area that lies immediately above the investing fascia of the abdominal wall musculature and immediately beneath the overlying subcutaneous fat. This potential space can be illustrated by a gentle dissecting finger that can lift the subcutaneous fat off of the investing fascia of the muscle. This space is avascular, and its anatomic limits are tissues (i.e. fascia and fat) that are equally poorly vascularized. When invasive infection gains access to the perifascial space, it can progress with necrosis of adjacent tissues because the space is relatively inaccessible to the protective effects of tissue inflammation. The rapidity of advancing infection will depend upon the bacterial inoculum, the virulence of the pathogen, and the integrity of the host. Thrombosis of the local tissue perfusion about the surgical incision, edema formation in a confined space, and toxic effects of microbial

Table 5.1 Risk factors for clinical failure and deaths in patients with severe peritonitis

Risk factor	Reference	Comments
Age > 50 years	Fry et al. 1980, Linder et al. 1987	Advancing age is associated with more chronic illnesses and an impairment of host responsiveness
Age > 65–70 years	Koperna and Schulz 2000, Lamme et al. 2004, Mulari and Leppäniemi 2004, Sartelli et al. 2012	
Female gender	Linder et al. 1987	A large experimental literature indicates males are more vulnerable to severe infection
Organ failure	Fry et al. 1980, Koperna and Schulz 2000, Linder et al. 1987	End-organ failure is likely a manifestation of severe systemic inflammatory response
Malignancy	Linder et al. 1987	Immunosuppression from cancer or concurrent cancer therapy is the likely association
Preoperative peritonitis >24 hours	Linder et al. 1987, Sartelli et al. 2012	The longer the active infection before the initial surgical intervention, the greater the likelihood of recurrent abscess
Preoperative peritonitis >60 hours	Kim et al. 2011	The longer the active infection before the initial surgical intervention, the greater the likelihood of recurrent abscess
Fecal peritonitis	Linder et al. 1987, Mulier et al. 2003	Very high microbial content in the peritoneal infection
APACHE (Acute Physiological and Chronic Health Evaluation) II > 20	Koperna and Schulz 2000, Lamme et al. 2004, Uggeri et al. 2004	Advanced systemic disease
Inadequate primary abscess drainage	Mulier et al. 2003	Persistent, undrained infection has systemic consequences
Diffuse peritonitis	Koperna and Schulz 2000, Linder et al. 1987	Failure of the host to contain infection is a grave sign
Bacteremia	Fry et al. 1980	This is an indicator of advanced, invasive infection
C-reactive protein	Mulari and Leppäniemi 2004	Indicates the severity of the inflammatory response
Septic shock at admission	Sartelli et al. 2012	Profound immune effects
Albumin < 30 g/L	Koperna and Schulz 2000	Likely reflects the severity of systemic inflammation
Peripheral vascular disease	Kim et al. 2011	Ischemia yields a poor host response
Alcohol abuse	Kim et al. 2011	Systemic immune suppression
Body mass index 29 kg/m^2	Kim et al. 2011	Immune suppression of obesity?
Ischemic bowel	Kim et al. 2011	Splanchnic ischemia
Primary abdominal closure	Holzheimer and Gathof 2003	Inadequate drainage

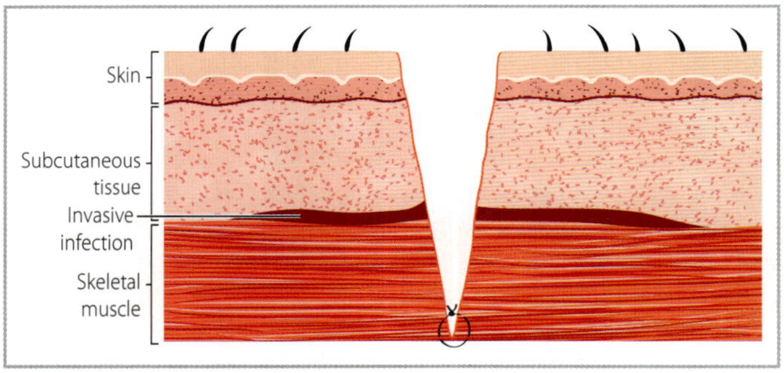

Figure 5.1 Illustration of the perifascial space, which is the potential space inferior to the subcutaneous fat and superior to the investing fascial of the abdominal wall musculature.

protein products leads to thrombosis of cutaneous and subcutaneous blood supply, myofascial necrosis, and dehiscence of the abdominal wall incision. Whether the sequel of massive microbial contamination is abdominal abscess, necrotizing fasciitis of the abdominal wall about the incision, or both, then additional interventions will be necessary for patient recovery.

DIAGNOSIS OF INFECTION REQUIRING REOPERATION

Abdominal abscess is a consideration in any postoperative laparotomy patient and has an array of specific and nonspecific signs and symptoms (**Table 5.2**). These findings include the typical observations of the systemic inflammatory response syndrome (American College of Chest Physicians 1992). Persistent postoperative ileus, poor systemic oxygenation, hyperglycemia, and early kidney injury may reflect other nonspecific manifestations of postoperative intra-abdominal abscess. Physical findings by examination of the abdomen are very difficult to evaluate in the postoperative patient since localized or rebound tenderness will be obscured by the recent abdominal incision (Bader et al. 2009). When this clinical constellation of findings that suggest postoperative infection are present, then it should always be a first order of priority to evaluate in the laparotomy patient 'where the hands of man' have been, specifically, the surgical wound and the intra-abdominal cavity.

Although examination of the abdomen for findings of abscess is equivocal, examination of the surgical incision will be useful in the identification of infection at that site. The classic signs of infection of erythema and induration are common preludes to actual drainage

Table 5.2 The signs and symptoms that are associated with postoperative abdominal abscess

Signs and symptoms	Pathophysiology
Abdominal pain	An inconsistent finding in postoperative patients because of the pain of incision, operative manipulation, drains, etc.
Abdominal mass	A positive finding when present, but abdominal guarding in the postoperative patients makes this infrequently seen
Hiccups	Gastric distention and poor gastric emptying may herald an inflammatory mass in proximity to the stomach
Kerr's sign	Referred pain to the apex of the shoulder may reflect an inflammatory lesion at the diaphragm
Diarrhea	Colonic irritation of a pelvic abscess may be associated with diarrhea
Tenesmus	Painful defecation may relate to a pelvic abscess
Increased/painful micturition	Inflammatory lesions about the urinary bladder may be seen in patients without urinary catheters
Fever/leukocytosis	A nonspecific finding of systemic inflammation that may be linked to other infectious and noninfectious events besides abscess
Pleural effusion	A unilateral effusion especially on the left side may be the consequence of subdiaphragmatic inflammation
Ileus/abdominal distention	Inflammatory collections will impair coordinated intestinal motility
Hyperglycemia	Hyperglycemia is a nonspecific response of systemic inflammation and hypermetabolism. This is often seen in abscess patients
Hypoalbuminemia	Most commonly reflects systemic changes in vascular permeability. This is a nonspecific finding of trauma, operations, and infections
Bacteremia	Bacteremia is uncommon with pyogenic abdominal infections, but anaerobic (e.g. B. fragilis) bacteremia means undrained pus!
Organ dysfunction	The end consequence of sustained and/or severe systemic inflammation. It has been most commonly associated with severe intra-abdominal infection

from the incision. Severe infection that requires prompt operating room debridement is customarily associated with pain and tenderness that extends well beyond those limits that will ordinarily be associated with incisional pain or pain from a well-contained wound abscess. When necrotizing infection is present, the patient will usually have evidence of the systemic inflammatory response.

The CT scan of the abdominal cavity becomes the diagnostic method of choice for abscess (**Figure 5.2**). When feasible, triple contrast should be employed to permit differentiation of fluid and air that is present in the intestinal tract from that in an extraluminal collection. Intravascular contrast may be associated with enhancement of the inflammatory perimeter about the abscess cavity. Intraluminal contrast may identify extravasation from leaking suture lines. The triple contrast becomes very important in defining anatomic landmarks for percutaneous drainage strategies. Accessible intra-abdominal abscesses should be percutaneously drained, and avoidance of re-exploration in the face of postsurgical and infectious inflammation is in the patient's best interest (**Figure 5.3**).

However, there remain circumstances when formal open re-exploration remains necessary. Extravasation of contrast with poor localization of the infection that is not amenable to percutaneous drainage or control of the source of the extravasation will require surgical management. Patients with multiple abscesses and those where the collection is perilously close to major vascular or other luminal structures may not be amenable to percutaneous drainage. Lesser sac collections particularly when associated with suppurative pancreatitis may need open drainage both because of poor percutaneous access but also because sloughed pancreatic tissue cannot be effectively drained by percutaneous methods. Finally, apparently successful percutaneous drainage that is associated with persistent signs of the systemic inflammatory response syndrome, bacteremia from enteric pathogens, evolving evidence of organ dysfunction syndrome when no alternative sites of infection can explain the persistent clinical state will require re-exploration. Recurrence of abscess may occur after apparently successful drainage of abscess (**Figure 5.4a** and **b**). Persistence of abscess may be the consequence of premature removal of the percutaneous drainage catheter. An algorithm for selecting percutaneous versus reoperative drainage is presented in **Figure 5.5**.

Infectious complications of the surgical incision are customarily managed by opening and drainage of the site and do not require a formal return to the operating room. Pus is evacuated, subcutaneous sutures and fibrinous debris are removed. Inadequate opening of the severely infected wound in the interest of preserving a partial segment of the original wound closure is flirting with necrotizing infection of the abdominal wall.

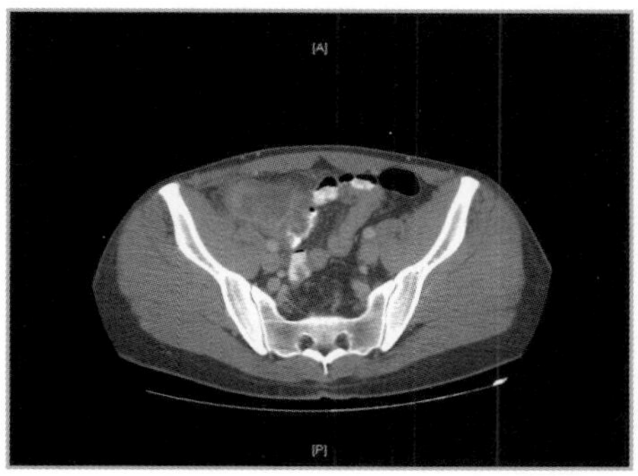

Figure 5.2 Demonstration of the excellent anatomic detail of an abdominal abscess in association with a perforated appendix.

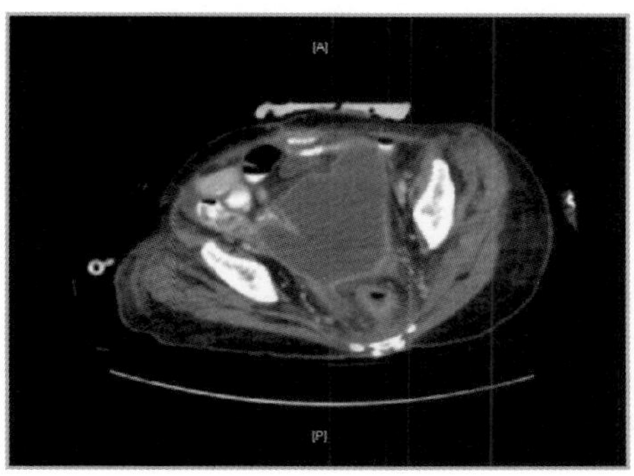

Figure 5.3 Illustration of an abdominal abscess that is readily accessible by percutaneous drainage.

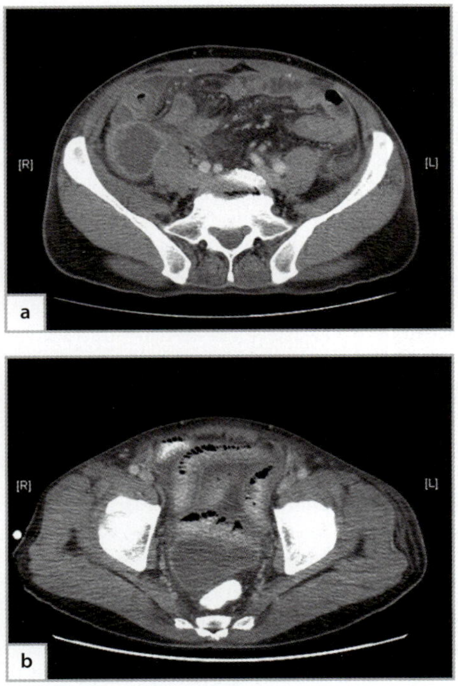

Figure 5.4 (a) An abscess after a perforated appendix that appears to be an ideal candidate for percutaneous drainage. (b) Recurrent pelvic abscess after the apparently successful percutaneous drainage of the abscess in (a) but recurrence after catheter removal.

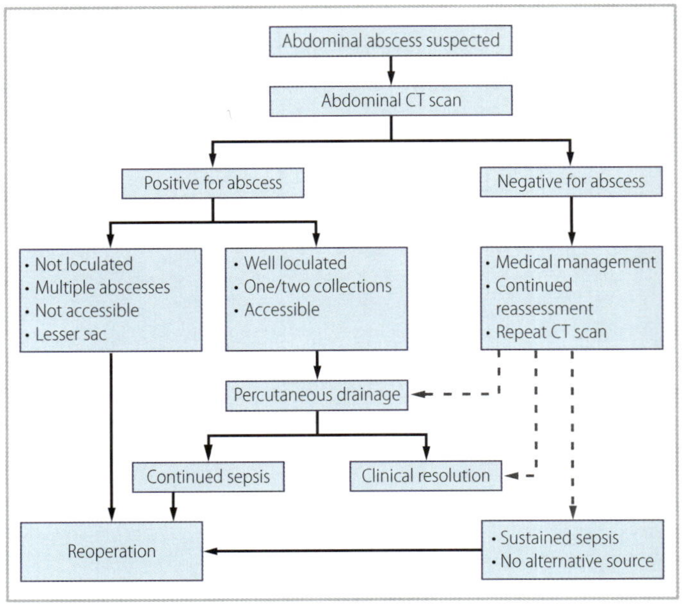

Figure 5.5 An algorithm for selecting percutaneous drainage or open surgical reoperation of the abdomen for abdominal abscess.

Once the wound is opened, careful physical examination is required to ensure that the fascial sutures from the prior operation are intact. The fascia is inspected and areas of suspicious viability of fascia or potential fascial separation from increased intra-abdominal pressure require vigilant monitoring for evidence of dehiscence. Dehiscence of the fascial closure, evidence of dissection of the infection into the perifascial space, or frank necrosis of fascia even without dehiscence means that a return to the operating room for debridement will be necessary. It is too easy to ascribe signs and symptoms to the surgical site infection and assume that all will be well with simple beside management. Severe surgical site infections may well be associated with necrotizing infection and need immediate attention. Furthermore, it is likely that the same high inoculum of bacteria that resulted in the incisional infection also existed within the abdominal cavity at the time of the original operation. Intra-abdominal abscess may well accompany the severe or necrotizing surgical site infection. Preoperative CT scans for the invasive incisional infection is necessary to provide guidance in the pursuit of a simultaneous exploration of the abdomen at the same time of abdominal wall debridement.

TIMING OF REOPERATION

In general, the patient with indications for re-exploration of the abdomen for abscess needs to have the reoperation promptly. With these severe infections there is no benefit for attempts to improve the patient's condition with exaggerated supportive efforts of a day or longer. Sometimes, patients are too sick to not be reoperated! Sustained systemic inflammation damages the functional reserve of critical organs, exhausts the effectiveness of both the innate and adaptive host response, and extinguishes opportunity for patient recovery.

The clinical evidence in postoperative patients with severe intra-abdominal infection may not be clearly definable until rapidly advancing systemic sepsis evolves. This observation has led to considerable debate about whether reoperation should be 'on-demand' when the clinical evidence indicates that reoperation is necessary, or whether reoperation should be 'planned' and proceed in 36–48 hours after the index intervention (van Goor 2002). Planned reoperation is advocated when the initial index procedure is viewed as being suboptimal in terms of source control, when fecal peritonitis if diffuse in character, when hemodynamic instability is present at the initial procedure, or when tenuous suture lines are present and need reassessment (Ordoñez & Puyana 2006). There have been numerous clinical reports, which have examined this issue. All publications from before 2000 were summarized in a meta-analysis where no evidence was convincing in favor of either option because of the heterogeneity of the study populations and the nonrandomized nature of the patients (Lamme et al 2002). In **Table 5.3**, the more recent studies have been summarized. Only the study by van Ruler et al. (2007) represents a randomized controlled trial of some 225 evaluable patients. This study showed no advantage to either approach but presented evidence that significant numbers of negative operations occurred in the planned laparotomy group. Thus, the prevailing attitude at this time would support reoperation on-demand, but planned re-exploration may be justified in extraordinarily severe circumstances.

Similarly with abdominal wall necrotizing infection, debridement in the operating room should proceed promptly (Ustin & Malangoni 2011). The magnitude of fascial infections can bridge a vast continuum of mild to extremely severe. Polymicrobial fascial infection can evolve in a more indolent fashion than Group A streptococcal or staphylococcal necrotizing infection, but inattention to the progressive necrosis of fascia, muscle, and subcutaneous tissue will lead to more tissue loss and severe future problems of management and reconstruction. There is the temptation to attempt bedside debridement and to 'cheat' on the magnitude of debrided tissues. Bedside debridements usually prove ineffective and inadequate, and only delay the return for comprehensive debridement of the abdominal wall.

Table 5.3 Summarizes studies since 2000 that have compared planned versus on-demand laparotomy for severe intra-abdominal infection

Authors (year)	Country	Results	Commentary
Koperna and Schulz 2000	Austria	105 Reoperations; 51% mortality rate; authors favored early (<48 hours) reoperation on- demand	Retrospective review; Early reoperation on demand for age > 70 years, APACHE > 20, albumin < 30 g/L, emerging organ failure
Lamme et al. 2004	Netherlands	278 peritonitis patients; overall 37% mortality rate at 2 years; no difference in planned reoperation vs reoperation on demand	Patients in the planned reoperation group were clearly higher risk of requiring reoperation
Uggeri et al. 2004	Italy	94 reoperations; 40% mortality rate; authors favored planned reoperation for high-risk cases	Retrospective review; authors considered diffuse peritonitis, APACHE > 20, primary infection > 72 hours as indications for planned reoperation
Rakić et al. 2005	Croatia	65 reoperations; 45% mortality; no difference in planned vs on-demand reoperation	Severity of illness appears to be most important factor in survival and not planned vs on-demand reoperation
van Ruler et al. 2007	Netherlands	225 randomized patients; Overall 32% mortality rate; no difference between on-demand vs timed relaparotomy	Planned reoperations were twice as likely (66%) as on-demand cases (31%) had negative reoperations

PREOPERATIVE PREPARATION FOR REOPERATION

The preoperative preparation of the patient for relaparotomy needs to focus upon the optimization of key physiologic parameters. Adequate volume resuscitation is essential and is best validated by the patient with an appropriate mean arterial pressure, a pulse < 100, respiratory rate that is <20, and a urine output of 50 mL/h. Central venous pressure (CVP) monitoring is usually employed with pressures of 10 mmHg necessary. Adequate systemic oxygenation requires pulse oximetry monitoring that approaches 100% saturation and arterial blood gases with appropriate Po_2, Pco_2, and pH. Many of these patients will already be receiving ventilator support to achieve goals of satisfactory oxygenation, or will require ventilator support in expectation of needed support of oxygenation. Ventilatory support particularly with in postexpiratory end-tidal pressure support may make use of CVP tenuous, and may require overall clinical assessment of the patient to ensure adequate perfusion.

An appropriate hemoglobin concentration is always a controversial issue for the relaparotomy patient with intra-abdominal infection. Even without blood loss, the postoperative patient with infection will have a progressive decline in the hemoglobin from normal values to <100 g/L (10 g/dL). Transfusion is usually withheld in the preoperative period unless hemoglobin values are ≤ 80 g/L (8 g/dL) (Carson et al. 2012). At least four units of packed red cells should be available for the operation itself, and the blood bank alerted to the possibility that additional units may be necessary. Once reoperation has begun, an assessment of the technical severity of the anticipated operation is made, and it is frequently prudent to begin transfusion early in the patient who had < 100 g/L (10 g/dL) at the outset of the procedure when measurable blood loss is expected.

Intraoperative blood loss is always a source of concern in the relaparotomy patient. The patient and family should be made aware of this issue so that transfusion and even reoperation for bleeding are understood risks. The acute to subacute inflammatory environment of the abdominal cavity makes blood loss a major issue from weeping surfaces, not to mention vascular disruptions from distorted anatomy within the omentum and mesentery of the abdomen. Fresh frozen plasma should be administered preoperatively for abnormal coagulation studies and intraoperative administration may be necessary if clinical bleeding from dissection surfaces is recognized. Vitamin K is usually administered to the patients with an abnormal INR (International Normalized Ratio), but the liver cannot be expected to produce significant clotting proteins within a few hours of time, especially when the patient is experiencing a systemic septic response.

Because of bleeding risks in the patient undergoing relaparotomy, the prevention of deep venous thrombophlebitis (DVT) and pulmonary embolism (PE) become difficult. Clinical sepsis is perceived as being a greater risk of microcirculatory thrombosis, DVT, and even PE in laparotomy (Semeraro et al. 2012). Large abdominal abscesses in the pelvis or adjacent to large venous structures can readily be appreciated for increasing this risk. The use of a heparin preparation as would be done in elective laparotomy assumes special risks in the septic relaparotomy patient with abscess or a necrotic wound because of bleeding. Sequential compression devices are important intraoperative preventive measures that should be used in all patients. Because the magnitude of bleeding from dissection and exploration are not known until the abdomen has been opened, the use of a low molecular weight or conventional heparin preparation from prevention might be deferred until surgical assessment of conditions within the abdomen. A sensible practice would be to defer heparin utilization until the threat of bleeding within the abdomen has passed in the postoperative period. If a patient has already had DVT or PE on the hospitalization, strong consideration should be given to placement of a vena cava filter prior to relaparotomy.

A particularly difficult issue leading up to the relaparotomy or major abdominal wall debridement is the use of perioperative systemic antibiotics. All patients undergoing relaparotomy for intra-abdominal abscess or invasive abdominal surgical wound infection will already be on one or more antibiotics. If the clinician is satisfied with the antibiotic choices for the treatment of the bacterial infection, then redosing should be undertaken immediately prior to the reoperation. While the intra-abdominal or necrotizing surgical wound infection may not have evidence of methicillin-resistant *Staphylococcus aureus* (MRSA), the patient who has been in the intensive care unit and has been receiving broad-spectrum antibiotics is likely to have cutaneous MRSA colonization. Prudent behavior might add a systemic dose of vancomycin to cover this risk but discontinue the drug after the operation in the absence of clinical evidence for continuation (Fry & Barie 2011).

Intraoperative hypothermia is a significant consideration for the relaparotomy patient and its management should be planned before the reoperation. These operations can prove to be lengthy with sizable blood loss, and hypothermia is associated with both coagulopathy (Dirkman et al. 2008) and increased infections (Qadan et al. 2009) after abdominal operations. Circulating water blankets or forced air devices are applied to the patient and employed throughout the procedure to maintain core body temperature as close to 37°C as possible. Warming devices for fluid administration may also be used. Importantly, maintaining core temperature is far more successful than trying to rewarm patients who have already developed clinically relevant hypothermia (<35°C).

INTRAOPERATIVE MANAGEMENT

The reoperation begins with positioning of the patient on the operating room table. Supine positioning is appropriate for most all patients with both arms extended for access by anesthesiology. Peripheral intravenous sites and arterial lines are usually employed, and their maintenance during the procedure is best achieved by having both arms extended. An occasional patient may need to be positioned in a lithotomy position if pelvic pathology is anticipated and either perineal drainage or flexible endoscopy is needed. In patients with necrotizing infections at the abdominal incision, then positioning may require a bias by tilting the patient to one side in anticipation of debridement.

The abdominal wall is prepped with an antiseptic solution. MRSA or other hospital-acquired bacterial colonization of the skin of the abdomen wall can assume significance in the patient's subsequent course. The entire anterior abdominal wall is first scrubbed with an antiseptic soap. This is followed by the application of the topical antiseptic solution. Chlorhexidine is the preferred antiseptic and is applied in a circular fashion beginning about the previous incision and moving far laterally to include any area that may be chosen for a subsequent stoma. Some evidence has supported the use of chlorhexidine-isopropyl alcohol together (Darouiche et al. 2010) when compared with povidone iodine alone, but the use of the electrocautery may make the risk of fire undesirable for this antiseptic combination. If the wound is already open, it is generally not desirable to place antiseptics on subcutaneous and fascial tissues.

The abdomen is re-entered through the prior incision, whether it was a midline or a transverse incision. In the past before the advent of percutaneous drainage methods, limited incisions were made to access abscess without going back through the original wound. However, abscesses that are amenable to limited incisions are those that are easily accessed by percutaneous drainage. Hence, the prior incision is generally the choice of re-entry into the abdomen.

The initial goal is to re-enter the abdominal cavity without an iatrogenic injury to intestinal structures. The prior wound is extended into new fascia in a superior or inferior direction from the original incision. It is not appropriate to crosshatch a new incision that is perpendicular to the prior incision. In a midline incision, extending the fascial incision in a cephalad direction within the linea alba permits re-entry into the abdomen in an area that will ordinarily had limited or no adherence of intestine or omentum to the parietal peritoneum of the anterior abdominal wall. Retractors (not crushing instrument clamps) are then used to enhance direct visualization, and the blunt dissection process is initiated to tease the abdominal contents away from the undersurface of the incision.

The preoperative imaging studies will provide direction for surgical identification and drainage of the abscess cavity. With pelvic abscesses, the gentle digital dissection of abdominal contents away from the peritoneal surface is systemically achieved, and a plane is established over the surface of the urinary bladder. Similar dissection styles are employed if the subphrenic, subhepatic, or pericolic gutters are the goal of the dissection. It is advised to maintain the dissection plane over the posterior peritoneum as the dissection proceeds. Deep sharp dissection at this early phase risks intestinal injury. Mobilizing the abdominal contents away from the anterior abdominal wall also minimizes blood loss during this early phase of the procedure.

Marked induration and edema is usually identified as the area of suppuration is encountered. The abscess is approached from the lateral direction to minimize risks of intestinal injury. Entering and draining the abscess away from the intestine also have advantages in the placement of drains through the abdominal wall and directly into the abscess cavity without contact with intestine that can be a cause of delayed fistula.

The lesser sac is a common objective for pancreatic abscess or for complications of biliary or gastric operations. The lesser sac is best approached by identification of the great curve of the stomach, and sequentially dividing the omental attachments to expose the retrogastric potential spaces. Care is taken to not mechanically injure the gastric wall when exposing the lesser sac. These are potential spaces because severe inflammation and suppuration in the lesser sac makes dissection in this area very difficult. Pus pockets are identified and drained, fibrinous debris is removed, and sloughed pancreatic tissue is excised. Care is taken in the lesser sac to avoid the major vascular structures that lie posterior and about the pancreas.

Many abcesses will be interloop pyogenic collections that will have the wall of intestinal structures that comprise a major boundary of the abscess wall. Dissection of edematous and acute inflamed intestine has considerable attendant risk of bowel injury. Sometimes the bowel loops can be easily separated with light digital dissection and other times tedious sharp dissection is necessary. The bowel will tear easily or perforate when sharp dissection wonders from the serosal plane between adjacent loops. Usually with interloop abscesses, the intestinal loops are completely separated, and the abscess cavity is completely disrupted.

The management of suture line leaks that account for the abscess in many cases, or management of the iatrogenic perforation requires individualized judgment. With small bowel injury or leaks, it is desirable to resect the diseased segment back to uninflammed or minimally inflamed bowel and do a primary anastomosis. These may be done with stapling instruments, but subacutely inflamed bowel may be best repaired by a traditional hand-sewn method. Attempts at oversewing leaking anastomoses or mechanical injury of inflamed bowel simply leads to recurrent abscesses or enterocutaneous fistulas. Colonic leaking anastomoses in the middle of an abscessed abdominal field are best handled by colostomy. Iatrogenic injuries in a field of pus are often repaired by oversewing but may require colostomy.

An important component of open drainage is to collect appropriate culture material. These infections occur after several days of systemic antibiotics, intensive care unit time, and after drains have been initially placed. All of these variables lead to hospital-acquired resistant bacteria as participants in the infection. Cultures are commonly collected by the surgeon by simply passing a cotton-tipped swab into the area of infection and sending it off for culture. A preferred method is to aspirate pus, which will have a better chance of recovering anaerobic pathogens. Tissue or 'rind' sampling for culture from the wall of the abscess will commonly yield the best overall recovery of pathogens. Broad-spectrum antibiotics are employed after drainage of the abscess, and therapy is then de-escalated as the culture and sensitivity data are available.

Management of the aggressive abdominal wall infection in these patients similarly requires surgical management. All apparent necrosis of subcutaneous fat, fascia, and abdominal wall muscle requires excision to normal bleeding tissue. These are most commonly polymicrobial infections, and they will burrow over the surface and beneath the anterior and posterior fascia of the rectus muscle. Failure to recognize, unroof, and debride this burrowing effect will result in the identification of more necrosis at the next dressing changes and the progressive loss of additional abdominal wall tissue.

Adequate abdominal wall debridement commonly leads to the inability to primarily close the abdominal wall. In the face of ongoing infection in the abdominal wall or in the abdominal cavity, only temporary methods should be used for closing the abdomen. The objective of the temporary closures is to avoid dessication or injury of the intra-abdominal contents. Temporary plastic or silicone partitions, moist towels, and absorbable mesh on-lays are used until the infection has resolved. Permanent reconstruction remains a controversial subject of using separation of parts (Kanaan et al. 2011), synthetic mesh (Vrijland & Jeekel 2003), or biological materials for wound closure, but only after complete resolution of infection and the local inflammatory response.

POSTRELAPAROTOMY MANAGEMENT

The relaparotomy patient has sustained sequential physiologic insults that require extraordinary diligence in postoperative management. Postrelaparotomy management is focused on overall physiologic support of the patient and avoidance of additional complications of care. Maintenance of oxygenation and intravascular volume are essential as would be required in any postoperative laparotomy patient. Monitoring the hemoglobin concentration is equally important as blood loss during the re-exploration of the abdomen is commonly underestimated. Transfusion is usually employed to keep the hemoglobin above 80–90 g/L (8–9 g/dL). Vitamin K is used to support the INR, and fresh frozen plasma may be used as clinical (not surgical) blood loss is identified from dissected wounds. Acute kidney injury must be avoided by maintenance of urine output with appropriate volume and cardiac output support (not diuretics). The sequential compression devices are used for prevention of DVT/PE. Elevation of the feet and legs, and early mobilization of the patient as clinical improvement permits are also important in the prevention of thromboembolic complications.

Effective antibiotic management is important after reoperation for abscess or debridement of the abdominal wall from invasive infection. The results of intraoperative cultures will be important since the influences of exposure to the hospitalization environment, critical illness, and prior antibiotic therapy will increase the probability of hospital-acquired resistant organisms. Antibiotic recommendations of the Surgical Infection Society should be followed (Solomkin et al. 2010), and drug selections should be carefully matched to the sensitivities of cultured pathogens. MRSA, enterococci, resistant gram negatives, and even fungi can be anticipated. The multiply operated intra-abdominal infection patient or those patients with severe invasive soft tissue infection of the abdominal wall will have an increased volume of distribution and more aggressive dosing may be necessary (Adnan et al. 2012). Antibiotics are continued until clinical resolution of infection is identified. Fever and leukocytosis that continues 3–5 days beyond the relaparotomy is not likely to be antibiotic failure but raises the question of recurrent abscess, intestinal leakage, or impending fistula formation as causes. Failure to respond after reoperation means that continued intra-abdominal or abdominal wall infection is an issue, and additional imaging studies or reoperation again will be necessary.

Unfortunately, the abdominal abscess patient commonly has a difficult postrelaparotomy course with fever and leukocytosis. The question is always whether recurrent abscess or an alternative site is responsible for the infection. While infection of the surgical site and the intra-abdominal compartment are always of concern after relaparotomy, other sites of infection require evaluation. Postoperative pneumonia especially in ventilator-supported patients must be considered for these patients (Sachdev & Napolitano 2012). Daily chest roentgenograms are performed but may be deceptive and will require bronchoalveolar lavage to document the presence of pneumonia. All relaparotomy patients will have had urinary tract drainage catheters, and this source is always a potential suspect in continued postoperative fever and leukocytosis (Owen et al. 2012). Intravascular catheters are also sources of suspected infection (McHugh et al. 2011), particularly if the patient has documented positive blood cultures for either *Staphylococcus aureus* or *Candida albicans*. Positive *Candida* cultures may reflect the accumulated consequences of severe illness and sustained broad-spectrum antibiotic therapy and will require antifungal antimicrobial treatment (Kourkoumpetis et al. 2010).

Nutritional support of the relaparotomy patient is another important consideration (Braga et al. 2009). Relaparotomy confers a severe catabolic state with attendant immunosuppression. Placement of a gastrostomy or jejunostomy for feeding has been employed during the relaparotomy but can be problematic with diffuse gastrointestinal inflammatory changes, or can be logistically difficult with severe necrotizing infection of the abdominal wall. Nasointestinal feeding tube technology has advanced and is commonly used early for feeding when intestinal motility permits. With sustained ileus and in patients with fistula complications, there still remains a role for parenteral nutrition.

The post-relaparotomy management of the open abdomen either because of the damage-control option or because of debridement of infected tissue requires clinical judgment. In the damage-control option it is desirable to reoperate on these patients at about 24 hours to remove abdominal packs, and to hopefully close the abdominal fascia (Fabian 2007). When several days have passed without an opportunity to close the open abdomen, then delayed reconstruction generally becomes the pathway for closure. Whether the open abdomen is from the damage control option, or from extended debridement, attempts at a permanent closure cannot be undertaken until the patient is cleared of all infectious complications and has assumed a trajectory of clinical recovery.

REFERENCES

Adnan S, Paterson DL, Lipman J, et al. Pharmacokinetics of beta-lactam antibiotics in patients with intra-abdominal disease: a structured review. Surg Infect 2012; 13:9–17.

American College of Chest Physicians/Society of Critical Care Medicine Consensus Conference: definition for sepsis and organ failure and guidelines for the use of innovative therapies in sepsis. Crit Care Med 1992; 20:864–874.

Bader FG, Schröder M, Kujath P, et al. Diffuse postoperative peritonitis – value of diagnostic parameters and impact of early indication for relaparotomy. Eur J Med Res 2009; 14:491–496.

Braga M, Ljungqvist O, Soeters P, et al. ESPEN guidelines on parenteral nutrition: surgery. Clin Nutr 2009; 28:378–386.

Carson JL, Grossman BJ, Kleinman S, et al. Red blood cell transfusion: a clinical practice guideline from the AABB. Ann Intern Med 2012; 157:49–58.

Darouiche RO, Wall MJ Jr, Itani KM, et al. Chlorhexidine-alcohol versus povidone-iodine for surgical-site antisepsis. N Engl J Med 2010; 362:18–26.

Dirkman D, Hanke AA, Görlinger K, Peters J. Hypothermia and acidosis significantly impair coagulation in human whole blood. Anesth Analg 2008; 106:1627–1632.

Fabian TC. Damage control in trauma: laparotomy wound management acute to chronic. Surg Clin N Am 2007; 87:73–93.

Fry DE. Pathogenesis and management of postoperative intra- abdominal abscess. In: Fry DE (ed.), Reoperative surgery of the abdomen. New York: Marcel Dekker, Inc, 1986: 31–51.

Fry DE, Barie PS. The changing face of *Staphylococcus aureus*: a continuing surgical challenge. Surg Infect 2011; 12:191–203.

Fry DE, Clevenger FW. Reoperation for intra-abdominal abscess. Surg Clin N Am 1991; 71:159–174.

Fry DE, Garrison RN, Heitch RC, et al. Determinants of death in patients with intra-abdominal abscess. Surgery 1980; 89:517–523.

Holzheimer RG, Gathof B. Re-operation for complicated secondary peritonitis-how to identify patients at risk for persistent sepsis. Eur J Med Res 2003; 8:125–134.

Kanaan Z, Hicks N, Weller C, et al. Abdominal wall component release is a sensible choice for patients requiring complicated closure of abdominal defects. Langenbecks Arch Surg 2011; 396:1263–1270.

Kim JJ, Liang MK, Subramanian A, et al. Predictors of relaparotomy after nontrauma emergency general surgery with initial fascial closure. Am J Surg 2011; 202:549–552.

Koperna T, Schulz F. Relaparotomy in peritonitis: prognosis and treatment of patients with persisting intra-abdominal infection. World J Surg 2000; 24:32–37.

Kourkoumpetis T, Manolakaki D, Velmahos G, et al. Candida infection and colonization among non-trauma emergency surgery patients. Virulence 2010; 1:359–366.

Lamme B, Boermeester MA, Belt EJT, et al. Mortality and morbidity of planned relaparotomy versus relaparotomy on demand for secondary peritonitis. Brit J Surg 2004; 91:1046–1054.

Lamme B, Boermeester MA, Reitsma JB, et al. Meta-analysis of relaparotomy for secondary peritonitis. Brit J Surg 2002; 89:1516–1524.

Linder MM, Wacha H, Feldmann U, et al. The Mannheim peritonitis index. An instrument for the intraoperative prognosis of peritonitis. Chirurg (German) 1987; 58:84–92.

McHugh SM, Corrigan MA, Dimitrov BD, et al. Preventing infection in general surgery: improvements through education of surgeons by surgeons. J Hosp Infect 2011; 78:312–316.

Mulari K, Leppäniemi A. Severe secondary peritonitis following gastrointestinal tract perforation. Scand J Surg 2004; 93:204–208.

Mulier S, Penninckx F, Verwaest C, et al. Factors affecting mortality in generalized postoperative peritonitis: multivariate analysis in 96 patients. World J Surg 2003; 27:379–384.

Ordoñez CA, Puyana JC. Management of peritonitis in the critically ill patient. Surg Clin North Am 2006; 86:1323–1349.

Owen RM, Perez SD, Bornstein WA, Sweeney JF. Impact of surgical care improvement project inf-9 on postoperative urinary tract infections: do exemptions interfere with quality patient care? Arch Surg 2012; 147:946–953.

Qadan M, Gardner SA, Vitale DS, et al. Hypothermia and surgery: immunologic mechanisms for current practice. Ann Surg 2009; 250:134–140.

Rakić M, Popović D, Rakić M, et al. Comparison of on-demand vs planned relaparotomy for treatment of severe intra-abdominal infections. Croat Med J 2005; 46:957–963.

Sachdev G, Napolitano LM. Postoperative pulmonary complications: pneumonia and acute respiratory failure. Surg Clin North Am 2012; 92:321–344.

Sartelli M, Catena F, Ansaloni L, et al. Complicated intra-abdominal infections in Europe: a comprehensive review of the CIAO study. World J Emerg Surg 2012; 7:36.

Sartelli M, Catena F, Ansaloni L, et al. Complicated intra-abdominal infections in a worldwide context: an observational prospective study (CIAOW Study). World J Emerg Surg 2013; 8:1.

Semeraro N, Ammollo CT, Semeraro F, Colucci M. Sepsis, thrombosis and organ dysfunction. Thromb Res 2012; 129:290–295.

Solomkin JS, Mazuski JE, Bradley JS, et al. Diagnosis and management of complicated intra-abdominal infection in adults and children: guidelines by the Surgical Infection Society and the Infectious Diseases Society of America. Surg Infect 2010; 11:79–109.

Uggeri FR, Perego E, Franciosi C, Uggeri FA. Surgical approach to the intra-abdominal infections. Minerva Anestesiol 2004; 70:175–179.

Ustin JS, Malangoni MA. Necrotizing soft-tissue infections. Crit Care Med 2011; 39:2156–2162.

van Goor H. Interventional management of abdominal sepsis: when and how. Langenbeck's Arch Surg 2002; 387:191–200.

van Ruler O, Mahler CW, Boer KR, et al. Comparison of on-demand vs planned relaparotomy strategy in patients with severe peritonitis. A randomized trial. JAMA 2007; 298:865–873.

Vrijland WW, Jeekel J. Prosthetic mesh repair should be used for any defect in the abdominal wall. Curr Med Res Opin 2003; 19:1–3.

Chapter 6 The modern approach to the open abdomen and abdominal compartment syndrome

William P. Schecter, Asher Hirshberg

INTRODUCTION

Leaving the abdomen open, an almost unthinkable surgical sin as recently as 25 years ago has become a routine part of emergency laparotomy for trauma, infection, and intestinal ischemia. This shift in surgical culture is based on improved understanding of increased intra-abdominal pressure (IAP) and the physiology of the critically ill surgical patient. The abdomen is left open either to facilitate planned reoperation or to prevent or treat the abdominal compartment syndrome, a lethal clinical entity that was virtually unknown until the mid-1990s. While this approach improves outcome in critically ill patients, it also creates new challenges related to management of the exposed viscera, the need for multiple operations in a hostile abdomen, and difficulty in achieving definitive closure.

Acute care surgery is now emerging as a distinct specialty that includes critical care, trauma, and emergency general surgery. One of the hallmarks of this subspecialty is expertise in the management of all aspects of the open abdomen. The aim of this chapter is to review the modern approach to the open abdomen with special attention to intra-abdominal hypertension (IAH), abdominal compartment syndrome, and abdominal wall reconstruction.

HISTORY

Sir William Heneage Ogilvie first described the use of sterilized light canvas or 'stout' cotton cloth to cover the open abdomen in the treatment of severe wounds during World War II (Ogilvie 1940). However, this concept was not widely practiced until the 1980s when French and German surgeons began using an open abdomen approach ('laparostomy') combined with planned reoperations for peritoneal toilet in patients with severe abdominal infection (Teichmann et al. 1986).

At the same time, American trauma surgeons began using abdominal packing for major liver injuries and other types of abdominal trauma. Packing, by definition, requires a reoperation to remove the packs. In 1992, Burch et al. (1992) reported a series of 200 patients who underwent 'abbreviated' laparotomies for severe trauma with temporary abdominal closure. This was followed by resuscitation and stabilization in the intensive care unit and later a planned return to the operating room for definitive repair of the injuries. A year later, Rotondo et al. (1993) coined the term 'damage control laparotomy' to describe this new operative strategy. This term emphasizes the urgent nature of the abbreviated laparotomy, which addresses only life-threatening hemorrhage and control of intestinal spillage. Prolonged visceral reconstruction and definitive abdominal closure are deliberately delayed to avoid the 'lethal triad' of hypothermia, coagulopathy, and acidosis (Kashuk et al. 1982).

Patients undergoing damage control laparotomy required massive resuscitation typically resulting in generalized edema and continuous oozing for hours after the operation. Despite heroic resuscitation efforts in the intensive care unit, many of these patients died of 'irreversible shock' within hours of the abbreviated laparotomy. In retrospect, this 'irreversible shock' was, in fact, abdominal compartment syndrome (ACS).

Although the experimental physiology of IAH was described by Emerson as early as 1911 (Emerson 1911), the first clinical description did not appear until 1984 (Kron et al. 1984) and the term 'abdominal compartment syndrome' was not coined until 1989 (Fietsam et al. 1989). The close association between the need for damage control laparotomy and the development of ACS led to the realization that any attempt to close the abdomen could set the stage for the syndrome. The safest course of action was therefore to leave the abdomen open and cover the viscera with some form of temporary closure device that is sutured to the skin, such as an absorbable mesh or the famous 'Bogota bag,' an empty 3-L genitourinary irrigation fluid bag that is unfolded by cutting the seam (Rutherford et al. 2004).

By the dawn of the new millennium, the critically ill patient with an open abdomen became a common sight in surgical intensive care units. This led to better understanding of the physiology of the open abdomen and stimulated the development of innovative techniques to contain and protect the exposed bowel, prevent and control enteroatmospheric fistulae (EAF) and achieve delayed primary fascial closure in the majority of these patients.

INDICATIONS FOR LEAVING THE ABDOMEN OPEN (BOX 6.1)

The classic indications for damage control surgery are based on physiological parameters such as hypothermia, acidosis, or massive blood loss. However, experienced trauma surgeons make their decision to bail out much earlier. They rely on three major considerations: the pattern of injury, the overall trauma burden,

Box 6.1 Indications for open abdomen management

1. Damage control laparotomy
2. Abdominal compartment syndrome
3. Severe peritonitis
4. Mesenteric ischemia
5. Loss of abdominal wall due to infection or injury

and the quality of the system supporting the surgeon. For example, the combination of vascular and hollow viscous injuries usually means that by the time the bleeding is controlled, the patient is in no condition to undergo an elaborate intestinal resection and reconstruction. The presence of serious injuries outside the operative field (e.g. ongoing bleeding from a chest tube) is another indication to abbreviate the laparotomy. A realistic assessment of available operative resources and surgical support is also crucial. Operating with limited resources, an inexperienced surgical team, or in an austere environment is a situation where damage control for severe trauma is the best option.

In gauging the patient's physiology, the surgeon focuses on variables that reflect the cumulative physiologic insult over time such as the estimated total blood loss and the duration of hypotension. Both metabolic acidosis (pH < 7.30) and hypothermia (<35°C) are useful but late indicators; the surgeon should ideally make the decision to bail out well before their onset.

Decompressive laparotomy is indicated in patients with increased IAP who fail to respond to nonoperative management (see below), and in all patients with IAP > 25 mmHg with associated organ dysfunction (Cheatham et al. 2007). The clinical picture of full-blown ACS is rarely seen nowadays because increased IAP is routinely monitored, and the tense abdomen typically decompressed well before the clinical signs of the syndrome become obvious. Delay in surgical decompression is associated with an increased risk of death (Cheatham et al. 2000).

Open abdomen management is often used in severe abdominal infection when a single laparotomy does not achieve effective source control. Examples are dehiscence after an anastomotic leak, infected pancreatic necrosis, or severe peritonitis. Leaving the abdomen open permits repeated access to the site of infection for irrigation, drainage, and debridement (Ivatury et al. 1989, 1990, Wittmann et al. 1990). Despite the lack of prospective supporting evidence (Adkins et al. 2004), open abdomen management of severe abdominal infection remains an integral part of the surgical armamentarium of the acute care surgeon.

A 'second look' to assess bowel viability is mandatory after laparotomy for mesenteric ischemia. The open abdomen permits monitoring of intestinal viability (Oida et al., 2011, Ward et al., 1995] and allows the surgeon to be more conservative during the initial operation, resecting only clearly necrotic bowel and leaving segments of questionable viability for reassessment later.

On rare occasions, a patient may lose a major portion of the abdominal wall after debridement of a necrotizing soft tissue infection (Bertram et al., 2000, Levy et al., 1988) or massive injury. In this situation, open abdomen management is the only realistic option until the abdominal wound heals and is covered with skin, since an early prosthetic closure of the contaminated wound is likely to fail.

INTRA-ABDOMINAL HYPERTENSION AND THE ABDOMINAL COMPARTMENT SYNDROME

Normal IAP ranges from 1–6.5 mmHg. Pressure in excess of 12 mmHg is defined as IAH and is graded as shown in **Table 6.1**. The modern definition of ACS is a sustained IAP of > 20 mmHg associated with new organ dysfunction or failure (Malbrain et al. 2006).

The IAH has severe deleterious effects in and outside the abdomen. It decreases the perfusion of the intra-abdominal organs increasing the risk of renal failure (Doty et al. 1999, 2000), intestinal ischemia (Caldwell & Ricotta 1987), and liver dysfunction, particularly in patients with pre-existing liver disease (Luca et al. 1993). Furthermore, ACS occurring in postoperative patients increases the risk of wound infection, dehiscence, and subsequent ventral hernia (Diebel et al. 1992).

As in other types of compartment syndromes in the extremities or the brain, the perfusion pressure within the abdomen can be calculated by subtracting the IAP from the mean arterial pressure. Although values > 60 mmHg indicate good visceral perfusion and a favorable prognosis (Malbrain et al. 2006), most surgeons continue to use IAP as their guide to clinical decision making.

The adverse effects of IAH extend far beyond the abdomen: it increases intrathoracic pressure resulting in diminished venous return, ventricular compliance, cardiac output, and increased systemic vascular resistance (Kashtan et al., 1981, Ridings et al., 1995, Richardson and Trinkle 1976). IAH also limits diaphragmatic excursion causing decreased pulmonary compliance and very high airway pressures with their detrimental effects on lung physiology and ventilation (Bloomfield et al. 1997). Not surprisingly, IAH is also closely associated with increased intracranial pressure (Bloomfield et al. 1997, Citerio et al. 2001, Deeren et al. 2005). In fact, a series of patients with increased intracranial pressure as a result of ACS was reported in 2004, with a sustained decrease in intracranial pressure in 11 of the 17 patients after decompressive laparotomy (Joseph et al. 2004).

Routine measurement and monitoring of IAP is recommended in the presence of two or more risk factors for ACS (Papavramidis et al. 2011) because clinical examination is frequently inaccurate (Lambert et al. 2005, Sanchez et al. 2001). If IAH is present, IAP should be monitored throughout the course of the critical illness.

The standard technique for measuring IAP is through the bladder, since the compliant bladder wall reliably transmits the IAP. Some 50 mL of saline are instilled into the bladder through a Foley catheter, to separate the bladder walls and create a cushion that will transmit IAP. The main port of the Foley catheter is clamped, and a transducer (zeroed to the level of the patient's right atrium) is attached to the side port of the catheter filled with saline. The intravesicular pressure is then recorded on a standard pressure monitor and is assumed to reflect the IAP (Carlotti & Carvalho 2009).

The ACS is classified as primary, secondary, or recurrent. Primary ACS is caused by conditions originating within the abdomen; secondary ACS is caused by conditions outside of this region. When ACS recurs after either medical or surgical treatment, it is classified as recurrent (Malbrain et al. 2006).

Although acute ACS was originally recognized in patients with abdominal injury, any critically ill patient with a systemic inflammatory response and a massive capillary leak is at risk. Over-resuscitation with large volumes of crystalloids increases the risk of ACS in burns (Saffle 2007) and other medical and surgical conditions (Britt et al. 2005, Daugherty et al. 2007, Sugrue & Buhkari 2009). Patients with high venous pressures due to chronic cardiac, pulmonary, and renal disease or morbid obesity may also be more susceptible (Cheatham et al. 2000).

Nonoperative management of IAH is based on reduction of the volume of the intra-abdominal contents and/or improvement of abdominal wall compliance. Decompressing the GI tract (e.g. nasogastric decompression of the foregut or colonoscopic decompression of a distended colon) is an example of the former. Limiting crystalloid administration in patients with a systemic inflammatory response may help limit visceral and bowel edema, thereby either reducing or at least stabilizing the IAP. Patients with the systemic inflammatory response syndrome who develop acute renal failure are at a particular risk to develop IAH due to the combination of fluid overload, capillary leak, and visceral edema. Colloid and hypertonic saline fluid resuscitation protocols may decrease the volume of fluid administered (Azzopardi et al. 2009) as well as the risk of ACS and death (Cotton et al. 2006). Percutaneous catheter drainage of the peritoneal cavity in patients with large volumes of ascites, blood, or pus can sometimes be effective in reducing IAP and associated organ dysfunction thus eliminating the need for decompressive laparotomy (Cheatham et al., 2007, Corcos & Sherman 2001, Latenser et al., 2002, Reckard et al., 2005).

Suggested methods to improve abdominal wall compliance in patients with IAH include sedation and analgesia, neuromuscular blockade, and nursing the patient in the supine as opposed to the elevated head position (Cheatham et al. 2007, Papavramidis et al. 2011). These measures make intuitive sense, but there are no prospective trials evaluating their efficacy.

Decompressive laparotomy is indicated in patients with ACS unresponsive to nonoperative management (Cheatham et al. 2007). It is a surgical emergency that should be performed in the operating room with careful attention to the patient's respiratory and hemodynamic status. Occasionally, hemodynamic collapse can accompany a decompressive laparotomy because of systemic reperfusion. This has led to the classic recommendation to have two teams of anesthesiologists, one managing hemodynamics and the other rapidly responding to the swift changes in the patient's ventilatory needs before and after decompression (Morris et al. 1993).

Very rarely, the situation is so dire that a decompressive laparotomy may be necessary in the ICU in a patient with rapid decompensation who is too unstable to be transferred to the operating room. However, routine monitoring of IAP should identify most patients with IAH prior to hemodynamic collapse thereby allowing a more controlled laparotomy in the operating room. Although a minimally invasive subcutaneous linea alba fasciotomy has been described to treat ACS patients with acute pancreatitis (Cheatham et al. 2008, Leppaniemi et al. 2011), most patients needing decompression will require a formal laparotomy followed by open abdomen management.

INITIAL CARE OF THE OPEN ABDOMEN

At the end of the index operation, the open abdomen is covered with a temporary closure device to contain and protect the viscera, yet spare the fascia for the definitive closure. The options for temporary closure are listed in **Box 6.2**. The specific choice is often a matter of personal preference or institutional tradition. A running monofilament skin – only closure above the open fascia may be feasible when there is no concern about IAH, but these cases are rare. Typically some form of coverage is needed to contain and protect the bulging bowel. A soft absorbable mesh or plastic 'silo' sutured to the skin edges were popular solutions in the 1990s. Subsequently, Barker et al. (Barker et al., 2000, Brock et al. 1995) introduced the vacuum pack, a 3-layer 'sandwich' in which the visceral block is wrapped in a polyethylene sheet, then covered with a surgical towel to absorb fluids and finally sealed to the skin with a plastic adhesive drape over suction drains. This technique is rapid, sutureless, and provides continuous controlled drainage of the peritoneal fluid. The vacuum pack has become the leading temporary coverage technique in trauma surgery (**Figure 6.1**).

The open abdomen cannot just be covered and left to heal. It must be maintained and washed out by planned re-exploration every 24–48 hours with careful attention to the healing wound. Every reoperation is an opportunity to identify and drain new infected fluid collections, optimally reposition previously placed drains, and – very importantly – gently separate the granulating visceral block from the inner aspect of the abdominal wall thereby extending the window of opportunity for delayed primary closure (see below). The integrity of suture lines, the viability of the abdominal viscera, and the possibility of missed injury should be assessed at each re-exploration.

Box 6.2 Options for temporary abdominal closure

1. Skin only closure
2. Mesh or plastic silo
3. Vacuum packed dressing
4. Vacuum assisted wound management

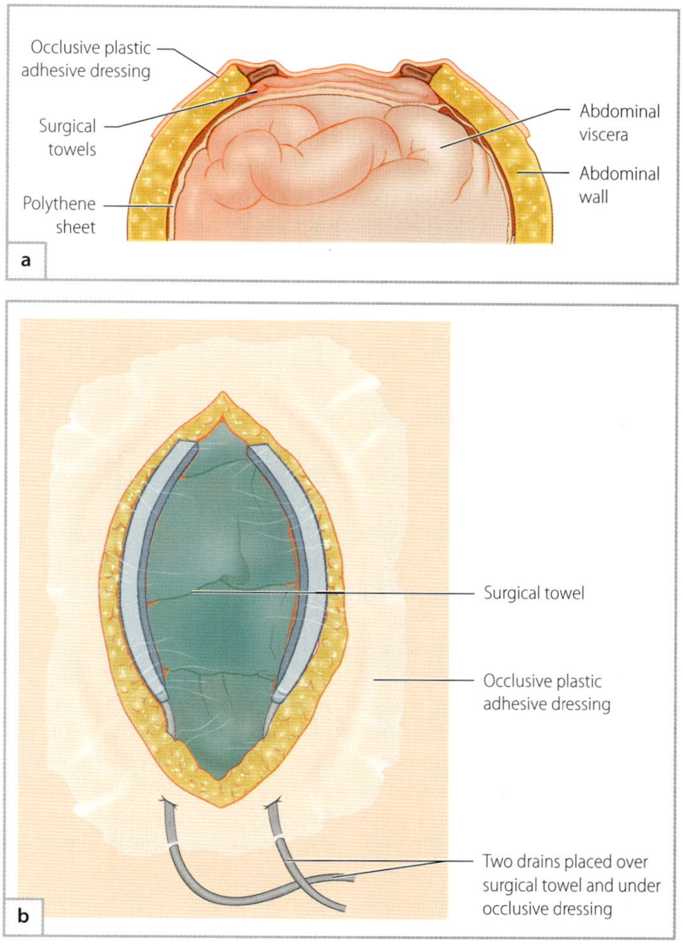

Figure 6.1 (a) Vacuum pack dressing. A polyethelene sheet is placed between the abdominal wall and the underlying viscera. (b) Surgical towel placed over polyethelene sheet. Two drains placed over the towel followed by an occlusive plastic adhesive dressing creating a watertight seal. Images redrawn and adapted from Hirshberg A, Mattox KL. Top knife: the art & craft of trauma surgery. Copyright © January 2005. With permission from TFM Publishing Ltd (www.tfmpublishing.com).

If packs have been used to control hemorrhage (usually around the liver), pre-emptive angioembolization will often precede the reoperation to prevent bleeding after pack removal. As a general rule, packs should be removed no later than 72 hours after placement (usually within 48 hours), because the risk of infection increases with time (Granchi et al. 2004). The surgeon should also be prepared to definitively control rebleeding or even repack the bleeding area, although this is rarely necessary. If gut continuity has been interrupted during the index operation, it should be restored prior to pack removal since rebleeding from the packed area may curtail the reoperation, forcing the surgeon to abandon intestinal reconstruction.

When re-exploring the open abdomen for severe intra-abdominal infection, a careful washout of the peritoneal cavity is crucial. Pus tends to accumulate in the subphrenic spaces bilaterally, as well as the subhepatic space, the lesser sac, both paracolic gutters and in the pelvis. A key principle with severe infection is the need to determine the need for another reoperation during the preceding one, regardless of the patient's subsequent clinical course. The patient should be returned to the operating theater every 36–48 hours until a clean peritoneal cavity has been achieved. As the open abdomen granulates, adhesiolysis become more dangerous, progressively restricting the explored space. If the patient's clinical trajectory points to the possibility of occult abdominal sepsis, it is prudent to obtain a computed tomographic scan prior to re-exploration, to identify inaccessible abscesses that may be amenable to percutaneous drainage.

If an intestinal stoma is needed, thoughtful placement can save hours of work during definitive closure. Temporary stomas should be placed as laterally as possible to allow maximal medial mobility of the abdominal wall during closure (Jernigan et al. 2003). It is often prudent to defer stoma formation during the initial laparotomy because progressive bowel and abdominal wall edema may cause stoma retraction and necrosis. A better alternative is to leave the stapled ends of intestine in the peritoneal cavity until the first re-exploration, when a good stoma can be safely fashioned. It is also prudent to oversew the staple lines to prevent dehiscence due to bowel wall edema.

When possible, a loop stoma protecting a distal anastomosis is preferable to an end stoma with a remote mucous fistula or a Hartmann pouch, because the former can be taken down without the need to re-enter a hostile peritoneal cavity. If a loop stoma is not possible, bringing both ends of the bowel out through the same incision and suturing their posterior walls together over a rubber catheter creates a loop stoma (Gosain et al. 1987).

On rare occasions, in morbidly obese patients or in massively edematous patients with a foreshortened mesentery, a primary anastomosis without proximal diversion may actually be safer than trying to exteriorize what is likely to become an ischemic bowel segment under tension. Any compromise of the anastomosis will be identified at reoperation.

The open abdomen as a healing wound

Understanding the healing process of the open abdomen is the key to modern management. Like any other wound, the open abdomen can either heal by delayed primary closure or granulate and close by secondary intention.

Immediately after the index laparotomy, the gut and other abdominal organs are usually massively distended and edematous, and the abdominal wall is swollen and noncompliant. Edema increases over the next 36–48 hours, often involving the mesentery. Then, as the inflammatory process subsides (either after definitive repair of the injuries or effective control of infection), edema and distension progressively diminish, whereas the bowel begins to granulate and adhere to the inner aspect of the abdominal wall. In other words, the open abdomen granulates just like any other wound. In the absence of ongoing peritoneal infection, this process becomes clearly visible during the second week after the index operation: the loops of bowel are fused and covered by granulation tissue. Individual loops cannot be identified or separated, and the entire abdominal content becomes a solid visceral block. By the end of the second week, this visceral block is completely fused and tightly adherent to the inner aspect of the abdominal wall, precluding delayed primary closure of the fascia.

It is clear from the above description that after a damage control laparotomy and subsequent definitive repair, there is a window of opportunity for wound closure. This window begins some 3–5 days after the index operation and lasts for about a week. By the end of the second week, it is usually too late, since the visceral block is fused to the abdominal wall and the abdomen is 'frozen.'

PLANNED VENTRAL HERNIA

Until the late 1990s, the window of opportunity for delayed primary closure of the open abdomen was missed in more than half the cases. In these patients, the granulating abdominal wound was accepted as a successful result, and attention was focused on atraumatic containment and protection of the exposed bowel. This traditional approach to the healing open abdomen was described by Fabian et al. in 1994 (Fabian et al. 1994).

During the period or repeated operations, the open abdomen was covered with a temporary closure device such as a polyethylene sheet. When further laparotomies were no longer required, the granulating wound was covered with an absorbable mesh (Fabian et al. 1994, Greene et al., 1993). As the wound continued to heal, the granulations grew through the interstices of the mesh and were subsequently covered with a skin graft. The patient was sent home with a 'planned ventral hernia,' a giant defect in the anterior abdominal wall (**Figure 6.2**). Definitive repair of this hernia was undertaken 6–12 months later, after the abdominal wound was completely healed, the visceral block was no longer 'frozen,' and the dense granulation tissue had matured into filmy adhesions.

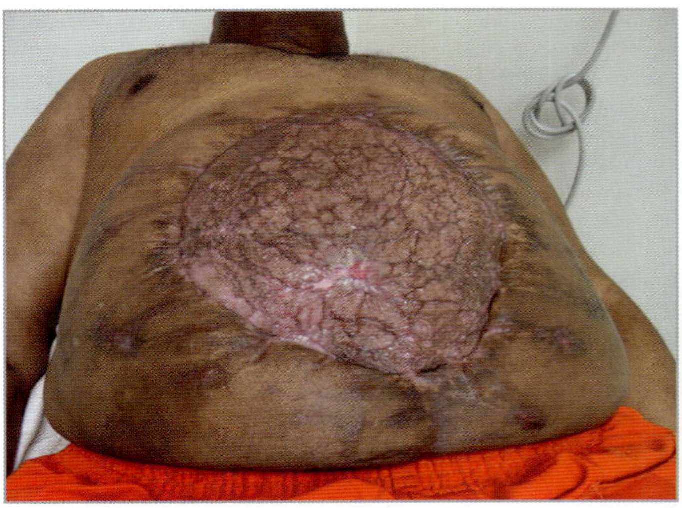

Figure 6.2 A 'planned ventral hernia.'

Repair of these very large ventral hernias is a lengthy procedure fraught with potential complications, because the bowel must be dissected off the skin graft and separated from the inner aspect of the abdominal wall. The timing of reconstruction is critical. As a basic principle, it is impossible to operate on these patients too late, only too early. The definitive reconstruction is often performed a year or more after the index operation. The patient and the family frequently urge hernia repair as soon as possible. However, the surgeon will regret an ill-advised elective procedure in an abdomen still in the throes of active inflammation. Reconstruction should be delayed until the skin graft can be pinched off the bowel between the thumb and the index finger, the so-called 'pinch test' (Jernigan et al. 2003). This simple bedside test indicates that the abdominal wound has 'matured,' and therefore the dense granulations that characterize the healing open abdomen (and cause a 'frozen abdomen') have been replaced with filmy adhesions that are amenable to adhesiolysis. The skin graft can now be safely dissected off the underlying bowel with a much lower risk of enterotomy.

Definitive abdominal closure begins with a circumferential incision along the edges of the fascial defect. The skin graft is then sharply dissected off the bowel. Patient adhesiolysis frees both sides of the fascia from bowel and other viscera that are adherent to the inner aspect of the abdominal wall. The defect is usually too large for side-to-side closure and requires a reconstructive solution, as discussed below.

The planned ventral hernia approach is associated with significant morbidity. During the healing process, the bowel is at risk of forming EAF, the most lethal complication of the open abdomen as described below. On occasion, even a bout of coughing can cause a tear in the exposed bowel, creating a technically challenging emergency. Delayed return to work and depression related to altered body image and abdominal wall instability are other concerns (Zarzaur et al. 2011). In view of these difficulties, it is not surprising that surgeons have searched for technical solutions that allow them to perform delayed primary closure in these patients, thus avoiding the planned ventral hernia altogether. In the past decade, we have witnessed a quiet revolution that nowadays enables surgeons to achieve delayed primary closure in the majority of trauma patients with an open abdomen. Planned ventral hernia remains a feasible solution for those patients in whom the preferred option of delayed primary closure is not possible.

THE REVOLUTION

During the late 1990s, three innovative concepts converged to greatly facilitate definitive closure of the open abdomen. These new concepts are preservation of the peritoneal space, progressive approximation of the fascia, and vacuum-assisted wound management (Scott et al. 2005).

The discovery that surgeons can alter the healing process of the open abdomen was fortuitous – an unintended consequence of Barker's vacuum pack. It soon became evident that the polyethylene sheet that is used as the inner layer of the vacuum pack creates a physical barrier between the granulating visceral mass and the inner aspect of the abdominal wall. When properly placed all the way down to the paracolic gutters and deep into the pelvis, the polyethylene sheet prevents adhesion of the visceral block to the inner aspect of the abdominal wall, thereby maintaining medial mobility of the fascia. The healing process of the open abdominal wound continues – but the visceral block granulates separately from the abdominal wall. This separation delays the onset of the 'frozen abdomen' and extends the window of opportunity for delayed primary closure from around a week to as long as a month from the index operation (Miller et al. 2002).

The second new concept was gradual progressive approximation of the fascial edges. Lateral retraction of the fascia is a surprisingly aggressive process in the open abdomen. If not counteracted, it results within a few days in a gaping wound that cannot be closed. Many creative devices have been described to achieve progressive fascial closure by exerting ongoing medial traction on the fascial edges between reoperations (Atweh et al., 2002, Kafie et al., 2003, Koniaris et al., 2001, Losanoff et al., 2003, Paran et al., 2001, Regner et al., 2012, Wittmann et al., 1990). The best known (which also yielded a popular commercial product) is the burr closure device (Wittmann et al. 1990). Velcro-based flaps sutured to the fascia allow daily progressive approximation of the wound edges at the bedside as well as at the end of each re-exploration.

An alternative to the burr device is to use mesh sutured to the fascia, to re-enter the abdomen through a longitudinal midline incision in the mesh and to 'reef' the edges of the mesh progressively at each subsequent reoperation until the fascia can be closed.

Regardless of the specific technique chosen, the key principles are firm but gentle traction to prevent fascial necrosis, and placement of an atraumatic nonadherent layer (e.g. a polyethylene sheet and a thin sponge) between the fascial bridge and the underlying bowel to keep them separate and preserve the peritoneal space. It is critical to prevent any contact between the bridging material and the viscera to reduce the risk of erosion into the bowel.

The third conceptual innovation is vacuum-assisted wound management. The concept was introduced for soft tissue wounds in 1997 by Argenta et al. from Wake Forest University (Argenta & Morykwas 1997) and then rapidly applied to the open abdomen by trauma surgeons from the same institution. Vacuum-assisted wound management is a modification of Barker's vacuum pack whereby the middle layer of the original sandwich (a surgical towel) is replaced by a sponge. Under negative pressure, the sponge atraumatically pulls the edges of the fascia medially, counteracting their natural tendency to retract laterally (Garner et al. 2001). There is also evidence suggesting that the negative pressure has other beneficial effects on the healing wound by improving blood flow and lowering the bacterial count (Banwell et al. 1998, Morykwas et al. 1997).

Although the negative pressure sponge technique alone has been touted as a method to prevent lateral fascial retraction (Stevens 2009), some surgeons combine it with an additional device to bridge the gap in the fascia and allow progressive reapproximation of the defect (Verdam et al. 2011). We use a thin sponge over the polyethylene sheet covering the bowel and immediately below the fascial bridge. An additional sponge is placed above the fascial bridge. The negative pressure is applied to the most superficial sponge but transmitted through the mesh to the inner sponge as well.

An alarming report of fistula formation as a complication of the negative pressure (Rao et al. 2007) appeared soon after the widespread use of this technique. This report led to a call for caution applying negative pressure directly over bowel (Fischer 2008) especially if fresh suture or staple lines are present. Since these communications, three studies have addressed this issue. A literature review found no published evidence to suggest that the negative pressure sponge itself was the cause of the fistulas (Stevens 2009). A subsequent retrospective study of 49 secondary peritonitis patients treated with vacuum-assisted closure for >7 days demonstrated a fascial closure rate of only 22% (11 patients). Re-exploration after starting vacuum-assisted closure was associated with enterocutaneous fistula in 11 patients (22%), but no comment was made on the role of the sponge (Schmelzle et al. 2010). A prospective multicenter study of open abdomen management comparing vacuum-assisted wound management with mesh mediated fascial traction demonstrated a fascial closure rate of 76.6% in intention-to-treat analysis (Acosta et al. 2011). Eight fistulas occurred, seven of which were associated with bowel ischemia. At present, there is no prospective evidence proving that negative pressure per se increases the risk of fistula formation, but there is enough retrospective data to strongly advocate caution when using this very popular technology.

OPTIONS FOR DELAYED RECONSTRUCTION OF THE ABDOMINAL WALL

The goal of delayed abdominal wall reconstruction is to achieve a durable well-vascularized closure without tension. There are two categories of 'bridging' options: autologous tissue solutions and prosthetics. Sometimes the solution to a giant defect may involve a combination of both. Patients with very large defects also benefit from the timely involvement of a plastic surgeon in planning and executing the procedure. Preoperative assessment of the abdominal wall defect is important to determine which tissue components are missing or inadequate and which can be used for reconstruction. Autogenous tissue is obviously an ideal choice in a procedure requiring bowel resection or repair, because it reduces the risk of prosthetic infection.

The components separation technique introduced by Ramirez et al. (1990) is the workhorse of abdominal wall reconstruction. Its popularity stems from its simplicity: it can easily be performed by a general surgeon and does not involve complex tissue transfers. In essence, the procedure is a relaxing (or releasing) incision. It is based on the anatomical observation of Oscar Ramirez that the rectus abdominis myofascial unit is held laterally by the external oblique fascia, and therefore a releasing incision in this fascia will free the rectus and mobilize it medially across a considerable distance that can be as much as 10–12 cm on each side in the mid-abdomen.

The procedure starts by dissecting longitudinally just above the fascia along the entire length of the abdominal defect, on each side. Careful sharp dissection separates the abdominal wall elements (rectus muscles and fascia and external oblique fascia) from the overlaying skin and subcutaneous tissue, creating a large thick skin flap on each side of the abdominal defect. These flaps extend from the edge of the defect to well beyond the lateral border of the rectus sheath, fully exposing the rectus sheath. A longitudinal incision is then made in the external oblique fascia immediately lateral to the rectus sheath, and the avascular plane between the external oblique fascia and the internal oblique muscle is identified and entered. If the lateral border of the rectus is not easily identified, a short transverse incision in the fascia will allow the surgeon to see the interface between longitudinal muscle (rectus) and transverse fibers (internal oblique) and thus enter the correct plane. Bluntly developing this plane between the external and internal oblique is the key maneuver of components separation, and this is continued longitudinally for the entire length of the defect from the costal margin to the pelvis (**Figure 6.3**). This releasing incision gives the rectus myofascial unit considerable medial mobility. A similar procedure is repeated on the other side to free the contralateral rectus. Care is taken to preserve the attachment of the umbilicus to the rectus sheath to prevent ischemic necrosis of the skin.

After components separation, the abdominal wound is closed in the midline in the standard fashion, using a mass closure technique. Suction drains are left under the large flaps and brought out laterally, and the subcutaneous tissue and skin are closed in the midline to provide an air-tight seal. If the wound has been heavily contaminated, the surgeon can close the abdominal wall, put a negative pressure sponge underneath each of the large skin flaps, and perform a delayed primary closure of the skin 4–7 days later to reduce the risk of wound infection.

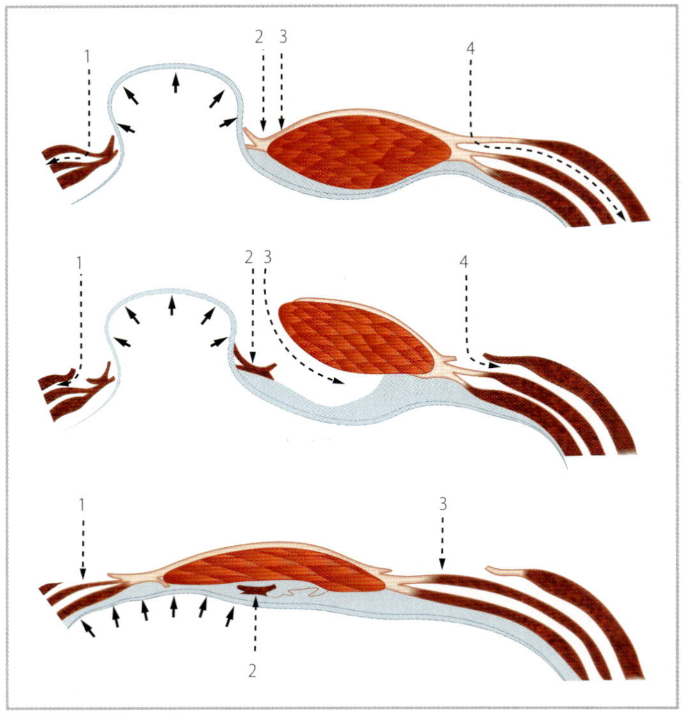

Figure 6.3 Cross-sectional schematic diagram of the dissection of the abdominal wall into its component sections and final flap reconstruction. Note planes of dissection and advancement of muscle layers. With permission from Ramirez et al. (1990).

Follow-up studies of ventral herniorrhaphy with the separation of parts technique report an incidence of hernia recurrence ranging from 2–32% (Candage et al. 2008, Jin et al. 2007). The use of a prosthetic device in these studies significantly increased the risk of recurrence.

However, when abdominal closure cannot be achieved with these releasing incisions, prosthetic mesh is an obvious alternative. Polypropylene mesh should never be placed in direct contact with the viscera because of the risk of bowel erosion. As a general rule, a prosthetic mesh should be used as an inlay, not onlay, whenever possible. The overlaying fascia should overlap the mesh for a distance of several centimeters on all sides. We favor use of a dual layer mesh composed of polypropylene and polyflourotetraethylene since the inner layer is unlikely to erode into the bowel.

Unfortunately, nonabsorbable mesh is contra-indicated if an intestinal stoma or enteral fistula is present because of the very high risk of infection. In this situation, bioprosthetic meshes such as acellular human (Maurice & Skeete 2009) or porcine (Hsu et al. 2008) dermal matrix and porcine intestinal submucosa (Johnson & Paquette 2007) can be considered. However, the initial enthusiasm for bioprosthetic materials has been tempered by reports of very high rates of hernia recurrence and abdominal wall laxity (Bluebond-Langner et al. 2008, Candage et al. 2008, de Moya et al. 2008, Jin et al. 2007). The indications for bioprosthetic meshes are a contaminated abdomen or insufficient skin for complete mesh coverage. In either case, the long-term results of biologic meshes are vastly inferior to the other options described above.

Complex plastic reconstructions of the abdominal wall should be considered depending upon the nature of the defect, comorbidities, and the degree of obesity. Examples of flaps useful in abdominal wall reconstruction include the tensor fascia lata (Williams et al. 1998), rectus femoris, (Koshima et al. 1999), and latissimus dorsi (de Weerd et al. 2007) muscle flaps. Microvascular techniques increase the scope of technical options available to the plastic surgeon. The use of tissue expanders to increase the surface area of skin flaps prior to definitive reconstruction is another useful adjunct (Livingston et al. 1992).

In everyday practice, the majority of patients with large abdominal wall defects can be closed by components separation. In especially large defects, a combination of components separation and a nonabsorbable prosthetic will typically bridge the gap. Sometimes a biological mesh has to be used because of contamination or compromised skin, but using it amounts to an admission of defeat. Complex plastic reconstructions are rarely needed. Referral to a center capable of providing optimal comprehensive care by a multispecialty team is prudent in these complex cases.

THE ENTEROATMOSPHERIC FISTULA

The wide adoption of open abdomen management has confronted surgeons with a new and especially vicious adversary: the EAF. This fistula, originally termed an 'exposed fistula' in the French literature, is a hole in the gut in the midst of an open abdominal wound. In contrast with an enterocutaneous fistula, here there is no overlying skin or soft tissue and therefore no realistic expectation of spontaneous closure (Visschers et al. 2008). EAFs are classified based on the status of the surrounding abdominal wound (Al-Khoury et al. 2008). A deep EAF occurs in the early stages of an open abdomen before the wound has a chance to granulate and heal. A deep fistula continuously spills intestinal content onto the peritoneal cavity causing ongoing diffuse peritonitis with its lethal physiological effects and dire metabolic consequences. In contrast, a superficial EAF occurs after the open abdominal wound has granulated. The opening in the gut drains atop a carpet of granulation tissue, whereas the peritoneal space, obliterated by the dense adhesions of a 'frozen abdomen,' no longer exists. A superficial EAF is therefore a completely extraperitoneal process. A deep EAF causes uncontrolled diffuse peritonitis, a life-threatening emergency. A superficial EAF is predominantly a wound management problem.

The EAF is very often a preventable complication (Schecter et al. 2006) and simple precautions reduce the risk that it will develop (**Box 6.3**). When a deep EAF is identified, the first priority is to control the ongoing peritonitis. After rapid resuscitation, the patient should undergo emergency surgery with the understanding that in most deep EAFs the hole in the gut cannot be closed with any hope of success. A more realistic goal is to gain temporary control of the fistula effluent to allow the patient to recover from the devastating consequences of ongoing peritonitis. The open abdominal wound will then granulate and heal around the hole in the gut, converting the deep fistula with time into a superficial one, in anticipation of definitive closure many months later.

In the operating room, achieving source control of a deep EAF is much easier said than done. Exteriorization or proximal diversion, both excellent options in theory, is often impossible due to massive edema of the viscera and abdominal wall, as well as foreshortening of the mesentery. Later, there is gradual fusion of the bowel into an impenetrable visceral block as described above (Scott et al. 2005). The patient's only hope rests in finding a way to somehow separate the open and exposed peritoneal cavity from the continuous stream of intestinal content (Subramaniam et al. 2002)

Tube drainage of a deep EAF is neither practical nor useful. Since there is no tract, a drainage tube will only serve to progressively enlarge the hole while intestinal content leaks around the tube. An improvised technique to achieve source control, the 'floating stoma' (Subramaniam et al. 2002), was the first attempt to gain control of a deep EAF based on an understanding of its unique pathophysiology. This entails covering the open abdomen with a plastic sheet (similar to the 'Bogota bag') sutured to the skin edges of the wound. A small opening is then created in the plastic sheet directly over the hole in the gut. The edges of the hole in the bowel are then sutured to the hole in the plastic sheet, creating a kind of 'floating stoma' in the middle of the sheet. The plastic sheet acts as a physical barrier between the intestinal effluent (above the sheet) and the peritoneal cavity (beneath it). An ostomy bag is applied to the plastic sheet around the improvised 'stoma,' collecting the effluent in a controlled fashion and allowing the protected peritoneal cavity to heal. In other words, the deep EAF is gradually converted into a superficial one over several weeks.

In recent years, vacuum-assisted wound management has simplified the approach to deep EAF (Boulanger et al. 2007). Applying negative pressure to the open abdominal wound continuously sucks the effluent from the peritoneal cavity and thus controls the fistula without the need for a physical barrier between it and the peritoneal cavity. A technical refinement of this concept is the 'tube vac' where the hole in the gut is intubated with an appropriately sized Malecot catheter that is then pulled out perpendicularly through the negative pressure sponge (Al-Khoury et al. 2008). The sponge thus serves as a 'rig' supporting the tube and preventing lateral motion that may enlarge the hole. Most of the intestinal effluent is drained by the tube, while the sponge absorbs any residual fluid that may leak around it. The negative pressure dressing also simplifies nursing care and protects the surrounding skin. Although the negative pressure sponge may be associated with an increased risk of fistula formation in the open abdomen (see above), it is an excellent option for management of an established fistula.

A central feature of a deep exposed fistula is the tremendous catabolism it generates. The ongoing peritonitis, an open abdominal wound (the metabolic equivalent of a large full-thickness burn), and protein losses from the GI tract all combine to create a catabolic 'black hole' in an already critically ill patient. While it is difficult to quantify all these losses, it is nevertheless becoming clear that conventional nutritional support often does not suffice. A combination of parenteral and enteral nutrition given simultaneously may be needed to fulfill the patient's nutritional needs and prevent a lethal catabolic meltdown.

Box 6.3 Steps to prevent an enteroatmospheric fistula

1. Cover exposed bowel with omentum
2. Apply a biological dressing early
3. Do not place non-absorbable mesh on exposed bowel
4. Do not place gauze on exposed bowel
5. Avoid negative pressure to suture lines
6. Restrict access to the open abdomen

A superficial EAF, though not a life-threatening emergency, presents a major wound management challenge. The surgeon faced with a fistula spilling intestinal content onto a large carpet of granulation tissue has to buy time until definitive closure can be undertaken, typically 6–12 months from the index operation. The two realistic options are, therefore, either to attempt direct closure of the fistula extraperitoneally or to convert it into a manageable stoma.

Direct closure of superficial 'bud' fistulae was first described by Sarfeh and Jakowatz (1992). The procedure entails very limited dissection to define the edges of the fistula opening, followed by extraperitoneal suture repair of the hole in the bowel. All this is done on the surface of the granulating abdominal wound. The key principle is to cover the suture line with a biological dressing (autologous or homologous skin graft or acellular dermal matrix), with or without a tissue adhesive. Sarfeh and Jakowatz(1992) reported a success rate of 50%, but the important point here is that these are local, low-risk procedures that can easily be repeated as necessary. We (Jamshidi & Schecter 2007) reported successful local closure of 5 of 7 EAFs but needed a mean of 4 attempts per patient.

If local closure fails or is not feasible, another option is to accept the fistula and approach it as a stoma. The aim is therefore to create a stable skin platform that will allow the application of a stoma appliance around the fistula opening. Split-thickness skin graft coverage of the granulating wound surrounding the fistula is often necessary to achieve stable wound coverage. A negative pressured sponge dressing with a hole fashioned in the center to allow free drainage through the sponge into an ostomy appliance can protect the fresh skin graft from the intestinal contents until the graft takes. After a successful skin graft, management of the superficial EAF becomes much simpler and follows standard lines of stoma management. A skilled stomal therapist and nursing staff are essential prerequisites to a successful outcome.

Once the wound matures (6–12 months later), take down of the superficial EAF is performed in conjunction with abdominal wall reconstruction as described above. The operative procedure entails complete mobilization of the small bowel from the Ligament of Treitz to the colon to clearly delineate the anatomy and relieve any potential points of obstruction distal the anastomosis. Meticulous adhesiolysis assisted by injection of normal saline into dense adhesions to separate tissue planes will reduce the risk of inadvertent enterotomy in these difficult cases. The procedure should be scheduled as the first and only case of the day as these are long operations. A two-team approach has considerable merit. The visceral team concentrates on the tedious intestinal dissection, fistula resection, and anastomosis. We prefer a hand-sewn anastomosis for abnormal bowel. After this, a well-rested reconstructive team can take over, focusing on abdominal wall reconstruction and closure.

CONCLUSION

The widespread use of damage control surgery, greater awareness of IAH, and better understanding of severe abdominal infection have all contributed to the proliferation of patients with an open abdomen. There is a wide range of methods to contain the bowel and manage the open wound. Amidst the array of new information, personal preference, and institutional tradition, it is easy to lose sight of the guiding principles.

Modern management is based on the realization that the open abdomen behaves like any other open wound. Current methods to modify the healing process have extended the window of opportunity to achieve delayed primary closure in most patients. Adherence to these basic principles will allow the surgeon to confidently manage the patient with the open abdomen and avoid or successfully manage complications such as an EAF.

REFERENCES

Acosta S, Bjarnason T, Petersson U, et al. Multicentre prospective study of fascial closure rate after open abdomen with vacuum and mesh-mediated fascial traction. Br J Surg 2011; 98:735–743.

Adkins AL, Robbins J, Villalba M, et al. Open abdomen management of intra-abdominal sepsis. Am Surg 2004; 70:137–140; discussion 140.

Al-Khoury G, Kaufman D, Hirshberg A. Improved control of exposed fistula in the open abdomen. J Am Coll Surg 2008; 206:397–398.

Argenta LC, Morykwas MJ. Vacuum-assisted closure: a new method for wound control and treatment: clinical experience. Ann Plast Surg 1997; 38:563–576; discussion 577.

Atweh NA, Lye KD, Kavic S, et al. Closure of large abdominal wounds with an adjustable suture-tension device. J Am Coll Surg 2002; 195:281–283.

Azzopardi EA, McWilliams B, Iyer S, et al. Fluid resuscitation in adults with severe burns at risk of secondary abdominal compartment syndrome – an evidence based systematic review. Burns 2009; 35:911–920.

Banwell P, Withey S, Holten I. The use of negative pressure to promote healing. Br J Plast Surg 1998; 51:79.

Barker DE, Kaufman HJ, Smith LA, et al. Vacuum pack technique of temporary abdominal closure: a 7-year experience with 112 patients. J Trauma 2000; 48:201–206; discussion 206–207.

Bertram P, Treutner KH, Stumpf M, et al. Postoperative necrotizing soft-tissue infections of the abdominal wall. Langenbecks Arch Surg 2000; 385:39–41.

Bloomfield GL, Ridings PC, Blocher CR, et al. A proposed relationship between increased intra-abdominal, intrathoracic, and intracranial pressure. Crit Care Med 1997; 25:496–503.

Bluebond-Langner R, Keifa ES, Mithani S, et al. Recurrent abdominal laxity following interpositional human acellular dermal matrix. Ann Plast Surg 2008; 60:76–80.

Boulanger K, Lemaire V, Jacquemin D. Vacuum-assisted closure of enterocutaneous fistula. Acta Chir Belg 2007; 107:703–705.

Britt RC, Gannon T, Collins JN, et al. Secondary abdominal compartment syndrome: risk factors and outcomes. Am Surg 2005; 71:982–985.

Brock WB, Barker DE, Burns RP. Temporary closure of open abdominal wounds: the vacuum pack. Am Surg 1995; 61:30–35.

Burch JM, Ortiz VB, Richardson RJ, et al. Abbreviated laparotomy and planned reoperation for critically injured patients. Ann Surg 1992; 215:476–483; discussion 483–474.

Caldwell CB, Ricotta JJ. Changes in visceral blood flow with elevated intra-abdominal pressure. J Surg Res 1987; 43:14–20.

Candage R, Jones K, Luchette FA, et al. Use of human acellular dermal matrix for hernia repair: friend or foe? Surgery 2008; 144:703–709; discussion 709–711.

Carlotti AP, Carvalho WB. Abdominal compartment syndrome: a review. Pediatr Crit Care Med 2009; 10:115–120.

Cheatham ML, Fowler J, Pappas P. Subcutaneous linea alba fasciotomy: a less morbid treatment for abdominal compartment syndrome. Am Surg 2008; 74:746–749.

Cheatham ML, Malbrain ML, Kirkpatrick A, et al. Results from the International Conference of Experts on Intra-abdominal Hypertension and Abdominal Compartment Syndrome. II. Recommendations. Intensive Care Med 2007; 33:951–962.

Cheatham ML, White MW, Sagraves SG, et al. Abdominal perfusion pressure: a superior parameter in the assessment of intra-abdominal hypertension. J Trauma 2000; 49:621–626; discussion 626–627.

Citerio G, Vascotto E, Villa F, et al. Induced abdominal compartment syndrome increases intracranial pressure in neurotrauma patients: a prospective study. Crit Care Med 2001; 29:1466–1471.

Corcos AC, Sherman HF. Percutaneous treatment of secondary abdominal compartment syndrome. J Trauma 2001; 51:1062–1064.

Cotton BA, Guy JS, Morris JA, Jr, et al. The cellular, metabolic, and systemic consequences of aggressive fluid resuscitation strategies. Shock 2006; 26:115–121.

Daugherty EL, Hongyan L, Taichman D, et al. Abdominal compartment syndrome is common in medical intensive care unit patients receiving large-volume resuscitation. J Intensive Care Med 2007; 22:294–299.

Deeren DH, Dits H, Malbrain ML. Correlation between intra-abdominal and intracranial pressure in nontraumatic brain injury. Intensive Care Med 2005; 31:1577–1581.

de Moya MA, Dunham M, Inaba K, et al. Long-term outcome of acellular dermal matrix when used for large traumatic open abdomen. J Trauma 2008; 65:349–353.

de Weerd L, Kjaeve J, Aghajani E, et al. The sandwich design: a new method to close a high-output enterocutaneous fistula and an associated abdominal wall defect. Ann Plast Surg 2007; 58:580–583.

Diebel L, Saxe J, Dulchavsky S. Effect of intra-abdominal pressure on abdominal wall blood flow. Am Surg 1992; 58:573–575; discussion 575–576.

Doty JM, Saggi BH, Blocher CR, et al. Effects of increased renal parenchymal pressure on renal function. J Trauma 2000; 48:874–877.

Doty JM, Saggi BH, Sugerman HJ, et al. Effect of increased renal venous pressure on renal function. J Trauma 1999; 47:1000–1003.

Emerson H. Intra-abdominal pressures. Arch Intern Med 1911; 7:754–784.

Fabian TC, Croce MA, Pritchard FE, et al. Planned ventral hernia. Staged management for acute abdominal wall defects. Ann Surg 1994; 219:643–650; discussion 651–643.

Fietsam R, Jr, Villalba M, Glover JL, et al. Intra-abdominal compartment syndrome as a complication of ruptured abdominal aortic aneurysm repair. Am Surg 1989; 55:396–402.

Fischer JE. A cautionary note: the use of vacuum-assisted closure systems in the treatment of gastrointestinal cutaneous fistula may be associated with higher mortality from subsequent fistula development. Am J Surg 2008; 196:1–2.

Garner GB, Ware DN, Cocanour CS, et al. Vacuum-assisted wound closure provides early fascial reapproximation in trauma patients with open abdomens. Am J Surg 2001; 182:630–638.

Gosain A, Markison RE, Schecter WP. Temporary colostomy for trauma. A new method to simplify colostomy closure. Dis Colon Rectum 1987; 30:220–222.

Granchi TS, Abikhaled JA, Hirshberg A, et al. Patterns of microbiology in intra-abdominal packing for trauma. J Trauma 2004; 56:45–51.

Greene MA, Mullins RJ, Malangoni MA, et al. Laparotomy wound closure with absorbable polyglycolic acid mesh. Surg Gynecol Obstet 1993; 176:213–218.

Hsu PW, Salgado CJ, Kent K et al. Evaluation of porcine dermal collagen (Permacol) used in abdominal wall reconstruction. J Plast Reconstr Aesthet Surg 2009; 62:1484–1489.

Ivatury RR, Nallathambi M, Rao PM, et al. Open management of the septic abdomen: therapeutic and prognostic considerations based on APACHE II. Crit Care Med 1989; 17:511–517.

Ivatury RR, Nallathambi M, Rohman M, et al. Open management of the posttraumatic septic abdomen. Am Surg 1990; 56:548–552.

Jamshidi R, Schecter WP. Biological dressings for the management of enteric fistulas in the open abdomen: a preliminary report. Arch Surg 2007; 142:793–796.

Jin J, Rosen MJ, Blatnik J, et al. Use of acellular dermal matrix for complicated ventral hernia repair: does technique affect outcomes? J Am Coll Surg 2007; 205:654–660.

Jernigan TW, Fabian TC, Croce MA, et al. Staged management of giant abdominal wall defects: acute and long-term results. Ann Surg 2003; 238:349–355; discussion 355–347.

Johnson EK, Paquette EL. Use of surgisis for abdominal wall reconstruction/closure in battlefield casualties during Operation Iraqi Freedom. Mil Med 2007; 172:1119–1124.

Joseph DK, Dutton RP, Aarabi B, et al. Decompressive laparotomy to treat intractable intracranial hypertension after traumatic brain injury. J Trauma 2004; 57:687–693; discussion 693–685.

Kafie FE, Tessier DJ, Williams RA, et al. Serial abdominal closure technique (the "SAC" procedure): a novel method for delayed closure of the abdominal wall. Am Surg 2003; 69:102–105.

Kashtan J, Green JF, Parsons EQ, et al. Hemodynamic effect of increased abdominal pressure. J Surg Res 1981; 30:249–255.

Kashuk JL, Moore EE, Millikan JS, et al. Major abdominal vascular trauma – a unified approach. J Trauma 1982; 22:672–679.

Koniaris LG, Hendrickson RJ, Drugas G, et al. Dynamic retention: a technique for closure of the complex abdomen in critically ill patients. Arch Surg 2001; 136:1359–1362; discussion 1363.

Koshima I, Moriguchi T, Inagawa K, et al. Dynamic reconstruction of the abdominal wall using a reinnervated free rectus femoris muscle transfer. Ann Plast Surg 1999; 43:199–203.

Kron IL, Harman PK, Nolan SP. The measurement of intra-abdominal pressure as a criterion for abdominal re-exploration. Ann Surg 1984; 199:28–30.

Lambert DM, Marceau S, Forse RA. Intra-abdominal pressure in the morbidly obese. Obes Surg 2005; 15:1225–1232.

Latenser BA, Kowal-Vern A, Kimball D, et al. A pilot study comparing percutaneous decompression with decompressive laparotomy for acute abdominal compartment syndrome in thermal injury. J Burn Care Rehabil 2002; 23:190–195.

Leppaniemi A, Hienonen P, Mentula P, et al. Subcutaneous linea alba fasciotomy, does it really work? Am Surg 2011; 77:99–102.

Levy E, Palmer DL, Frileux P, et al. Septic necrosis of the midline wound in postoperative peritonitis. Successful management by debridement, myocutaneous advancement, and primary skin closure. Ann Surg 1988; 207:470–479.

Livingston DH, Sharma PK, Glantz AI. Tissue expanders for abdominal wall reconstruction following severe trauma: technical note and case reports. J Trauma 1992; 32:82–86.

Losanoff JE, Richman BW, Jones JW. Adjustable suture-tension closure of the open abdomen. J Am Coll Surg 2003; 196:163–164.

Luca A, Cirera I, Garcia-Pagan JC, et al. Hemodynamic effects of acute changes in intra-abdominal pressure in patients with cirrhosis. Gastroenterology 1993; 104:222–227.

Malbrain ML, Cheatham ML, Kirkpatrick A, et al. Results from the International Conference of Experts on Intra-abdominal Hypertension and Abdominal Compartment Syndrome. I. Definitions. Intensive Care Med 2006; 32:1722–1732.

Maurice SM, Skeete DA. Use of human acellular dermal matrix for abdominal wall reconstructions. Am J Surg 2009; 197:35–42.

Miller PR, Croce MA, Bee TK, et al. Associated injuries in blunt solid organ trauma: implications for missed injury in nonoperative management. J Trauma 2002; 53:238–242; discussion 242–234.

Morris JA, Jr, Eddy VA, Blinman TA, et al. The staged celiotomy for trauma. Issues in unpacking and reconstruction. Ann Surg 1993; 217:576–584; discussion 584–576.

Morykwas MJ, Argenta LC, Shelton-Brown EI, et al. Vacuum-assisted closure: a new method for wound control and treatment: animal studies and basic foundation. Ann Plast Surg 1997; 38:553–562.

Ogilvie WH. The late complications of abdominal war-wounds. Lancet Infect Dis 1940; 2:253–256.

Oida T, Mimatsu K, Kawasaki A, et al. Open abdominal surgery with mesh and zipper for superior mesenteric artery occlusion. Hepatogastroenterology 2011; 58:1394–1397.

Papavramidis TS, Marinis AD, Pliakos I, et al. Abdominal compartment syndrome – intra-abdominal hypertension: defining, diagnosing, and managing. J Emerg Trauma Shock 2011; 4:279–291.

Paran H, Mayo A, Afanasiev A, et al. Staged primary closure of the abdominal wall in patients with abdominal compartment syndrome. J Trauma 2001; 51:1204–1206.

Ramirez OM, Ruas E, Dellon AL. "Components separation" method for closure of abdominal-wall defects: an anatomic and clinical study. Plast Reconstr Surg 1990; 86:519–526.

Rao M, Burke D, Finan PJ, et al. The use of vacuum-assisted closure of abdominal wounds: a word of caution. Colorectal Dis 2007; 9:266–268.

Reckard JM, Chung MH, Varma MK, et al. Management of intraabdominal hypertension by percutaneous catheter drainage. J Vasc Interv Radiol 2005; 16:1019–1021.

Regner JL, Kobayashi L, Coimbra R. Surgical strategies for management of the open abdomen. World J Surg 2012; 36:497–510.

Richardson JD, Trinkle JK. Hemodynamic and respiratory alterations with increased intra-abdominal pressure. J Surg Res 1976; 20:401–404.

Ridings PC, Bloomfield GL, Blocher CR, et al. Cardiopulmonary effects of raised intra-abdominal pressure before and after intravascular volume expansion. J Trauma 1995; 39:1071–1075.

Rotondo MF, Schwab CW, McGonigal MD, et al. 'Damage control': an approach for improved survival in exsanguinating penetrating abdominal injury. J Trauma 1993; 35:375–382; discussion 382–373.
Rutherford E, Skeete D, Brasel K. Management of the patient with an open abdomen: techniquest in temporary and definitive closure. Curr Probl Surg 2004; 41:815–876.
Saffle JI. The phenomenon of "fluid creep" in acute burn resuscitation. J Burn Care Res 2007; 28:382–395.
Sanchez NC, Tenofsky PL, Dort JM, et al. What is normal intra-abdominal pressure? Am Surg 2001; 67:243–248.
Sarfeh IJ, Jakowatz JG. Surgical treatment of enteric 'bud' fistulas in contaminated wounds. A riskless extraperitoneal method using split-thickness skin grafts. Arch Surg 1992; 127:1027–1030; discussion 1030–1021.
Schecter WP, Ivatury RR, Rotondo MF, et al. Open abdomen after trauma and abdominal sepsis: a strategy for management. J Am Coll Surg 2006; 203:390–396.
Schmelzle M, Alldinger I, Matthaei H, et al. Long-term vacuum-assisted closure in open abdomen due to secondary peritonitis: a retrospective evaluation of a selected group of patients. Dig Surg 2010; 27:272–278.
Scott BG, Feanny MA, Hirshberg A. Early definitive closure of the open abdomen: a quiet revolution. Scand J Surg 2005; 94:9–14.
Stevens P. Vacuum-assisted closure of laparostomy wounds: a critical review of the literature. Int Wound J 2009; 6:259–266.
Subramaniam MH, Liscum KR, Hirshberg A. The floating stoma: a new technique for controlling exposed fistulae in abdominal trauma. J Trauma 2002; 53:386–388.
Sugrue M, Buhkari Y. Intra-abdominal pressure and abdominal compartment syndrome in acute general surgery. World J Surg 2009; 33:1123–1127.
Teichmann W, Wittmann DH, Andreone PA. Scheduled reoperations (etappenlavage) for diffuse peritonitis. Arch Surg 1986; 121:147–152.
Verdam FJ, Dolmans DE, Loos MJ, et al. Delayed primary closure of the septic open abdomen with a dynamic closure system. World J Surg 2011; 35:2348–2355.
Visschers RG, Olde Damink SW, Winkens B, et al. Treatment strategies in 135 consecutive patients with enterocutaneous fistulas. World J Surg 2008; 32:445–453.
Ward D, Vernava AM, Kaminski DL, et al. Improved outcome by identification of high-risk nonocclusive mesenteric ischemia, aggressive reexploration, and delayed anastomosis. Am J Surg 1995; 170:577–580; discussion 580–571.
Williams JK, Carlson GW, deChalain T, et al. Role of tensor fasciae latae in abdominal wall reconstruction. Plast Reconstr Surg 1998; 101:713–718.
Wittmann DH, Aprahamian C, Bergstein JM. Etappenlavage: advanced diffuse peritonitis managed by planned multiple laparotomies utilizing zippers, slide fastener, and Velcro analogue for temporary abdominal closure. World J Surg 1990; 14:218–226.
Zarzaur BL, DiCocco JM, Shahan CP, et al. Quality of life after abdominal wall reconstruction following open abdomen. J Trauma 2011; 70:285–291.

Chapter 7 Laparoscopic reoperative surgery after open and laparoscopic abdominal operations

Petachia Reissman, Yair Edden

INTRODUCTION

The use of laparoscopic techniques for reoperation after previous abdominal surgery was, until recently, regarded as taboo. This may have been expected due to the fear of adhesions, inadvertent injury to the intestines or other adjacent organs, the expected limited exposure, and the difficulties in anatomical orientation and pathology identification. However, with increasing experience of complex, advanced procedures over the last two decades, the laparoscopic approach in reoperative surgery has gained increasing interest, and its use in a variety of acute and chronic conditions is feasible, with many advantages already apparent from primary laparoscopic procedures.

Obviously, laparoscopic procedures after previous abdominal surgery are challenging and should be practiced in high-volume centers by experienced surgeons late in their learning curve. This way, the many pitfalls may be safely handled to ensure the primary and most important goal, which is the patient's safety.

A thorough evaluation of the patient's condition, complete and detailed information regarding their previous surgical procedures and postoperative course, careful planning of the current surgical procedure including exact port positioning and establishing of pneumoperitoneum, and a low threshold for conversion are mandatory for a successful outcome.

The following chapter outlines the general laparoscopic surgery principles of reoperative laparoscopic abdominal surgery, elective procedures including colorectal cancer, inflammatory bowel disease, recurrent intestinal obstruction, recurrent adrenal and pancreatic tumors, redo foregut surgery for recurrent hiatal hernia, recurrent reflux, and recurrent achalasia. The management of reoperation for morbid obesity is discussed in a separate chapter in this book. As for the emergency setup, conditions such as postoperative bleeding, anastomotic leakage, and perforation are discussed. Contraindications for reoperative laparoscopy are detailed and a literature review with results of the various procedures followed by references concludes this chapter.

GENERAL PRINCIPLES (OR HOW TO AVOID PITFALLS)

After the diagnostic evaluation of the patient's condition and indication for reoperation are established, the first step is to obtain complete and detailed information about their previous operations. This information, obtained from medical charts and previous operative notes should focus on the following:

- Was this was an elective or emergency procedure.
- Were there any intraoperative unexpected problems?
- Was the postoperative course uneventful?
- When was the last procedure performed?

Such information may help the surgeon decide whether this patient is a good candidate for laparoscopic reoperation or whether an open surgery is preferable. An experienced surgeon may also use such information to visualize the expected intraoperative findings and better plan the surgical strategy. A history of peritonitis, excessive bleeding, prolonged ileus, or early postoperative bowel obstruction in the previous operation may indicate the presence of dense adhesions and limited exposure during the future planned procedure. In cases of previous intestinal or solid organ resection, anatomical orientation may be difficult and vascular anatomical changes have to be considered in the planning of the future procedure.

In most reoperative laparoscopic procedures, the patient's position and room setup should be planned to allow maximal flexibility for the surgical team. Both arms should be tucked in and a modified lithotomy position is very helpful. In cases of pelvic surgery, preoperative introduction of ureteral stents for easier and safer identification should be practiced.

Port placement is the initial and most critical step in any procedure. Principles such as avoiding previous surgery scars including laparoscopic scars and using an open technique for the creation of pneumoperitoneum should be followed. If needed, one simple and efficient trick is 'finger adhesiolysis,' when the surgeon's finger is introduced through the first port incision for gentle adhesiolysis and creation of an initial working space prior to insufflation. Use of an angled scope, gentle atraumatic graspers, and both sharp and blunt dissection are practiced to allow the placement of additional ports under vision, gradual identification of the anatomy, and confirmation of the pathology to be addressed. After a previous midline incision, one may expect dense omental and/or intestinal adhesions to the abdominal wall along the midline scar, and therefore plan the placement of the port site to be far enough from the midline to allow for safe and convenient dissection and adhesiolysis for gaining exposure. Placement of the camera or working ports too close to the midline scar will significantly limit the ability for lysis of abdominal wall adhesions.

Whenever the exposure remains limited and the procedure is not progressing within a reasonable amount of time, switching to a hand-assisted laparoscopic surgery technique should be considered as the next step prior to conversion. This technique is based on the use of one of the surgeon's hand introduced through a special 'hand port' requiring a 7–8 cm incision, keeping the preset intra-abdominal pressure and enabling dissection, retraction, and tactile sensation.

Such a 'hand port' may also be very useful for teaching purposes with the senior and junior surgeons switching hands. The incision for this port placement is then used at the end of the procedure for specimen removal as needed. However, the most important principle when performing reoperative laparoscopic surgery is sound judgment and a low threshold for conversion to ensure the patients' safety and favorable outcome.

ELECTIVE REOPERATIVE LAPAROSCOPIC SURGERY

Inflammatory bowel disease

Reoperative laparoscopy may be used for a variety of indications in both ulcerative colitis and Crohn's disease.

Ulcerative colitis

In ulcerative colitis, the main reoperative surgical procedure is completion proctectomy with the creation of an ileoanal pouch, in patients who initially underwent subtotal or total abdominal colectomy with end ileostomy, as an emergency or urgent procedure for severe fulminant colitis. In such conditions, the patient is often in a poor general and metabolic state, on high-dose steroids and in extreme cases peritonitis may even be present. Therefore, a salvage procedure with subtotal colectomy and end ileostomy without entering the pelvis is often required as the initial step, to be followed after several months by restorative proctectomy and the creation of an ileoanal pouch. The subtotal colectomy with end ileostomy procedure can be performed laparoscopically with avoidance of any incision as the entire abdominal colon is removed through the ileostomy opening. Such technique will result in decreased abdominal adhesions. However, if laparotomy is performed, future laparoscopic surgery may be more difficult. Therefore, the feasibility of performing a laparoscopic-assisted proctectomy and ileoanal pouch depends mainly, although not solely, on the technique used for the initial surgery. Depending on the surgeon's experience, laparoscopy may be attempted in most patients with careful reference to the principles of reoperative laparoscopic surgery mentioned above. The most challenging part of this procedure is the low division of the rectum about 1 cm from the dentate line when a double-stapled pouch is performed. Several techniques and devices were suggested including the use of angled endo staplers, an assistant's fist pushing the anal canal toward the surgical instruments used for the pelvic dissection, and even an inversion of the rectum through the anal canal with extracorporeal division close to the dentate line followed by double-stapled pouch anal anastomosis when the very short rectal stump is introduced back to the pelvis with the circular stapling device. Alternatively, if a hand-sewn anastomosis is desired, the lower rectum is transanally divided via a perineal approach, and later removed through the umbilical or suprapubic incision.

The other important step is the creation of a well-vascularized tension-free 'J' pouch from the terminal ileum and the previous ileostomy. The pouch can be easily constructed extracorporeally using a midline umbilical or a suprapubic incision, which is also usually used for the extraction of the rectal stump. Special attention should be given to maximal mobilization of the meso of the terminal ileum all the way to the duodenum and pancreas, and to consider 'mesenteric windows' to ensure tension-free reach of the pouch to the anus. The pouch itself should be constructed only after its reach has been confirmed. In the rare event when the mesoileum is short and the pouch does not appear to reach the anus, an 'S' pouch should be considered, as its efferent limb usually enables a tension-free pouch anal anastomosis. Temporary ileostomy is used in most cases and may be brought out through the site of the previous stoma.

Another condition where reoperative laparoscopic surgery may be needed is in patients who suffer from acute or recurrent adhesive small bowel obstruction following total proctocolectomy with ileoanal pouch. This subject is discussed later in this chapter.

Crohn's disease

One of the most frustrating findings in Crohn's disease is the high recurrence rate despite the many advances in medical treatment and surgical techniques. Hence, one of the surgical principles in primary as well as in reoperative surgery for Crohn's disease must be bowel sparing. Resection margins are defined by the macroscopic appearance only and not histology, and strictureplasty is often used in short strictures. Surgically challenging findings in recurrent Crohn's disease include various fistulae formation (enteroenteric, enterocutaneic, enterovesicle, enterovaginal, etc.) or an inflammatory mass involving several intestinal loops. Another problem is the often poor condition of the patients referred for surgery only after exhausting all medical options. Therefore, whenever reoperation (open or laparoscopic) is considered, the timing and preparation are of utmost importance to ensure a successful outcome. Patients with acute conditions such as abdominal collection, fistulae or an inflammatory mass should be 'cooled down' by using a combination of antibiotics, drainage [using computed tomography (CT) or ultrasound guidedtechniques], and elemental enteral nutrition for a period of several weeks at least. Total parenteral nutrition is rarely used in these patients due to the many formulae of elemental diet currently available. The reduction in the size of the inflammatory mass and in the extent of peri-intestinal inflammation will enable the surgeon to spare any normal 'innocent bystander' intestine, which may look inflamed because of its proximity to the diseased intestine, and after waiting until the end of the 'cooling down' period, such secondary inflammatory changes will often resolve in any case. In stricturing disease, when chronic obstruction is present with massive dilatation and wall thickening of the intestine proximal to the stricture, the use of elemental nutrition will result in a gradual decrease in bowel diameter and wall thickness, thus allowing for a safer anastomosis.

Periodic physical examination and laboratory tests, including albumin levels, weight measurements, and imaging studies [mainly magnetic resonance enterography (MRE) or ultrasound] following a collection, are used to determine the optimal timing for surgery. Colonoscopy is always mandatory to evaluate the previous anastomosis or any colonic disease. In addition, detailed information of the previous surgical procedure, including the extent and location of previous resection, is crucial before planning the reoperative intervention.

Of several anticipated technical difficulties in reoperative laparoscopic procedures for Crohn's disease, regaining the anatomical orientation may be the most difficult of all, especially in patients who have had more than one previous open resection. Fistulae formation commonly causes changes in the anatomical position of the intestine. After the initial obstacle of insufflation is overcome, tedious and time-consuming adhesiolysis should be expected. Such adhesions, including pelvic adhesions of the intestine to the female genitalia, may result not only from the previous operations but also from the inflammation and fistulae formation of the primary disease.

The initial step in Crohn's disease surgery is to fully inspect the small intestine before the planned procedure is carried out. It is not unusual for additional disease not seen on preoperative imaging to be found. Inspection may be safely performed by using gentle graspers running segment-by-segment, starting at the ligament of Treitz and moveing toward the ileum until the pathology is encountered. The use of clips or sutures applied to the mesentery at the site to be addressed will facilitate the later identification of this segment. Minor Crohn's disease intestinal changes should be documented but not surgically addressed.

Occasionally, fistulae connections may prevent exposure and intestinal assessment. In such cases, the fistula tract should be divided to regain anatomical orientation without the fear of bowel content spillage due to the patient's mechanical bowel preparation as well as the elemental nutrition often resulting in partial or complete obliteration of the fistula tract. However, if required, suture closing of the fistula opening may be used prior to the dissection and mobilization of the intestine. Another issue in Crohn's disease surgery is the presence of a short and very thick mesentery of the affected intestine, which requires the use of endovascular stapling rather than ordinary division and clipping or suturing techniques. Oversuturing of the stapling line for hemostasis is often required and recommended.

If multiple resections are needed, each segment is exteriorized sequentially through a small umbilical or suprapubic incision. The anastomosis following resection may be carried out extra- or intracorporeally. Strictureplasty may also be performed, but due to the multiple suturing required, an extracorporeal technique is preferred. As mentioned previously, a hand-assisted technique may facilitate dissection and definition of the pathology. In patients who have undergone multiple previous laparotomies, an initial short incision for adhesiolysis and then used for the insertion of the 'hand port' may be very useful. Unlike strictures in other portions of the intestine, where strictureplasty may be considered, anastomotic stricture recurrence always requires resection.

As the current surgical procedure may not be the last, it is mandatory to document the findings and the exact procedure performed. The inclusion of a schematic drawing in the operative report may be very helpful for future reference. Although challenging, and with many technical difficulties, the outcome for Crohn's disease patients who have a successful reoperative laparoscopic procedure is good. It is our experience that in 80% of patients with recurrent Crohn's disease, laparoscopic surgery can be safely performed (**Figures 7.1** and **7.2**).

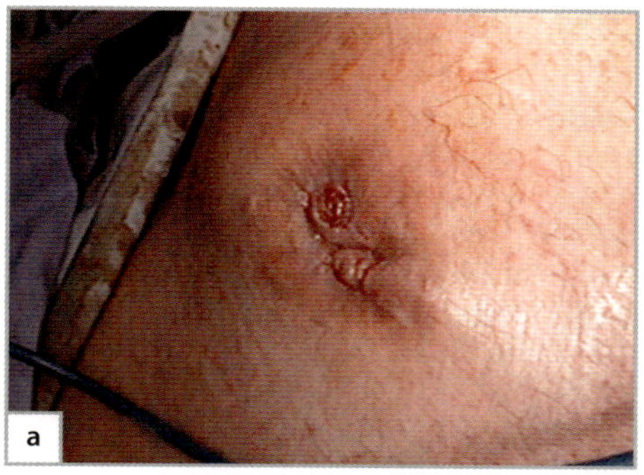

a

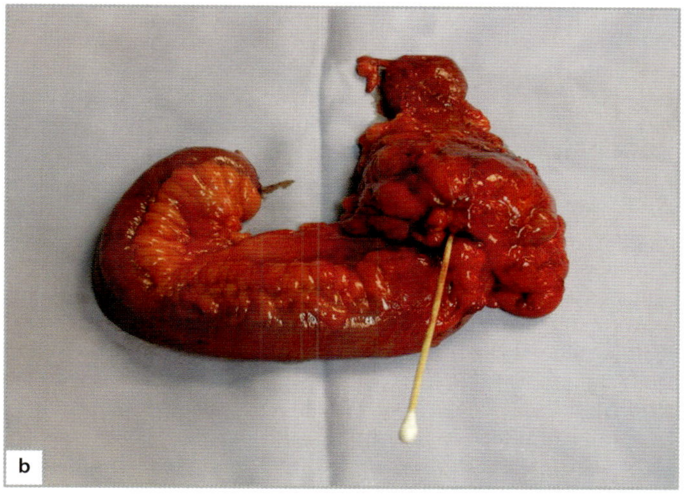

b

Figure 7.2
Enterocutaneic fistula after appendectomy. (a) View of the patient's abdomen with the fistula draining opening. (b) The specimen of terminal ileum and cecum with demonstration of the fistula opening.

Recurrent colon and rectal cancer

Laparoscopic surgery for recurrent colon cancer involves some special and unique considerations, which make it different from the surgery used to treat other benign colorectal disorders. The first and most important is the oncological safety of the procedure and the manda-

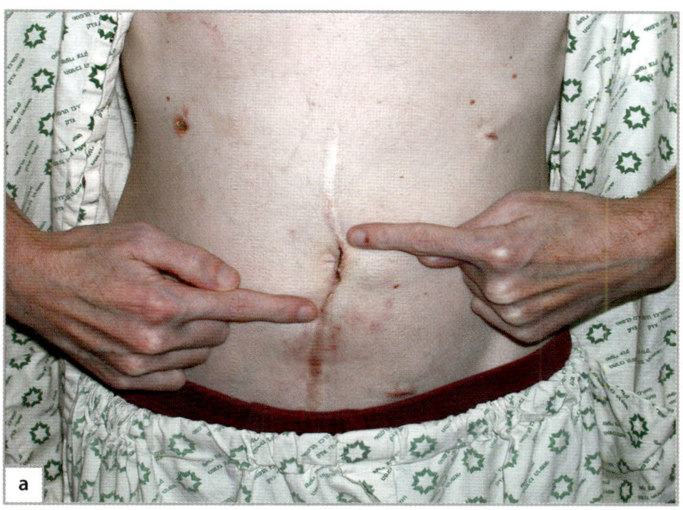

a

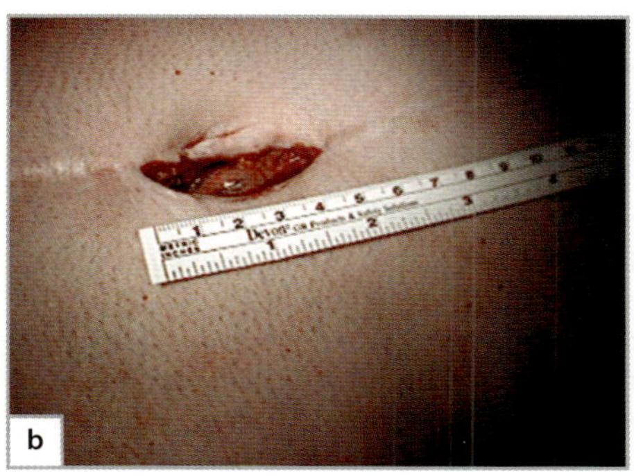

b

Figure 7.1
Reoperative ileocolic resection for recurrent Crohn's disease. (a) Note the current incision marked by the patient's fingers on the background of the previous midline scar used for open resection. Also, note the three port sites used: two in the upper abdomen and one in the left lower quadrant, which was the first port introduced using open technique. (b) The current umbilical incision for specimen extraction and extracorporeal anastomosis was made longitudinal and not transverse due to the previous scar.

tory principles of surgical oncology that must be followed. The current reoperative procedure will be based on the following factors:

- The exact previous procedure.
- The location of the recurrent tumor.
- Is this a potentially curative or purely palliative procedure?
- The patient's condition and comorbidity.

Such information will dictate the type of procedure required, ranging from extended/subtotal colectomy, through segmental colectomy, anterior or abdominoperineal rectal resection, to the performance of a palliation only such as a stoma or bypass. One of the major concerns is the alteration in vascular anatomy due to the previous resection, which has to be taken into account when additional resection and anastomosis is planned, to avoid the dire consequences of bowel ischemia and anastomotic leak. Laparoscopy may also be used initially as a diagnostic/staging step. Occasionally, peritoneal metastatic spread may not be detected on preoperative imaging, but may be encountered only during the laparoscopic exploration itself, and thus require a change in the surgical strategy.

In any event of previous left colectomy, sigmoidectomy, or anterior resection, the use of ureteral stents is highly recommended. In recurrent rectal cancer, a laparoscopic abdominoperineal resection is usually performed. Pelvic adhesions and fibrosis should be expected, with alterations in the normal rectal anatomy. Rigid intraoperative rectoscopy for better outlining the distal rectum and manual retraction of the posterior vaginal wall off the rectum are both helpful maneuvers. The laparoscopic pelvic dissection should be carried out to the level of the levators or beyond, to enable easier transperineal extraction of the specimen. The oncological principles of total mesorectal excision, nerve sparing, and radial margins should be strictly followed. Reoperative rectal resection is one of the most challenging and demanding procedures in colorectal surgery when performed in the open fashion, let alone when performed laparoscopically. Therefore, such an attempt should be made only late in the surgeon's 'learning curve', after they have gained wide experience in laparoscopic pelvic surgery and even then, a high conversion rate should be expected.

These are the reasons why some practitioners feel that reoperative laparoscopic resection of recurrent colon and rectal cancer should be further investigated before its safety and outcome can be established. In cases of pelvic recurrence, when pelvic exenteration is considered, the role of laparoscopy is limited due to the extent of the procedure. However, it may — and indeed should — be used as an initial staging procedure, after peritoneal adhesiolysis is completed and exposure of the peritoneal cavity is achieved, to exclude the presence of extrapelvic disease. The latter prohibits the performance of the planned major procedure, and leads to stoma creation as a palliation instead. This approach may avoid unnecessary laparotomy, similar to the widely accepted use of initial laparoscopy prior to any planned gastric or pancreatic surgery.

Laparoscopic reversal of Hartmann's procedure

Since it was originally described in 1921, Hartmann's procedure has been modified to include various procedures, which all result in either an end colostomy or ileostomy and a distal rectal or colonic stump. However, the majority of these procedures are performed as emergencies or urgent cases, and the role of laparoscopy may therefore be limited. Conversely, the laparoscopic reversal of Hartmann's procedure may have much wider applications.

The reversal procedure is always elective after the patient is thoroughly investigated and well prepared. Although technically challenging, laparoscopic reversal of Hartmann's procedure has proven to be feasible and safe. The results of this procedure have shown morbidity and mortality rates comparable to those of open procedures with the benefits of decreased postoperative pain, shorter duration of ileus and hospitalization, an earlier return to normal activity, and enhanced cosmesis.

When Hartmann's procedure was originally introduced, reversal with closure of the stoma at a later time was not considered. Since then, the majority of patients who undergo Hartmann's procedure are reoperated upon for reversal and establishment of intestinal continuity. The only patients who retain a permanent stoma are those with unresectable extensive malignancy, those with fecal incontinence who are not candidates for sphincter reconstruction, those with intractable irradiation or Crohn's proctitis, and debilitated patients who are in a generally poor condition. The optimal timing for stoma closure is controversial and varies from patient to patient: a period of 3–6 months is usually recommended but should be extended according to the patient's condition. Thorough investigations of both the rectal stump and the proximal colon are mandatory before reversal is considered.

These investigations aim to exclude any previously undiagnosed pathology such as concomitant malignancy, new pathology such as stricture formation, or residual pathology such as diverticulosis or inflammation. Care should be taken not to be misled by diversion colitis, which resolves after intestinal continuity has been re-established. These investigations should be performed by either endoscopic or contrast studies. Standard mechanical bowel preparation is undertaken prior to the reversal, including phosphate enemas of the rectal stump. The patient is placed in the modified lithotomy position. The legs are almost flat to avoid interference with the laparoscopic instruments during surgery. This position is important for several reasons:

- It enables the transanal introduction of a circular stapler.
- It provides the option for intraoperative rectoscopy.
- The rectoscope may also be used for identification and retraction of the rectal stump, which may be buried in the pelvis, thereby facilitating the dissection.
- If required, another assistant or the camera holder may be placed between the legs.

Intraoperative ureteral stent insertion is extremely helpful. The initial step is to dissect the stoma free of the abdominal wall using an ordinary surgical technique. Subsequently, any adhesions in the proximity of the fascia are lysed under direct vision to ensure a free space before the introduction of the laparoscope. After sufficient mobilization of the stoma is achieved, the segment of the stoma is resected and the anvil of a 29- or 33-mm circular stapler device is introduced and a purse string suture placed.

Subsequently, the proximal colon containing the anvil is placed into the abdominal cavity. Several fascial sutures are placed, but not tied. A 10–12 mm trocar is introduced through the incision, and some of the fascial sutures are tied to prevent CO_2 leak. The peritoneal cavity is now insufflated. As in any other laparoscopic procedure, the abdominal cavity and pelvis are inspected. Adhesions from the previous procedure are frequently present and should be carefully lysed using blunt and sharp dissection. At least three additional 10– 12-mm ports are placed under laparoscopic visualization. After adequate exposure is achieved by lysis of adhesions and retracting the small bowel out of the pelvis, attention is paid to both the proximal colon and the rectal stump. The proximal colon is inspected for sufficient mobilization to provide a tension-free anastomosis. Additional mobilization is frequently required by incising the lateral peritoneal attachments, including mobilization of the splenic flexure or left transverse colon.

Another resection may be required according to the preoperative or intraoperative findings.

The rectal stump must be clearly identified and freed from adhesions to other organs. Rigid rectoscopy may be performed to facilitate the rectal stump dissection. This step may be easier if the rectal stump is tagged by a long, non-absorbable stitch during the initial Hartmann's procedure. After both the rectal stump and the proximal colon are cleared and confirmed for a safe, well-vascularized and tension-free anastomosis, the anvil is grasped with a clamp, which is introduced through a right port. The circular stapler is introduced transanally and laparoscopically guided to reach the end of the rectal stump at the previous staple line. Occasionally, the upper edge of the rectal stump is contracted and deformed requiring resection with an angled endostapling device introduced through one of the 12-mm ports. In cases of a short rectal stump in women, special attention must be paid to prevent injury to the posterior vaginal wall. The skin at the colostomy site is left open. In the unique case of a long distal colonic stump (left or transverse) with a proximal end ileostomy or colostomy, a laparoscopic-assisted reversal procedure may be performed, with the anastomosis performed extracorporeally after the two ends (stoma and distal colon) have been mobilized and brought out of the abdominal wall through an incision. This incision may be carried out in continuity with the stoma incision or in a remote area, according to the anatomical findings.

Laparoscopic management of recurrent small bowel obstruction and abdominal adhesions

Intestinal or intra-abdominal adhesions are most commonly caused by previous abdominal surgery, although other rare causes include primary peritonitis or congenital conditions. Adhesions are the leading cause of chronic recurrent or acute intestinal obstruction. Previous abdominal surgery and suspected intestinal adhesions, along with dilated bowel, were initially considered a contraindication for laparoscopy due to the risk of bowel injury and limited visualization. However, both increased surgical experience and improved surgical instrumentation have led to a change, and bowel obstruction is now included as a potential indication for laparoscopic surgery.

Laparoscopic adhesiolysis is often performed as the initial step in patients who undergo a planned elective laparoscopic procedure after previous open or laparoscopic abdominal and pelvic operations. Less commonly, it is performed for recurrent small bowel obstruction as an elective or semielective procedure. It may also be a potential treatment for abdominal and pelvic pain when adhesions are suspected after other causes have been ruled out. Interestingly, there is a rich gynecologic literature concerning this issue in women after gynecologic procedures.

The indications for laparoscopic adhesiolysis include patients who have had previous abdominal surgery and present with transient recurrent episodes or an acute progressive onset of intestinal obstruction. Laparoscopic management of acute bowel obstruction is discussed later in this.

In chronic recurrent intestinal obstruction, when an elective or semielective procedure is planned, a thorough gastrointestinal (GI) evaluation should precede any planned intervention. MRE and CT enterography are currently the most common imaging studies used for surgical planning. Studies such as single or double balloon enteroscopy and video capsule endoscopy are relatively contraindicated unless a primary small bowel disorder is suspected.

As in other reoperative procedures, detailed information regarding the previous operation and postoperative course is crucial. Multiple laparotomies, previous pelvic sepsis, irradiation (no matter how long ago), leak, or postoperative hemorrhage are all risk factors for multiple dense adhesions and increased technical difficulty, whereas a single previous laparotomy with an uneventful recovery and with anticipation of a single band as a cause of the recurrent obstruction makes such a patient a much better candidate for laparoscopic adhesiolysis.

The preparation of the patient and creation of pneumoperitoneum are similar to the aforementioned principles of reoperative laparoscopy. Once the initial port and scope are placed, gradual insertion of additional ports is carried out while sharp lysis of adhesions is performed. Since no specimen is anticipated, 5-mm camera and ports may be used. Frequent repositioning of the camera and instruments through different ports is usually required when adhesions of omentum and bowel to the abdominal wall are divided. External manual compression of the abdominal wall will often allow the adhesions to be delivered into the operative field without requiring an additional port. Once the abdominal wall is free of adhesions, careful inspection of the bowel is undertaken. A two-hand (hand-over-hand) technique is used to perform the inspection, with an atraumatic bowel clamp, and frequent shifting of the operating table position according to the area inspected is very useful. Interloop adhesions are sharply divided as needed. Obviously, once surgery is performed, although the 'critical zone' may be clearly identified, any additional adhesions that may be a potential cause of future obstruction should be divided.

If a conglomerate of bowel is captured between a network of adhesive bands, careful, sharp dissection of the adhesions should be performed until the bowel is completely mobilized. Alternatively, a small midline incision may be used for exteriorizing this conglomerate and adhesiolysis performed extracorporeally.

After full enterolysis, care must be taken to carefully reinspect the entire small bowel. Individual areas, especially those sites from which adhesions were divided, must be inspected. Any questionable areas of seromyotomy and certainly any enterotomies should be repaired, preferably with intracorporeal sutures. Any persistent doubts warrant extracorporeal inspection. If a loop of bowel needs to be resected, the general principles of laparoscopic colorectal surgery should be applied. Careful selection of patients with recurrent small-bowel obstruction for laparoscopic adhesiolysis, along with a low threshold for conversion even by experienced surgeons, will ensure a safe outcome.

Recurrent adrenal tumors

Laparoscopic adrenalectomy for primary adrenal tumors has become the preferred standard of care since the mid-1990s, and there is no doubt that this is one of the procedures in which the advantages of laparoscopy as compared with open adrenalectomy are most impressive. However, in recurrent adrenal tumors the role of reoperation by laparoscopy has been debated due to the expected adhesions and the critical anatomic adherence of the recurrent adrenal mass to the adjacent major vessels such as the renal vein and artery, inferior vena cava (IVC), aorta, and to adjacent organs such as the liver, kidney, spleen, or pancreas, depending on the side. Occasionally, the recurrent mass may extend into adjacent retroperitoneal spaces such as the para-aortic and retrocaval space.

The etiology of recurrent adrenal tumors includes incomplete primary resection, the histology of the primary tumor (i.e. pheochromocytoma, adrenocortical carcinoma), and the underlying disorder (e.g.multiple endocrine neoplasia (MEN) type II, familial pheochromocytoma, and von Hippel–Lindau syndrome). Tumor recurrence may also be seen following cortical sparing adrenalectomy performed during bilateral adrenalectomy to avoid lifelong corticosteroid replacement therapy. Therefore, although previously more commonly practiced, the popularity of cortical sparing adrenalectomy has decreased due to the major technical difficulties encountered during redo adrenalectomy.

Another critical issue in laparoscopic adrenal surgery concerns the treatment of suspected adrenocortical carcinoma during redo adrenalectomy. Any violation of surgical oncology principles, such as inappropriate margins, inadequate lymph node dissection, or spillage of neoplastic cells during the initial operation, will shortly result in local recurrence and may remove at a stroke the patient's only chance for a cure.

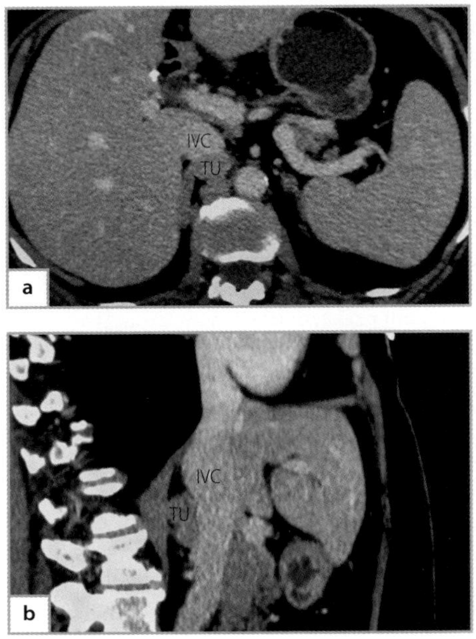

Figure 7.3 Retrocaval recurrence of a right adrenal pheochromocytoma. (a) Computed tomographic scan showing the relation of the tumor to the IVC and aorta. (b) Lateral view, the tumor (TU) is located between the IVC and the diaphragmatic crura.

Before attempting laparoscopic reoperation of an adrenal mass, it is of utmost importance to enrol a multidisciplinary team and to carefully plan the surgical strategy with 'bail out' options, as the margin for error is extremely narrow in these cases. A complete endocrine and biochemical workup is the first step, and medical control of blood pressure is essential in all patients with pheochromocytoma. It is important to keep in mind, however, that some of these tumors are intermittently secreting, and the fact that there is no increase in urine or serum catecholamines does not exclude the presence of such a tumor, which may cause excessive alterations in pulse rate and blood pressure during the operation. Anesthetic evaluation and preparation are therefore extremely important.

Imaging studies including high-resolution CT, CT angiography, and MRI are essential for planning the surgery to be undertaken. Formal angiography is rarely required due to the high resolution of the above studies and the currently available three-dimensional reconstruction software, which give the surgeon a clear anatomical view of the tumor and its relation to adjacent vessels and organs. In cases of MEN type II or von Hippel–Lindau syndrome, the recently introduced somatostatin receptor scintigraphy – PET – Gallium 68 DOTATOC scan is used to exclude systemic spread. Occasional partial resection of an adjacent solid organ may be needed and planned in collaboration with liver surgeons and urologists if, for instance, partial nephrectomy is considered. Similarly, for retrocaval or para-aortic masses, a vascular surgeon with experience of of grafting or reconstruction should be involved.

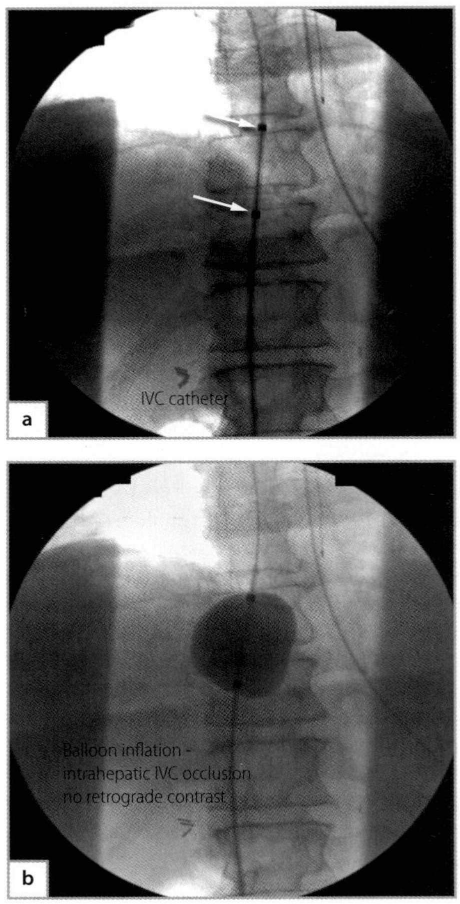

Figure 7.4 IVC balloon catheter inserted by fluoroscopy in the operating room. (a) The two small black markers on the catheter (arrows) show the balloon margins. Of note are the metal clips from the previous laparoscopic adrenalectomy seen in the right lower part of the picture. (b) The balloon is inflated and injection of contrast material through it shows no retrograde flow indicating complete occlusion of the IVC.

In left adrenal mass recurrence, due to the close proximity to the pancreas tail and possible difficulty in anatomical orientation, intraoperative laparoscopic ultrasound should be used for outlining the tumor margins and dissection plains. Unlike relatively small primary adrenal tumors, where the surgical approach may be retroperitoneal or posterior for recurrent adrenal lesions, only a transabdominal approach is used as it provides the best exposure and vascular control of major vessels. The patient is placed in the lateral position and the skin is marked for possible subcostal or thoracoabdominal incision. Such marking, along with the preparation of the nursing staff and room setting for quick conversion, may save precious time.

In the unique setup of retrocaval recurrence of a right adrenal mass (**Figure 7.3**), the major concern is control of the vena cava while dissecting the mass, and since proximal control at the level of the intrahepatic vena cava is virtually impossible, it is the authors' practice in such cases, prior to the operation, to introduce a trans-femoral balloon catheter to the IVC at a level just inferior to the hepatic veins. This catheter which is introduced by an invasive radiologist under fluoroscopy in the operating room is kept in place throughout the procedure, to be used in case of vena cava laceration when immediate proximal control should be gained (**Figure 7.4**). The exact volume of the balloon inflation required to completely occlude the retrograde flow of the IVC is measured, and a syringe containing this volume is kept connected for easy access and instant use during the operation. If bleeding occurs, this catheter may also be used as a high flow venous access for rapid transfusion or even used by the level one rapid transfusion system.

Regardless of the exact tumor location, a mandatory step during the dissection of the recurrent adrenal mass will be vascular isolation of the right renal vein, left renal vein at its origin from the IVC, and the infrarenal IVC. Vesseloops are used to encircle these vessels and thereby gain distal control if needed. When attempting such a highly challenging and complicated procedure, the surgeon should have a broad experience in laparoscopic adrenalectomy, master intracorporeal suturing, and be familiar with using laparoscopic vascular clamps and laparoscopic 'Bulldog' clamps requiring a specially designed laparoscopic introducer For the dissection, various sharp and blunt techniques with instruments of various energy sources may be used according to the intraoperative findings and surgeon›s preference. However, one of the most efficient hemostatic tools is the laparoscopic argon beam coagulator, which is used to gain hemostasis of raw surfaces such as the liver and retroperitoneum (**Figure 7.5**).

As in other complex procedures, only careful and detailed preoperative evaluation and planning with collaboration of multidisciplinary experts will ensure a favorable outcome. It is imperative that the surgeon should use sound judgment, and if surgical oncology principles cannot be strictly maintained by the laparoscopic technique, a controlled and safe conversion to an open procedure should take place.

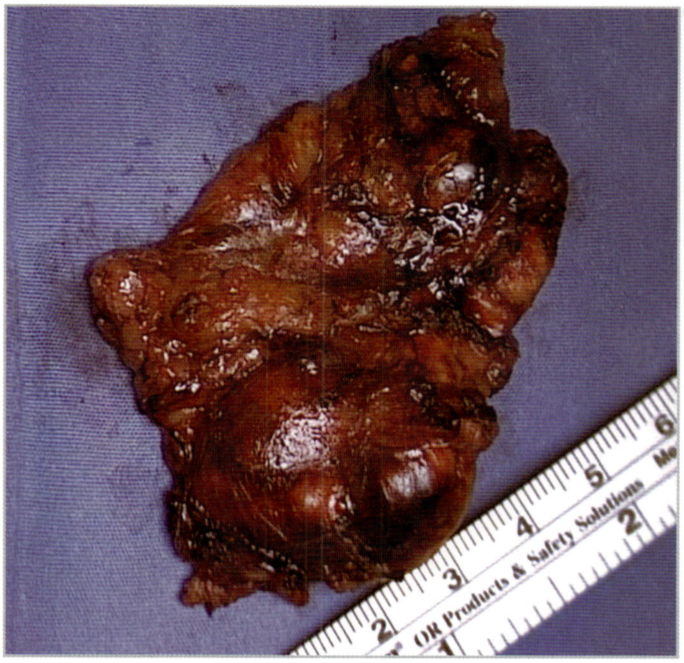

Figure 7.5 The complete resected specimen.

Recurrent pancreatic neuroendocrine tumors

Laparoscopic reoperation of pancreatic tumors may be considered in patients with a recurrent neuroendocrine tumor (NET) after a previous open or laparoscopic enucleation or partial pancreatectomy has been performed. This may be seen sporadically in MEN type I and in patients with von Hippel–Lindau syndrome. The commonly slow growing nature of these tumors along with their relatively low malignant potential probably makes them an indication for pancreatic reoperation. Therefore, all patients who undergo a primary resection of a pancreatic NET should be periodically followed-up to rule out recurrence.

Once recurrency is diagnosed, thorough investigations for systemic versus local recurrence should be carried out, and a multidisciplinary discussion with endocrinologists specializing in NET, radiologists, and pathologists should be undertaken before the optimal therapeutic approach is determined. Surgery remains the only curative treatment for these tumors, if complete resection is feasible (**Figure 7.6**). In specific cases, preoperative treatment with a somatostatin analog, or alternatively, protein receptor radiotherapy using radioactive labeled somatostatin, for downsizing tumors of borderline resectability is practiced.

As in other reoperative laparoscopic procedures, the current procedure can be planned only after gaining detailed information regarding the previous operation, and recent imaging including endoscopic ultrasound (EUS) has been performed. Currently, in experienced hands, EUS may provide the most accurate information regarding the size, anatomic relation (including vascular involvement), and histology, with determination of the proliferation index of the tumor cells.

The current procedure should be planned according to the following criteria:

- Tumor size, given the fact that tumors above 2 cm in diameter bear a higher risk of malignancy and therefore require a more radical procedure such as formal distal pancreatectomy or pancreaticoduodenectomy, rather than a local excision or enucleation.
- Involvement of major vessels such as the splenic, superior mesenteric, and portal vein and superior mesenteric artery. Of note, however, is the fact that these tumors are usually 'vessel respecting,' and true encasement of major vessels is rare.
- The anatomical changes due to the previous operation, with special attention whether total pancreatectomy is required (resulting in the severe consequences of insulin-dependent diabetes) or whether pancreatic sparing can be achieved with suspected endocrine function of the remaining pancreas even if the exocrine function is lost.

Of the different reoperative laparoscopic pancreas resection procedures, obviously, the relatively easier one is enucleation or limited resection of a small tumor with benign features in patients who have also previously had an enucleation or a limited resection. One of the current debates among endocrinologists concerns observation of small NET versus resection. Concern is based on recent reports of up to 7% incidence of malignancy even in tumors <1 cm in size. However, if a previous formal resection was performed, and the current tumor is large, a completion total pancreatectomy may be needed. Regardless of the previous procedure, obliteration of the lesser sac with adhesions of the stomach and transverse colon should be expected and carefully lysed. A full exposure of the pancreas is required with mobilization of the retroperitoneal attachments to allow for a complete inspection. For recurrent large tumors, special consideration should be given to the use of a hand port and hand-assisted technique, as this may facilitate the retraction and dissection.

One of the crucial modalities for any laparoscopic pancreas surgery is laparoscopic ultrasound, which is used intraoperatively to identify small intraparenchymal tumors, assess their resectability, and their relation to the major regional vessels and the pancreatic duct. Rarely, intraoperative ultrasound may detect an additional small tumor that was missed on the preoperative imaging studies. The laparoscopic ultrasound probe is introduced through a 10-mm port, and its flexible tip enables easy and complete scanning of the gland. Several laparoscopic ultrasound instruments are currently available: some are equipped with a working channel for intraoperative needle biopsy of an unclear mass, and some instruments even have software that provides a three-dimensional picture of the scanned organ. Color Doppler sonography is used to differentiate between vessels, common

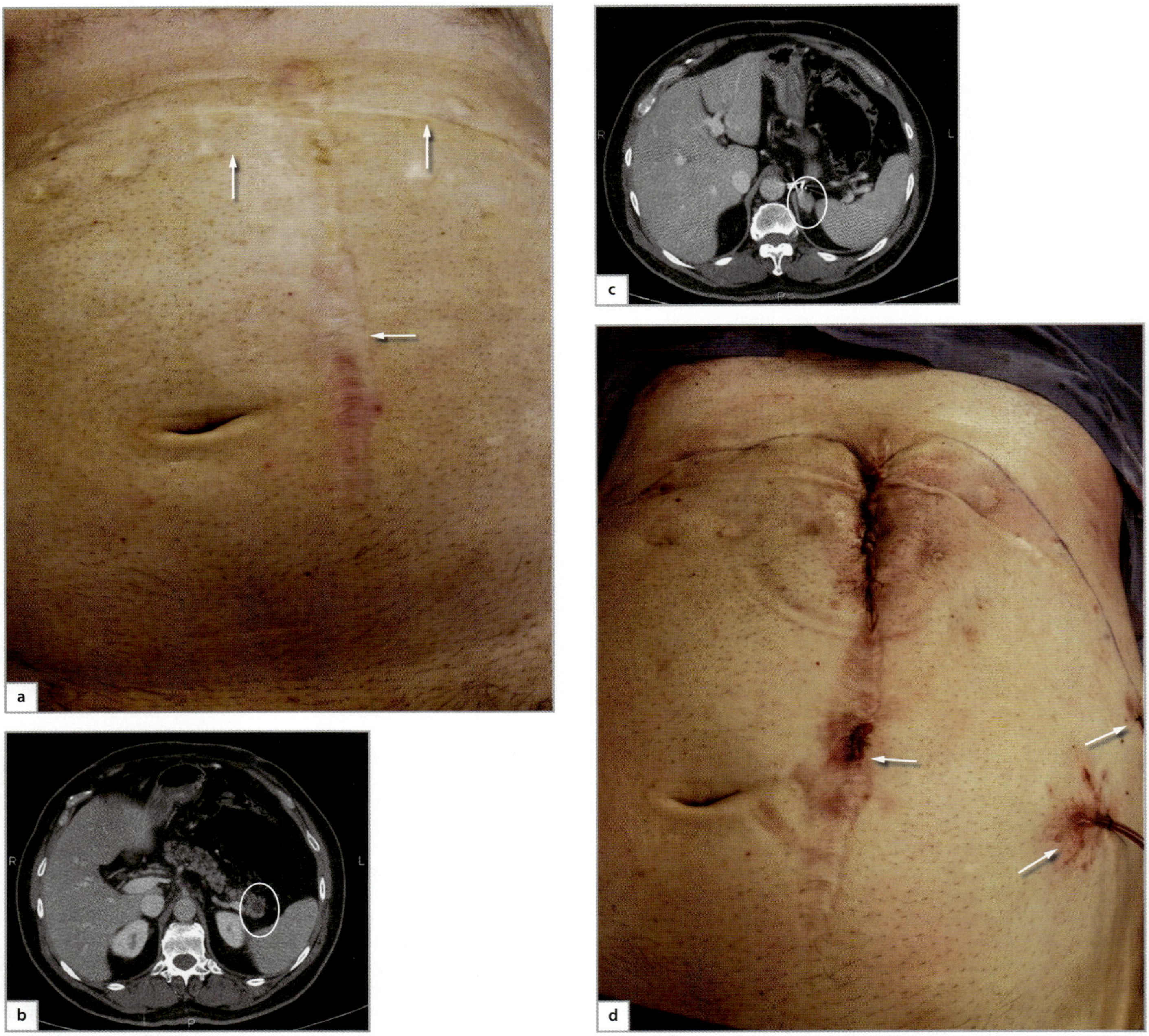

Figure 7.6 A 54-year-old patient with von Hippel–Lindau syndrome who had over the last 30 years three laparotomies for right open adrenalectomy, left open adrenalectomy, and laparotomy for bowel obstruction. (a) Two Chevron scars and one left paramedian scar can be seen (arrows). Due to elevated urine catecholamines, computed tomographic scan was obtained (b,c) showing recurrent left adrenal mass and a neuroendocrine tumor in the tail of the pancreas, both confirmed by endoscopic ultrasound and iodine-131-meta-iodobenzylguanidine (MIBG) scan. Note the pancreatic tail tumor and the recurrent left adrenal tumor next to metal clips from the previous open adrenalectomy. The patient underwent a laparoscopic hand-assisted distal pancreatectomy with spleen preservation and left readrenalectomy. Postoperative course was uneventful and he was discharged after 5 days. (d) The upper abdominal incision of 7.5 cm is seen with additional three port sites (arrows). The lower left one was used for drain placement.

duct, and pancreatic duct. The ultrasound view is shown on the major screen used by the principal surgeon (as a split screen), thus avoiding the need to use additional screens outside of the surgeon's visual field. If enucleation is planned, ultrasound is repeatedly used while the dissection is carried out to ensure that complete excision is performed, and injury to adjacent vessels and the pancreatic duct is avoided. If formal resection is planned, the ultrasound is used to determine that the resection margins are in a safe distance from the tumor.

Various energy sources can be used for hemostatic parenchymal dissection. Argon beam coagulation, biological glue, or other hemostatic agents may be used. If formal resection is performed, the division of the pancreas is usually performed by using a vascular endostapling device, with oversuturing of the stapled line with a nonabsorbable suture in an attempt to reduce the chance of pancreatic leakage and fistula formation.

Unfortunately, as in open pancreatic surgery, pancreatic leak with fistula formation or pancreatic collection is still one of the major morbidities associated with laparoscopic pancreatectomy. Its incidence ranges from 20 - 40%, with a higher incidence noted after enucleation compared with formal resection.

Therefore, soft closed suction drains should always be placed to control postoperative pancreatic fistula and to reduce the incidence of collection. Occasionally, such a drain may be kept in place for several weeks until a low output of 10–20 mL over 24 hours is confirmed. Various modalities, including the use of glue, postoperative somatostatin administration, preoperative pancreatic duct stenting, and the use of coated endo-staplers, still did not resolve this problem.

Reoperative laparoscopic foregut surgery

Antireflux procedure

Although many patients with gastroesophageal reflux disease (GERD) can be treated medically and recently endoscopically, laparoscopic antireflux surgery is still one of the most common laparoscopic foregut procedures performed. The most common procedure is a Nissen fundoplication with a floppy 360° wrap and crural repair. Indications for reoperative intervention include recurrence of reflux symptoms or dysphagia.

Recurrent reflux may occur in <10% of patients due to intrathoracic migration of the fundoplication, or slippage of the wrap toward the stomach. If such a condition is suspected, evaluation with endoscopy, contrast study, and 24-hour pH monitoring should be obtained. Laparoscopic management consists of mobilization of the stomach, which is commonly adhered to the left lobe of the liver, exposing the esophagogastric (EG) junction, taking down the previous wrap and performing a new but still loose fundoplication, preferably with one stitch going through the anterior muscular wall of the esophagus, closing the crura securely. In the authors' opinion, adding two fixating sutures on each side of the fundus wrap between the wrap and the crura is recommended. This should be performed over a 52–56 French bougie to avoid narrowing of the EG junction and postoperative dysphagia. To facilitate the identification of the esophagus during the dissection in the hiatus and lower mediastinum, a bougie (available in an illuminated version) or intraoperative endoscopy may be used. If esophageal or gastric integrity after this procedure is in doubt, air inflation and/or methylene blue saline injection to fill the distal esophagus and stomach should be carried out. In case of a defect being noted, laparoscopic repair using interrupted sutures with special attention for mucosal closure is performed. If possible, the wrap should cover the suture line. A nasogastric tube should be kept in place for 5–7 days and removed only after water-soluble contrast study showed complete healing.

The other most common indication for reoperation after a laparoscopic antireflux procedure is persistent dysphagia related to too tight a fundoplication, too tight a crural repair, or previously undetected achalasia. Dysphagia in the early postoperative period is commonly treated by endoscopic dilatation. However, if the problem persists for a long period of time and is not responding to endoscopic treatment, redo surgery should be considered. After defining the exact cause of dysphagia by performing contrast studies and manometry, appropriate treatment can be planned.

If achalasia is detected, laparoscopic transabdominal myotomy is performed, and partial or no fundoplication should be considered according to the intraoperative findings and the surgeon's preference. If the problem was too tight of a wrap or crural closure, these should be re-established ensuring the looseness of the wrap and the crura closed over the bougie, and allowing some additional space.

Recurrent hiatal hernia

The recurrence rate of laparoscopic as well as open hiatal hernia repair is relatively high and may range from 20 to 40%. Therefore, different techniques for the repair, including the use of felts, or absorbable and nonabsorbable mesh for the crural approximation were suggested.

Symptom recurrence, along with endoscopic and imaging findings, will confirm the diagnosis, which is always related to the failure of crural closure. However, it is important to realize that many recurrences are minor, with only a very small portion of the stomach migrated into the mediastinum, causing minor symptoms and not requiring any repeated surgical intervention. In cases of significant anatomical and symptomatic recurrence, surgical intervention is unavoidable, with several technical options depending on the patient's general condition, age, and anatomy.

In younger patients, a complete repair is warranted, following the same principles described for reoperative antireflux surgery, with the exception of clear evaluation of the length of the esophagus in order to be prepared for an esophageal elongation procedure if needed. After the repair is completed, fundoplication and anterior wall suture gastropexy are recommended to enhance gastric adherence to the upper abdominal wall and reduce the incidence of recurrent hernia. Conversely, when recurrence occurs in elderly or poor-risk patients, a minimal procedure such as laparoscopic gastrostomy with fixation of the stomach to the abdominal wall using a tube gastrostomy should be performed without any attempt at hiatal closure. The gastrostomy tube should be left in place for several months at least to ensure gastric fixation. Another advantage of this procedure is the potential use of this tube for enteral nutrition in debilitated patients. In addition, such a minor procedure may be performed under regional anesthesia, avoiding the consequences of general anesthesia in these patients.

As in many other surgical problems, prevention is easier than treating the complications, and although it is not within the scope of this chapter, mention should be made that during the initial repair of a hiatal hernia, all possible measures to prevent recurrence should be taken. This includes performing a fundoplication, suturing the wrap to the crura, performing an anterior gastric wall suture gastropexy or tube gastrostomy, and finally performing an esophageal elongation procedure if a short esophagus is encountered.

Recurrent achalasia

As in many other GI procedures, laparoscopic Heller's myotomy with or without an antireflux procedure became the standard of care for patients requiring surgical intervention for achalasia. The term 'recurrence' is not always accurate when dealing with achalasia, as the cause of persistent symptoms is often incomplete myotomy during the initial procedure. In addition to insufficient myotomy, other potential causes include esophageal stricture and a secondary motility disorder that may require a very long myotomy initially.

Evaluation of persistent or recurrent symptoms should again include all of the studies performed during the initial evaluation, including endoscopy, contrast studies, and manometry. The surgeon and the interventional gastroenterologist should discuss each case and decide collaboratively upon the preferred and safest approach. Medical treatment, balloon dilatation, or botulinum toxin injection should be considered, based on the patient's symptoms and general condition before surgery is pursued.

If the need for repeated myotomy is established, careful planning of the new myotomy site is mandatory, as adhesions to the mucosa at the previous site may lead to mucosal laceration if dissection is attempted. Therefore, it is recommended to expose the left side of the esophageal wall and perform a new myotomy in a 'virgin' zone. If transabdominal exposure of the esophagus is not feasible due to adhesions or is insufficient for performing the desired procedure, one should be prepared for left thoracoscopy and exposure of the lower esophagus via the left thorax, thus enabling the performance of a long myotomy at a previously untouched portion of the esophagus. Alternatively, many practitioners suggest an initial left thoracoscopic approach for recurrent achalasia, thereby dodging the expected adhesions and technical difficulties of a repeated abdominal approach. Such an approach does not usually require an antireflux procedure. In the extremely unusual event of the need for a very long myotomy, the right thorax should be used for access to the entire length of the thoracic esophagus. Intraoperative endoscopy is very helpful in determining the true anatomical EG junction, to outline the extent of the myotomy and, by air insufflation while the surgeon is irrigating the myotomized segment, to ensure mucosal integrity. Water-soluble contrast study is always performed on the first postoperative day, and if normal, a clear liquid diet is started. Reoperative laparoscopic surgery after morbid obesity operations are discussed in a separate chapter.

EMERGENCY REOPERATIVE LAPAROSCOPIC SURGERY

Reoperative laparoscopy in the emergency setting has a broad spectrum of indications after both open and laparoscopic abdominal procedures. These include diagnostic indications when other commonly used diagnostic tests fail to reveal the cause of the patient's condition deterioration, and as a result the appropriate treatment is unclear. Conditions such as anastomotic leakage following colorectal procedures, covered or obscure perforation following foregut procedures, and inadvertent bowel injury during any abdominal procedure may occasionally present with minor or unclear symptoms, and routine contrast studies (mainly CT) may fail to demonstrate the pathology. Diagnostic laparoscopy under such circumstances has the highest accuracy and can often be used not only as a diagnostic tool, but also as a therapeutic tool when peritoneal and pelvic irrigation, anastomotic or hollow viscus repair, or diverting stoma is warranted. Peritoneal cavity irrigation including the pelvis and subphrenic spaces can be efficiently performed with placement of drains under direct vision. If esophageal or gastric perforation is encountered in the early postoperative period, primary repair, irrigation, and drainage of the mediastinum and creation of gastrostomy and feeding jejunostomy may be all performed by laparoscopy, and relaparotomy thus avoided. If desired (although of limited benefit), cervical esophageal diversion may be added. In experienced hands, the laparoscopic technique can often achieve the same surgical results as a formal laparotomy. Obviously, if the extent of dissection, exposure, and surgical goals cannot be fully obtained by laparoscopy, conversion to a formal laparotomy should be promptly performed.

Moreover, it is the common practice of many surgeons to take the patient back to the operating room for a diagnostic/therapeutic laparoscopy rather than to perform a time-consuming contrast-enhanced abdominal CT in the event of any adverse postoperative course. In many acute surgical conditions diagnosed during the postoperative course (after either open or laparoscopic procedures), such as bleeding, inadvertent injury of an adjacent organ, abdominal abscess in a location inaccessible to CT or ultrasound-guided percutaneous drainage, or early bowel obstruction, laparoscopy may be used for definite treatment as mentioned above. Compared with laparotomy, the clear vision, scope placement flexibility, and exposure of the entire peritoneal cavity may be superior and allow for better decision-making when laparoscopy is practiced.

Postoperative bleeding in the abdominal cavity may be related to failure of major mesenteric vessels during the initial procedure, inadvertent solid organ injury, such as the spleen, during left colectomy or foregut surgery, bleeding from retroperitoneal vascular bed, or rarely due to laceration of one of the abdominal wall vessels during trocar placement. In the majority of these conditions, provided the patient is stable, laparoscopy may be an excellent tool for the evacuation of abdominal cavity blood and clots followed by diagnosing and controlling the source of bleeding using clips, sutures, vascular staples, or hemostatic agents as required.

In any laparoscopic intervention during the early postoperative period, following open and obviously laparoscopic surgery, adhesions are usually not a prohibiting factor for performing the planned procedure as they are filmy and not yet dense. Obviously, in cases of severe abdominal distension, hemodynamic instability or coagulopathy, time-consuming laparoscopy should not be considered, and prompt laparotomy should be carried out instead. A more detailed discussion of the contraindications for reoperative laparoscopy appears later in this chapter.

Adhesive acute small bowel obstruction

The criteria for laparoscopic surgical treatment of an acute intestinal obstruction are identical to the indications for laparotomy and include failure of conservative treatment with increasing pain, progressive dilatation of bowel loops on repeated radiographs, leukocytosis, fever, or the development of localized tenderness with localized peritoneal signs.

Laparoscopy in the setting of an acute bowel obstruction may pose certain hazards to the patient. The dilated bowel increases the risk of bowel injury at any entry site, especially at the first entry port. Manipulation of thin-walled friable bowel may cause bowel perforation and spillage of large amounts of contaminated bowel content into the abdominal cavity, and manipulation of gangrenous bowel without rapid vascular control may lead to endotoxic sepsis. These problems can be limited by the use of the open technique for the first trocar insertion, by handling the bowel loops gently with specifically designed atraumatic instruments and by frequent changes in the table's position using gravity to facilitate exposure.

Once the scope is in the peritoneal cavity, an initial general inspection is performed to detect any obvious bowel ischemia or gangrene, perforation, or fecal content in the peritoneal cavity, all of which require prompt laparotomy. This should also be the case if the distended bowel loops appear massively dilated, very thin-walled, friable, and difficult to safely manipulate. As described in the section discussing laparoscopic adhesiolysis for recurrent bowel obstruction, additional ports are placed while adhesions to the abdominal wall are lysed. Once adequate exposure of the peritoneal cavity is achieved, the small bowel loops are carefully inspected in a retrograde fashion, starting at the ileocecal valve where the intestines are normal and collapsed, and moving proximally toward the dilated loops in an attempt to reach the transition zone and obstruction often caused by a single dense fibrotic band or as an internal hernia with one or more loops involved. If intestinal viability is in doubt after its release, warm saline may be applied with observation until it regains color and peristalsis. Once the transition zone is reached and the cause of obstruction eliminated, further inspection of the proximally dilated loops is contraindicated due to the risk of bowel perforation. If, however, a conglomerate of multiple loops surrounded by a net of dense adhesions is found, either laparotomy or exteriorization through a limited incision should be carried out. In addition to the expected short-term benefits of the laparoscopic management of acute bowel obstruction, it seems that the laparoscopic technique may have a significant long-term effect of reduced reformation of abdominal adhesions when compared with conventional laparotomy.

Although it is not within the scope of this chapter, the authors would like to mention the use of laparoscopy in the management of acute small bowel obstruction without any previous laparotomy, not related to colonic pathology, when preoperative imaging did not reveal the cause of obstruction. Laparoscopy under such conditions may easily reveal the cause of obstruction, such as a primary small bowel or mesenteric mass, internal hernia including paraduodenal, Winslow foramen and right gutter, adhesive band, short segment Crohn's disease, bezoar, or a functional diffuse dilatation of the small intestine without any mechanical obstruction. Laparoscopy may be efficiently used for the definitive treatment of the underlying cause with the many known advantages of minimally invasive surgery.

CONTRAINDICATIONS FOR REOPERATIVE ABDOMINAL LAPAROSCOPY

The historical contraindications such as previous laparotomy, bowel obstruction, or even peritonitis and hollow viscus perforation are no longer valid as more experience has been gained and major laparoscopic procedures are routinely and successfully performed in patients who have undergone previous open and laparoscopic abdominal surgery. However, although this chapter outlined some of the common indications for reoperative laparoscopy, there are also some absolute and relative contraindications to be considered, all based on common sense and sound judgment.

Hemodynamic instability due to postoperative bleeding or severe sepsis is the first and most important contraindication for laparoscopy. This is due to the time-consuming laparoscopic technique and to the expected deterioration of the patient, when the intra-abdominal pressure is increased during the creation of pneumoperitoneum. The increased intra-abdominal pressure reduces the venous return from the lower part of the body and may lead to reduced cardiac output. The reduction in mesenteric and splanchnic blood flow may also have hazardous consequences, as demonstrated in several animal studies. Another absolute contraindication is coagulopathy in a patient requiring an emergency intervention. The expected obscured surgical field and uncontrolled bleeding should lead to formal laparotomy.

Other relative contraindications include (a) multiple laparotomies performed for peritonitis and abdominal sepsis or multiple bowel resections due to the expected multiple dense adhesions with distorted anatomy, and (b) large/complex postoperative ventral hernia involving most of the abdominal wall, when significant portions of the intestine are located in the hernia sac and and are irreducible. Such conditions will not permit abdominal insufflation and creation of pneumoperitoneum will be impossible. However, depending on the currently planned procedure, the surgeon's experience and level of comfort in performing reoperative abdominal laparoscopy, and most importantly, a low threshold for conversion, laparoscopy may be attempted.

RESULTS OF REOPERATIVE LAPAROSCOPIC SURGERY FOLLOWING LAPAROSCOPIC AND OPEN ABDOMINAL OPERATIONS

A laparoscopic approach following previous surgery was originally considered a complete contraindication (Partensky 1992). However, as surgeons increased their experience and strengthened their confidence in the minimally invasive approach, it became evident that re-entering the abdominal cavity exercising this approach was comparable and even superior to open surgery (Awais et al. 2011, Canin-Endres et al. 1999, Edden et al. 2008, James et al. 2012, Pointner et al. 1999).

Reoperative laparoscopic surgery is used for most parts of the GI tract, such as foregut antireflux and achalasia procedures, morbid obesity, recurrent colorectal cancer, inflammatory bowel disease, and intestinal obstruction (Reissman et al. 1995, Reissman et al. 2003, Cirocchi et al. 2010). It is successfully applied for both benign and malignant indications and may be practiced in the immediate and in the delayed postoperative period following either laparoscopic or open procedures (Awais et al. 2011, Canin-Endres et al. 1999, Frantzides & Carlson 1997, Edden et al. 2008, James et al. 2012, McCormick & Simmang 2006, Pointner et al. 1999).

Foregut surgery has contributed a significant part of the accumulated knowledge and established pivotal experience with redo laparoscopy. One of the first series reported in 1997 described nine patients who were failed by a primary laparoscopic antireflux procedure. All patients underwent successful laparoscopic repair, and the authors concluded that reoperative laparoscopic Nissen fundoplication was both feasible and effective (Frantzides & Carlson 1997). In another study, Pointner et al. (1999) described 30 patients who underwent redo laparoscopic antireflux procedure. The authors compared two groups of patients: one group had a primary open procedure and the other had initial minimally invasive surgery. There were no significant differences between the groups, and the authors summarized that laparoscopic refundoplication was a feasible and effective procedure with excellent postoperative results, independent of whether the primary procedure was done by the open or laparoscopic technique (Pointner et al. 1999). Recently, an outcome analysis of 275 patients with a failed antireflux procedure was published. In that series, there was no perioperative mortality, and the quality of life, based on a validated score, was excellent to satisfactory in over 85% of the patients. The authors concluded that redo antireflux surgery could be performed safely in experienced centers and that minimally invasive, complex redo esophageal antireflux procedures were safe, with good results (Awais et al. 2011).

A similar perspective is held toward redo Heller's myotomy for recurrent achalasia, as it was demonstrated by James et al. (2012) in a meta-analysis of seven studies reporting outcomes in 54 patients. Once again, their conclusion was that laparoscopic reoperation for recurrent achalasia was feasible and safe, with complication rates comparable with the primary laparoscopic operation (James et al. 2012).

Crohn's disease, due to its recurrent pattern and the frequent necessity for reoperations over the patient's lifetime combined with the benign basic pathology, has motivated many surgeons to attempt minimally invasive surgery in redo cases. One of the first reports by Canin-Endres et al. was published in 1999. The authors described laparoscopic experience with intestinal resections for Crohn's disease in 88 patients. One of the subsets of patients included 28 cases of secondary or tertiary ileocolic resection. All procedures were performed and concluded laparoscopically with results comparable with open surgery (Canin-Endres et al. 1999). Another series, from the same institution, of 168 patients included 34 patients who had a previous ileocolic resection. The conversion rate to laparotomy in patients who underwent laparoscopic redo as secondary or even tertiary resection was not statistically different from the conversion rate in patients who underwent primary laparoscopic surgery (Edden et al. 2008).

As may be expected, results of reoperative laparoscopy are variable. McCormick and Simmang (2006) reviewed different indications for reoperation following minimally invasive surgery. In this review, the authors discussed acute indications for surgical intervention such as bowel obstruction or anastomotic leak as well as delayed procedures for Crohn's disease or staged surgery for ulcerative colitis. They concluded that laparoscopic reoperative surgery was feasible for the treatment of many complications following laparoscopic major abdominal surgery and bowel resection. However, concerning cancer recurrence, based on limited literature and their personal experience, the authors commented that most recurrent colorectal carcinomas were not amenable to a laparoscopic approach regardless of the initial approach (McCormick & Simmang 2006).

SUMMARY

Reoperative laparoscopy after previous open and laparoscopic abdominal surgery may be safely used for a broad spectrum of elective and emergency conditions outlined in this chapter. Its role is still not ascertained, however, in recurrent colorectal cancer, and further investigation is needed.

Whenever reoperative laparoscopy is planned, the importance of careful patient selection, gaining detailed information regarding the previous procedures and the postoperative course, thorough evaluation of the current condition, careful planning of the operative strategy in collaboration with multidisciplinary specialists, large experience in advanced and complex laparoscopic procedures, adherence to sound surgical, oncological, and laparoscopic principles, and above all, keeping the patient's safety as the primary goal at all times, cannot be overemphasized. Only strict fulfillment of all of these principles will be key to a successful outcome.

REFERENCES

Awais O, Luketich JD, Schuchert MJ, et al. Reoperative antireflux surgery for failed fundoplication: an analysis of outcomes in 275 patients. Ann Thorac Surg 2011; 92:1083–1089; discussion 1089–1090.

Canin-Endres J, Salky B, Gattorno F, Edye M. Laparoscopically assisted intestinal resection in 88 patients with Crohn's disease. Surg Endosc 1999; 13:595–599.

Cirocchi R, Abraha I, Farinella E, Montedori A, Sciannameo F. Laparoscopic versus open surgery in small bowel obstruction. Cochrane Database Syst Rev 2010; 1469–493.

Edden Y, Ciardullo J, Sherafgan K, et al. Laparoscopic-assisted ileocolic resection for Crohn's disease. JSLS 2008; 12:139–142.

Frantzides CT, Carlson MA. Laparoscopic redo Nissen fundoplication. J Laparoendosc Adv Surg Tech A 1997; 7:235–239.

James DR, Purkayastha S, Aziz O, et al. The feasibility, safety and outcomes of laparoscopic re-operation for achalasia. Minim Invasive Ther Allied Technol 2012; 21:161–167.

McCormick JT, Simmang CL. Reoperation following minimally invasive surgery: are the "rules" different? Clin Colon Rectal Surg 2006; 19:217–222.

Partensky C. Indications for classical surgery and celiosurgery evaluation. Rev Prat 1992; 42:1509–1515.

Pointner R, Bammer T, Then P, Kamolz T. Laparoscopic refundoplications after failed antireflux surgery. Am J Surg 1999; 178:541–544.

Reissman P, Spira RM. Laparoscopy for adhesions. Serninars in laparoscopic surgery 2003; 10:185–190.

Reissman P, Wexner SD. Laparoscopic Hartmann's and Hartmann's reversal procedures. In: Phillips EH, Rosenthal R (eds), Operative strategies in laparoscopic surgery. New York: Springer Verlag, 1995:251–257.

Chapter 8 Resuscitation and intervention for postoperative hemorrhage after abdominal surgery

Ronald V. Maier, Scott C. Brakenridge

INTRODUCTION

The most important complication that should be on the mind of the surgeon in the immediate postoperative period following any abdominal procedure is the possibility of postoperative hemorrhage. From the onset of surgical training, a high index of suspicion for postoperative bleeding is engrained into the surgeon's mindset, no matter how minor the procedure. Bleeding after any surgical procedure, even with apparent technical perfection, is undeniably due to the surgeon's act of operative intervention. It is therefore incumbent upon the operating surgeon to remain actively involved in the ongoing postoperative care, be able to recognize the clinical signs of postoperative bleeding, and quickly determine its etiology so that resuscitation and subsequent intervention for hemorrhage control can be initiated in a timely fashion. The diagnostic and management decision algorithms for postoperative bleeding after abdominal surgery can be complex depending on the situation and require thoughtful but expedient deliberation. This chapter focuses on the prompt clinical diagnosis and treatment of postoperative abdominal hemorrhage.

INITIAL DIAGNOSIS OF POSTOPERATIVE HEMORRHAGE

Patient history

A thorough knowledge of the patient's history, including details of the procedure just completed in the operating room, is required to help guide the physician caring for the surgical patient in the immediate postoperative period (**Table 8.1**). This information includes technical difficulties encountered during the procedure, significant intraoperative hemorrhage, any abnormal coagulation test results, and the requirement for transfusion of blood products in the operating room. Although this information would seem obvious to the operative surgeon, one must remember that the care of the postoperative patient is often shared with surgical intensivists, anesthesiologists, or resident trainees who may not have been present in the operating room during the procedure. This is especially true in academic training institutions where trainee work hour restrictions can lead to frequent patient handoffs and transitions of care. In these circumstances, it is incumbent upon the operating surgeon to clearly communicate the relevant details of the operative procedure to the other members of the multidisciplinary care team. It must not be forgotten that this includes the patient's bedside nurse, as this key member of the patient care team is most often the provider that first detects clinical findings suggestive of postoperative hemorrhage.

Apart from the details of the operation, a thorough knowledge of the patient's underlying medical comorbidities is key to elucidating the differential diagnosis of a postoperative patient with signs concerning hemorrhage. Every surgical patient should have a complete and adequately documented preoperative history and physical placed in the medical record and available for review by all providers. In addition to the surgical history and active medical problems, the operating surgeon should document any history of coagulation disorders, recent or current administration of anticoagulants or antiplatelet agents, and any history of bleeding complications with previous operations. It should be remembered that a surgeon's preoperative assessment is useless if it is not adequately documented, is illegible, or is not interpretable by other providers. This history may provide critical assistance in narrowing the differential diagnosis when the patient's postoperative clinical status changes. For example, myocardial infarction may present with similar clinical findings to hemorrhagic shock in the immediate postoperative period in a patient with known cardiac atherosclerotic disease. Findings of postoperative tachycardia may not be due to hypovolemia from blood loss, but rather a failure to continue perioperative beta-blockade, because the patient's medication profile

Table 8.1 Perioperative information

Patient comorbidities	Cardiovascular disease
	Pulmonary disease
	Renal disease
	Previous surgical procedures
	Hereditary bleeding disorders
	History of bleeding complications with surgery
Preoperative medications	Oral anticoagulants (warfarin, dabigatran, rivaroxaban)
	Antiplatelet agents (aspirin, clopidogrel, dipyridamole)
	Beta-blockers
	Chronic analgesic/narcotic use
	HMG-CoA reductase inhibitors (statins)
Operative procedure	Details of operative procedure
	Technical difficulties
	Significant intraoperative hemorrhage
	Blood product transfusions
	Vasopressor requirements
	Oxygenation/ventilation difficulties
	Use of systemic anticoagulation
	Intraoperative coagulation test abnormalities

was not adequately reviewed. In addition, several studies in surgical and trauma patients have shown that appropriate continuation of baseline medications (i.e. statins) postoperatively is associated with improved outcomes (Gomez Sandoval et al. 2011, Le Manach et al. 2007). This suggests that it is important to restore the patient's physiologic homeostasis, which is affected by chronic medications, as soon as possible after surgery. Overall, it must be remembered that a complete knowledge of the patient's medical, operative, and medication history is required to be able to correctly, and expediently, diagnose postoperative hemorrhage as the cause of clinical deterioration in the surgical patient.

Clinical signs

Abnormal clinical findings are usually the first sign of ongoing hemorrhage in the immediate postoperative period (**Table 8.2**). Occasionally, findings such as blood-soaked surgical dressings, the rapid development of abdominal distention, or continuous sanguineous output from surgical drains quickly point to the fact that the patient has ongoing cavitary hemorrhage. In the setting of hypotension, findings such as these make the diagnosis of postoperative hemorrhagic shock obvious. However, more commonly the initial clinical findings associated with ongoing intra-abdominal bleeding are subtle. A narrowed pulse pressure (a decrease in the difference between systolic and diastolic blood pressures as diastolic pressure rises with increased adrenergic arteriolar tone) is often the first detectable clinical sign of hypovolemia secondary to hemorrhage. Persistent tachycardia and transient episodes of hypotension are often signs of ongoing hemorrhage as hypovolemia progresses beyond 30% of normal circulating blood volume. Compensatory tachycardia is common as an attempt to maintain cardiac output in the setting of decreased cardiac preload. However, shock states are often associated with decreased cardiac compliance and contractility, which lead to a decrease in stroke volume and cardiac output even when ventricular preload is adequate or 'normal.' The end-result is an overall reduction in end-organ tissue perfusion. Adequate postoperative pain control is mandatory, not only for ethically appropriate patient comfort, but also to remove pain as a background stimulus of tachycardia and hemodynamic lability.

Table 8.2 Classification and clinical signs of hypovolemic shock

Shock class	I	II	III	IV
Blood loss (cm³)	≤750	750–1500	1500–2000	≥2000
Blood loss (% volume)	≤15%	15–30%	30–40%	≥40%
Blood pressure	NL	NL	↓	↓
Pulse rate	NL	>100	>120	≥140
Pulse pressure	NL	↓	↓	↓
Capillary refill	NL	↓	↓	↓
Respiratory rate	14–20	20–30	30–40	>35
Urine output (mL/h)*	>30	20–30	5–15	Minimal
Mental status	NL	Anxious	Confused	Lethargic

Advanced Trauma Life Support for Doctors. Student Course Manual, 8th Edition. American College of Surgeons, Chicago, 2008.

*Approximately 80-kg person; cm³, cubic centimeters; h, hour; NL, normal.

Other systemic mechanisms for compensation of hypovolemic shock include adrenal release of vasoconstrictive catecholamines and activation of the renin-angiotensin-aldosterone system. The resulting rise in systemic vascular tone preferentially affects splanchnic and renal vascular beds to preserve cerebral perfusion. A decrease in the quantity of urine output is one of the first signs of end-organ dysfunction secondary to hypovolemia, although this often requires several hours to trend and identify. The attempt by the kidneys to maintain circulating volume at the expense of urine excretion and metabolic toxin clearance should actually be considered acute 'renal success' rather than renal failure. However, if a hypovolemic state is not promptly treated, acute tubular necrosis will develop and true physiologic renal failure will subsequently follow. Complete cessation of UOP and an acute decrease in mental status are late signs of hemorrhagic shock, indicative of critical end-organ dysfunction, and require immediate resuscitative intervention.

INITIAL DIAGNOSTIC EVALUATION AND RESUSCITATION

Initial evaluation and therapy

Occasionally, bedside evaluation of the postoperative patient will reveal obvious signs of significant hemorrhage and clinical instability that should trigger immediate mobilization of operative resources and a return to the operating room. More commonly, there will be subtle clinical signs suggestive of ongoing bleeding that must be further investigated before committing a return to the operating room or other invasive interventions such as angiographic embolization. When a hypovolemic state secondary to postoperative hemorrhage is suspected, the patient should be examined by the treating physician at the bedside and an initial fluid bolus of 1–2 L of crystalloid solution should be administered. The focused physical examination should look for obvious signs of hemorrhage, and a cardiopulmonary examination to rule out tension pneumothorax. A chest radiograph and electrocardiogram and cardiac enzymes should be ordered immediately. Lactated ringers solution is generally preferred over normal saline to avoid the hyperchloremic metabolic acidosis associated with large volume saline administration. A rapid and sustained improvement in vital signs and/or urine output with initial fluid bolus may suggest that the patient's hypovolemia was secondary to inadequate intraoperative volume resuscitation required to compensate for interstitial 'third-spacing' and intravascular fluid shifts. However, a transient or complete lack of response to fluid challenge should immediately increase the index of suspicion for ongoing hemorrhage and warrant further timely investigation and consideration for either immediate return to the operating room or transfer to the intensive care unit for increased monitoring and higher level of care. Non-hemorrhagic causes of circulatory shock should be considered based on the patient's history, operative procedure, and clinical picture and expediently ruled out. These include cardiogenic, obstructive, distributive, and endocrine etiologies (**Table 8.3**). Initial laboratory testing should include a complete cell count, serum chemistry, cardiac enzymes, and a full coagulation panel, including prothrombin (PT/INR), activated partial thromboplastin time (aPTT), and fibrinogen levels.

If ongoing hemorrhage is suspected, adequate intravenous access should be assured with preference for two large bore (≥18 gauge) peripheral venous catheters. In addition to peripheral access, consideration may be given for placement of a central venous catheter.

Central venous catheters offer the benefit of central access for drug administration as well as central venous pressure (CVP) measurement. While only a crude surrogate for intravascular volume status, a measured CVP of <5 mmHg is highly supportive of decreased intravascular volume. It should be remembered that standard multilumen central venous catheters usually have small gauge channels (18–23 gauge), which when combined with long catheter lengths lead to high flow resistances and are not conducive to rapid volume infusion. If the need for rapid, large volume resuscitation is anticipated, placement of a large caliber percutaneous introducer sheath into a central vein should be considered. Internal jugular or subclavian vein access is preferred; however, femoral venous access is acceptable and easily obtained in emergent circumstances. Following stabilization and control of hemorrhage, alternative access should be obtained and femoral venous introducers and/or catheters should be removed as soon as possible as they are associated with increased incidence of deep venous thrombosis and catheter-based bloodstream infections (Hamilton & Foxcroft 2007, Parienti et al. 2012). Invasive hemodynamic monitoring should also be considered, including a peripheral arterial catheter for real-time blood pressure monitoring. In addition to providing more accurate and continuous hemodynamic information, arterial lines are a convenient access for serial laboratory blood drawing and arterial blood gas samples to monitor adequacy of ventilation and resolution of any base deficit with resuscitation.

Figure 8.3 Etiologies of shock states in the postoperative patient

Shock classification	Etiology	Evaluation
Hypovolemic	Hemorrhage, third-space volume shifts, inadequate intraoperative resuscitation	Physical examination, fluid volume challenge, CVP, echocardiography, evaluate potential sources of bleeding
Cardiogenic	Myocardial infarction, acute congestive heart failure, cardiac arrhythmias	Physical examination, electrocardiogram, serum cardiac enzymes, CVP, echocardiography
Obstructive	Tension pneumothorax, pulmonary embolus, pericardial tamponade	Physical examination, CVP, CXR, CT angiography, echocardiology
Distributive	Sepsis, anaphylaxis	Physical examination, CVP, fluid volume challenge, vasopressor test dose, CXR blood/urine cultures, evaluate sources of infection
Endocrine	Adrenal insufficiency	Patient history, empiric corticosteroid administration, basal and ACTH-stimulated serum cortisol levels.

ACTH, adrenocorticotrophic hormone (cosyntropin); CT, computed tomography; CVP, central venous pressure; CXR, chest radiograph.

Resuscitation for hemorrhagic shock

If the clinical response to crystalloid infusion is transient, hemoglobin (Hgb) or hematocrit (Hct) levels have decreased significantly, and ongoing bleeding is strongly suspected, and the prompt administration of blood products is initiated. Continued infusion of isotonic crystalloid solution until 'salt water drowning' occurs is not the goal of resuscitation. It should be remembered that in the early phases of acute hemorrhage, Hgb and Hct levels may not decrease until intravascular volume has been repleted with crystalloid solution or enough time has transpired for compensatory fluid shifts from the interstitium. Early administration of two units of cross-matched packed red blood cells (PRBCs) is preferred. However, type O negative units may be administered if no cross-match is available and the patient's clinical status is rapidly deteriorating. If initial laboratory results suggest the presence of a significant coagulopathy, this may be a cause of nonsurgical bleeding and should be rapidly treated with appropriate blood component therapy (**Table 8.4**). Fresh frozen plasma (FFP) may be administered to treat increased PT/INR and aPTT values. Platelet levels <50,000/mm^3 should be treated with pooled platelet concentrates. In addition, fibrinogen levels <5.6 mmol/L (100 mg/dL) should be treated with cryoprecipitate.

Table 8.4 Blood component therapy in surgical/traumatic bleeding and coagulopathy

Component	Approximate dose volume (mL)	Coagulation constituents	Indication
Packed red blood cells (pRBC)	300–350	RBCs	Acute blood loss, anemia (Hgb<7, Hct<21), MTP
Fresh frozen plasma (FFP)	200–250	Factors II, V, VII, IX, X, XI; fibrinogen	Active bleeding and increase in PT/PTT >3x normal, INR >1.6, MTP
Cryoprecipitate	90–150 (15 mL/unit)	Fibrinogen, von Willebrand factor (vWF), factor VIII, factor XIII, fibronectin	Hypofibrinogenemia (<100 mg/dL), MTP
Platelet	200–400 (60 mL/unit)	Platelets	Thrombocytopenia (Plt <50,000/mm3), MTP
PCC (3-factor)	20–60 (25U/kg)	Factors II, IX, X	Warfarin-associated coagulopathy
rVIIa	<10 (90 mg/kg)	Factor VII	Hemophilia A- or B-associated bleeding, massive hemorrhage*, MTP

Adapted from Puget Sound Blood Center guidelines, www.pbsc.org.

PCC, prothrombin complex concentrate; rVIIa, recombinant activated factor VII; MTP, massive transfusion protocol.

*Recombinant activated VIIa use for nonhemophilia-associated massive hemorrhage is for compassionate and investigational use on an institutional basis in the USA.

Thromboelastography (TEG, Haemonetics Corporation, Braintree, MA, USA) has shown promise in guiding component therapy for postoperative and traumatic coagulopathy (Kashuk et al. 2010). Although the concept of TEG to describe the functionality of the clotting cascade was first described in the 1940s, its utility as a practical clinical tool is only recently being realized. A whole blood sample is placed into a heated (37°C) specimen cuvette into which a sensor piston is inserted (**Figure 8.1**). Depending on the type of system, the cuvette (TEG) or piston (ROTEM, Tem Innovations GmbH, Munich) is rotated and clot strength is transmitted to the sensing piston via rotational forces and recorded as a time-dependent tracing. Significantly, TEG is the only single test able to describe the functionality of the entire thrombotic cascade from initial enzymatic function, through the generation of thrombin and clot formation, and finally fibrinolysis. This allows targeted therapy with blood products to treat specific abnormalities within the coagulation cascade. The development of rapid TEG (rTEG) now allows point-of-care testing in the emergency department, operating room, or intensive care unit, with results available within minutes. However, there remain limitations to the routine clinical utilization of TEG. These include the fact that accurate interpretation of TEG waveform tracings is user dependent, training provider and additional logistics are required, and the availability of TEG hardware for routine clinical use is still not widespread.

If there is ongoing clinical instability and evidence of major ongoing blood loss, early activation of a massive transfusion protocol (MTP) should occur, if available. MTPs have been widely incorporated in both military and civilian trauma centers (Cotton et al. 2009). It is becoming more common for MTPs to also be utilized in situations outside of traumatic injury such as operative cardiac and obstetric hemorrhage. In situations where transfusion of large volumes of blood products is required, the use of these protocols ensures that appropriate ratios of blood product components are systematically administered to prevent increased dilution of coagulation factors required for adequate hemostasis. Several recent studies from both military and civilian trauma populations suggest that MTPs utilizing blood component resuscitation in ratios approaching that of whole blood best prevent the development of coagulopathy, decrease overall resuscitation requirements, and have been shown to be associated with improved survival (Spinella et al. 2008, Zink et al. 2009). Currently, the administration of PRBC, FFP, and platelets in ratios approaching 1:1:1 (one unit PRBC, one Unit FFP, one 6-pack pooled platelets) is advocated. However, the optimal ratio of blood products administered in MTPs is controversial and remains an active area of prospective investigation. In addition, other coagulation adjuncts such as tranexamic acid (TXA) and active recombinant factor VII (rVIIa) are often included in MTPs. TXA is a low-cost, synthetic inhibitor of plasminogen activation and excessive fibrinolysis. A recent large multinational, randomized controlled trial showed that TXA administration to trauma patients at risk of significant hemorrhage within 8 hours of injury showed a modest but statistically significant decrease in all-cause and hemorrhage-related mortality (CRASH-2 Trial Collaborators 2010.). The results of several randomized controlled trials regarding the safety and efficacy of rVIIa in the setting of massive transfusion have been mixed (Neal et al. 1960). However, in select patients it appears to improve control of severe coagulopathy. Its use remains controversial given the high cost and concern for thrombotic complications. Currently, the use of rVIIa for hemorrhage is approved for investigational and compassionate use only in the United States on an institution-specific basis.

Although restoration of adequate circulating volume is key to survival of patients in hemorrhagic shock, overresuscitation can also be detrimental to patient outcomes. During the Vietnam War, it was noted that aggressive, large volume crystalloid resuscitation for hemorrhagic shock succeeded at preventing acute renal failure secondary to hypovolemia but led to massive pulmonary edema. Initially labeled 'DaNang lung,' this entity is now known as an etiology of acute respiratory distress syndrome (ARDS). Along with the implementation of MTPs, the broader concept of 'damage control resuscitation' is now considered a key overall strategy in the resuscitation of hemorrhagic shock (Holcomb et al. 2007). This includes limiting isotonic crystalloid solution resuscitation, the early utilization of blood component volume resuscitation in ratios approaching those of whole blood, and limited or 'balanced' goal-directed volume administration. The

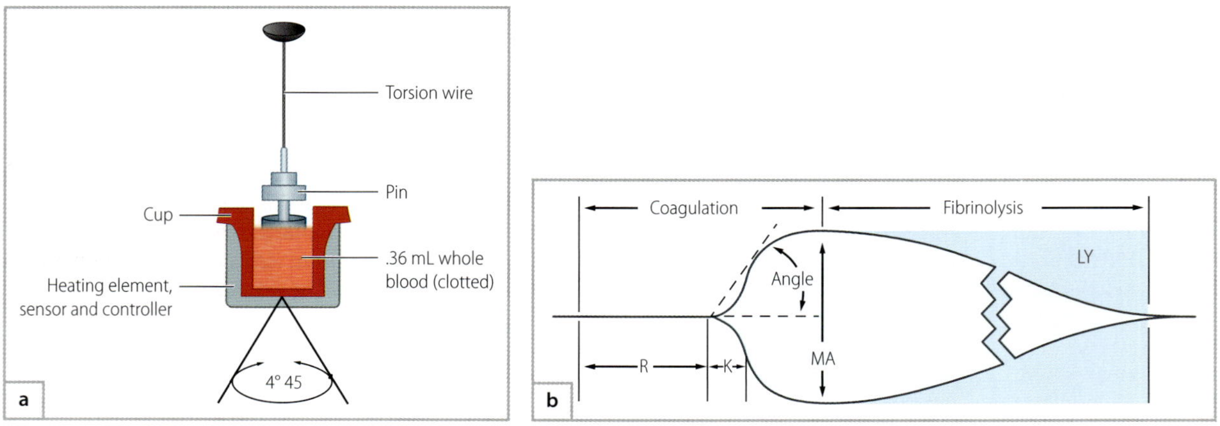

Figure 8.1 Technique of thromboelastography (TEG). (a) The TEG analyzer measures the clot's physical properties via a stationary cylindrical cup, which holds the blood sample and is oscillated through an angle of approximately 4°. A pin is suspended in the blood by a sensing torsion wire whose magnitude of motion is sensed and directly proportional to clot strength. The rotational movement of the pin is converted to an electrical signal and displayed as a hemostasis profile tracing. (b) The TEG tracing has four primary coagulation parameters (R, K, a, MA), which can be combined to yield other indices of coagulability. Reaction time (R) is the time until first detection of significant clot formation and represents the enzymatic portion of coagulation. K-time (K) and the 'angle' (a) reflect the speed of clot formation and primarily reflects fibrinogen level. Maximum amplitude (MA) is a measurement of the maximum fibrin/platelet clot strength. The clot lysis time and amplitude at 30 minutes (A30) represent fibrinolytic activity. With permission of Haemonetics Corporation, Braintree, MA, USA: TEG and Thromboelastograph are registered trademarks of Haemonetics in the United States, other countries, or both.

goal of limited resuscitation is to maintain low-normal systolic pressure (80–90 mmHg) until definitive hemorrhage control is obtained. The minimization of crystalloid administration and early utilization of blood products helps prevent the dilution of coagulation factors, reduces acute hemorrhage-related mortality, and may decrease pulmonary edema and the incidence of ARDS and multiple organ failure (Cotton et al. 2009, Holcomb et al. 2008).

Diagnostic imaging

The need for intervention to control ongoing surgical hemorrhage is usually determined by the patient's clinical status and their response to initial resuscitation. Within the first few days after surgery, if the index of suspicion is high, diagnostic confirmation and control of hemorrhage are usually best obtained simultaneously in the operating room. However, there are instances where diagnostic imaging prior to intervention may be appropriate. Confirmation and further characterization of the location of ongoing hemorrhage via intravenous contrast-enhanced computed tomography or diagnostic angiography may be preferable in circumstances where the diagnosis of hemorrhage is in question and tenuous patient physiology renders significant risk to a return to the operating room. However, remember that if the patient's life is imminently at risk of death from exsanguination, no patient is 'too sick' for an operation. The amount of time passed since the index procedure can also be an important factor in deciding whether or not to obtain diagnostic imaging prior to intervention. If >7–10 days has elapsed, intra-abdominal inflammation and the development of highly vascular adhesions can make re-entry into the abdomen a proposition not without risk. In this time period, intra-abdominal anatomy can be unclear, structures are adherent and difficult to mobilize, and inflamed, friable tissues are prone to further bleeding and injury.

Differentiating between several different potential sources of hemorrhage is another scenario where further diagnostic information prior to intervention may be prudent. For example, in the severely injured trauma patient, there can be multiple sources of hemorrhage, some of which may be difficult to control by open surgical techniques. In addition to its diagnostic utility, angiography has the additional benefit of offering the possibility of simultaneous intervention via vessel embolization. This may be of significant benefit, especially in areas where surgical control of hemorrhage may be difficult, such as the retroperitoneum, severe pelvic fractures with arterial bleeding, or areas where severe inflammation leaves tissues friable and not easily amenable to control with suture ligature. Specific scenarios where angiography and embolization are most appropriate will be discussed in the following sections.

The use of gastrointestinal (GI) endoscopy may also be an appropriate first step in certain situations and disease processes. Postoperative GI bleeding may be due to culprit lesions, which are surgery related (anastomotic line mucosal bleeding), surgery associated (anastomotic ulcer, gastric stress ulcer), or related to comorbidities (esophageal/rectal variceal bleeding) and may best be diagnostically evaluated with upper or lower endoscopy. Similar to angiography, endoscopy offers the potential of simultaneous diagnostic and therapeutic value in these situations. Endoscopy may be most helpful when there is evidence of slow but persistent GI hemorrhage. Endoscopic interventions, such as injection of submucosal epinephrine and the application of endoscopic clips, have been shown to be effective in controlling postoperative anastomotic bleeding (Mayer et al. 2004). Upper endoscopy has also become the first-line treatment of acute hemorrhage from gastric and duodenal ulcers. The endoscopic diagnosis and treatment of bleeding from a surgery-associated gastric stress ulcer may spare a patient from unnecessary reoperation. This is especially salient when there are patient comorbidities that significantly raise the perioperative risk of reoperation. For example, in a postoperative patient with significant cirrhosis and a history of previous GI hemorrhage, it would be an unfortunate and unnecessary physiologic stress to undergo reoperation for a rapidly dropping Hct and subsequently discover esophageal or hemorrhoidal variceal bleeding as the cause of postoperative hemorrhage. Conversely, there are situations where time should not be wasted on endoscopic maneuvers. Although endoscopic techniques continue to advance rapidly, most small bowel anastomotic bleeding of any significant quantity will be difficult to visualize and/or treat via this modality and, if not self-limited, will ultimately need operative revision.

INTERVENTION FOR POSTOPERATIVE HEMORRHAGE

Once initial resuscitation has begun and attempts at correcting any postoperative coagulopathy have been implemented, if it becomes apparent that there continues to be ongoing bleeding, the method and timing of intervention to control hemorrhage must quickly be determined. The choice of intervention is driven not only by the disease process and index procedure but also by the available resources and expertise of the institution. Ultimately, it is the responsibility of the operating surgeon to decide the safest and most expedient method of hemorrhage control for the patient under their care.

Reoperative surgery

A return to the operating room for direct surgical control of hemorrhage should remain the primary option on the mind of the surgeon to treat bleeding in the perioperative period. The multiple options that are available to approach hemorrhage should not distract the surgeon when direct operative control is indicated. A return to the operating room should not be avoided due to the surgeon's ego and perception of failure. A bleeding patient is never too sick for a necessary operation. Under most circumstances, mobilization of operating room resources can be performed rapidly. In many large institutions and most high-volume trauma centers, bleeding patients can be on the operating table within minutes after making the decision to operate. From a systems and logistical standpoint, the operating room also has many advantages as the primary location for the treatment of the bleeding patient. The operating room is often the best place in the hospital for the initial resuscitation of the unstable surgical patient. In the operating room, the surgeon is able to maintain leadership of the situation, operating room staff is accustomed to deal with urgent situations (specifically hemorrhage), and transfer of the patient to the operating room automatically mobilizes manpower and resources. By default, available human resources are increased by the presence of the anesthesia team, as well as circulating and scrub nurses. In addition, the blood bank usually has well-formed protocols for rapid transfer of blood products to the operating suite, and most necessary equipment, drugs, and adjuncts are present or easily obtainable by operating room staff. The presence of adequate resources to optimally 'rescue' the patient has been shown to significantly improve survival in the critically ill patient (Haupt et al. 2003).

When performing reoperative abdominal surgery for postoperative hemorrhage, the patient should be broadly prepped, preferably with topical chlorhexidine. Alternatively, an iodine-based agent may be used. Similar to a trauma laparotomy, the surgical prep should range from chin to knees to allow rapid proximal or distal exposure if necessary. The chest should always be included within the prep boundary to allow for emergent thoracotomy in case of the rare need for proximal aortic control or open-chest resuscitative cardiac compressions. Bilateral thighs should also be included to allow for saphenous vein harvest if vascular bypass or reconstruction is required. Initial exposure is obtained by reopening the incision utilized during the index operation. Hemoperitoneum and clot, which is encountered, is expediently, but gently, evacuated by hand and the use of laparotomy pads and suction. In reoperative surgery, attention can then often be turned directly to the area of suspicion based on the index procedure. If the source of hemorrhage is initially unclear, it may be best to pack the area of blood welling with laparotomy pads. The abdomen may then be systematically evaluated to determine the culprit area.

It should be remembered that there is no bleeding in the human body that cannot be controlled, at least temporarily, by the surgeon's hand. If brisk arterial or venous bleeding is encountered, often the most effective initial maneuver to control active hemorrhage is with latex, via direct manual pressure. This allows time to evaluate the situation, determine what further exposure may be required, and formulate an initial operative plan. This can also allow the anesthesiology team to catch up on volume resuscitation if the patient is hemodynamically unstable. After many abdominal procedures, a single small arterial vessel that was transected during the initial dissection, and in vasospasm at the completion of the index procedure, is the culprit. In these cases, direct control via suture ligature is all that is required. Other approaches to control of hemorrhage will be specific to the individual patient and index procedure. Bleeding from a GI anastomosis that is not self-limited frequently is best treated by anastomotic revision. Failure to divide the falciform or triangular ligaments in situations where liver mobilization is required during the initial procedure may result in liver capsule tears that can bleed insidiously. Bleeding from raw organ surface areas is often best treated with the application of hemostatic agents such as cellulose-based matrices (Surgicel, Ethicon Inc., Somerville, NJ, USA) or topical thrombin formulations. Occasionally, even when a significant amount of hemoperitoneum is present, no source of active hemorrhage will be found. Most commonly in these cases, a transected small arterial vessel was responsible, and bleeding was self-limited by vasoconstriction and subsequent vessel thrombosis. In addition, with raw surface areas, removal of clot and its ongoing endogenous fibrinolytic process will lead to a hemostatic bed. Although unsettling, if a careful and thorough exploration with removal of all clot has been performed and no source of active bleeding identified, it is usually best to close the patient before hypothermia and coagulopathy develops in the operating room. In some circumstances, diffuse nonsurgical bleeding will be encountered that cannot be controlled by any intraoperative maneuver. Careful communication with the anesthesia team should reveal any onset or worsening of hypothermia and acidosis. In these cases, it is often best to perform a damage control procedure, pack oozing areas with laparotomy pads, perform a temporary open abdominal closure, and return to the intensive care unit as quickly as possible to further resuscitate and rewarm the patient, and correct any coagulopathy with appropriate blood products. In all cases, patients should be monitored postoperatively in the surgical intensive care unit until hemostasis and stability are ensured.

Angiography and endovascular embolization

Under certain circumstances, angiography-based endovascular techniques offer an effective, lower-risk approach to hemorrhage control than reoperative abdominal surgery. When local expertise and resources are available, these techniques may be a useful adjunct in cases where anatomy or patient disease makes open surgical control of hemorrhage problematic. Bleeding from small- and medium-sized arteries, such as pelvic and retroperitoneal vessels, can often be controlled by transcatheter vessel embolization. Percutaneous endovascular access is obtained, most commonly via the femoral artery, and wire-directed selective catheters are utilized to deliver metal coils or gelatin-based bioabsorbable particulate matter (Gelfoam, Pharmacia & Upjohn Co., Kalamazoo, MI) into target vessels. While coils provide permanent vessel occlusion, Gelfoam will ultimately be resorbed and allow potential recanalization of critical vascular beds. These agents achieve hemostasis by a combination of direct mechanical obstruction of arterial flow and by acting as a framework for thrombus formation.

The timing of bleeding onset after the index abdominal operation is an important factor that may assist in choosing between operative and endovascular approaches to hemorrhage control. In the time period from 7–10 days to 3–6 months after the initial operation, a diffuse network of dense and highly vascular intra-abdominal adhesions often develops, which can make re-exploration challenging and high risk. This is especially likely to be true after open procedures that require extensive dissection and mobilization, or after reoperative procedures. During this time period, the risk of bowel injury during dissection is high, and the subsequent formation of enterocutaneous fistulae is a devastating complication for the patient. Avoiding re-entry into a 'hostile' abdomen by utilizing angiography to locate and embolize sources of postoperative bleeding may be the easiest and safest approach.

Embolization can also be especially useful to control bleeding from challenging anatomic locations or in the setting of certain disease processes. Arterial bleeding from the retroperitoneum or deep in the pelvis can be extremely difficult to control with open surgery, and operative exploration of these areas often causes more bleeding than it can solve. Obtaining surgical control of hemorrhage that is associated with inflammatory disease processes can also be challenging. For example, in the postoperative period after operating for complications associated with chronic gastroduodenal ulcer disease or chronic pancreatitis, tissues are inflamed, friable, tear easily with manipulation, and will not securely hold suture ligatures. Afngiographic embolization of the gastroduodenal or splenic artery is well tolerated, and may offer a safer approach than trying to reoperate to control bleeding in the vicinity of a severely inflamed duodenum or pancreatic bed. Bleeding from deep within an open, 'frozen abdomen' is another situation where identifying and controlling a source of hemorrhage via embolization avoids the risks associated with re-exploration of the chronically inflamed and hostile abdomen.

Another scenario where angiographic techniques can be a key adjunct is in severely injured blunt trauma patients who have already undergone damage control surgery. Arterial bleeding from severe pelvic fractures that persists after reduction in the pelvic ring with a sheet, pelvic binder, or external fixation is extremely difficult to control with open surgical techniques and is often best managed with angiographic embolization. Similarly, in select circumstances, embolization can be a useful adjunct in bleeding from abdominal solid organ injury. This is especially true of liver injuries that exhibit continued arterial bleeding after compressive packing and failed surgical attempts at control. These injury-specific indications will be elaborated in the following section.

ORGAN/DISEASE-SPECIFIC CONSIDERATIONS

Trauma/damage control surgery

The concept of damage control surgery is now accepted as the preferred surgical option for severely injured patients who present with severe physiologic derangement and require operative control of abdominal hemorrhage (Gruen et al. 2012, Rotondo et al. 1993). Patients in hemorrhagic shock with a high injury burden often present with the 'lethal triad' of hypothermia, acidosis, and coagulopathy, which has been shown to be associated with increased mortality (Niles et al. 2008). To prevent death in these critically ill patients, the surgeon's top priorities should be to control hemorrhage and restore physiologic homeostasis. The concept of damage control surgery consists of limiting the initial surgical procedure to life-saving, temporizing maneuvers, to expedite transfer to the surgical intensive care unit for definitive physiologic resuscitation. The goals of the damage control operation are to stop bleeding, control enteric spill, and resect grossly nonviable tissues. Small arterial bleeders are controlled via suture ligature. Temporary vascular shunts may be utilized to restore distal perfusion if complex vascular reconstruction of major named arteries is needed (Aucar & Hirshberg 1997). Venous bleeding and oozing from solid organ injuries are controlled by packing with laparotomy pads. If bowel resection is required, rapid stapling and resection are performed and patients are left in intestinal discontinuity with nasogastric tube decompression. When the goals of damage control have been achieved, a temporary abdominal closure is performed. Commercially available vacuum-assisted temporary abdominal closure dressings are available. However, another easy and cost-effective alternative is the Parkland/Harborview 'vac-pack' closure (**Figure 8.2**). A standard plastic 'bowel-bag' is used to protect the viscera and is tucked into the gutters to prevent adhesion to the abdominal wall. The bowel bag's standard cloth ties are cut and removed, and a few small slits are cut into the plastic bag to allow the underlying fluid to drain. A sterile X-ray cassette cover is an easy to utilize and commonly available alternative. Large compressible ('burn-fluff') Kerlix gauze dressings are then placed in the midline over the bowel bag with two Jackson-Pratt drains within the gauze layers for application of suction. Finally, the dressing is secured with a large sheet of Ioban (3M, St Paul, MN, USA) with moderate tension and the drains are placed to low-pressure continuous suction. The application of suction controls buildup of fluid collections and aids in maintaining apposition of the anterior abdominal wall for subsequent closure. Once the patient has been resuscitated, rewarmed, and any coagulopathy has been corrected, the patient may then be taken back to the operating room. At this time, usually 24–48 hours after the damage control procedure, definitive surgical repairs may be performed such as bowel anastomoses, vascular reconstruction, and, if possible, abdominal closure. Delay >72 hours risks the onset of an excessive inflammatory response to the dressing that makes follow-up procedures considerably more difficult and causes other systemic physiologic derangements.

Evidence of ongoing postoperative hemorrhage after damage control laparotomy for trauma presents a vexing challenge to the surgeon. This most often manifests as continuous sanguineous drainage from abdominal drains or a vacuum-type temporary abdominal closure.

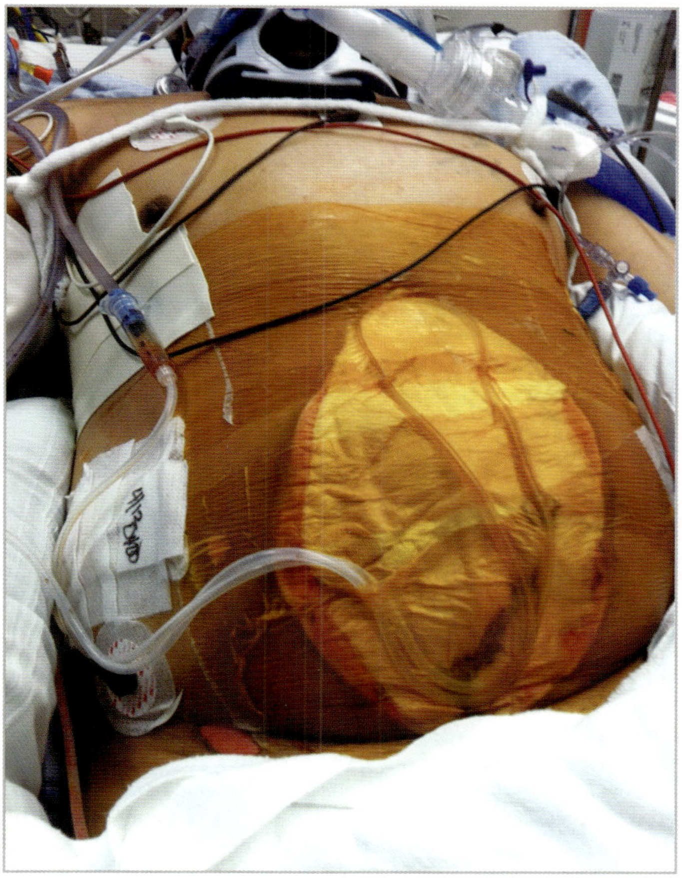

Figure 8.2 Parkland/Harborview 'vac-pack' temporary abdominal closure dressing. Photograph by S. Brakenridge.

The surgeon may be tempted to return immediately to the operating room. However, patients who are best served by initial damage control surgery are, by definition, hypothermic and coagulopathic. If possible, these patients should be rewarmed to >36°C and have coagulopathy corrected with blood products prior to return to the operating room for re-exploration. A surgeon who takes a cold and coagulopathic patient back to the operating room in search of surgically correctable hemorrhage is likely to find the experience unsatisfying, with only diffuse coagulopathic oozing from every raw surface. However, if the patient cannot be rewarmed or coagulopathy corrected due to significant ongoing blood loss, intervention by angiography or reoperation must occur without delay to avoid attempting to achieve the impossible. Similarly, if evidence of bleeding persists once normothermia and normal coagulation parameters have been achieved, then a return to the operating room is necessary.

As mentioned previously, angiography can be a useful adjunct with associated severe pelvic fracture, or in select cases of solid organ injury. Hepatic artery embolization is indicated in severe liver injuries that continue to exhibit arterial bleeding despite compressive packing and surgical attempts at hemorrhage control (Stassen et al. 2012a). Similarly, difficult-to-explore areas are best treated angiographically, such as persistent blood loss following dissection with or without resection of the pancreaticoduodenal complex, or other retroperitoneal structures such as the renal/adrenal organs or paraspinous tissues. There is also evidence to support the selective use of splenic artery embolization for the nonoperative management of blunt splenic injury (Stassen et al. 2012b). However, ongoing bleeding after an attempt of splenic salvage at the initial trauma laparotomy is best addressed by returning to the operating room for completion splenectomy.

Liver

Hepatic bleeding after surgery is best addressed, at least initially, in the operating room. Bleeding from capsular tears is a common source of postoperative abdominal hemorrhage and can be surprisingly voluminous. These tears often occur due to inadequate mobilization of the falciform and triangular ligaments during the index procedure. This bleeding can usually be controlled with electrocautery, compression, and topical hemostatic agents. Argon beam coagulation can also be a useful adjunct for diffuse capsular and parenchymal bleeding. Large subcapsular hematomas should not be unroofed, as they are almost universally self-limited by capsular tamponade. If there is evidence of significant ongoing parenchymal hemorrhage, with blood continuously welling up in the right upper quadrant, careful compressive 'sandwich' packing above and below the liver with minimally unfolded laparotomy pads should be the first maneuver. Initial vascular control can then be obtained via a Pringle maneuver. The Pringle maneuver occludes portal vein and hepatic artery inflow by isolating and securing the gastroduodenal ligament with a vessel loop, Rummel tourniquet, or vascular clamp. This allows for identification and control of bleeding vessels fed by the portal venous and hepatic artery distributions, which can usually be controlled with targeted suture ligatures. If necessary, partial hepatic resections can be accomplished with limited blood loss by the use of newer compression/coagulation dissectors such as the LigaSure device (Covidien, Mansfield, MA, USA) or a surgical stapler with vascular loads. In trauma, nonanatomic 'completion' resections to control hemorrhage are usually reserved for when the injury has already performed most of the resection.

Occasionally, attempts at control of arterial parenchymal bleeding, often from within deep lacerations, will not be successful. In these circumstances, selective ligation of the right or left hepatic artery has been described. However, if angiography resources are available, hepatic angiography and embolization can be a useful and more targeted adjunct. Selective embolization minimizes the potential risk and ultimate extent of subsequent hepatic necrosis. In the operating room, compressive liver packing is performed and a temporary open abdominal closure is placed. The patient is then taken to the angiography suite for identification and selective embolization of bleeding branches of the hepatic artery. The patient is taken back to the operating room 24–36 hours later. At this time, if the patient has stabilized, the liver is usually hemostatic and the compressive packs can be carefully removed without recurrence of significant bleeding.

Venous bleeding from deep behind the liver that is not controlled with application of the Pringle maneuver likely originates from the retrohepatic inferior vena cava (IVC) or major hepatic veins. These injuries are challenging to repair. Full mobilization of the liver by completely dividing the ligamentous attachments of the liver to the diaphragm and retroperitoneum is the key maneuver to gain adequate access to repair these injuries. Severe lacerations or disruption of the retrohepatic IVC may necessitate total hepatic isolation for successful repair. This consists of a Pringle maneuver and obtaining control of the suprarenal and intrapericardial IVC. To achieve this, a sternotomy must be performed to obtain proximal control of the vena cava intrapericardially at the atrial–caval junction. Although with significant risks, patients can tolerate clamping of the intrapericardial IVC. Careful coordination with the anesthesia team and adequate volume loading is required to compensate for the decrease in venous return and cardiac preload. Total inflow and outflow occlusion should not persist for >30 minutes to minimize the risk of irreversible ischemic liver injury. If more time is required to complete the repair, control of bleeding should be maintained via direct compression and the Pringle should be released for 5–10 minutes to allow the liver to be reperfused. After 'ischemic preconditioning,' total hepatic isolation can be re-established to complete the repair. The use of makeshift atriocaval shunts is often quoted, but rarely successfully utilized, and is therefore not recommended.

Spleen

The robust arterial flow and collateralization of the spleen offer many potential bleeding sources following elective or emergent splenic surgery. Sources of hemorrhage after open or laparoscopic splenectomy include an unidentified short gastric artery during division of the gastrosplenic ligament, bleeding from the raw retroperitoneal bed beneath the splenic attachments, or failure of the splenic artery ligature or staple line. In the immediate postoperative period, prompt operative re-exploration should be the definitive intervention of choice. Although splenic artery embolization has been described preoperatively in preparation for elective splenectomy and in the nonoperative management of blunt splenic injury, it has little role in the management of postsplenectomy hemorrhage. Either open or laparoscopic exploration to identify and control the culprit vessel is appropriate depending on the index procedure, surgeon comfort, and patient stability. As described in the previous section, bleeding after partial splenectomy or attempted salvage of an injured spleen is best treated definitively with a return to the operating room for explant of the remaining spleen into a surgical basin.

Pancreas/duodenum

The retroperitoneal area containing the pancreaticoduodenal structures is known as the 'surgical soul' for good reason. The management of injuries, inflammatory processes, and malignancies within this area are amongst the most challenging of all surgical procedures. Many vital structures are contained within, or pass through this area, including the duodenum, pancreas, common bile duct, portal vein, hepatic artery, and superior mesenteric artery and vein. The pancreaticoduodenal arcades based on the gastroduodenal and superior mesenteric arteries provide the area with a robust and redundant collateral blood supply. It is this dense network of small, fragile vessels that is usually the culprit for postoperative bleeding following operations involving the pancreas and duodenum.

If hemorrhage is apparent in the immediate postoperative period after elective pancreatic, duodenal, or biliary tract surgery, a return to the operating room is the usual approach to identify and control the source of bleeding. However, there are situations where alternative approaches to hemorrhage control may be appropriate. Evidence of intraluminal upper GI bleeding after distal gastric or duodenal resection and reconstruction may be successfully approached with upper endoscopy. Mucosal or anastomotic sources of bleeding can be both identified and treated via this approach. In the setting of a severe inflammatory process, such as after procedures for obstructed or perforated gastroduodenal ulcer disease and severe necrotizing pancreatitis, hemorrhage within the severely inflamed retroperitoneal bed may be extremely difficult to control with open surgical techniques. Bleeding in these situations is commonly from the vascularized and friable inflammatory tissues of the initial operative bed. Undergoing reoperation in an attempt to obtain surgical control carries a significant risk of causing further bleeding, as well as causing injury to other vital structures such as the common bile duct, portal vein, and superior mesenteric artery and vein due to distorted anatomy. In these cases, angiographic embolization of the gastroduodenal or splenic arteries may be easier and more effective than trying to obtain adequate purchase with further dissection and suture ligatures in these friable tissues. The robust arterial supply to this area is both a boon and bane regarding the use of embolization to control postoperative hemorrhage. The rich collateralization significantly reduces the risk of incurring ischemia to surrounding structures. However, it can also make control of all inflow to the bleeding area extremely difficult.

Pelvis

Managing hemorrhage associated with pelvic surgery or severe pelvic fracture can be extremely challenging and requires a cautious and thoughtful approach to avoid worsening the situation. Arterial bleeding can be from small lacerated or transected branches of the internal iliac, middle sacral, or superior rectal arteries. However, hemorrhage after pelvic surgery most likely stems from tearing of branches of the robust pelvic venous plexus. Extreme care and patience must be wielded when significant pelvic venous bleeding is encountered. Desperate, blind throws of suture ligatures into the nonflexible and frail presacral tissues most often lead to further tearing of the venous plexus, and cause more bleeding than it can solve. The initial approach to deep pelvic venous hemorrhage is with careful packing of the posterior and lateral true pelvis with laparotomy pads and assuring that the anesthesia team initiates appropriate resuscitation, including correction of any coagulation abnormalities with appropriate blood products. The placement of sterile thumbtacks into the sacrum to control venous plexus tears is another technique that is often quoted but mostly of historic interest. Manual compression, the use of hemostatic adjuncts, such as topical thrombin solutions, and a large dose of patience are much more likely to yield success. A patient who is cold and coagulopathic with ongoing pelvic venous hemorrhage is best served with a damage control approach including packing the pelvis and utilizing a temporary abdominal closure, with a planned return to the operating room after the patient has been appropriately resuscitated, as previously described.

A large pelvic hematoma found during trauma laparotomy, indicative of hemorrhage from a severe pelvic fracture, should not be approached intraperitoneally. Most bleeding associated with pelvic fractures is venous, low pressure, and self-limited. Unroofing of a contained pelvic hematoma will release any effective tamponade already present, leading to copious, diffuse bleeding into the pelvic cavity that is nearly impossible to identify and control by surgical means. If the patient remains hemodynamically unstable after completion of the trauma laparotomy or damage control procedure, the patient should undergo pelvic angiography to identify and embolize any bleeding arterial vessels. Operative retroperitoneal packing has been described as an alternative, effective measure to temporize bleeding associated with pelvic fractures when endovascular resources or expertise are unavailable (Osborn et al. 2009). A transverse suprapubic approach and midline splitting of the fascia and muscles gain access to the preperitoneal space. Blunt dissection bilaterally displaces the bladder medially and permits packing of the pelvis bilaterally to the posterior midline to tamponade and control bleeding. The packs are cautiously removed, after resuscitation, at 24–48 hours. Prolonged pack retention or need for repacking, most commonly associated with 'open' pelvic fractures, has a significant rate of infectious complications.

Gastrointestinal bleeding

The surgical control of intraluminal GI bleeding necessitates localization of the source of hemorrhage. The index procedure may, or may not, make this localization intuitively obvious. In some cases, such as in the setting of an isolated small bowel resection and anastomosis, bleeding is likely from the mucosa of the anastomotic line. In these circumstances, bleeding is usually self-limited. However, if bleeding persists, current endoscopic techniques have limited ability to obtain access to this portion of the GI tract, and operative revision will be necessary. In contrast, when in the setting of gastric or colorectal surgery, endoscopy offers the potential for both diagnostic and therapeutic effectiveness (Mayer et al. 2004).

GI hemorrhage after abdominal surgery that does not include resection and/or anastomosis of the GI tract necessitates localization before any surgical action is undertaken. The diagnostic algorithm is the same as GI bleeding outside the context of recent surgery. Upper and lower endoscopy should be the first maneuver in these situations. Endoscopy may reveal known, or unknown, comorbid sources of hemorrhage including gastroduodenal ulcer disease, diverticulosis, or bleeding gastroesophageal varices. GI hemorrhage in the setting of an aortic tube graft or endograft is to be considered a result of an aortoenteric fistula until proven otherwise. However, this life-threatening complication is most often associated with a chronic graft infection and is therefore an unlikely source of GI hemorrhage in the acute postoperative setting after vascular surgery. If suspected, upper endoscopy is diagnostic in these circumstances and emergent graft excision or temporization with an aortic endograft is required.

Vascular

Bleeding after any vascular procedure should be considered a technical failure until proven otherwise. The most common causes of postoperative bleeding after open vascular procedures include residual anticoagulation from systemic heparinization, needle holes within grafts, or technical error in the vascular anastomosis, particularly at an anastomotic 'crotch' or 'heel.' If systemic heparinization was utilized during the procedure, it is important to know whether reversal with protamine was performed at the conclusion of the case. If protamine reversal was not administered, an activated clotting time (ACT) is a quick and readily available point-of-care testing modality to monitor the anticoagulant effect of administered unfractionated heparin. A patient with evidence of bleeding and an ACT value of >180–200 seconds should be given a reversal dose of protamine sulfate (1–1.5 mg IV/100 units of heparin). Administration of FFP will also reverse the effects of heparinization if protamine is contraindicated due to previous adverse reaction. If the ACT is <180, the patient is normothermic, and PT/INR values are within normal limits, the patient should be taken back to the operating room. If re-exploration is needed after open vascular procedures, the placement of a single suture or the application of topical hemostatics such as thrombin-soaked Gelfoam (Pharmacia & Upjohn Co., Kalamazoo, MI, USA) is often all that is required. Otherwise, revision of the anastomosis or other reconstruction may be required.

The explosive growth in endovascular techniques and technology now allows for the possibility of a minimally invasive approach to many index and reoperative vascular procedures. This includes endovascular approaches to emergent conditions such as ruptured abdominal aortic aneurysms, aortic dissection, and traumatic blunt aortic or subclavian artery injury (Starnes et al. 2010). Bleeding after endovascular procedures can be from access site complications, angioplasty-related vessel rupture, stent complications, and residual systemic heparinization.

Access site bleeding is the most common bleeding complication following endovascular procedures and is usually identified in the postoperative holding area as a large groin hematoma. Initial treatment depends on the size of access sheath used for the procedure. Percutaneous suture closure devices are commonly utilized for sheath sizes > 6–8 French. Bleeding associated with sheath sizes < 8–10 French usually is self-limited when further pressure is applied. Any groin hematoma after percutaneous femoral access should be assessed with duplex ultrasonography. If a pseudoaneurysm is subsequently identified, it can usually be successfully treated with ultrasound-guided thrombin injection. Access site bleeding that is not controlled after manual compression requires operative exploration and repair. Bleeding associated with large caliber access sheaths used for endovascular aortic procedures (10–24 French) is more likely to require operative repair.

When intervention for bleeding is required after open or endovascular procedures, the utilization of an endovascular approach may offer simultaneous diagnosis and treatment, via angiography and the placement of endovascular stents. Given the significant comorbidities often present in this patient population, this minimally invasive approach may offer the easiest and least morbid option for hemorrhage control, depending on the index procedure and surgeon expertise.

Damage control for elective surgery misadventures

It should be remembered that the concepts of damage control surgery are applicable outside the scope of trauma. Damage control techniques should be utilized when significant bleeding from an elective or reoperative procedure causes the rapid physiologic deterioration of the patient. When significant and unexpected bleeding occurs during an elective procedure, it can be difficult for the primary surgeon to change their mindset of an elective operation, to that of an urgent/emergent situation. The element of 'summit fever' that tempts the surgeon to push on and complete the operation can be even stronger during reoperative procedures where much time and effort is often invested in the difficult re-exploration of the target area.

A common scenario is to receive a consultation to assist a colleague in the operating room when an elective case has gone awry. In situations such as this, a significant amount of time (and blood loss) has elapsed in an attempt to deal with the problem before calling for assistance or deciding to abort the procedure. It is important to re-establish a sense of calm to what is usually a stress-filled environment, and to mentally take a step back to gain a wider perspective of the situation. First, it is crucial to establish an understanding of the physiologic status and stability of the patient. If communication with the anesthesia team reveals hypothermia, acidosis, and coagulopathy, the goals of the procedure must immediately switch from the completion of a technically perfect operation to expediently get the patient out of the operating room to 'live to fight another day.' It is crucial to reassure the primary surgeon, or oneself, that aborting an elective procedure and taking a damage control approach in these situations is not a failure. As described previously in the setting of trauma, temporizing measures are taken to control bleeding and enteric spill, a temporary open abdominal closure is applied, and the patient is taken to the intensive care unit for resuscitation. Once normal physiology has been re-established, and the surgeon is well rested, the patient can then be taken back to the operating room for completion of the procedure.

POSTINTERVENTION RESUSCITATION AND SUPPORTIVE CARE

Any patient requiring intervention for significant postoperative bleeding should subsequently be managed in the surgical intensive care unit for continued resuscitation, supportive care, and monitoring. Often, these patients will require continued ventilator support for decreased pulmonary compliance and inadequate tidal volumes, acidosis, or pulmonary edema. In addition, ongoing mechanical ventilation may be required if there is plan for a second look, or if there are adverse effects on respiratory mechanics secondary to the temporary abdominal closure and open abdomen. Vigilant clinical monitoring is required to ensure that hemostasis is maintained. Serial Hgb/Hct levels should be obtained initially every 2–4 hours. Many patients who have required reoperation or other procedural intervention for ongoing hemorrhage will require further volume resuscitation, even after hemostasis is achieved and blood count levels stabilize. This is due to the systemic inflammatory response that occurs in response to hemorrhagic shock, ischemia, and tissue damage. These stimuli provoke a dramatic increase in the expression of a wide range of proinflammatory genes leading to a surge in serum levels of inflammatory cytokines such as interleukin (IL)-1, IL-6, and tumor necrosis factor-α (Xiao et al. 2011). The systemic effects of these inflammatory processes include activation of endothelium and increased capillary permeability, which leads to interstitial third spacing that can require significant ongoing volume replacement.

If not already initiated in the operating room for the initial resuscitation, most patients with significant blood loss and hemorrhagic shock should have access for invasive hemodynamic monitoring in place, including an arterial line and central venous catheter. Devices that calculate pulse pressure variation and stroke volume variation from standard arterial line pressure measurements, such as the LiDCO (LidCo Ltd, Cambridge, UK) or FlowTrac (Edwards Lifesciences, Irvine, CA, USA) systems, are better predictors of preload status and responsiveness to volume challenge than CVP measured from a central venous catheter in mechanically ventilated patients (Belloni et al. 2008). Pulse pressure variation > 10–13% has been shown to be a reliable indicator of decreased preload and positive response to fluid bolus administration (Benes et al. 2010).

Pulmonary artery catheters (PACs) have fallen out of favor in the management of critically ill patients based on the findings of several randomized controlled trials (Harvey et al. 2005, Rajaram et al. 2013). However, it is not clear whether these trials are translatable to acutely unstable surgical and trauma patients. Although a full discussion on the use and interpretation of PACs is beyond the scope of this chapter, it should be noted that their use may be helpful in select patients who present with more than one possible etiology of shock. For example, hemodynamic parameters obtained via PAC may assist in determining the primary cause of persistent hypotension in a severely injured blunt trauma patient who is postoperative day one after splenectomy who also has a severe pelvic fracture (hemorrhagic shock), possible cardiac contusion (cardiogenic shock), and complete cervical spinal cord injury (neurogenic shock). Despite their limitations and decreasing utilization, PACs remain a valuable tool in the surgeon and surgical intensivist's armamentarium. Point of care, limited echocardiography is another method to gain information regarding the patient's cardiac function and intravascular volume status. This modality has been shown to accurately obtain multiple hemodynamic variables in a noninvasive manner, and many argue that bedside echocardiography should routinely replace PAC placement in the intensive care unit (Noritomi et al. 2010). While its use is increasing the critical care setting, interpretation of point-of-care ultrasound is user dependent and appropriate training is required to ensure accurate and reproducible results.

As delineated in previous sections, patients who have undergone multiple procedures and large volume resuscitation for hemorrhagic shock secondary to postoperative bleeding are likely to be hypothermic, coagulopathic, and acidotic. All three factors of this 'lethal triad' must be treated simultaneously as severe hypothermia and acidosis contribute to the development of a refractory coagulopathy that will cause continued nonsurgical bleeding and is associated with high mortality (Niles et al. 2008). Hypothermia must be corrected to allow for proper platelet and coagulation factor enzymatic function. Mild hypothermia (35–37°C) often can be corrected with passive maneuvers such as warm blankets and increasing room temperature. Active, noninvasive measures such as forced air rewarming devices – the Bair Hugger – (Arizant Inc, Eden Prarie, MN, USA), resistive heating blankets, and intravenous fluid warmers/infusers should also be ubiquitously utilized and carry little risk. Hypothermia below 35°C needs aggressive correction and frequently requires active invasive warming measures such as continuous venovenous rewarming or intravascular rewarming catheters. Active rewarming catheter systems like the Arctic Sun system (Medivance Inc, Louisville, CO, USA) allow for the rapid correction of severe hypothermia (1.5–3°C/h), are self-contained, and can be performed with standard femoral central venous access techniques. Acidosis after hemorrhagic shock is usually secondary to increased serum lactic acid levels from anaerobic tissue metabolism. Treatment of acidosis should focus on correction of the underlying cause (i.e. shock and tissue ischemia). In the setting of hemorrhagic shock, this consists of intravascular volume resuscitation and the judicious use of vasopressive agents to maintain adequate mean arterial pressure to provide adequate tissue perfusion. However, vasopressors should only be added after adequate repletion of intravascular volume is achieved and proven insufficient. Bicarbonate administration should not be considered as primary treatment of acidosis in this setting and should be administered only with severe, persistent acidosis (pH < 7.15) to allow for adequate enzymatic function while treatment of the underlying shock state continues.

Once surgical control of hemorrhage has been obtained and the patient's condition has stabilized with initial resuscitation, serial laboratory evaluation of coagulation parameters allows for targeted administration of blood product components to treat any remaining coagulopathic bleeding. Coagulation parameters including PT/INR, aPTT, platelet, and fibrinogen levels should be repeated every 1–2 hours until corrected and then monitored serially. At this point, administration of FFP, platelets, and cryoprecipitate should be individually tailored to correct specific deficits. As mentioned previously, if the equipment and expertise is available, TEG may be utilized to further characterize and titrate individualized treatment of any coagulation abnormalities.

Conversely, critically ill trauma and surgical patients are simultaneously at high-risk of venous thromboembolic (VTE) complications (Knudson et al. 2004). This increased risk of these complications is thought to be secondary to inflammation and coagulation abnormalities present in these patients. It is now known that deep venous thrombosis and pulmonary embolus often occur within the first few hours to days after the initial insult in these patients; therefore, timely initiation of VTE prophylactic measures is warranted as soon as possible following hemostasis (Brakenridge et al. 2011). Pneumatic compression devices should be utilized immediately, and initiation of heparin-based pharmacologic VTE prophylaxis should be considered when the patient is stable and without signs of further bleeding for 24 hours. Currently, low-molecular weight fractionated heparins are preferred to unfractionated whole heparins.

CONCLUSION

The diagnosis and treatment of postoperative hemorrhage after abdominal surgery must proceed promptly but with appropriate thoughtfulness and planning. Reoperative surgery remains the gold standard for both definitive diagnosis and treatment of postoperative hemorrhage in the immediate postoperative period. However, there are situations where alternative diagnostic and therapeutic modalities, such as surgical endoscopy and angiography-based endovascular techniques, may offer a safer and more effective approach to hemorrhage. Regardless of the modality, the surgeon's top priority remains the prompt control of hemorrhage and the appropriate resuscitation of any associated abnormal physiology. This should include the early use of blood products during initial volume resuscitation, the liberal use of damage control surgical techniques, and close postoperative monitoring along with continued resuscitation and supportive care in the surgical intensive care unit to re-establish physiologic homeostasis.

REFERENCES

Aucar JA, Hirshberg A. Damage control for vascular injuries. Surg Clin North Am 1997; 77:853–862.

Belloni L, Pisano A, Natale A, et al. Assessment of fluid-responsiveness parameters for off-pump coronary artery bypass surgery: a comparison among LiDCO, transesophageal echocardiography, and pulmonary artery catheter. J Cardiothor Vasc Anesth 2008; 22:243–248.

Benes J, Chytra I, Altmann P, et al. Intraoperative fluid optimization using stroke volume variation in high risk surgical patients: results of prospective randomized study. Crit care (London, England) 2010; 14:R118.

Brakenridge SC, Toomay SM, Sheng JL, Gentilello LM, Shafi S. Predictors of early versus late timing of pulmonary embolus after traumatic injury. Am J Surg 2011; 201:209–215.

CRASH-2 trial collaborators. Effects of tranexamic acid on death, vascular occlusive events, and blood transfusion in trauma patients with significant haemorrhage (CRASH-2): a randomised, placebo-controlled trial. Lancet 2010; 376:23–32.

Cotton BA, Au BK, Nunez TC, et al. Predefined massive transfusion protocols are associated with a reduction in organ failure and postinjury complications. J Trauma 2009; 66:41–48; discussion 8–9.

Gomez Sandoval YH, Braganza MV, Daskalopoulou SS. Statin discontinuation in high-risk patients: a systematic review of the evidence. Curr Pharm Des 2011; 17:3669–3689.

Gruen RL, Brohi K, Schreiber M, et al. Haemorrhage control in severely injured patients. Lancet 2012; 380:1099–1108.

Hamilton HC, Foxcroft DR. Central venous access sites for the prevention of venous thrombosis, stenosis and infection in patients requiring long-term intravenous therapy. Cochrane Database Syst Rev (Online) 2007:CD004084.

Harvey S, Harrison DA, Singer M, et al. Assessment of the clinical effectiveness of pulmonary artery catheters in management of patients in intensive care (PAC-Man): a randomised controlled trial. Lancet 2005; 366:472–477.

Haupt MT, Bekes CE, Brilli RJ, et al. Guidelines on critical care services and personnel: Recommendations based on a system of categorization of three levels of care. Crit Care Med 2003; 31:2677–2683.

Holcomb JB, Jenkins D, Rhee P, et al. Damage control resuscitation: directly addressing the early coagulopathy of trauma. J Trauma 2007; 62:307–310.

Holcomb JB, Wade CE, Michalek JE, et al. Increased plasma and platelet to red blood cell ratios improves outcome in 466 massively transfused civilian trauma patients. Ann Surg 2008; 248:447–458.

Kashuk JL, Moore EE, Sawyer M, et al. Postinjury coagulopathy management: goal directed resuscitation via POC thrombelastography. Ann Surg 2010; 251:604–614.

Knudson MM, Ikossi DG, Khaw L, Morabito D, Speetzen LS. Thromboembolism after trauma: an analysis of 1602 episodes from the American College of Surgeons National Trauma Data Bank. Ann Surg 2004; 240:490–496; discussion 6–8.

Le Manach Y, Godet G, Coriat P, et al. The impact of postoperative discontinuation or continuation of chronic statin therapy on cardiac outcome after major vascular surgery. Anesth Analg 2007; 104:1326–1333, table of contents.

Mayer G, Lingenfelser T, Ell C. The role of endoscopy in early postoperative haemorrhage. Best Pract Res Clin Gastroenterol 2004; 18:799–807.

Neal MD, Marsh A, Marino R, et al. Massive transfusion: an evidence-based review of recent developments. Archives of surgery (Chicago, IL: 1960) 2012; 147:563–571.

Niles SE, McLaughlin DF, Perkins JG, et al. Increased mortality associated with the early coagulopathy of trauma in combat casualties. J Trauma 2008; 64:1459–1463; discussion 63–65.

Noritomi DT, Vieira ML, Mohovic T, et al. Echocardiography for hemodynamic evaluation in the intensive care unit. Shock (Augusta, Ga) 2010; 34:59–62.

Osborn PM, Smith WR, Moore EE, et al. Direct retroperitoneal pelvic packing versus pelvic angiography: A comparison of two management protocols for haemodynamically unstable pelvic fractures. Injury 2009; 40:54–60.

Parienti JJ, du Cheyron D, Timsit JF, et al. Meta-analysis of subclavian insertion and nontunneled central venous catheter-associated infection risk reduction in critically ill adults. Crit Care Med 2012; 40:1627–1634.

Rajaram SS, Desai NK, Kalra A, et al. Pulmonary artery catheters for adult patients in intensive care. Cochrane Database Syst Rev (Online) 2013; 2:CD003408.

Rotondo MF, Schwab CW, McGonigal MD, et al. 'Damage control': an approach for improved survival in exsanguinating penetrating abdominal injury. J Trauma 1993; 35:375–382; discussion 82–83.

Spinella PC, Perkins JG, Grathwohl KW, et al. Effect of plasma and red blood cell transfusions on survival in patients with combat related traumatic injuries. J Trauma 2008; 64:S69–77; discussion S-8.

Starnes BW, Quiroga E, Hutter C, et al. Management of ruptured abdominal aortic aneurysm in the endovascular era. J Vasc Surg 2010; 51:9–17; discussion 8.

Stassen NA, Bhullar I, Cheng JD, et al. Nonoperative management of blunt hepatic injury: an Eastern Association for the Surgery of Trauma practice management guideline. J Trauma Acute Care Surg 2012a; 73:S288–S293.

Stassen NA, Bhullar I, Cheng JD, et al. Selective nonoperative management of blunt splenic injury: an Eastern Association for the Surgery of Trauma practice management guideline. J Trauma Acute Care Surg 2012b; 73:S294–S300.

Xiao W, Mindrinos MN, Seok J, et al. A genomic storm in critically injured humans. J Experim Med 2011; 208:2581–2590.

Zink KA, Sambasivan CN, Holcomb JB, Chisholm G, Schreiber MA. A high ratio of plasma and platelets to packed red blood cells in the first 6 hours of massive transfusion improves outcomes in a large multicenter study. Am J Surg 2009; 197:565–570; discussion 70.

Chapter 9 Reoperative surgery in trauma

Joyce I. Kaufman, Howard M. Lieberman, Mauricio Lynn

INTRODUCTION

The Center for Disease Control reported 2,437,163 American deaths in 2009. Of these, 4.8% died of trauma-related injuries, making trauma the fifth overall and the leading cause of death among patients between the ages of 1-44 in the USA (WISQARS 2012). Worldwide, injuries account for 1 in every 10 deaths and are estimated to account for 11% of the global burden of disease as measured by the number of disability-adjusted life years experienced by the world's population (Murray & Lopez 1996). Thus, trauma and trauma-related injuries are not limited to developed nations but pose a worldwide public health problem. From a global burden of disease perspective, it has been projected that by 2020 road-related injuries will rise to third place, violence is expected to rise to twelfth place, and self-inflicted injuries to rise up to fourteenth (Murray & Lopez 1996). These shocking statistics underscore the severity of trauma as a major cause of death and disability both now and in the future.

Trauma surgery is unique from every other type of surgery. Unlike the vast majority of operations, the surgeon does not have the luxury of meeting patients preoperatively to discuss the surgical plan in detail, nor to propose alternative treatment modalities. Too often, patients and their trauma surgeons meet only once the patient has severe and profound metabolic and physiologic derangements. Finally, the need for planned reoperations is becoming common practice in the management of the multiply injured trauma patient and this decision is frequently required before even reaching the operating room for the first time (Hirshberg & Mattox 1995).

STAGED SURGERY

Historically, one of the earliest and best known examples of staged surgery is the resection of the pancreatic head for ampullary cancer as described by A.O. Whipple in 1930s (Whipple 1938). The more modern history of two-stage laparotomy arose from experiences gained in dealing with major hepatic trauma (Lucas & Ledgerwood 1976, Walt 1978). The next chapter in the history of staged laparotomy began with a seminal report from Stone et al (1983) in 1982. He described the survival of 65% (11/17) of patients who sustained predominately penetrating wounds and had abdominal packing compared with only 7% (1/14) survival of patients undergoing definitive management of their injuries. The original description of staged laparotomy for trauma stated: '...major vessels were repaired, ends of resected bowel were ligated, and holes in other GI segments and bladder were closed by purse-string sutures.' In addition, the authors envisioned the fundamental objective of staged operations: 'this technique of initial abortion of laparotomy, establishment of intra-abdominal pack tamponade, and then completion of the surgical procedure once coagulation has returned to acceptable level has proven to be life saving.'

THE TRAUMA LAPAROTOMY

Although the exact history of trauma laparotomy cannot be accurately traced, there are writings discussing abdominal trauma and intestinal surgery for trauma from Celsus in the 1st century AD and from the Greek physician Galen in AD 130–200. Significant progress in the management of penetrating abdominal trauma was made in 1847 by the discovery of chloroform by Simpson and thus the introduction of general anesthesia. The concept further evolved over the decades and with the introduction of blood transfusions, it became standard practice to explore all penetrating abdominal injuries in both civilian and military personnel. However, this policy was challenged in the 1960s–1970s when selective nonoperative management of penetrating abdominal injuries was slowly introduced. It is now widespread and an acceptable practice in today's modern approach to trauma surgery.

A midline laparotomy incision is the standard incision for trauma surgery. The incision itself can be made using the electrocautery or with a scalpel. Earlier concerns that the cautery would lead to impaired wound healing or increased infection rates have proven unfounded. Kearns et al. (2001) showed that cautery incision was associated with less blood loss with a similar rate of wound infection in both groups. In the hemodynamically unstable patient, the abdomen should be entered as rapidly and as safely as possible but without the concern of meticulously controlling every small subcutaneous bleeding vessel.

The main tenets of the trauma laparotomy can be divided into four components: (1) control of bleeding, (2) identification of injuries, (3) control of contamination, and (4) reconstruction (if patient's physiology allows). These were the foundation of the first 'damage control' laparotomy or 'abbreviated laparotomy.' This principle is designed to manage life-threatening injuries first, stabilize the patient's physiology in the intensive care unit (ICU), and allow for a return to the operating room at which time definitive procedures can be safely and effectively performed.

Trauma patients who ultimately succumb to their injuries do so by several mechanisms, the most common include head injury, exsanguination, sepsis, and multiple organ failure. Another cause of death was only recognized in the late 1970s and early 1980s once the capability of transfusing large quantities of blood was introduced. This new modality allowed trauma surgeons to continue operating until patients developed profound metabolic derangements such as coagulopathy, metabolic acidosis, and hypothermia (Feliciano et al. 1981), currently known as the 'triad of death' (Mikhail 1999). Although the actions of this triad at the cellular and microbiological levels are complex, it can be simplified as follows: evaporative and conductive heat loss combined with blood loss lead to hypothermia. Metabolic acidosis arises from shock that can be further exacerbated by aortic cross clamping and ongoing blood loss. Coagulopathy occurs due to hemodilution, consumption of clotting factors, hypothermia, and acidosis. All three components interact in a circular fashion to exacerbate one another, thus forming a potentially endless cycle that will result in the ultimate demise of the patient, unless something is done to end the cycle (Kashuk et al. 1982). Hence, the introduction of the abbreviated trauma laparotomy.

There are preoperative as well as intraoperative clues regarding which patients will require abbreviated trauma laparotomy. Waiting until the appearance of the 'death triad' of hypothermia, coagulopathy, and acidosis is almost invariably too late. The patients who most likely will need a damaged control trauma operation are listed below (Feliciano et al. 2008):

Thoracic trauma
- Penetrating thoracic wound and systolic blood pressure (SBP) <90 mmHg
- Pericardial fluid on the focused abdominal sonography for trauma (FAST)
- S/P emergency department thoracotomy for penetrating trauma

Abdominal or pelvic trauma
- Penetrating abdominal wound and SBP <90 mmHg
- Blunt abdominal trauma, SBP <90 mmHg and peritoneal fluid seen on FAST examination or gross blood on a diagnostic peritoneal lavage
- Closed pelvic fracture, SBP <90 mmHg and peritoneal fluid seen on FAST examination or gross blood on a diagnostic peritoneal lavage
- Open pelvic fracture

Trauma to an extremity
- Penetrating wound to femoral triangle
- Mangled extremity from blunt trauma

The above subset of patients should be kept in the trauma bay or emergency department just long enough to secure an airway, decompress an obvious pneumothorax, and have blood drawn for type and cross and then be taken immediately to the operating room.

Once in the operating room following steps can be taken to prevent hypothermia:
- Increasing the room temperature to >29.4°C
- Infusion of IV fluid through a warming device
- Covering patient's body parts with a warming device
- Irrigation of the nasogastric tube and thoracotomy tubes with warm saline
- Irrigation of the peritoneal and any other open cavity with warm fluids

HYPOTHERMIA

Older literature reviews show that 66% of severely injured patients had body temperatures <36°C, including 23% who were severely hypothermic with a temperature <34°C (Jurkovich et al. 1987). Many factors and mechanisms are involved in the development of hypothermia in trauma patients including hypovolemic shock, which leads to an adverse affect on oxygen delivery at the tissue level, thus leading to a decrease in oxygen consumption and therefore less production of heat (Chaudry 1983, Durham et al. 1999, Weg 1991). The effect of hypothermia on mortality in severely injured patients is no longer controversial and thus the practice of damage-control surgery seems logical in patients whose temperature is <35°C. Of note, hypothermia will not resolve until the thoracic or abdominal cavity is closed.

ACIDEMIA

Prolonged hypovolemic shock leads to anaerobic metabolism and a state of acidemia. This acidotic state in turn leads to a decrease in cardiac output, worsening hypotension, and an ongoing viscous circle of events. In this state, the patient becomes susceptible to cardiac arrhythmias, which may be irreversible despite volume replacement. In addition, acidosis is usually coupled to coagulopathy and hypothermia.

COAGULOPATHY

Nonmechanical bleeding is commonly encountered during emergency trauma laparotomies and thoracotomies. Coagulopathy resulting in irreversible bleeding is a significant cause of morbidity and mortality in the immediate postoperative period and thus requires aggressive therapy (Kauvar et al. 2006). The traditional replacement of blood loss with large volumes of crystalloid solutions and cold packed red blood cells (pRBC) causes clotting dysfunction due to dilution of clotting factors and hypothermia. In particular, hypothermia has adverse effects on enzymes associated with platelet function and the coagulation cascade (Reed et al. 1992, Watts et al. 1998). Traditionally, one unit of fresh frozen plasma was transfused for every four units of pRBC. However, current literature suggests that a ratio of 2:3 or even 1:1 is favored in the severely injured trauma patient (Ketchum et al. 2006). In severely coagulopathic patients, characterized by an international normalized ratio (INR) or partial thromboplastin time 50% greater than normal after major sources of hemorrhage have been controlled, damage-control laparotomy should be undertaken.
Intraoperative objective indications for abbreviated/damage-control laparotomy are as follows:
- Initial body temperature <35°C
- Initial pH <7.2
- Initial base deficit of –15 in a patient <55 years old or <–6 in patient >55 years old
- INR or PTT >50% of normal

Intraoperative subjective signs of adverse physiology (Hirshberg & Mattox 2008) are as follows:
- Edema of bowel mucosa
- Midgut distention
- Dusky serosal surfaces
- Tissue that is cold to touch
- Swollen noncompliant abdominal wall
- Diffuse oozing from surgical incision and surfaces

The trauma surgeon should always be thinking several moves ahead. The decision to implement the 'damage control laparotomy' concept should be made before entering the operating room and the decision to leave the operating room should be made well before encountering the 'triad of death.' Patients who are best suited for the abbreviated laparotomy were outlined above and can be further categorized into the following six groups (Moore 1996):
- Inability to achieve hemostasis due to intractable coagulopathy, i.e. the 'triad of death'
- Inaccessible major venous injury such as retrohepatic vena cava
- Anticipated need for lengthy and time*consuming procedures such as pancreaticoduodenectomy
- The need for nonsurgical control of extra-abdominal bleeding such as that seen in pelvic fractures requiring angiography and embolization
- Inability to close the abdominal wall or the fear of adnominal compartment syndrome
- The need to reassess abdominal organs

The technical aspects of the damage-control laparotomy are primarily dictated by the injury pattern. The main objectives are to stop bleeding, limit contamination, temporarily close the abdomen, and transfer the patient to the ICU as quickly as possible for ongoing resuscitative efforts that include reversing hypothermia, coagulopathy, and hemodynamic support.

PHYSIOLOGICAL RESUSCITATION IN THE ICU

Once the decision has been made to perform a damage-control laparotomy, the patient should be promptly transported to the ICU for ongoing resuscitative efforts and hemodynamic support. Priorities in the ICU are focused on restoring the physiological status of the patient and stopping the cycle of acidosis, hypothermia, and coagulopathy. Patients need restoration of volume with either crystalloid fluids or blood and blood products; inotropic or vasopressor support may be needed but should be short until volume replacement has been completed. Rewarming is paramount in helping to reverse coagulopathy.

PLANNED REOPERATION

The exact timing of a planned return to the operating room after abbreviated laparotomy is not well defined and still remains controversial. In some reported series, reoperation was done within 24–48 hours (Burch et al. 1992, Rotondo et al. 1993, Stone et al. 1983), while others prefer to wait for 48–96 hours (Carrillo et al. 1993). The timing of the return to the operating room is more often dictated by clinical circumstances rather than absolute parameters. An example may be the salvage of an ischemic limb after major artery ligation, where a suboptimal vascular repair or the use of temporary intraluminal shunts that may rapidly clot off with restoration of normal coagulation. Once the patient becomes normothermic, evidence of ischemia becomes more apparent with a reliable comparison to the contralateral limb. This circumstance would demand a more urgent return to the operating room. Other examples of earlier return to the operating room may be seen in cases where bowel interruption at several sites was required at the initial operation, thereby creating a closed loop bowel obstruction, which threatens bowel viability. Also, suboptimal control of enteric spillage and contamination at the time of the initial laparotomy may require earlier return to the operating room (Hirshberg et al. 1997). Patients who develop elevated bladder pressure and abdominal compartment syndrome may require immediate intervention (Moore 1996).

Conversely, in other clinical settings, delaying the return to the operating room may be in the patient's best interest. If the goal is to perform definitive abdominal closure, it is best to wait for bowel edema and large fluid shifts to resolve, which usually occurs at 72–96 hours (Smith et al. 1992). The patient should be in a negative fluid balance, off any inotropic support and with a more compliant abdominal wall.

Delaying the reoperation may also be indicated in patients who remain unstable from a cardiopulmonary perspective. The transport of a patient on high ventilator support and on high doses of vasopressors may be extremely risky thus making any trip to the operating room contraindicated. Often, the decision when to return to the operating room for a planned reoperation is a complex decision and good clinical judgment is paramount. It is essential that the initial operating surgeon should be the one making the decisions and he should also be the one who performs the planned reoperative surgery.

Re-exploration

The return to the operating room may often be as challenging as the initial surgery. The abdomen that has seen significant tissue destruction, gross spillage of intestinal content, possible contamination, as well as significant inflammatory reaction throughout the peritoneum may be extremely hostile.

Prior to returning to the operating room, a preoperative check list should be in place and should include:

- Notification and discussion with anesthesia with respect to the patient's physiologic status and planned procedures. The anesthesiologist should examine the patient in the ICU prior to the operation
- Warming of the operating room should be started prior to patient arrival
- Notification of all consulting services for potential simultaneous or sequential interventions
- Notification of the blood bank to ensure availability of blood and blood products
- Discussion with the operating room nursing staff with respect to anticipated procedures to be performed and if unique equipment will be required
- Consideration for the need of a tracheostomy and/or gastrostomy, jejunostomy, or other feeding access

Although the goal of the reoperation is definitive hemostasis and organ repair, the concept of damage control still applies, even upon return to the operating room, and a bailout strategy should be kept in mind. Survivors of an initial laparotomy often undergo more than just one reoperation. A mean of 1.7 reoperations were required before definitive repair was achieved in one series of 124 patients (Hirshberg et al. 1994). Just like the initial trauma laparotomy, the planned reoperation follows the same meticulous principles. The reoperation begins with meticulous exploration and irrigation of the abdominal cavity to help better visualize the surgical field. Missed injuries in these patients are common (Hirshberg et al. 1994). It is therefore the responsibility of the surgeon to carefully trace the trajectory of the missile in the case of penetrating abdominal injuries. A discontinuous trajectory or an odd number of gastrointestinal perforations are classic markers for missed injury at the time of initial laparotomy (Hirshberg et al. 1994). Packs are not removed first due to the risk of resumption of uncontrollable hemorrhage, which would require an interruption of the procedure, repacking, and for needing a second bailout procedure (Martin, Byrne 1997). Bleeding vessels are ligated as they are encountered and major vascular reconstruction usually precedes gastrointestinal repair.

A fundamental principle during reoperative trauma surgery is the removal of packs and other temporary hemostatic devices. The technique for packing removal is usually poorly performed and is an underrated skill. Packs should be removed after having been thoroughly soaked in normal saline allowing for the fluid to soak through the packs. Some surgeons have advocated the use of a syringe with normal saline, providing a constant stream of water to further facilitate pack removal. Additionally, the surrounding tissue or organ should also be well soaked or 'under water.' If an organ or vascular pedicle has been packed, it is prudent to obtain appropriate vascular control before beginning the unpacking process. Hemostatic agents should be available on the surgical field should bleeding restart. A full complement of vascular instruments should be available in case major bleeding is uncovered at the time of pack removal. The argon-beam coagulator may be a valuable tool to help facilitate hemostasis during pack removal. If bleeding is encountered, pack removal should be stopped and appropriate hemostasis becomes the focus. After this is achieved, pack removal can again be resumed keeping in mind that if uncontrollable bleeding is encountered repacking and bailout may be needed.

RECONSTRUCTION

Reconstructive work immediately follows exploration. Gastrointestinal reconstruction follows major vascular repair. The principals are simple. High-risk and complex gastrointestinal reconstructions should be avoided. A host of factors have been implicated in the healing process of an anastomosis. There are patient-related factors that cannot be altered, such as body mass index (BMI) and comorbid conditions like diabetes, hypertension, heart disease, cancer, anemia, and malnutrition. There are preoperative factors, such as prior history of chemotherapy and chronic steroid use. Finally, there are the surgery-related factors that include duration of surgery, blood loss and transfusion requirements, contamination of the surgical field, blood supply to the anastomosis, and tension-free repair (Kingham & Pachter 2009). Leak rates after abbreviated laparotomy have been reported in the literature ranging from 0.5% to 30% (Nasirkhan et al. 2006).

GASTROINTESTINAL INJURIES

Gastric repair

Due to the nature of its rich vascular supply, the stomach is almost always amenable to repair during the initial laparotomy under almost any circumstance (Behran et al. 1998). If an anterior hole is found on the stomach, a careful search must be done to find the second hole, which is usually apparent. However, there are locations where a second hole can be hard to find and thus missed or not found until reoperative laparotomy. The greater and lesser curvatures and the posterior wall of the stomach can conceal a gastric perforation. If a missed injury is suspected but not visualized, the anesthesiologist may insufflate the stomach with air through the nasogastric tube, while the stomach is submerged in saline. The presence of air bubbles in the water indicates a missed perforation. Also, infusion of dye such as methylene blue can also help but will cover the field in a blue color potentially making other injuries difficult to detect. Most injuries to the stomach can be repaired in one or two layers. A single layer of silk Lembert sutures can be used or if a two-layer repair is desired, an inner running layer of absorbable suture is placed with an outer layer of interrupted silk sutures. Larger injuries can be repaired using a two-layer technique or a GIA stapler, which is less time consuming.

Small bowel repair

During the initial laparotomy, the small bowel should have been eviscerated and inspected loop by loop. The plan for resection versus repair should be delayed until the entire bowel has been inspected. A range of techniques exist to control spillage from the use of temporizing Babcock clamps to quickly suturing the perforation, if that segment maybe resected at a later time. The use of staples for a temporary closure has also been described. Finally, the use of a GIA stapler to remove the injured segment(s) is a commonly used technique. Definitive repair depends on the grade of injury. Small serosal tears can be left alone or repaired with a single layer of silk Lembert sutures. Full-thickness injuries that involve <50% of the circumference should undergo debridement to clean edges and then closed in two layers with an inner running layer of Vicryl and an outer layer of interrupted silk sutures. A transverse closure is always preferred as it allows for the widest lumen while reducing the risk of bowel stricture. Large segments of bowel with multiple injuries or perforations as well as complete transections are treated with resection. Areas that have mesenteric injuries with compromised blood supply should also be resected.

During reoperative surgery, the entire length of bowel must be inspected fully again, using the utmost care since it is usually edematous and friable. Previous repairs are re-examined to ensure viability and the absence of leaks. Areas that were questionably viable during the initial surgery, such as serosal tears or areas of ischemia, are also reinspected to ensure healthy bowel integrity. Gentle handling of the bowel and early abdominal closure is advised to prevent fistula formation (Miller & Morris 2005, Scott et al 2006). There still remains some controversy over the safety of a stapled anastomosis versus hand-sewn anastomosis in the setting of traumatic bowel injuries. Most of the data is retrospective in nature and there are no controlled clinical trials comparing the two techniques. Nonetheless, the general consensus is that the complication rates are similar (Brundage et al. 1999). There are several points that should be evaluated before doing an anastomosis in the setting of trauma. The surgeon should rely on the technique with which he is most familiar and experienced. Markedly edematous or thickened bowel should be either hand sewn or stapled with a stapler cartridge better suited for thick tissue. Finally, there are certain conditions that will make an anastomosis a high risk procedure, such as shock, massive transfusion, or volume resuscitation and associated pancreatic injuries.

Colonic repair

The colon is anatomically defined at its proximal margin by the ileocolic valve and distally by the rectosigmoid junction. When confronted with a colonic injury, two main strategies can be utilized: primary repair or colostomy. Similar to injuries of the small intestine, primary repair can be accomplished with suture repair of the colotomy or resection with primary anastomosis. Again, surgical decision will be based on multiple factors but starts with the injury severity as defined by the American Association for the Surgery of Trauma (AAST) (**Table 9.1**).

The patient's physiology, their hemodynamics, and associated injuries additionally will be factors in the surgeon's decision-making algorithm. For AAST grade I–III injuries, primary repair is the preferred method of treatment. This can involve resection and primary anastomosis with the GIA and TA staplers. Another acceptable option for grade I–III injuries is primary repair using a one or two-layer technique of absorbable monofilament. For more severe and complex injures, including grade IV and V injuries, the consideration of colostomy becomes a viable and valuable option; however, primary repair has been established as the optimal treatment of destructive colon injuries (Asensio & Trunkey 2008). Again hemodynamics, physiology, and associated injuries cannot be overemphasized in the surgical decision-making process as it pertains to management. Injuries involving the ascending and proximal transverse colon (proximal to the middle colic artery) are treated with a right hemicolectomy with ileocolic anastomosis. Injuries that are distal to the middle colic artery can also be treated with segmental resection and primary anastomosis. During the initial damage-control laparotomy, stapling or tying off the ends after resecting the injured area can be employed as a means to simply yet effectively manage colonic contamination. Anastomosis or colostomy is not necessary or needed during the initial surgery. An abundance of retrospective and prospective studies exist that both support and advocate colonic resection with primary anastomosis providing evidence of equal if not superior results to colostomy with respect to postoperative complications (Nelson & Singer 2003, Murray

Table 9.1 AAST colon injury scale

Grade	Injury	Description
I	Hematoma	Contusion/hematoma; no devascularization
	Laceration	Partial thickness, no perforation
II	Laceration	<50% of circumference
III	Laceration	>50% of circumference without transection
IV	Laceration	Transection of colon
V	Laceration/vascular	Transection of colon with segmental tissue loss/devascularized segment

AAST, American Association for the Surgery of Trauma

et al. 1999). Most trauma surgeons are in agreement when it comes to primary repair versus diverting ostomy, and evaluating the amount of bowel edema is crucial. Edematous bowel, which is usually secondary to large volume resuscitation, increases tension on an anastomosis and adds to the uncertainty in terms of healing. Colon repair performed 1–3 days later is felt to be safe and appropriate by most if the surgeon adheres to the principles and techniques outlined above.

Rectal repair

Anatomically, the rectum begins at the rectosigmoid junction and terminates distally at the dentate line, at which point the anus begins. The rectum can then be further divided into intraperitoneal or extraperitoneal segments. For extraperitoneal penetrating rectal injuries, much of the literature supports diverting colostomy without repair of the rectal injury itself as a safe and effective option (Navsaria et al. 2004, Velmahos et al. 2000). Another option to consider for extraperitoneal rectal injuries is primary repair via a transanal approach. This technique likewise does not require a diverting ostomy (Machado et al. 2005).

Intraperitoneal rectal injuries are managed similarly to colonic injuries thus the treatment of choice is primary repair without an ostomy (McGrath et al. 1998).

PANCREATIC INJURIES

Both blunt and penetrating pancreatic injuries are associated with a high rate of morbidity and mortality. Furthermore, early and accurate diagnosis can be challenging from either etiology. Fortunately, pancreatic injuries are rather rare when compared with other injuries, estimated to be the 10th most injured organ when compared with other abdominal organs. Thus, a pancreatic injury is quite uncommon especially in patients with blunt abdominal trauma. It is estimated that fewer than 10% will sustain a pancreatic injury. This number does become slightly higher in penetrating abdominal trauma where it is estimated to range from 20% to 30% (Nikeghbalian et al. 2012) for all grades of injury.

Pancreatic injuries are classified not only based on their location within the gland itself but also whether or not there is ductal injury (**Table 9.2**). Fortunately, as mentioned above, injuries to the pancreas itself are rare and ductal injury is rarer still and usually only results from penetrating trauma.

In the setting of a pancreatic injury, the principles of damage-control laparotomy remain unchanged. However, the intraoperative diagnosis of a pancreatic injury may not be obvious and does require careful inspection of the pancreas in its entirety. This involves opening of the lesser sac, a Kocher maneuver, and mobilization of the hepatic and splenic flexures. Once a pancreatic injury is identified, treatment is based on the AAST injury classification scale. Grade I and II injuries account for approximately 50% and 25% of all pancreatic injuries, respectively. These injuries that do not involve the pancreatic duct are best managed by sump drainage. Balasegaram et al. reviewed 91 pancreatic injuries of which 47 were blunt and 44 penetrating, deriving two major conclusions from their retrospective review. First, all mortality and the majority of morbidity resulted from pancreatic injuries grade III or higher. Second, of the 17 grade I and 15 grade II injuries that received drainage alone (either in the form of a Penrose or sump), or those who had suture repair, no deaths were noted. One mortality (1/35) was seen in a patient who had pancreatectomy. Furthermore, most postoperative complications were observed in patients who had undergone pancreatoduodenectomy or primary repair of a ductal injury. Thus, concluding that suture repair of an injured pancreatic duct should be abandoned in favor of resection (Balasegaram & Lumpur 1976).

Stone et al. looked at 283 trauma patients (227 penetrating) with a diagnosis of pancreatic injury made at the time of laparotomy and their subsequent management over 30 years (Stone et al. 1981). Eighty-seven percent of patients were managed by drainage alone and 11% with resection. Those patients who had undergone resection had injuries in which the injury itself had performed the majority of the resection. Penrose drainage was used in 41 patients, while sump drainage was utilized in 198 patients. Pancreatic morbidity decreased from 46% to 2% with the change to sump drainage. They concluded that drainage without debridement is adequate for minor injuries and that sump (rather than Penrose) drains should be used. Of note, it is unclear what the grades of injuries were in this investigation; however, the implication is that they are referring to the management of grades I and II injuries. Leppaniemi et al. examined 43 patients with acute blunt pancreatic injury (Leppaniemi & Haapiainen 1994). There were 21 AAST grade I/II injuries and the remainder were AAST grades III or higher. Drainage or drainage and suture were used in 19/21 grade I patients with a low complication rate. When pancreatic injuries that involved the duct were not resected but simply treated with sump drainage alone, the fistula rate was 80% compared with 18%, furthering the idea that pancreatic injuries of grades III or higher require more than drainage alone.

From the above we can conclude that pancreatic AAST grade I/II injuries require adequate sump drainage, which yields very good results with low morbidity. For grade III and higher injuries, or those that explicitly involve the duct, drainage alone is not adequate. Resection with drainage is the procedure of choice for these injuries. Furthermore, distal parenchymal transection with disruption of pancreatic duct is best treated by distal pancreatectomy. The remaining proximal duct if normal (which can be confirmed with an intraoperative pancreatography) is identified and closed with a nonabsorbable monofilament 'U'-stitch suture ligature (Fitzgibbons and Yellin 1982).

The pancreatic parenchyma itself can be closed with the 4.8 mm TA-55 stapler (Andersen & Bolman 1980). However, some have found that this method excessively crushes the residual pancreas. Alternatively, a full-thickness mattress suture can be placed from the anterior to the posterior aspects of the capsule. This technique helps to minimize leaking from the parenchyma. Transected pancreatic parenchyma can be buttressed with an omental patch with a drain placed near the transection line.

An injury to the proximal pancreas in which duct involvement has occurred presents a very challenging scenario. The hallmarks of

Table 9.2 AAST pancreatic injury scale

Grade	Injury	Description
I	Hematoma/laceration	Minor contusion/superficial laceration. No ductal injury
II	Laceration/hematoma	Major contusion/laceration. No ductal injury
III	Laceration	Distal transection or parenchymal injury and duct injury
IV	Laceration	Proximal transection or parenchymal injury
V	Laceration	Massive injury to pancreatic head

AAST, American Association for the Surgery of Trauma

damage-control laparotomy still apply; however, the duct anatomy must be clearly identified in order to devise the best treatment strategy. This can be done simply by visually inspecting the area of injury or it can require more advanced techniques of intraoperative pancreatography. Most trauma surgeons would agree that a duodenotomy is not the procedure of choice, but rather a cholecystocholangiopancreatography that allows simultaneous visualization of the distal common bile and pancreatic ducts. If the duct cannot be seen and its anatomy cannot be defined, the procedure of choice is wide external drainage via placement of several closed suction drains.

This should be followed by early postoperative endoscopic retrograde cholangiopancreatography (ERCP). In the event that ERCP reveals a proximal duct injury, stenting should be the first option rather than a subtotal pancreatectomy (Huckfeldt & Agee 1996). If the ampulla and duodenum remain uninjured, two options are available: a subtotal pancreatectomy with wide drainage or a Roux-en-Y pancreaticojejunostomy using the uninjured tail of the pancreas. The latter remains exceedingly rare and only a handful of cases exist in the literature. Both Patton and Duchesne have demonstrated persuasive evidence for the efficiency of drainage as the sole modality of treatment instead of an extended pancreatectomy, in particular for suspected proximal pancreatic gland injury when the duct status is unclear (Duchesne & Schmieg 2008, Patton & Lyden 1997). It is important to note that in the Patton study of 37 patients, a pancreatography was never performed so the status of the duct was never known. He also had an acceptable 13.5% fistula/abscess rate.

LIVER INJURIES

'Rupture of the liver is fortunately an accident not often met with, but one that, when it is seen, may be associated with a condition of the patient as serious as any one can meet with in surgical practice.' So wrote J. Hogarth Pringle in his 1908 article, 'Notes on the Arrest of Hepatic Hemorrhage due to Trauma,' in which he described the now eponymous Pringle maneuver (Pringle 1908). In the intervening century since Pringle wrote this seminal work and the 140 years since Bruns reported the first hepatic resection for the treatment of a gunshot wound to the liver (Ackroyd & Pollard 1969), much debate has ensued about the optimal method of treating hepatic injuries as they remain some of the most formidable and potentially lethal injuries.

Tilton, in 1904, reviewed the literature and reported on 189 liver injuries. With respect to nonoperative management of liver injuries, he wrote, 'This seems a wrong principle to work on. Many cases might recover without interference but others will prove fatal from oversight, an intestinal perforation or foreign body or from insufficient drainage of the wound in the liver.' However, with the introduction of diagnostic peritoneal lavage by Root in 1965 and the advent of CT scanning in 1981, it was recognized that not all liver injuries required operative intervention. Indeed, hepatic injuries grade I and II in the absence of other injuries do not mandate surgery. Consequently, there has been a considerable shift in the management of these injuries over the past 40 years. It is estimated that 80% of blunt liver trauma is now managed nonoperatively (Polanco & Leon 2008).

Grade III, IV, and V liver injuries, collectively referred to as complex or devastating, generally do require surgery as risk of exsanguination increases with increasing injury grade (**Table 9.3**). World War II marked a shift in the treatment of these injuries, as prior to the war surgeons often employed either expectant management or perihepatic packing for the treatment of liver injury. However, due to the high rates of perihepatic abscesses and hepatic necrosis that frequently occurred with this treatment, more aggressive strategies, including ligation, hepatorrhaphy, and anatomic resection, were adopted and mortality rates dropped significantly from 1944 through the end of the war (Trunkey 2004).

Through the 1960s, anatomic hepatic resection was widely used but eventually abandoned because of persistently, unacceptably high morbidity and mortality (Strong & Lynch 1998). Over the next half century, despite improved antibiotics, hemostatic adjuncts and greater understanding and manipulation of physiology and critical care death secondary to complex liver trauma remained high. Some even continue to propose that the lack of progress with respect to liver injuries may be because the pathophysiology of liver injury may itself be too devastating or because 'We have the difficult circumstance as trauma surgeons of infrequently needing to operate on the liver for trauma, but when operation is required, it is technically challenging with high mortality' (Polanco et al. 2008). Stone made significant strides in the management of complex liver injuries after the introduction of the damage-control laparotomy in 1983.

Rotondo and Schwab subsequently described a three-phase procedure for patients with devastating abdominal injuries and coined

Table 9.3 AAST liver injury scale*

Grade	Injury	Description
I	Hematoma	Subcapsular (<10% surface area)
	Laceration	Capsular (<1 cm parenchymal depth)
II	Hematoma	Subcapsular (10–50% surface area) or intraparenchymal (<10 cm diameter)
	Laceration	1–3 cm parenchymal depth, <10 cm length
III	Hematoma	Subcapsular: >50% surface area or expanding or ruptured. Parenchymal: ruptured. Intraparenchymal: >10 cm or expanding
	Laceration	>3 cm parenchymal depth
IV	Laceration	Parenchymal disruption involving 25–75% of a lobe or 1–3 segments of a lobe
V	Laceration	Parenchymal disruption involving >75% of a lobe or >3 segments of a lobe
	Vascular	Juxtahepatic veins: retrohepatic vena cava or central major hepatic veins
VI	Vascular	Hepatic avulsion

*Advance one grade for multiple injuries to same organ up to Grade III (Polanco et al. 2008).

AAST, American Association for the Surgery of Trauma.

it 'damage control surgery.' 'Damage control surgery' or 'abbreviated laparotomy' is perhaps most suitable for patients with liver injuries, who frequently present in shock and already with the lethal triad of acidosis, coagulopathy, and hypothermia. By 1985, there were ringing endorsements for the packing of hepatic injuries from Moore and Feliciano. In the paper, 'Nonresectional Management of Major Hepatic Trauma – An Evolving Concept,' Moore et al. continued to recognize an 'alarming' 70% mortality rate for patients treated with lobectomy and advocated a shift to packing hepatic wounds. He concluded that there were no instances of death from exsanguination in his series of patients treated with packing and no increase in delayed death from sepsis.

Feliciano in a discussion response at the end of the article wrote, '...we are absolutely convinced that this is the correct procedure when a patient is hypothermic, acidotic and has nonmechanical bleeding' (Moore et al. 1985). Definitive repair of complex hepatic injuries, which even in the most experienced and surgically adept hands is always time consuming, can exacerbate an unstable patient's condition and therefore generally should not be attempted during an initial surgery, unless abdominal packing does not stop the hemorrhage. One prospective study of 293 polytrauma patients between 1996 and 2008 found revised trauma score, hemodynamic instability, and pH and base excess to be prognostic for morbidity and mortality, concluding that 'fast and effective' damage-control surgery with perihepatic packing and early ICU admission is associated with lower complication rates and shorter ICU stays (Di Saverio & Catena 2014).

The decision of when to take a patient back for pack removal has been debated for some time and was looked at by Caruso et al. in a study comparing pack removal at 36 and 72 hours post-op. Though the characteristics were not significantly different between the two groups, they found complication rates to be similar. The group that had shorter intervals to pack removal did have higher rates of rebleeding (Caruso & Battistella 1999). Other studies have corroborated their findings and similarly found no increased rates of intra-abdominal infection for those patients with packs left in longer. As such, the corollary can be drawn that patients should be taken for pack removal and definitive repair, only once they have been fully resuscitated with complete correction of acidosis, coagulopathy, and hypothermia.

In preparation for a second-look procedure, the operating room should be warmed, equipped with an adequate retraction system such as a Rochard rib retractor, an argon-beam coagulator, or ultrasonic dissector as well as hemostatic agents such as gelfoam, surgicel, and fibrin glue. Blood products should be available on standby, if not already in the operating room, in case transfusion is needed. In addition, a cell saver for autotransfusion can be used, provided that the patient does not have any concomitant hollow viscous injury.

Upon judicial removal of abdominal packing, with care not to disturb any adherent clots, the liver should be inspected for ongoing hemorrhage. Bleeding that has not been controlled by packing is usually suggestive of a complex hepatic injury. If not already done so in the first procedure, the falciform, coronary, and triangular ligaments should be taken down. After these peritoneal attachments have been taken down, a Pringle maneuver to gain control of the hepatic arterial and venous inflow should be performed. Although prospective studies looking at maximal inflow occlusion time have not to our knowledge been reported, several authors suggest that in the case of trauma an hour of vascular occlusion is generally acceptable. Focus can then be turned to control of any injured vessels, bile ducts, and nonviable tissue. One of the advantages of delayed definitive repair of hepatic injury during second-look procedures is that time allows for the delineation of nonviable hepatic tissue, which can then be easily debrided manually or with the assistance of an electrocautery or argon beam. Strong makes the distinction between 'partial resection' that removes the injured, devascularized liver peripheral to the fracture line and 'resectional debridement' that is limited to the removal of nonviable liver that borders the injured site (Strong et al. 1998). Access to injured vessels and bile ducts can be gained via finger fracture through the injury tract or tractotomy. Simple suture ligature or clips in combination with electrocautery can be employed to control the injured structures. Alternatively, a GIA stapler can be used for injuries on the liver's edge. It is generally recommended to avoid deep parenchymal sutures because of the risk of tissue necrosis and injuring nondamaged vessels and bile ducts. If bleeding has been controlled with these simple measures, but a deep recess remains in the body of the liver, omentum can be buttressed into the dead space.

In the event that these maneuvers do not control bleeding, Trunkey advocates using the Heaney technique to gain additional vascular control. This involves complete mobilization of the right lobe of the liver, placing a Satinsky clamp across the suprahepatic vena cava and a Rummel tourniquet around the porta hepatis. Although there have been many descriptions of atrial-caval shunts or veno-veno bypass for the repair of devastating hepatic injuries, outcomes remain dismal for these procedures. If bleeding is noted from the confluence of the hepatic veins and vena cava, it may be necessary to perform a sternotomy and control the inferior vena cava from within the pericardium. Trunkey further stresses that clamping the aorta is not beneficial in this instance, unless there is a suspected concomitant injury to the abdominal aorta. Clamping of the aorta does not control bleeding from the liver and only serves to exacerbate acidosis and reperfusion injury (Trunkey 2004).

Finally, no discussion about the management of hepatic trauma would be completed with acknowledging the debate between formal lobectomy and resectional debridement. In 1979, Mays reported 'major resection should be done only when an entire lobe of the liver is reduced to pulp' (Kozar & Feliciano 2014). However, some advocates of formal lobectomy claim that when performed by specialists, mortality is significantly reduced with anatomic lobectomy. Strong et al. reported a series of 287 trauma patients, 37 with severe liver trauma, who underwent anatomic resection with an overall mortality of 8.1%. and liver-related morbidity of 19% (Strong et al. 1998). Trunkey touts this outcome as a 'gold standard.' Following Strong's recommendation that severe liver trauma be managed by hepatobiliary specialists or transplant surgeons, a referral system has been set up in Birmingham, England, to shift management of complex liver injures to specialized facilities. In a prospective audit of 99 patients treated for liver injury between 2001 and 2008, they achieved successful perihepatic packing in 77% of patients and overall mortality between 10% and 15% (Ramkumar & Perera 2014), on par with Strong's results. These same rates of success however are being achieved by trauma surgeons in the United States. Polanco et al. reported a 15-year retrospective observational study of grade III, IV, and V complex liver injuries in 216 patients at the University of Pittsburgh. Trauma surgeons performed the hepatic resection 77% of the time. They utilized a range of techniques including segmentectomies, nonatomic resections, lobectomies, and total hepatectomy with liver transplant and achieved an admirable 9% liver mortality rate (Polanco et al. 2008). While the debate will continue to ensue, each of these studies corroborate that the most important determinant in outcome of hepatic injuries is not who or which surgeons perform the intervention, but familiarity and facility with treating them.

URINARY RECONSTRUCTION

Ureter repair

Ureteral injury is a rare phenomenon, accounting for only 1% of all genitourinary trauma. Genitourinary tract injuries overall account for <5% of all trauma and <10% of penetrating trauma injuries (Pereira & Ogilvie 2014). However, missed ureter injuries can be a significant source of morbidity and mortality in the multiply injured patient, including retroperitoneal abscesses, infected urinomas, and fistulae, and even pancreaticoureteral fistulas have been reported (Wolf & Miller 2007). Fortunately, the ureters are highly amenable to delayed repair (function is not compromised by delayed repair) and therefore conducive to attention during second-look or reoperative procedures after damage-control laparotomy, allowing the trauma surgeon to focus on more life-threatening injuries during the initial operative procedure (Azimuddin & Ivatury 1997). Furthermore, because the extent of damage and the viability of ureteral tissue may only become apparent after a time has elapsed from the initial traumatic event, by controlling urine extravastation, ureteral functional integrity can be maintained by addressing the injury only after a patient is stabilized and taken for reoperation.

Tucked away in the retroperitoneum, the ureters are protected by the bony pelvis, psoas muscle, and vertebrae, which help account for their low rate of injury. However, their relationship to the duodenum, tail of the pancreas, and inferior vena cava should raise the suspicion of a ureteral injury when any of these other structures are compromised by trauma. In a comprehensive literature review of 81 articles about trauma-related ureteral injuries, 90.4% of patients had associated injuries (Wolf et al. 2007). The key to successful recognition, repair, and preservation of function is a high index of suspicion for injury based on force, trajectory, and mechanism. **Table 9.4** outlines grading for ureteral injuries (Fraga & Borges 2007).

If a ureteral injury is obvious during an initial damage-control surgery, immediate diversion should be employed, provided that the surgeon is familiar with the technique. A temporizing 'single-J' stent can be utilized to externalize the flow of urine (Coburn 1997). This is accomplished by placing the stent through the transected or lacerated ureter and passing it proximally to the level of the kidney. The internal guidewire is removed and the stent is tied in place with a 3-0 silk, incorporating 1–2 mm of ureteral tissue within the tie. Care must be taken not to cause further trauma to the ureter. The stent is then brought out through a separate stab incision. It is important not to ligate the distal ureteral stump and to avoid handling, debriding, or ligating the remainder of the ureter. This will be addressed during the subsequent procedure.

Alternatively, the proximal ureter can be ligated with placement of a nephrostomy tube either intraoperatively during the abbreviated laparotomy for trauma or postoperatively by radiology, once the patient has been stabilized. Unlike with bowel injuries, as a worst-case scenario, the injured ureter can be left alone and although urine will collect intra-abdominally, it can be dealt with during an interval procedure. In this event, patients should be covered with broad-spectrum antibiotics (Brandes & Coburn 2004).

Definitive repair of the ureters during reoperative surgery focuses on key elements that include debridement, mobilization, spatulation, creation of a tension-free, and watertight anastomosis, isolation from other intra-abdominal injuries, and drainage of the retroperitoneum (Ahn & Loughlin 2001). Reconstruction of damaged ureters depends on the location of the injury. Injuries to the upper third may be repaired with a uretero-ureterostomy or a ureteropyelostomy; injuries to the middle third may be repaired with uretero-ureterostomy, transuretero-ureterostomy, or a Baori flap. Transuretero-ureterostomy has fallen out of favor as a repair option since the popular consensus is that it jeopardizes the integrity of the contralateral kidney. For this reason, the technique will not be described further. Finally, injuries to the lower third of the ureter may be repaired with a ureteroneocystostomy (via direct reimplantation) or via a psoas hitch (ureteroneocystostomy). **Table 9.5** represents the reconstructive options, based on location of ureter injury (Wolf et al. 2007).

For the creation of a direct uretero-ureterostomy in either the upper or middle third of the ureter, following steps are simple (**Figure 9.1**):

1. Debride devitalized tissue with great care not to injure the fragile surrounding tissue
2. Spatulate the ends to prevent stricture formation or stenosis
3. Place a double J stent
4. Use absorbable sutures to form the anastomosis and place stay sutures on either side of the injury
5. Check to ensure the anastomosis is tension free
6. Isolate the repair from other injuries with omentum
7. Place a closed suction drain

For middle third injuries to the ureter, the Baori flap, is utilized by trauma surgeons if it can be completed efficiently and without tension on the anastomosis (**Figure 9.2**). This involves distal ureter resection

Table 9.4 AAST ureteral injury scale

Grade	Injury
I	Contusion or hematoma
II	Laceration: <50% transection
III	Laceration: <50% transection
IV	Laceration: 100% transection, <2 cm devascularization
V	Laceration: avulsion with >2 cm devascularization

AAST, American Association for the Surgery of Trauma.

Table 9.5 Reconstructive options based on injury location

Upper third	Uretero-ureterostomy (**Figure 9.1**)
	Ureteropyelostomy
Middle third	Uretero-ureterostomy
	Transuretero-ureterostomy
	Anterior wall bladder flap (Baori) (**Figure 9.2**)
Lower third	Ureteroneocystostomy (direct reimplantation)
	Ureteroneocystostomy (psoas hitch) (**Figure 9.3**)

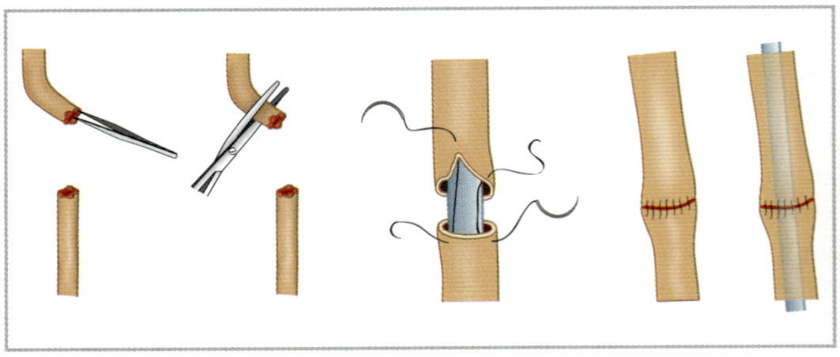

Figure 9.1 Uretero-uretostomy. Courtesy of Wolf et al. (2007).

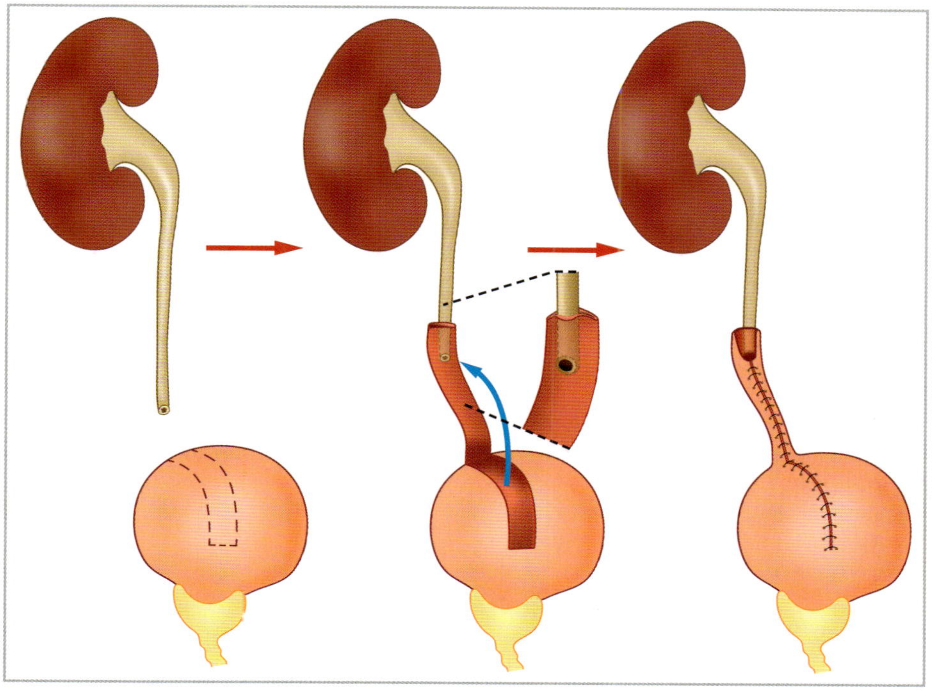

Figure 9.2 Baori flap. Courtesy of Wolf et al. (2007).

down to the level of the retrovesicular junction and creation of a rectangular flap of bladder tissue. The bladder is closed primarily, while the flap is fashioned into a tube, allowing for deep implantation of the distal ureter into the tube (Jacobs et al. 2004).

The psoas hitch ureteral reimplantation, used for lower third injuries to the ureters, was first described by Zimmerman et al. in 1960, though several modifications have since been described (**Figure 9.3**) (Jacobs et al. 2004). When there is loss of ureteral domain due to trauma to the lowest part of the ureter or in the event that there is too much tension on a Baori flap, the psoas hitch may be employed. This technique requires mobilization of the bladder, often by ligating the obliterated umbilical vein contralateral to the side of injury. The bladder is then sutured to the psoas tendon with a 2-0 Vicryl stitch, with care not to injure the surrounding neurovascular structures. The distal portion of the injured ureter is resected to viable tissue and the distal healthy end of ureter is implanted into the bladder. Some advocate positioning away from the dome of the bladder, while others advocate implanting it squarely on the anterior surface of the bladder. Whichever location is chosen for the anastomosis, the ureterovesicular junction must be ligated. Finally, a closed-suction drain is placed before abdominal closure.

Other procedures to repair ureters, specifically when there is significant loss of ureteral length, including ileal and appendiceal conduits are beyond the scope of this chapter.

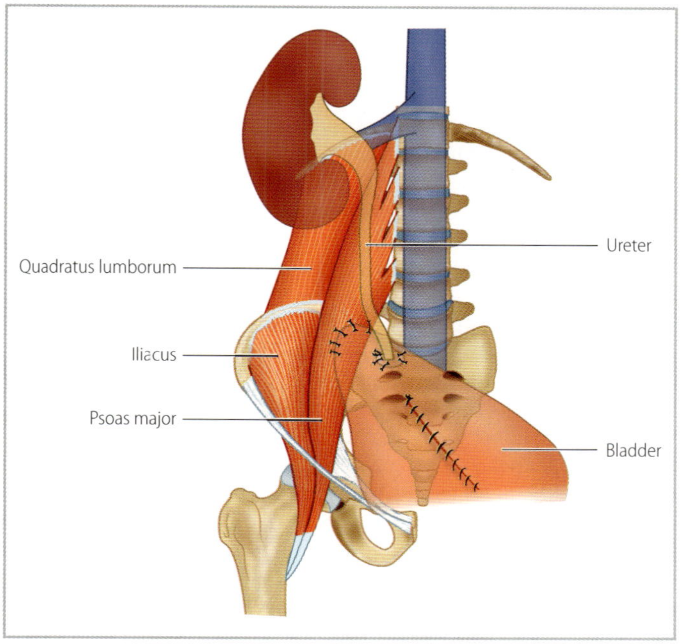

Figure 9.3 Psoas hitch. Courtesy of Wolf et al. (2007).

Kidney repair

Massive hemorrhage from a kidney injury accompanied with hemodynamic instability mandates immediate nephrectomy during the initial procedure (Brandes et al. 2004). However, Gerota's fascia acts as a natural anatomic tamponade and therefore unless the perinephric hematoma is pulsatile, expanding, or there is active blood extruding from the fascia, the injury needs not to be explored during the initial procedure, especially if the patient is too unstable due to bleeding from other injuries. If there is concern about the viability of a kidney and there is no risk of compromising a tamponaded hematoma, a small incision in Gerota's fascia can be made to confirm perfusion. Traditionally, urologists are taught to preoperatively confirm the presence of two functioning kidneys prior to performing a nephrectomy. In the critically injured hemodynamically unstable patient undergoing a damage-control procedure, this is a luxury not available. Palpating for a contralateral kidney or the administration of methylene blue, while occluding the ureter on the injured side, can confirm the presence of a functioning second kidney. However, nephrectomizing a solitary kidney is still preferred in a critical patient exsanguinating from a solitary kidney injury.

The salient points to renal exploration and repair are adequate exposure and control of the vascular pedicle. The latter avoids an unnecessary nephrectomy. Most authors recommend stenting or nephrostomy diversion when delayed reconstruction is necessary. The risk of postoperative urinary extravasation is higher than in primary repairs since tissues are more edematous, friable, and collecting systems (if not previously diverted) are more congested. Whenever a nephrectomy is performed, a ureterectomy is mandated as well, in theory to decrease the future risk of developing transitional cell carcinoma and ureteral calculi. However, this can be performed after the patient has been stabilized and brought to operating room for a second definitive procedure. This can be accomplished simply by following the ureter down from the kidney or alternatively locating its position as it crosses the common iliac artery. The ureter passes anteriorly to the artery and can be traced proximally. Upon completion of the ureterectomy, the vesicoureteral junction must be ligated.

To obtain maximal renal exposure, a medial visceral rotation on the left or right is mandated. Performing a Kocher maneuver facilitates exposure of the right kidney. For immediate vascular control, a vascular clamp can be placed across both the artery and vein, although digital dissection may be utilized to deliver the kidney more quickly. Once the kidney is elevated, manual compression can be applied, followed by clamping of the renal pedicle. This is then followed by debridement and evaluation of the extent of injury. Options for definitive repair can be based on the AAST's organ injury scale (**Table 9.6**) (http://www.trauma.org/index.php/main/article/809/).

Grade I injuries, if isolated, are usually managed nonoperatively. Grade V injuries generally necessitate nephrectomy, the technique for which has already been described. It is therefore grade II–IV injuries that will be addressed.

Grade II and III injuries are cortical lacerations <1 cm or >1 cm, respectively, with an intact calyx. A renorrhaphy is appropriate for this type of injury and can be accomplished with absorbable, interrupted sutures that are both hemostatic and hydrostatic. Pledgets are used for renal parenchyma. Some authors recommend a mesh wrap, though the pledgeted repair is more commonly performed (http://www.trauma.org/index.php/main/article/809/). The retroperitoneum should be drained with a closed-suction drain following repair.

Finally, grade IV injuries are those that involve injury to the collecting system. Repair should only be undertaken once the patient is fully stabilized, which is why the vast majority of these injuries are treated with nephrectomy. If attempt at calyceal repair is to be made, only fine, absorbable sutures should be used so the sutures do not become a nidus for calculus formation. The repair must be watertight to prevent development of a urinoma. As with all of the previous repairs, upon completion, a drain should be placed.

As with all surgical procedures, outcome is highly dependent on the surgeon's familiarity with the operative procedure. In trauma even more so, success and patient survival are dependent on surgical skill. In the event that the surgeon is unfamiliar with renal or ureteral injury repair, it is strongly recommended to collaborate with urologists, who may be able to assist in both the planning and execution of the repair procedure.

Table 9.6 AAST renal injury scale

Grade	Injury	Description
I	Contusion	Microscopic/gross hematuria. Normal urological studies
	Hematoma	Subcapsular, nonexpanding; no parenchymal laceration
II	Hematoma	Nonexpanding perirenal,confined to renal retroperitoneum
	Laceration	Parenchymal, <1 cm depth of cortex; no urinary extravasation
III	Laceration	Parenchymal, >1 cm depth of cortex; no collecting system rupture or urinary extravasation
IV	Laceration	Parenchymal, extending through cortex, medulla, and collecting system
	Vascular	Injury to main renal artery/vein, with contained hemorrhage
V	Laceration	Shattered kidney
	Vascular	Avulsion of renal hilum, devascularizing kidney

AAST, American Association for the Surgery of Trauma.

REFERENCES

Ackroyd FW, Pollard J, McDermott WV Jr. Massive hepatic resection in the treatment of severe liver trauma. Am J Surg 1969; 117:442–448.

Ahn M, Loughlin KR. Psoas hitch ureteral reimplantation in adults–analysis of a modified technique and timing of repair. Urology 2001; 58:184–187.

Andersen DK, Bolman RM 3rd, Moylan JA Jr. Management of penetrating pancreatic injuries: subtotal pancreatectomy using the auto suture stapler. J Trauma 1980; 20:347–349.

Asensio JA, Trunkey DD. Current therapy of trauma and surgical critical care Philadelphia, PA: Mosby Elsevier, 2008.

Azimuddin KR, Ivatury R, Porter J, Allman DB. Damage control in a trauma patient with ureteric injury. J Trauma 1997; 43:977–979.

Balasegaram M, Lumpur K. Surgical management of pancreatic trauma. Am J Surg 1976; 131:536–540.

Behran SW, Bertken KA, Stefanacci HA, Parks SN. Breakdown of intestinal repair after laparotomy for trauma: Incidence, risk factors and strategies for prevention. J Trauma 1998; 45:227–233.

Brandes S, Coburn M, Armenakas N, McAninch J. Diagnosis and management of ureteric injury: an evidence-based analysis. BJU Int 2004; 94:277–289.

Brundage SI, Jurkovich GJ, Hoyt DB, et al. Stapled versus sutured gastrointestinal anastomosis in the trauma patient. J Trauma 1999; 3:500.

Burch JM, Ortiz VB, Richardson RJ, et al. Abbreviated laparotomy and planned reoperation for critically injured patients. Ann Surg 1992; 215:476–482.

Carrillo C, Fogler RJ, Shaftan GW. Delayed gastrointestinal reconstruction following massive abdominal trauma. J Trauma 1993; 34:233–235.

Caruso DM, Battistella FD, Owings JT, et al. Perihepatic packing of major liver injuries: complications and mortality. Arch Surg 1999; 134:958–962; discussion 962-3.

Chaudry CH. Cellular mechanisms in shock and ischemia and their correction. Am J Physiol 1983; 245:R117.

Coburn M. Damage control for urologic injuries. Surg Clin North Am 1997; 77:821–834.

Di Saverio S, Catena F, Filicori F, et al. Predictive factors of morbidity and mortality in grade IV and V liver trauma undergoing perihepatic packing: single institution 14 years experience at European trauma centre. Injury 2012; 43:1347–1354.
Duchesne JC, Schmieg R, Islam S, et al. Selective nonoperative management of low-grade blunt pancreatic injury: are we there yet? J Trauma 2008; 65:49–53.
Durham CM, Siegel JH, Weireter LJ, et al. Oxygen debt and the metabolic academia as quantitative predictors of mortality and the severity of the ischemic insult in hemorrhagic shock. Crit Care Med 1999; 19:231.
Feliciano DV, Mattox KL, Jordan GL. Intra-abdominal packing for control of hepatic hemorrhage: a reappraisal. J Trauma 1981; 21:285–290.
Feliciano DV, Mattox KL, Moore EE. Trauma, 7th edition New York: McGraw Hill Companies, 2012.
Fitzgibbons TJ, Yellin AE, Maruyama MM, Donovan AJ. Management of the transected pancreas following distal pancreatectomy. Surg Gynecol Obstet 1982; 154:225–231.
Fraga GP, Borges GM, Mantovani M, et al. Penetrating ureteral trauma. Int Braz J Urol 2007; 33:142–148, discussion 149–150.
Hirshberg, A, Mattox KL. Planned reoperation for severe trauma. Ann Surg 1995; 222:3–8.
Hirshberg A, Mattox KL. Top Knife . Harley, UK: TFM Publishing Ltd, 2004.
Hirshberg A, Stein M, Adar R. Damage control surgery. Surg Clin North America 1997; 77:4.
Hirshberg A, Wall MJ, Allen MK, et al. Causes and patterns of missed injuries in trauma. Am J Surg 1994; 168:229.
Hirshberg A, Wall MJ, Mattox KL. Planned reoperation for trauma: a two year experience with 124 consecutive patients. J Trauma 1994; 37:365–369.
Huckfeldt R, Agee C, Nichols WK, Barthel J. Nonoperative treatment of traumatic pancreatic duct disruption using endoscopically placed stent. J Trauma 1996; 41:143–144.
Jacobs L, Gross RI, Luk SS. Advanced trauma operative management. Woodbury, CT, Cine-Med, Inc, 2004.
Jurkovich GJ, Greiser WB, Luterman A, et al. Hypothermia in trauma victims: An ominous predictor of survival. J Trauma 1987; 27:1019.
Kashuk JL, Moore EE, Millikan JS, Moore JB. Major abdominal vascular trauma: a unified approach. J Trauma 1982; 22:672–679.
Kauvar DS, Lefering R, Wade CE. Impact of hemorrhage on trauma outcome: An overview of epidemiology, clinical presentations, and therapeutic considerations. J Trauma 2006; 60:S3–S11.
Kearns SR, Connoly EM, McNally S, et al. Randomized clinical trial of diathermy versus scalpel incision in elective midline laparotomy. Br J Surg 2001; 88:41.
Ketchum L, Hess JR, Hiippala S. Indications for early fresh frozen plasma, cryoprecipitate, and plate et transfusion in trauma. J Trauma 2006; 60:S51.
AAST Organ Injury Scale Scores for the Kidney. Trauma.org 2009. www.trauma.org/index.php/main/article/809/ (accessed 8 May 2014)
Kingham TP, Pachter HL. Colonic anastomotic leak: risk factors, diagnosis and treatment. J Am Coll Surg 2009; 208:269–278.
Kozar RA, Feliciano DV, Moore EE, et al. Western Trauma Association/critical decisions in trauma: operative management of adult blunt hepatic trauma. J Trauma 2011; 71:1–5.
Leppaniemi AK, Haapiainen RK. Pancreatic trauma with proximal duct injury. Ann Chir Gynaecol 1994; 83:191–195.
Lucas CE, Ledgerwood AM. Prospective evaluation of hemostatic techniques for liver injuries. J Trauma 1976; 16:442–451.
Machado GR, Bojalia MO, Reeves ME. Transanal endoscopic repair of rectal anastomotic defect. Arch Surg 2005; 140:1219.
Martin RR, Byrne M. Postoperative care and complications of damage control surgery. Surg Clin of North Am 1997; 77:929–942.
McGrath V, Fabian TC, Croce MA, et al.: Rectal trauma: Management based on anatomic distinctions. Am Surg 1998; 64:1136.
Mikhail J. The trauma triad of death: Hypothermia, acidosis and coagulopathy. AACN Clinical Issues. 1999; 10:85–94.
Miller RS, Morris JA Jr. , Diaz J Jr, Complications after 344 damage-control early celiotomies. J Trauma 2005; 59:1365.
Moore EE. Staged laparotomy for hypothermia, acidosis and coagulopathy syndrome. Am J Surg 1996; 172:405–410.
Moore FA, Moore EE, Seagraves AA. Nonresectional management of major hepatic trauma. An evolving concept. Am J Surg 1985; 150:725–729.
Murray JA, Demetriades D, Colson M, et al. Colonic resection in trauma: colostomy versus anastomosis. J Trauma 1999; 46:250.
Murray CJL, Lopez AD (eds). The global burden of disease. Geneva, Switzerland: World Health Organization, 1996.
Nasirkhan MU, Abir F, Longo W, Kozol R. Anastomotic disruption after large bowel resection. World J Gastroenterol 2006; 12:2497–2504.
Navsaria PH, Shae JM, Sellweger R, et al. Diagnostic laparoscopy and diverting sigmoid loop colostomy in the management of civilian extraperitoneal rectal gunshot injuries. Br J Surg 2004; 91:460.
Nelson R, Singer M. Primary repair for penetrating colon injuries. Cochrane Database Syst Rev 2003; 3:CD002247.
Nikeghbalian S, Akrami M, Fazelzadeh A. Late development of pancreatitis following gunshot trauma, a case report. Iran Red Crescent Med J. 2012; 14:584–586
Patton JH Jr, Lyden SP, Croce MA, et al. Pancreatic trauma: a simplified management guideline. J Trauma 1997; 43:234–239; discussion 239–241.
Pereira BM, Ogilvie MP, Gomez-Rodriguez JC, et al. A review of ureteral injuries after external trauma. Scand J Trauma Resusc Emerg Med 2010; 18:6.
Polanco P, Leon S, Pineda J, et al. Hepatic resection in the management of complex injury to the liver. J Trauma 2008; 65:1264–1269; discussion 1269–1270.
Pringle JH. V. Notes on the Arrest of Hepatic Hemorrhage Due to Trauma. Ann Surg 1908; 48:541–549.
Ramkumar K, Perera MT, Marudanayagam R, et al. A reaudit of specialist-managed liver trauma after establishment of regional referral and management guidelines. J Trauma 2010; 68:84–89.
Reed RL, Johnston TD, Hudson JD, et al. The disparity between hypothermic coagulopathy and clotting studies. J Trauma 1992; 33:465.
Rotondo MF, Schwab CW, McGonigal MD, et al. Damage control: an approach for improved survival in exsanguinating penetrating abdominal in jury. J Trauma 1993; 35:375–382.
Scott BJ, Welsh FJ, Pham HQ, et al. Early aggressive closure of the open abdomen. J Trauma 2006; 60:17.
Smith PC, Tweddell JS, Bessey PQ. Alternative approaches to abdominal wound closure in severely injured patients with massive visceral edema. J Trauma 1992; 32:16–20.
Stone HH, Fabian TC, Satiani B, Turkleson ML. Experiences in the management of pancreatic trauma. JOT 1981; 21:257–262.
Stone HH, Strom PR, Mullins RJ. Management of the major coagulopathy with onset during laparotomy. Ann Surg 1983; 197:532–535.
Strong RW, Lynch SV, Wall DR, Liu CL. Anatomic resection for severe liver trauma. Surgery 1998; 123:251–257.
Trunkey DD. Hepatic trauma: contemporary management. Surg Clin North Am 2004; 84:437–450.
Velmahos GC, Gomez H, Falabella A, et al. Operative management of civilian rectal gunshot wounds: simpler is better. Worl J Surg 2000; 24:114.
Walt AJ. The mythology of hepatic trauma – or Babel revisited. Am J Surg 1978; 135:12–18.
Watts DD, Trask A, Soeken K, et al. Hypothermic coagulopathy in trauma: effect of varying levels of hypothermia on enzyme speed, platelet function, and fibrinolytic activity. J Trauma 1998; 44:846.
Weg JG. Oxygen transport in adult respiratory distress syndrome and other acute circulatory problems: relationship of oxygen delivery and oxygen consumption. Crit Care Med 1991; 19:650.
Whipple AO. Surgical treatment of carcinoma of the ampullary region and head of the pancreas. Am J Surg 1938; 40:260–263.
WISQARS (Web-based Injury Statistics Query and Reporting System) fatal injuries: mortality reports. www.cdc.gov/injury/wisqars/fatal.html (accessed 8 May 2014)
Wolf JH, Miller G, Ashinoff R, et al. Pancreaticoureteral fistula following penetrating abdominal trauma. JOP 2007; 8:613–616.

Chapter 10 Urgent reoperative vascular surgery

Jessica L. Secor, K. Craig Kent

INTRODUCTION

As in every surgical specialty, reoperation for vascular procedural-related complications is sometimes an unavoidable occurrence. This is in part due to the complexity of the disease and a patient population with long-standing hypertension, diabetes mellitus, and widespread atherosclerosis. Despite aggressive medical management, vascular disease is progressive and reoperation for return of symptoms is also common. Although for many years traditional open surgery was the mainstay for the treatment of vascular disease, there is a growing number of endovascular techniques now available for initial disease treatment as well as for reintervention for complications or disease progression. The aim of this chapter is to highlight three of the most common arterial problems treated by vascular surgeons: carotid artery stenosis, abdominal aortic aneurysm (AAA), and lower extremity occlusive disease. Complications requiring reoperation related to both traditional surgical techniques and endovascular methods will be discussed as well as optimal approaches to treatment. In keeping with this book's intent, we begin with AAAs.

ABDOMINAL AORTIC ANEURYSM

Open surgical repair

Elective open surgical repair of AAAs has a well-established track record for being a durable procedure with a relatively low rate of surgical complication in appropriate surgical candidates. However, when complications do occur, many require immediate surgical reintervention.

Hemorrhage

In the early postoperative period, hemodynamic instability along with a falling hematocrit and poor response to transfusion should raise concern for ongoing hemorrhage. Emergent surgical exploration should be performed. Radiological imaging is not required and can delay a return to the operating room in an unstable patient. Upon reoperation, bleeding as the result of a technical error with an unligated lumbar vessel or anastomotic hemorrhage is the likely cause.

Ischemic colitis

The incidence of ischemic colitis following open AAA repair ranges from 1% to 3% (Miller et al. 2009). Patients may develop abdominal pain or rectal bleeding; however, fever, leukocytosis, or sepsis may be the initial manifestation. In patients for whom this diagnosis is suspected, colonoscopy is indicated. Mild cases can be treated with bowel rest and antibiotics. If full-thickness necrosis or perforation is suspected, return to the operating room for colonic resection is mandatory. There is generally no role for arterial reconstruction in these cases as the colonic damage is not reversible. The mortality associated with this complication is high, particularly if the diagnosis is made after the onset of perforation and peritonitis.

Infection and aortoenteric fistula

The incidence of infection after placement of a prosthetic aortic graft for AAA ranges from approximately 0.6% to 3% (Vogel et al. 2008). Patients often present in the first year after aneurysm repair with fever and leukocytosis; however, infection may also occur remotely from the initial surgery. Patients who develop nosocomial or surgical site infections are at increased risk of developing graft infection (Vogel et al. 2008). Patients with groin incisions are particularly predisposed and the presentation may include a wound infection or a draining sinus. Radiologic evidence supporting a graft infection includes perigraft fluid and air or focal thickening and tethering of the bowel immediately adjacent to the aorta. An example of a patient with infection after AAA repair is shown in **Figure 10.1**. An indium-labeled white blood cell scan may be positive in addition to positive blood cultures. Patients with an aortoenteric fistula often present with massive gastrointestinal bleeding. In addition to perigraft fluid and air, a computed tomography (CT) scan may demonstrate extravasation of contrast into a loop of bowel (Raman et al. 2012).

Operative management of graft infection typically involves one or two strategies: extra-anatomic bypass followed by graft explantation or inline reconstruction. The choice of procedure is made based on anatomical considerations and surgeon preference. For extra-anatomic bypass, usually an axillofemoral/femoral–femoral bypass is chosen. This is typically performed prior to graft explantation. If the patient is stable, over the next day or several days the graft is explanted with aggressive debridement (Reilly et al. 1987). The aortic stump is closed in two layers and should be covered with omentum if possible to help prevent stump disruption. Options for inline reconstruction include cryopreserved allografts, antibiotic-soaked prosthetic grafts, or autologous vein grafts. Inline reconstruction avoids the need for multiple operations and eliminates the issue of aortic stump blowout (Vogt 2011). However, the trade-off is the potential for the new graft/conduit that is placed through an infected field to also become infected.

Anastomotic aneurysms

Another complication requiring reintervention after open AAA repair is an anastomotic aneurysm. The reported incidence of anastomotic aneurysms ranges from 1% to 5%. These aneurysms may develop as a result of suturing to an already aneurysmal artery, tension on the anastomosis, progressive aneurysmal disease, or graft infection. An example of an anastomotic aneurysm that developed after AAA repair is shown in **Figure 10.2**. The majority of anastomotic aneurysms will develop late. The risk of rupture is relatively high, in that a pseudoaneurysm is a full-thickness defect in the arterial wall. Anastomotic aneurysms can also thrombose, embolize, or erode into adjacent structures. The recommendation is to intervene regardless of size.

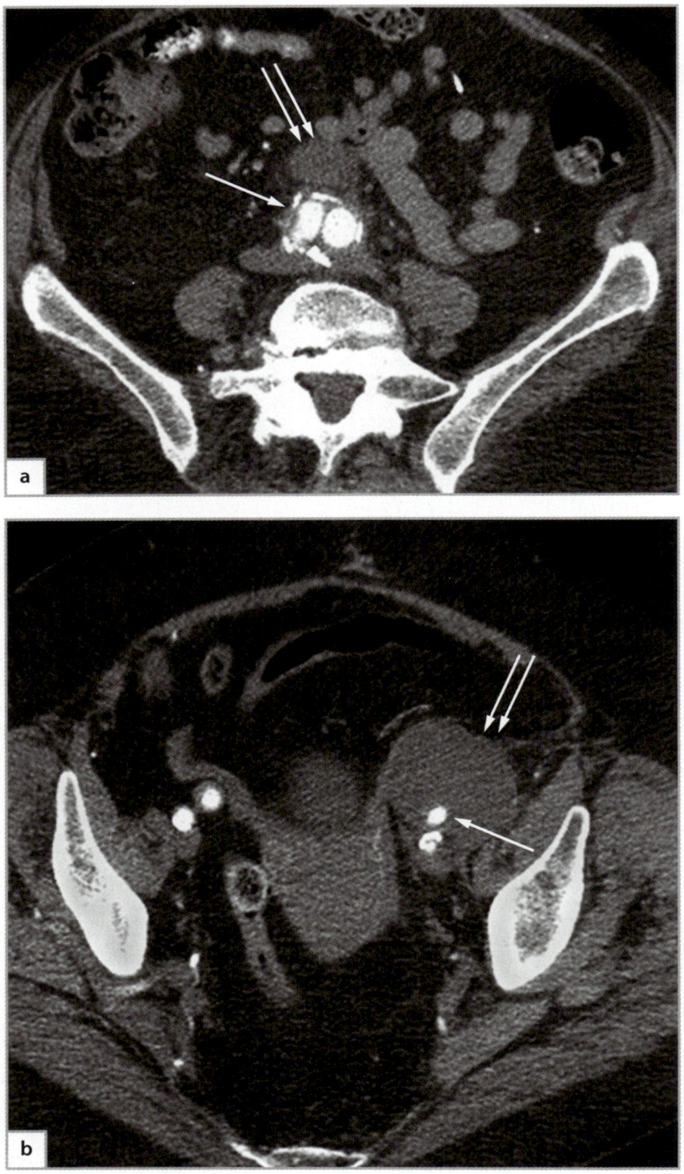

Figure 10.1 Patient with a history of prior abdominal aortic aneurysm repair presenting with fevers and abdominal pain and found to have large fluid collections adjacent to the graft in the abdomen (a) and pelvis (b) (one arrow = aortic graft, two arrows = abscess).

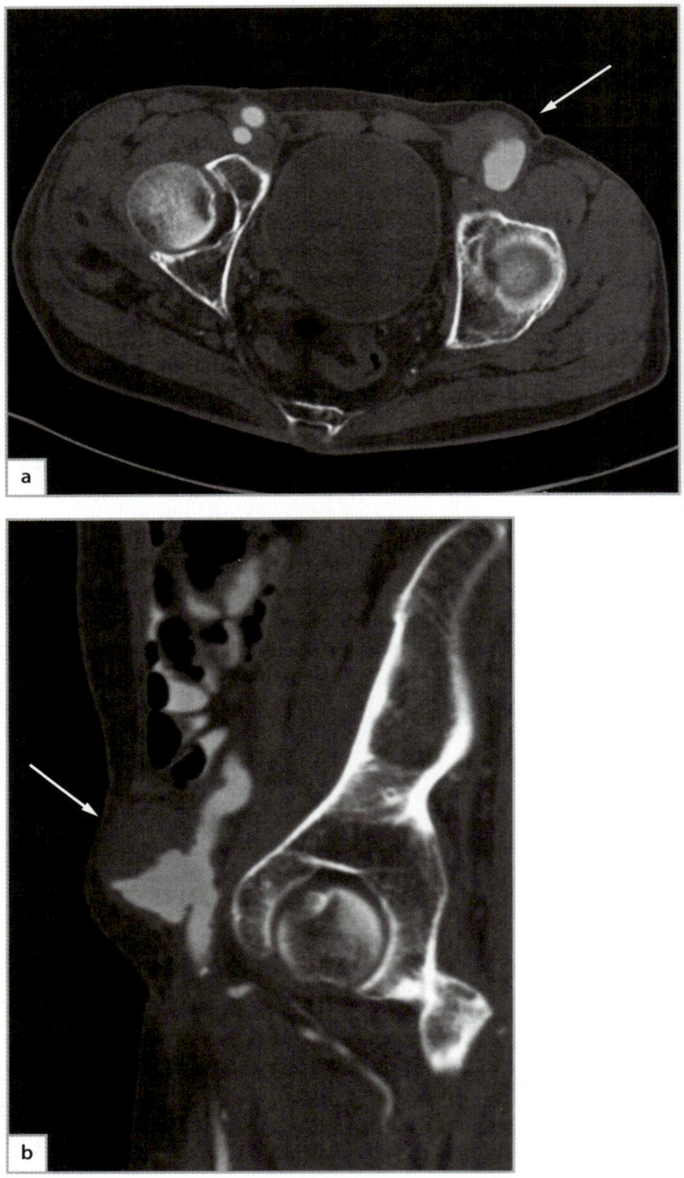

Figure 10.2 Patient with a history of prior abdominal aortic aneurysm repair who later developed an anastomotic aneurysm (arrow) at the distal anastomosis of the graft and the left iliac artery (a) Axial image and (b) sagittal image.

Open surgical repair can be accomplished with an interposition graft; however, the morbidity and mortality related to open surgical repair are not insignificant. There are also multiple reports of successful endovascular repair of anastomotic aneurysms with a low periprocedural morbidity and mortality (Di Tommaso et al. 2007, Nayeemuddin et al. 2012, Piffaretti et al. 2007, Tiesenhausen et al. 2001, van Herwaarden et al. 2004). Endovascular approaches have included aortic cuffs, bifurcated endografts, aortoiliac grafts with femoral–femoral bypass, and iliac limbs. A careful anatomical assessment is required to choose the appropriate strategy. The decision between open surgery and endovascular repair should be made after carefully considering patient anatomy and the patient's individual risk. Anastomotic aneurysms that develop as a consequence of infection are most often treated by removal of the infected graft and extra-anatomic bypass.

Graft thrombosis or embolization

Patients with graft thrombosis after open AAA may manifest symptoms of acute or chronic lower extremity ischemia. Overall, thrombosis is relatively uncommon (<1% of patients undergoing AAA repair) particularly when a tube graft is used for reconstruction of an aneurysm confined to the aorta. Nevertheless, severe iliac disease or impaired distal runoff predisposes to graft thrombosis. Lower extremity ischemia can also result from periprocedural embolization. Techniques for the treatment of either condition include embolectomy or thrombectomy, endarterectomy or bypass. Treatment may also be via endovascular interventions such as thrombolysis, angioplasty, or stent.

Additional complications requiring reoperation

Although open surgical repair of AAA is durable, long-term complications requiring reintervention related to laparotomy also occur. These include ventral hernias or small bowel obstruction (Kieffer et al. 2012). Recent comparative studies of open versus endovascular aneurysm repair (EVAR) suggest that the rate of reintervention for laparotomy-related complications in the cohort of open patients can be as high as 20%.

Endovascular aneurysm repair

Endovascular repair of AAA is being performed with increasing frequency; currently almost 70% of AAA repairs are with this technique. However, the durability of these repairs is less than with traditional surgery. Although the full array of surgical complications can occur, a host of reinterventions is required for graft-related issues and device failure.

Hemorrhage

Hemorrhage after EVAR may be a result of arterial rupture anywhere from the proximal neck of the aneurysm to the femoral access sites. The most common site of hemorrhage is the iliac arteries, particularly in patients with small or diseased vessels. Hypotension may develop intraoperatively at the time of sheath removal. Balloon occlusion of the iliac artery can temporize until a covered stent is placed across the site of arterial rupture. Postoperatively, persistent hypotension should raise high suspicion of a delayed manifestation of an intraprocedural arterial rupture. This should be addressed by a rapid return to the operating room with endovascular treatment of the site of rupture if possible.

Maldeployment

Intraoperative misadventure leading to graft maldeployment has become exceedingly rare with current EVAR technology. Nevertheless, successful EVAR requires careful preoperative planning to determine the appropriate type and sizing of the graft. Inaccurate planning can lead to improper device deployment, resulting in aortic or iliac artery thrombosis or failure to exclude the aneurysm. Removal of a maldeployed endograft is often difficult, particularly after the device has been completely released; therefore, conversion to open repair is often required in these cases.

Endoleaks

One of the most common reasons for reintervention after EVAR is an endoleak, resulting in aneurysm sac expansion. Endoleaks can be classified into several types (see **Table 10.1**). Type I endoleaks result from lack of apposition of the graft within the proximal or distal landing zones. These always require reintervention as direct flow of blood persists in the aneurysm sac placing patients at high risk of rupture. Often type I endoleaks can be repaired via endovascular means with extension cuffs or limbs; however, if these methods fail, then conversion to open repair is required. Type II endoleaks develop as a consequence of back flow into the aneurysm sac from patent lumbar, mesenteric, or accessory renal vessels. An example of this is shown in **Figure 10.3**. The current standard of care is to observe type II leaks, which often close spontaneously. However, if there is persistence of a type II leak and associated aneurysm sac expansion, treatment is advised. Minimally invasive options for treatment include embolization of the culprit vessels with coils or glue, or endoscopic ligation. These interventions are often successful in treating type II leaks; however, surgical explantation and reconstruction may occasionally be necessary. Type III endoleaks, which represent disruption within the body of the graft, also require repair; this can be accomplished by relining the endograft with an additional device. A type V endoleak represents continued aneurysm sac growth without direct evidence of an endoleak. In patients with type V leaks, if there is persistent and significant sac expansion, conversion to an open surgical repair will be required.

Explantation of an endograft can be complex and mortality and morbidity are increased compared with a primary open repair. Either a transperitoneal or retroperitoneal approach can be used. A disadvantage of the retroperitoneal approach is that exposure of the distal right iliac artery can be difficult. For endografts that have suprarenal fixation, proximal control requires a supraceliac cross-clamp. Techniques for explantation of an endograft may involve complete or partial removal of the graft. In some cases, the device

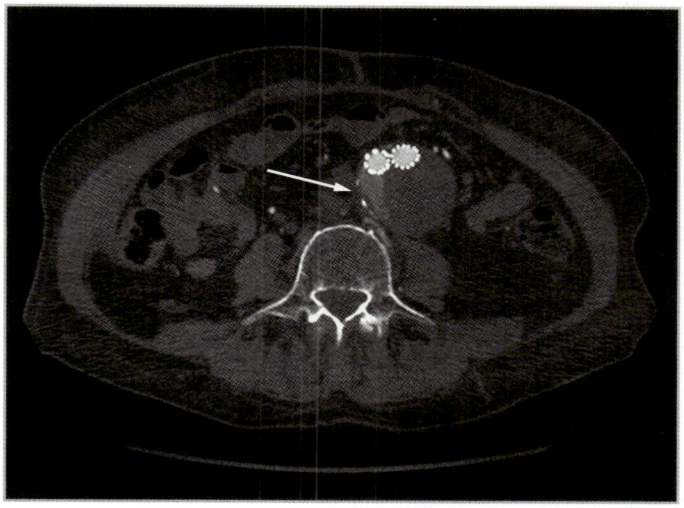

Figure 10.3 Example of a type II endoleak following endovascular aneurysm repair. Contrast extravasation is visualized in the aneurysm sac (arrow). Retrograde flow through a lumbar artery is the cause.

Table 10.1 Classification of endoleaks

Type	Definition	Initial management
I	Lack of seal at the proximal or distal sealing zones	Placement of extension cuffs or limbs
II	Retrograde flow into the aneurysm from patent lumbar, mesenteric, or accessory renal arteries	Observation, most resolve
III	Separation of graft components or graft fabric defect	Reline with additional components
IV	Fabric porosity leading to diffuse leakage through wall of endograft	Observation, most resolve
V	Continued aneurysm sac growth without observation of an endoleak	Observation until size reaches threshold for intervention

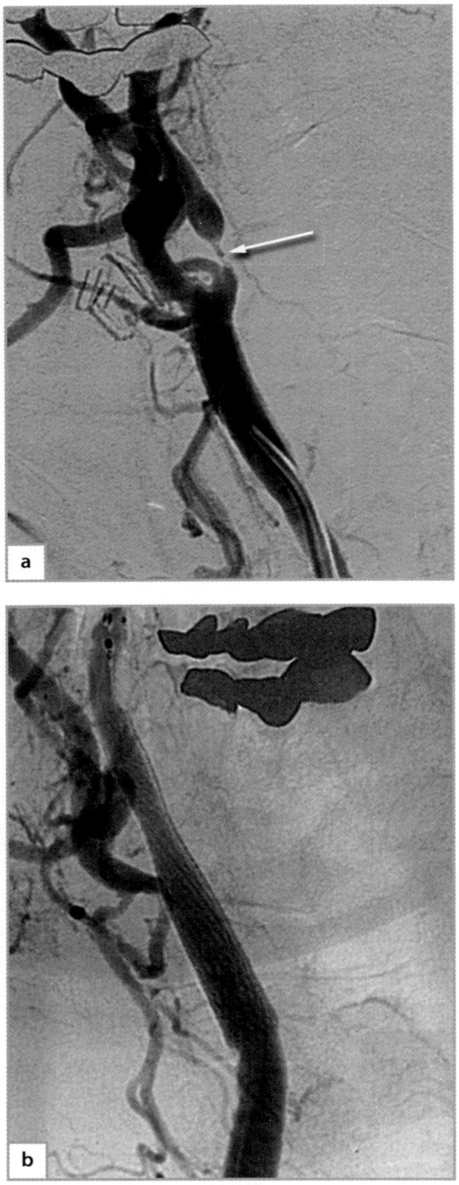

Figure 10.4 (a) Example of a high-grade (arrow) restenosis after a prior carotid endarterectomy. (b) Patient subsequently treated with a carotid stent resulting in resolution of stenosis.

can be removed by simply pulling it out. However, if the device is well incorporated, a hybrid approach can be taken in which the adhered portion of the endograft is left in place and the new graft is anastomosed to this remnant (Brinster et al. 2011, Kelso et al. 2009). Distal control during reconstruction can be difficult because of the inability to place clamps on the iliac stents. An alternative is to use balloon catheters to occlude the iliac arteries.

Graft thrombosis

Early thrombosis is usually the consequence of placing a graft in tortuous or diseased iliac arteries or alternatively from a defect created at the site of the femoral arteriotomy. Late graft thrombosis can occur as a consequence of remodeling of the aneurysm sac with kinking of the iliac limbs. Limb thrombosis, which occurs in 1% of cases, can be asymptomatic, result in claudication-like symptoms, or lead to limb-threatening ischemia. Early thrombosis can be prevented by stenting the graft in narrowed iliac vessels at the time of initial graft placement and by careful closure of femoral arteriotomies. Late thrombosis can be treated by thrombolysis and stenting or alternatively a cross-femoral bypass.

Infection

Infection of an endograft is quite rare with a reported incidence <1%. Similar to infections that develop following open repair, the morbidity and mortality associated with endograft infections are quite high. The clinical presentation of an infected endograft is similar to that of graft infection following open repair. After EVAR the most common presentations are low-grade sepsis (52%), abdominal or back pain (43%), or aortoenteric fistula (41%). Less common modes of presentations include a psoas abscess, emboli, or a pseudoaneurysm (Numan et al. 2011). Management of an infected endograft consists of endograft explantation, debridement of infected tissue, and arterial reconstruction. Endograft components should not be left in place. The reconstruction can be extra-anatomic and precede endograft removal or an in situ reconstruction can be used as previously described.

CAROTID ARTERY STENOSIS

Carotid endarterectomy

Carotid endarterectomy (CEA) is a well-established intervention shown to reduce the risk of stroke in patients with carotid artery stenosis, specifically in patients presenting with neurologic symptoms. This procedure is widely performed with a relatively low rate of complication. However, when complications do occur, they often have serious consequence. Patients who require reoperative carotid artery surgery can be divided into those who are in need of immediate intervention, often secondary to a technical failure, and those who require treatment of progressive disease.

Hemorrhage

One of the feared postoperative complications after CEA is bleeding, leading to a hematoma that may compromise a patient's airway. This may occur from a diffuse slow ooze from heparinization or the use of antiplatelet agents, or there may be brisk bleeding from a disrupted repair. Fortunately, the incidence of hematoma requiring reoperation is low, on the order of 1–2%. Drains have not been found to be helpful in preventing hematoma. Hematoma can lead to airway compromise, which can only be treated by the immediate opening of the wound; this may need to be accomplished before the patient can return to the operating room. Any evidence of respiratory distress or stridor following CEA requires prompt attention.

Stroke

Another postoperative complication often requiring reoperation is stroke. Despite careful monitoring in the operating room and precautions including electroencephalogram, measurement of stump pressures, and shunting, patients may awaken from anesthesia with a new neurologic deficit or develop a deficit soon after surgery. The three main causes of stroke after CEA are embolization during dissection, diminished cerebral perfusion during clamping, and technical defects in the final reconstruction, leading to embolization or arterial thrombosis.

Immediate reoperation is required in the case of a technical defect or acute thrombosis; however, reoperation is not able to alter the course in patients who suffer from embolization or intraoperative hypoperfusion. The difficulty then becomes identifying the cause in a patient with a postoperative defect. Waiting for imaging to evaluate the carotid artery wastes precious time. Bedside ultrasound is not always reliable, takes time, and can be hampered by normal postoperative swelling and surgical dressings. The accepted and most rapid option is to return to the operating room for re-exploration. In the setting of an angio-operating room, a quickly performed on-table angiogram as the patient is being prepped can be helpful. If the repair is patent, re-exploration might be avoided.

Time is the critical factor in that a neurologic defect can be reversed if flow is promptly restored. Thus, urgent reoperation is the most efficient strategy. Upon re-exploration, if the carotid artery is patent, an intraoperative angiogram can be useful. Causes of postoperative thrombosis include an intimal flap, platelet debris, or a kinked carotid artery. Fortunately, approximately two-thirds of patients with postoperative stroke who undergo re-exploration and repair can be expected to have a favorable neurologic outcome. There is a small subset of patients with postoperative strokes that may have intracranial embolization of thrombus as the cause of a postoperative neurologic deficit. In these patients, urgent thrombolysis can be effective in re-establishing flow.

Restenosis

The incidence of restenosis following CEA ranges from 10% to 34%, although reoperation is necessary in only 5% of patients (AbuRahma et al. 1998, Ballinger et al. 1997, Civil et al., 1988, Mansour et al. 1997, Ouriel & Green 1987, Rosenthal et al. 1996). Early restenosis (<2 years) after CEA is often a result of intimal hyperplasia, while late recurrent disease is generally a consequence of progression of atherosclerosis (Attigah et al. 2010, Bettendorf et al. 2007, Das et al. 1985, Moore et al. 1998, Stoney & String 1976). Generally, reintervention is warranted in patients who become symptomatic. However, in asymptomatic patients, the threshold for reintervention is great for restenosis compared with primary atherosclerosis. This is because hyperplastic plaque that typifies restenosis is less likely to embolize. Alternatively, lesions that are preocclusive should undergo repair as the risk of subsequent thrombosis and embolization is high.

Once the decision to reintervene has been made, optimal treatment is controversial and includes either repeat CEA or carotid artery stenting (CAS). Over time, CAS has emerged as the preferred approach (Aburahma et al. 2001, Bowser et al. 2003, Chakhtoura et al. 2001, Gable et al. 2003, Hobson et al. 1999, Lanzino et al. 1999, New et al. 2000). An example case is shown in **Figure 10.4**. Arguments in favor of CAS include a perceived increase in perioperative stroke and a higher rate of wound complication and cranial nerve injury following CEA. In addition, the smooth and nonembolic nature of intimal hyperplasia reduces the potential of stroke following CAS. Nevertheless, redo CEA remains an option, particularly in patients who develop late restenosis with complex plaque related to recurrent atherosclerotic disease (Cho et al. 2004, Coscas et al. 2010, de Borst et al. 2008, O'Hara et al. 2001, Mansour et al. 2001, 1997, Zhou et al. 2006). The decision regarding which procedure to perform should include consideration of multiple patient-specific factors including aortic arch anatomy, lesion type, location and complexity, existing cranial nerve defects, anesthesia risks, and surgeon experience.

Infectious complications after CEA

Infection following CEA is an exceedingly rare complication that occurs in <1% of patients and can develop in the early perioperative period as well as remotely from the initial surgery. Manifestations of infection include cellulitis, drainage, abscess, sepsis, pseudoaneurysm, or hemorrhage. These sequelae can lead to dire consequences. A patient presenting with infection should undergo operative exploration. If the infection does not extend to the carotid artery, treatment should include a washout and closure followed by treatment with appropriate antibiotics. However, if there is concern that the infection extends to the artery, or if there is a pseudoaneurysm or septicemia, a more definitive approach is required. Multiple operative strategies have been reported; perhaps most common is debridement to healthy tissue and autologous reconstruction. Options for reconstruction include a vein or bovine pericardial patch or an interposition vein or arterial graft. If there is a significant amount of debridement required, a muscle flap for coverage should also be considered (Mann et al. 2012).

Carotid artery stenting

Over the past several years, carotid stenting has been performed with increasing frequency. Despite significant differences in technique, complications requiring reintervention are quite similar to those for CEA, namely hemorrhage, stroke, and restenosis.

Hemorrhage

Hemorrhage after CAS is most often confined to the access site (usually the groin) and can result in hematoma or pseudoaneurysm. Occasionally operative intervention is required for an expanding hematoma. Pseudoaneurysms can be treated with expectant management or thrombin injection. Occasionally, a retroperitoneal hemorrhage can result in femoral nerve injury from compression. Rarely, hemorrhage may be the result of perforation of the carotid artery during stent deployment and emergent operative repair is most often required.

Stroke

The rate of periprocedural stroke after CAS has been reported to range from 2% to 7% (Gurm et al. 2008, Eskandari et al. 2010, Mantese et al. 2010). The main etiologies of stroke in the periprocedural period are atheroemboli, air emboli, thrombosis, or intracranial hemorrhage. To determine the course of action, emergent angiography should be performed to evaluate for patency of the carotid artery. Treatments include reversal of spasm, clot extraction, thrombolysis, treatment of a technical defect, or hyperbaric oxygen therapy for an air embolus (Gupta et al. 2007). The response to these treatments is variable, depending on the etiology of the neurologic event.

Maldeployment

Technical difficulties requiring emergent conversion to CEA are rare but might include misplacement of the stent, the inability to adequately dilate the stent, or a limitation in flow due to kinking. An additional technical problem that requires immediate conversion to CEA is failure to recover the distal embolic protection device. This can result when a large amount of thrombus or debris is entrapped in the device preventing its closure and extraction. Moreover, the device may potentially become entangled in the stent struts preventing removal. An extremely tortuous internal or common carotid artery may increase the potential for complication. If endovascular bailout techniques are not successful, an emergent CEA will need to be performed (Eskandari 2008).

Restenosis

The incidence of restenosis following CAS requiring reintervention is approximately 5% and similar to that of CEA. As with restenosis after CEA, reintervention is typically recommended in symptomatic patients or when the degree of stenosis exceeds 80%. In-stent restenosis is primarily the consequence of neointimal hyperplasia (Lal et al. 2007). Treatment options include angioplasty, balloon-cutting angioplasty, or angioplasty and stent. Surgical reconstruction is rarely required.

Ultrasound often overgrades stenosis, thus a CT angiography can be useful in definitively measuring the degree of arterial narrowing.

LOWER EXTREMITY OCCLUSIVE DISEASE

There are a wide variety of treatment options for patients with lower extremity occlusive disease, including surgical and endovascular interventions. For both approaches, the ultimate goal is to improve patient quality of life and avoid amputation. Reoperation or reintervention in these patients is for perioperative complications or the development of recurrent disease.

Lower extremity bypass

Hemorrhage

As with other vascular procedures, hemorrhage after lower extremity bypass has many causes including failure of an anastomosis, or an injured artery or vein. A common cause of bleeding after bypass with a vein conduit is bleeding from an inadequately ligated vein tributary. Reoperation is required for an expanding hematoma. However, even in a stable patient, a moderate-to-severe hematoma should be evacuated to reduce the level of discomfort, promote healing, and reduce the risk of subsequent infection.

Graft occlusion and restenosis

Early occlusion (within 30 days) after lower extremity bypass occurs is 3–5% of patients. Causes of early graft thrombosis are most often technical. For example, occlusion of in situ vein bypass grafts is often the consequence of a retained valve leaflet; or the graft could be twisted, kinked, or compressed through its tunnel. Angiography can help identify residual defects at the time of operation. Other more rare causes of graft occlusion include postoperative hypotension, inadequate inflow or outflow, or a prothrombotic state. The approach to these patients should be immediate re-exploration, with thrombectomy and graft revision as necessary. Revision of an anastomosis can be accomplished by creating a vein patch between the graft and the native artery.

Restenosis or late graft occlusion can be the result of multiple causes. A prosthetic graft can thrombose, particularly if a joint is crossed. Intimal hyperplasia or recurrent disease can form throughout a vein bypass or at the anastomoses of a prosthetic or autogenous graft. Progression of atherosclerotic disease can affect inflow or outflow leading to occlusion. Intimal hyperplasia is felt to be the most prominent cause of restenosis during the first 2 years. After this time, recurrent atherosclerosis is the primary etiology. Patients typically present with a recurrence of their original symptoms of claudication, rest pain, or a nonhealing wound. **Figure 10.5** illustrates an example of a stenosis within a lower extremity bypass graft.

Treatment must be designed to correct the causative defect and to remove thrombus if necessary. Options include open surgical revision versus an endovascular approach. Endovascular procedures are usually tried first. Endovascular alternatives include angioplasty with or without stenting, cutting-balloon angioplasty, cryoplasty, catheter-directed thrombolysis, and rheolytic thrombectomy. The latter two techniques are used for freshly thrombosed grafts. Surgical revision can include thrombectomy with correction of the causative problem such as patch angioplasty or bypass of a restenotic segment or a jump graft below a segment of recurrent disease. Unusually a completely new bypass will be required.

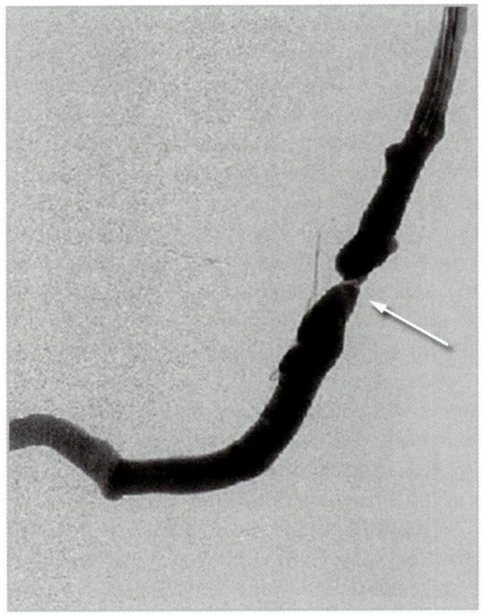

Figure 10.5 Illustration of a patient with a prior femoral–popliteal vein bypass who developed a high-grade stenosis (arrow) within the graft. Intervention was required to reduce the risk of graft thrombosis.

Infection

Infection of lower extremity bypass grafts most commonly occurs in the early postoperative period. Risk factors include a postoperative hematoma or seroma or an ongoing infection concurrent with performance of the bypass. Groin incisions are particularly vulnerable to infection due to an increased bacterial load. Management of graft infection depends on the extent of the infection and the condition of the patient. Operative options are limited in patients with systemic sepsis or hemodynamic instability. In these circumstances, emergent operation is undertaken to control infection and amputation if often the unfortunate result. In a stable patient, the reoperative approach to infection consists of excision and debridement of infected tissue and graft, rerouting blood flow to attempt limb preservation, and coverage of exposed areas with noninfected soft tissue and/or muscle. Ideally, a new vein graft can be anastomosed proximal and distal to the original graft. Partial graft excision is possible in cases where infection is clearly localized to a specific area. If possible, the new graft should lie in uninfected tissue, and if prosthetic graft is used this is mandatory.

Percutaneous endovascular intervention

Hemorrhage

As is the case with carotid stenting, significant hemorrhage after endovascular treatment of lower extremity occlusive disease is usually at the access site. Although bleeding can be the consequence of arterial injury at the time of sheath placement or maldeployment of a closure device, inadequate hemostasis is often the consequence of poor technique when holding manual pressure over the punctured artery. Arterial rupture at the site of an angioplasty is rare and can often be treated with endovascular means but occasionally requires surgical repair.

Arterial embolization and occlusion

Another complication of intraluminal therapy is the development of distal ischemia from micro- or macroembolization. Ideally, macroembolic lesions are recognized during the primary intervention and can be managed with suction thrombectomy or thrombolysis. To assure identification of distal emboli, it is important to perform a completion angiogram, demonstrating the runoff vessels following every intervention. Microembolization is a more difficult problem where microparticles of plaque block small arterioles of the muscle and skin. The consequences can be devastating and there is no treatment that can reverse this complication.

Acute thrombosis, which can develop as a consequence of an endovascular intervention, may result from arterial dissection, inadequate anticoagulation, a prothrombotic state, or spasm. Correction with endovascular techniques should be attempted first and are often successful. Rarely a surgical 'bailout' is required.

Restenosis

The advantage of percutaneous therapy for lower extremity vascular disease is its minimally invasive nature; however, the trade-off is durability. Restenosis is the consequence of intimal hyperplasia or hypercellular plaque. The frequency of restenosis is inversely proportional to the size of the treated vessel with rates as high as 70–80% at 1 year for the treatments of the tibial circulation. Fortunately, recurrent disease is usually amenable to repeated endovascular intervention. In addition to angioplasty and stent, techniques have been designed to address hyperplastic plaque such as a cold balloon (cryotherapy) or atherectomy. Patients will often prefer repeated percutaneous interventions performed under local anesthesia to a major surgical bypass. Alternatively, repeated percutaneous failures should lead to a surgical bypass. Surgical bypass should be considered before amputation.

CONCLUSION

Reinterventions, both early and late, following vascular reconstructions are common. Vascular interventions are technically demanding, and inattention to detail can lead to early failure. Moreover, atherosclerosis is a chronic and diffuse process often requiring late reinterventions for recurrent disease. The forgoing is a broad outline of three arterial processes treated by both open surgical and endovascular means. We present important principles regarding reoperative management of these patients with an emphasis beginning with AAAs. However, our survey has been superficial, and for individual reintervention the reader is encouraged to consult more detailed descriptions.

REFERENCES

Aburahma AF, Bates MC, Stone PA, Wulu JT. Comparative study of operative treatment and percutaneous transluminal angioplasty/stenting for recurrent carotid disease. J Vasc Surg 2001; 34:831–838.

AbuRahma AF, Robinson PA, Saiedy S, Kahn JH, Boland JP. Prospective randomized trial of carotid endarterectomy with primary closure and patch angioplasty with saphenous vein, jugular vein, and polytetrafluoroethylene: long-term follow-up. J Vasc Surg 1998; 27:222–232; discussion 33–34.

Attigah N, Külkens S, Deyle C, et al. Redo surgery or carotid stenting for restenosis after carotid endarterectomy: results of two different treatment strategies. Ann Vasc Surg 2010; 24:190–195.

Ballinger BA, Money SR, Chatman DM, Bowen JC, Ochsner JL. Sites of recurrence and long-term results of redo surgery. Ann Surg 1997; 225:512–515; discussion 6–7.

Bettendorf MJ, Mansour MA, Davis AT, et al. Carotid angioplasty and stenting versus redo endarterectomy for recurrent stenosis. Am J Surg 2007; 193:356–359; discussion 9.

Bowser AN, Bandyk DF, Evans A, et al. Outcome of carotid stent-assisted angioplasty versus open surgical repair of recurrent carotid stenosis. J Vasc Surg 2003; 38:432–438.

Brinster CJ, Fairman RM, Woo EY, et al. Late open conversion and explantation of abdominal aortic stent grafts. J Vasc Surg 2011; 54:42–46.

Chakhtoura EY, Hobson RW Goldstein J, et al. In-stent restenosis after carotid angioplasty-stenting: incidence and management. J Vasc Surg 2001; 33:220–225; discussion 5–6.

Cho JS, Pandurangi K, Conrad MF, et al. Safety and durability of redo carotid operation: an 11-year experience. J Vasc Surg 2004; 39:155–161.

Civil ID, O'Hara PJ, Hertzer NR, Krajewski LP, Beven EG. Late patency of the carotid artery after endarterectomy. Problems of definition, follow-up methodology, and data analysis. J Vasc Surg 1988; 8:79–85.

Coscas R, Rhissassi B, Gruet-Coquet N, et al. Open surgery remains a valid option for the treatment of recurrent carotid stenosis. J Vasc Surg 2010; 51:1124–1132.

Das MB, Hertzer NR, Ratliff NB, O'Hara PJ, Beven EG. Recurrent carotid stenosis. A five-year series of 65 reoperations. Ann Surg 1985; 202:28–35.

de Borst GJ, Zanen P, de Vries JP, et al. Durability of surgery for restenosis after carotid endarterectomy. J Vasc Surg 2008; 47:363–371.

Di Tommaso L, Monaco M, Piscione F, Sarno G, Iannelli G. Endovascular stent grafts as a safe secondary option for para-anastomotic abdominal aortic aneurysm. Eur J Vasc Endovasc Surg 2007; 33:91–93.

Eskandari MK. Preventable complications of carotid stenting. Perspect Vasc Surg Endovasc Ther 2008; 20:17–25.

Eskandari MK, Usman AA, Garcia-Toca M, et al. Eight-year institutional review of carotid artery stenting. J Vasc Surg 2010; 51:1145–1151.

Gable DR, Bergamini T, Garrett WV, et al. Intermediate follow-up of carotid artery stent placement. Am J Surg 2003; 185:183–187.

Gupta R, Vora N, Thomas A, et al. Symptomatic cerebral air embolism during neuro-angiographic procedures: incidence and problem avoidance. Neurocrit Care 2007; 7:241–246.

Gurm HS, Yadav JS, Fayad P, et al. Long-term results of carotid stenting versus endarterectomy in high-risk patients. N Engl J Med 2008; 358:1572–1579.

Hobson RW, Goldstein JE, Jamil Z, et al. Carotid restenosis: operative and endovascular management. J Vasc Surg 1999; 29:228–235; discussion 35–38.

Kelso RL, Lyden SP, Butler B, et al. Late conversion of aortic stent grafts. J Vasc Surg 2009; 49:589–595.

Kieffer WK, Sonnenberg S, Windhaber RA, Pal N, Pemberton RM. Complications and reintervention following elective open abdominal aortic aneurysm repair: a 10-year retrospective analysis. Ann R Coll Surg Engl 2012; 94:177–180.

Lal BK, Kaperonis EA, Cuadra S, Kapadia I, Hobson RW. Patterns of in-stent restenosis after carotid artery stenting: classification and implications for long-term outcome. J Vasc Surg 2007; 46:833–840.

Lanzino G, Mericle RA, Lopes DK, et al. Percutaneous transluminal angioplasty and stent placement for recurrent carotid artery stenosis. J Neurosurg 1999; 90:688–694.

Mann CD, McCarthy M, Nasim A, et al. Management and outcome of prosthetic patch infection after carotid endarterectomy: a single-centre series and systematic review of the literature. Eur J Vasc Endovasc Surg 2012; 44:20–26.

Mansour MA, Kang SS, Baker WH, et al. Carotid endarterectomy for recurrent stenosis. J Vasc Surg 1997; 25:877–883.

Mantese VA, Timaran CH, Chiu D, et al. The Carotid Revascularization Endarterectomy versus Stenting Trial (CREST): stenting versus carotid endarterectomy for carotid disease. Stroke 2010; 41:S31–S34.

Miller A, Marotta M, Scordi-Bello I, et al. Ischemic colitis after endovascular aortoiliac aneurysm repair: a 10-year retrospective study. Arch Surg 2009; 144:900–903.

Moore WS, Kempczinski RF, Nelson JJ, Toole JF. Recurrent carotid stenosis: results of the asymptomatic carotid atherosclerosis study. Stroke 1998; 29:2018–2125.

Nayeemuddin M, Pherwani AD, Asquith JR. Imaging and management of complications of open surgical repair of abdominal aortic aneurysms. Clin Radiol 2012; 67:802–814.
New G, Roubin GS, Iyer SS, et al. Safety, efficacy, and durability of carotid artery stenting for restenosis following carotid endarterectomy: a multicenter study. J Endovasc Ther 2000; 7:345–352.
Numan F, Gulsen F, Solak S, Cantasdemir M. Management of endograft infections. J Cardiovasc Surg (Torino) 2011; 52:205–223.
Ouriel K, Green RM. Clinical and technical factors influencing recurrent carotid stenosis and occlusion after endarterectomy. J Vasc Surg 1987; 5:702–706.
O'Hara PJ, Hertzer NR, Karafa MT, et al. Reoperation for recurrent carotid stenosis: early results and late outcome in 199 patients. J Vasc Surg 2001; 34:5–12.
Piffaretti G, Tozzi M, Lomazzi C, et al. Endovascular treatment for para-anastomotic abdominal aortic and iliac aneurysms following aortic surgery. J Cardiovasc Surg (Torino) 2007; 48:711–717.
Raman SP, Kamaya A, Federle M, Fishman EK. Aortoenteric fistulas: spectrum of CT findings. Abdom Imaging 2013; 38:367–75.
Reilly LM, Stoney RJ, Goldstone J, Ehrenfeld WK. Improved management of aortic graft infection: the influence of operation sequence and staging. J Vasc Surg 1987; 5:421–431.
Rosenthal D, Archie JP, Avila MH, et al. Secondary recurrent carotid stenosis. J Vasc Surg 1996; 24:424–428; discussion 8–9.
Stoney RJ, String ST. Recurrent carotid stenosis. Surgery 1976; 80:705–710.
Tiesenhausen K, Hausegger KA, Tauss J, Amann W, Koch G. Endovascular treatment of proximal anastomotic aneurysms after aortic prosthetic reconstruction. Cardiovasc Intervent Radiol 2001; 24:49–52.
van Herwaarden JA, Waasdorp EJ, Bendermacher BL, et al. Endovascular repair of paraanastomotic aneurysms after previous open aortic prosthetic reconstruction. Ann Vasc Surg 2004; 18:280–286.
Vogel TR, Symons R, Flum DR. The incidence and factors associated with graft infection after aortic aneurysm repair. J Vasc Surg 2008; 47:264–269.
Vogt PR. Arterial allografts in treating aortic graft infections: something old, something new. Semin Vasc Surg 2011; 24:227–233.
Zhou W, Lin PH, Bush RL, et al. Management of in-sent restenosis after carotid artery stenting in high-risk patients. J Vasc Surg 2006; 43:305–312.

Chapter 11 Postoperative intestinal anastomotic leak and enterocutaneous fistula

Solly Mizrahi

SCOPE OF THE PROBLEM

Postoperative bowel leaks are the most devastating consequences of small bowel and colorectal surgery, and are associated with increased morbidity, mortality, and prolonged hospital stay (Bruce et al. 2001, Lujan et al. 2011).

The intestinal leak varies between early disruption of anastomosis resulting in life-threatening diffuse peritonitis and sepsis with the mortality ranging between 1% and 15% (Leichtle et al. 2012) on one hand, and a late radiologically-demonstrated leakage of limited significance on the other hand. The outcome of intra-abdominal bowel leakage depends on the length of the contamination period, the amount, and the type of the bowel outflow content and its intra-abdominal degree of dispersion. The early detection of intestinal leakage reduces the contamination period, controls the violent effluent output and thereby improves the clinical outcome (McArdle et al. 2005).

The reported incidence of intestinal leakage ranges from 1% to 19%, depending on the location of the anastomosis (Manilich et al. 2003, Park et al. 2013, Ruggiero et al. 2011, Slieker et al. 2012). There are numerous reasons for anastomotic failure and leakage. The first sub-group of these relates to technical operative faults, including inadequate anastomotic blood supply, improper alignment of the anastomosis, tension on the bowel ends, inappropriate intestinal ends of approximation, and stapling device malfunction. The second sub-group relates to patient-specific etiology, including age >60 years, morbid obesity, obstructive pulmonary disease, heavy smoking and decreased oxygen saturation, malnutrition, hypoalbuminemia, anemia, extensive weight loss, and the overall physiological status of the patient. The third sub-group relates to delayed wound healing due to an immunodeficienct state, including the chronic use of steroids, malignancy, postirradiation state, chemotherapy or immunosuppressive treatment, the extensiveness of the intra-abdominal infection, and sepsis (Branagan & Finnis 2005).

Enterocutaneous fistula most often develops after abdominal bowel surgery and is mainly caused by operative complications either due to injury of the intestine during the surgical intervention or a leakage developed at the anastomotic site. The occurrence of postoperative enterocutaneous fistula is an unfortunate complication that inevitably happens in the most expert hands, requiring careful assessment and thoughtful treatment (Campos et al. 1999). Its management consumes substantial healthcare resources and is associated with significant morbidity and mortality. Enterocutaneous fistula has become more common since the use of the 'open abdomen' technique, damage control surgery, and the aggressive treatment of abdominal compartment syndrome (Ramsay & Mejia 2010).

Enterocutaneous fistula is a nonanatomical connection between the intestinal lumen and the skin with or without continuity of the intestinal mucosa, which is reinforced by the surrounded fibrous tissue. When the fistula is opened over an exposed intestinal loop, it is referred to as an enteroatmospheric fistula. This condition is extremely difficult to manage and almost never seals off spontaneously.

The fistula can be classified according to its daily effluent output: a low output fistula drains <200 mL/day and a high output one drains >500 mL/day. The latter is associated with higher morbidity and mortality due to malnutrition, volume depletion, electrolyte disturbances, and acid–base imbalance.

About two-thirds of enterocutaneous fistulae will close spontaneously with proper supportive care, control of sepsis, and adequate nutritive supply. The main barriers to spontaneous closure include distal obstruction, epithelialized mucocutaneous continuity, inflammatory bowel disease, postirradiation condition, a fistula course of <2 cm, and malignancy along the course of the fistula (Schien 2008).

History corner

In times past, enterocutaneous fistulae invariably had a fatal outcome, as reported by Von Cackovic at the beginning of the twentieth century (Von Cackovic 1903). Advocating conservative management in acute cases and an operative approach in chronic cases with 'maintenance of chemical balance' became the milestone in the management of this condition that remains valid today. The introduction of antibiotics in the mid-twentieth century did not make a critical difference. The improved results were reported during the 1960s when total parenteral nutrition (TPN), became part of patient management and was initiated concurrently with correction of volume imbalance and electrolyte and acid–base disturbances. Irving et al. demonstrated a significant decrease in the mortality rate to 20% during a 3-year period by referring patients to a center of excellence for extracellular fluid (ECF) management (Irving et al. 1985, Sepehripour & Papagrigoriadis 2010).

PRESENTATIONS AND DIAGNOSIS

A common presentation of a patient with intestinal leakage early after bowel surgery may begin dramatically, with peritoneal signs, abdominal distention, and failure to thrive, concomitant with septic syndrome including persistent high fever, tachycardia, and leukocytosis. This may progress to acute renal failure. Without an urgent surgical intervention, it can often deteriorate into multi-organ dysfunction and death.

A progressive fistula formation through the surgical wound may masquerade initially as a simple wound infection. The unhealed incision leads to an inflammatory collection in the subcutaneous space. The 'truth' is revealed when pus, followed a day later by typical intestinal content with bile staining, drained from the surgical incision, occasionally accompanied by intestinal gas. The fistula may become apparent at first only after postoperative percutaneous intra-abdominal abscess drainage. Occasionally, in spite of an uneventful recovery, drainage of 'suspicious' materials, usually preceded by pus, through a drain placed during the surgery may be the first sign of fistula (Wainstein et al. 2011).

When the persistence of the fistula is uncertain, methylene blue ingestion by mouth and inspection of the draining material may confirm the diagnosis but provides little information about its location or its cause. Fistulography may confirm the existence of a fistula and is safe to perform even in a sick patient. Computed tomography (CT) and ultrasound scans may identify an abscess cavity that may be accompanied by significant perianastomotic air bubbles, and these imaging modalities are instrumental for the minimally invasive drainage of such an abscess.

A small number of patients with a fistula manifest relatively late in the postoperative course with non-specific presentation: a careful CT scan with oral and rectal contrast material is indispensable. Delayed images after the progress of the contrast material through the small bowel are helpful to distinguish postoperative abscess or leakage from the unopacified segment of bowel. When a distal colorectal anastomotic leak is suspected, some studies have supported the superiority of a water-soluble enema to CT scan imaging (Nicksa et al. 2007).

CONSEQUENCES AND TREATMENT

The basic principles of management of bowel leakage and enterocutaneous fistula include fluid resuscitation, control of the fistula output, drainage of infection, nutrition support, skin and wound care, and closure of the fistula (**Figure 11.1**).

Bowel leakage is relatively infrequent and associated with a rather heterogeneous spectrum of presentations, and the surgical decision-making process is often complex as a result. Anastomotic leakage that occurs in the early phase after bowel surgery with septic syndrome and acute peritoneal signs mandates immediate abdominal re-exploration without any delay for diagnostic imaging: too often, radiological studies are obtained in the hope that there is another explanation for the patient's deterioration.

When the clinical findings are equivocal or misleading, but with high index of suspicion, an abdominal CT should be ordered. Contrast enema alone is often falsely negative. However, in patients with enterocutaneous fistula appearing more than 30 days postoperatively, a small intestinal leak is usually present, with a controlled low-output fistula that mostly resolves spontaneously.

The management of bowel leakage and enterocutaneous fistula is divided into three phases:

1. The diagnosis and early recognition
2. Stabilization of the patient and investigation
3. The patient's care

Successful management requires a coordinated effort by an experienced surgical and nursing team.

The major goal of the stabilization phase is aggressive resuscitation, correcting any fluid loses, re-establishing acid–base balance, and correcting electrolyte abnormalities (especially hypokalemia). A knowledge of the electrolyte contents and acid–base levels of the various secretions from the gastrointestinal tract is vital for calculating their replacement doses (Drause et al. 2006).

The cardinal point in the early treatment phase of anastomotic leakage or perforated damaged bowel is to surgically divert an uncontrolled fistula associated with generalized peritonitis and sepsis into a controlled one by taking down the anastomosis and creating a temporary Brook's ileostomy or exteriorization of the damaged bowel loop as a temporary stoma in order to avoid ongoing intra-abdominal

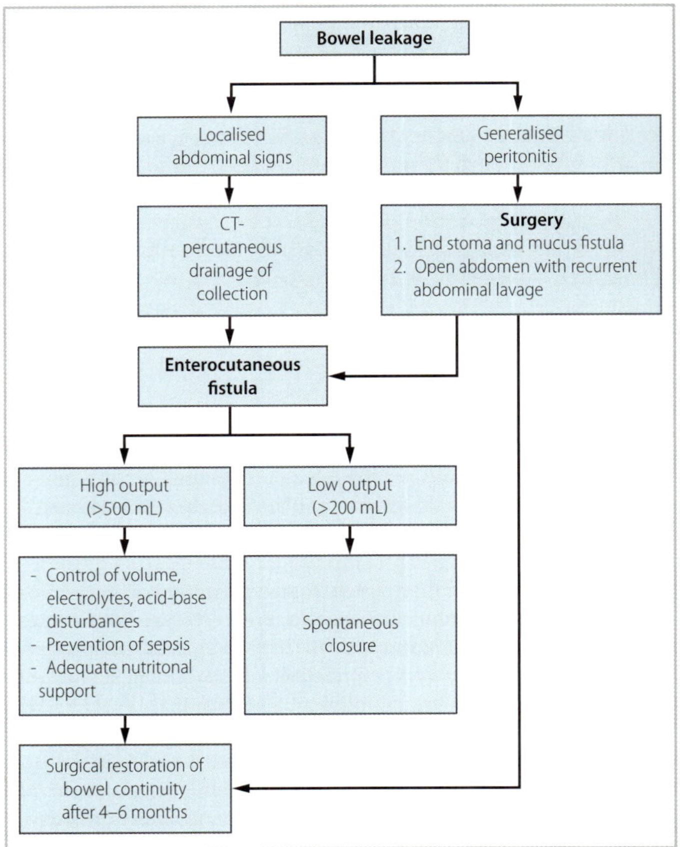

Figure 11.1 Treatment of bowel leakage and enterocutaneous fistula.

spillage of infected intestinal content. When a major disruption of colonic anastomosis is found, dividing it and creating an end anastomosis is often wise. Patients with a minor colonic leak of an otherwise healthy anastomosis may be treated by proximal diversion and local drainage. Direct suture often makes the disruption larger. Proximal diversion is particularly applicable to extraperitoneal and pelvic anastomotic leak, since later restoration of intestinal continuity to a short anorectal stump can be especially challenging (Fraccalvieri et al. 2012). When local peritonitis and abscess cavities are detected long after the initial bowel surgery, percutaneous image-guided drainage should be accomplished.

When a fistula develops, as soon as the electrolyte and any acid–base abnormalities are balanced, TPN should be instituted. Its effluent drainage should be collected and measured and a disposable ileostomy bag should be adhered to the surrounding skin, thereby protecting the patient from excoriations and erosions. In cases where the fistula is of low output/effluent and is located in the large bowel or at the end of the small bowel with no evidence of distal obstruction, elemental enteral feeding may be initiated. When enteral feeding is well tolerated and provides adequate calories, TPN should be withdrawn.

A subtype of enterocutaneous fistula is the enteroatmospheric fistula, which has a high morbidity and mortality and requires a much more challenging level of nursing care . The development of enteroatmospheric fistula may occur in patients with 'open abdomen' and exposed bowel loops due to various pathologies including acute compartment syndrome, severe abdominal trauma, or (rarely) necrotizing abdominal wall soft tissue catastrophe. In these cases, when closure of the abdominal wall is impossible and while waiting until the optimal time for closure, the exposed 'frozen' intestinal loops may 'fistulize.' The enteroatmospheric fistula is extremely difficult to manage and the use of a vacuum pack technique appears to be the preferred nursing approach at present.

The development of postoperative enterocutaneous fistula remains a serious problem and usually extends a patient's hospital stay by 2–3 months, associated with extensive expenditure on TPN, reoperations, intensive care unit admissions, and ongoing nursing care. Further surgery will be required at a later date to restore intestinal continuity and repair the abdominal wall defect. Even with the optimal therapy available, mortality still averages 20%.

A re-entry into the peritoneal cavity 2–3 weeks or more after a major abdominal surgery is usually ill-advised unless the procedure is deemed to be lifesaving. When operative management is required to control sepsis, a thoughtful and careful preoperative plan is critical. A laparoscopic penetration through a non-violated zone of the abdominal wall is always recommended. Unnecessary dissection should be avoided, especially in the anastomotic vicinity, where the surrounding structures are adhered and any attempt to isolate them may cause major bleeding or injury to 'innocent bystander' organs. A proximal diversion and adequate drainage is therefore usually a prudent approach.

The worst time to re-enter the abdomen, especially in a patient with a loss of abdominal wall domain associated with a fistula or a stoma, is between 3 weeks and 3 months postoperatively, due to the obliterative peritonitis that has developed as a consequence of severe intra-abdominal infection during the early phase of the bowel leakage (Latifi et al. 2012). Most surgeons wait 4–6 months after the major surgical event to address the fistula or the stoma unless a life-threatening high-output fistula or stoma develops. These cases should be handled exceptionally early (after 3–4 weeks).

When preparing to take down a fistula or establish gastrointestinal continuity, the open approach should be chosen. The surgical team should assume that all patients with enterocutaneous or enteroatmospheric fistula have a frozen abdomen and that entry into the abdominal cavity will be extremely challenging. Wherever possible, the surgeon should choose a healthy domain on the abdominal wall. In patients with a healed, skin-grafted open abdominal wall, the author prefers to use a transverse incision beginning away from the old skin graft area and progressing toward its indurate rim.

The separation of the skin from the underlying bowel loops may detach it from its nourishing vessels and may cause skin necrosis.

Even after an appropriate time interval, surgical reintervention to take down a fistula or establish bowel continuity may encounter inadvertent enterotomies or injuries during the challenging separation of the bowel loops. Although the surgeon may recognize and repair the damaged bowel, the procedure itself may take the patient back to 'square-one,' with resulting intra-abdominal recontamination, sepsis, stoma formation, and a significantly higher rate of morbidity and mortality. In the author's opinion, some high-risk patients with controlled protective stoma after fistula repair or healed anastomotic leak should carefully consider whether the benefits of such a dangerous procedure outweigh the costs.

CONCLUSIONS AND CLOSURE

Anastomotic leakage is the most common cause of enterocutaneous fistula developed after bowel surgery, and in second place stand the often overlooked enterotomies of small bowel during enterolysis. The consequence of intra-abdominal contamination with intestinal effluent is fibrinous peritonitis abscess formation and uncontrolled skin drainage through the 'weakest link' —the recent surgical incision or the radiologist's abscess-draining catheter. The worst mortality rate for enterocutaneous fistula is in older patients and when presentation occurs very early in the postoperative period (Visschers et al. 2012). The major cause of death is uncontrolled sepsis secondary to massive intraoperative infection, abscess formation, and ultimately, multiorgan failure. Intravenous nutritional support has proved to be a great breakthrough in reducing morbidity and mortality in the last 30 years of the twentieth century.

Once there is no sepsis, appropriate nutritional support has been initiated, the exit site of the fistula is protected and there are volume, electrolyte and acid–base disturbances, controlled, temporary non-operative management should be practiced.

The key principles of management of enterocutaneous fistula are as follows:

1. The best form of clinical practice is prevention
2. The most common reason for multiorgan malfunction after bowel surgery, until proven otherwise, is anastomotic leak: do not try to blame other sources of infection
3. Early recognition of anastomotic leakage is a key principle
4. Exteriorization of the feeding source of infection by a stoma formation or a proximal loop diversion is an excellent options
5. Tube drainage of the bowel fistula is ill advised and will only progressively enlarge the bowel opening, with consequent effluent leakage around the tube
6. Over-sewing attempts at the injured intestinal opening are always subject to failure
7. The hazard of pulling out the vulnerable and injured bowel loop during the period where it is edematous, with shortened mesentery and gradual fusion peritonitis (the 'no man's land' interval) is both dangerous and unnecessary
8. The definitive operation should be considered 4–6 months after the initial 'stormy' event
9. The goal of the final surgical procedure is to take down the fistula tract, to resect the encountered bowel loop, and to establish a hand-sewn anastomotic continuity of the remaining healthy bowel
10. Successful spontaneous closure of enterocutaneous fistula occurs in two-thirds of cases, especially when they are low-output and located in the distal gastrointestinal tract (Wainstein et al. 2011)

REFERENCES

Branagan G, Finnis D. Prognosis after anastomotic leak in colorectal surgery. Dis Colon Rectum 2005; 48:1021–1026.

Bruce J, Krukowski ZH, Al-Khairy G, Russell EM, Park KGM. Systematic review of the definitions and measurements of anastomotic leak after gastrointestinal surgery. Br J Surg 2001; 88:1157–1168.

Campos AC, Andrade DF, Campos GM, Matias JE, Coelho JC. A multivariate model to determine prognostic factors in gastrointestinal fistula. J Am Coll Surg 1999; 188:483–490.

Drause JM, Huss BS, Harty NJ, et al. Enterocutaneous fistula: are treatment improving? Surgery 2006; 140:570–576.

Fraccalvieri D, Biondo S, Saez J, et al. Management of colorectal anastomotic leakage: difference between salvage and anastomotic takedown. Am J Surg 2012; 204:671–676.
Irving M, White R, Tresadern J. Three years' experience with an intestinal failure unit. Ann R Coll Surg Engl 1985; 67:2–5.
Latifi R, Joseph B, Kulvatunyou N, et al. Enterocutaneous fistula and hostile abdomen: reoperative surgical approaches. World J Surgery 2012; 36:516–523.
Leichtle SW, Mouawad NJ, Welch KB, et al. Risk factors for anastomotic leakage after colectomy. Dis colon Rectum 2012; 55:569–575.
Lujan JJ, Nemeth ZH, Barratt-Stopper PA, et al. Factors influencing the outcome of intestinal anastomosis. Am Surg 2011; 77:1169–1175.
Manilich E, Vogel JD, Kiram RP, et al. Key factors associated with postoperative complications in patients undergoing colorectal surgery. Dis Colon Rectum 2003; 56:64–71.
McArdle CS, McMillan DC, Hole DJ. Impact of anastomotic leakage on long term survival of patients undergoing curative resection of colorectal cancer. Br J Surg 2005; 92:1150–1154.
Nicksa GA, Dring RV, Johnson KH, et al. Anastomotic leak: what is the best diagnostic imaging study? Dis Colon Rectum 2007; 50:197–203.
Park JS, Choi GS, Kim SH, et al. Multicenter analysis of risk factors of anastomotic leakage after laparoscopic rectal cancer excision: The Korean laparoscopic colorectal surgery study group. Ann Surg 2013; 257:665–671.
Ramsay PT, Mejia VA. Management of enterocutaneous fistula in the open abdomen. Am Surg 2010; 76:637–639.
Ruggiero R, Sparavigna L, Docimo A, et al. Postoperative peritonitis due to anastomotic dehiscence after colonic resections. Multicentric experience retrospective analysis of risk factors and review of the literature. Ann Intal Chir 2011; 82:369–375.
Schien M. What's new in post-operative enterocutaneous fistula? World J Surg 2008; 32:336–338.
Slieker JC, Koman N, Mannaerts GH, et al. Long term and perioperative corticosteroids in anastomotic leakage: a prospective study of 259 left sided colorectal anastomosis. Arch Surg 2012; 147:447–452.
Sepehripour S, Papagrigoriadis S. A systematic review of the benefit of total parenteral nutrition in the management of enterocutaneous fistula. Minerva Chir 2010; 65:577–585.
Wainstein DE, Tungler V, Ravazzola C, Chara O. Management of external small bowel fistulae: challenges and controversies confronting the general surgeon. Int J Surg 2011; 9:198–203.
Von Cackovic M. Ueber fistula des duodenum. Arc L Klin Chir 1903; 69:643.
Visschers RG, Van Gemert WG, Winkens B, et al. Guided treatment improves outcome of patients with enterocutaneous fistula. World J Surg 2012; 36:2341–2348.

Chapter 12 Reoperation for open and laparoscopic groin hernia

Shahzad M. Ali, David R. Farley

INTRODUCTION

With over 770,000 procedures performed annually, groin hernia repairs are among the most commonly performed general surgical procedures in the United States (Rutkow 2003). While a majority of these repairs are performed for primary inguinal and femoral hernias, secondary repairs or 'redo' surgery constitute approximately 10–20% of operations (Bisgaard et al. 2008, Sevonius et al. 2011). Although recent data from a large epidemiologic study suggests that this number is dropping (Bemdsen & Sevonius 2002); more than 100,000 recurrent inguinal and femoral hernias will be repaired this year in the United States.

HISTORY

Hernias have been repaired in a variety of manners, but it was not until Bassini laid the groundwork for anatomically based repairs in 1883 that the era of modern hernia repair began (Lau 2002). With his careful research, analysis, and effort on repairing inguinal hernias, patients of the late nineteenth century in Padua, Italy, were afforded a truly viable and dependable option for repair. However, hernia recurrences after a Bassini repair were not uncommon, and it being the sole technique of repair, surgeons had no other dependable options for re-do operations. Over time, in order to tackle the problem of recurrence and achieve higher success rates, new techniques were devised. McVay (1948) used the iliopectineal ligament in repair of primary and recurrent groin hernia as an alternative option for the treatment of hernias. Similarly, Shouldice (2010) with the proposed imbrication of the transversalis fascia and strengthening of the posterior wall of the inguinal canal with a continuous suture in layers was able to decrease the recurrence rate considerably. However, as most of these techniques involved some modification or improvement in Bassini's original repair, surgeons continued to see frequent recurrences after primary or recurrent groin hernia operations. It was not until the practice of implanting mesh within the groin in the late 1980s, either through an anterior approach, championed by Lichtenstein (**Figure 12.1a** and **b**), or via a retroperitoneal approach, described by Stoppa, were patients afforded a dependable and realistic option for curative procedures in a reoperative setting. Furthermore, over the last several decades, laparoscopic approaches have offered additional methods to repair difficult and problematic primary or recurrent inguinal hernia. Given the diversity and complexity in our patient population, an individualized approach should be adopted for patients with recurrent inguinal hernia.

ANATOMICAL ISSUES

While the most important assessment of a patient with recurrent inguinal hernia is the history and physical examination, a thorough evaluation of the previous operative report is critical for surgical planning. Patients who have undergone an open repair, either with a Bassini, McVay, Shouldice, or mesh repair, are important to differentiate from those who underwent a laparoscopic or posterior repair with or without mesh. The previous operative report and the current physical examination with a history of associated symptoms will lead the surgeon to an optimal surgical procedure. As a rule of thumb, attempting to avoid dissection in previously operated fields or areas of scarring is advantageous (**Figure 12.2**). Our own bias is to repair recurrences that were previously fixed via an open anterior

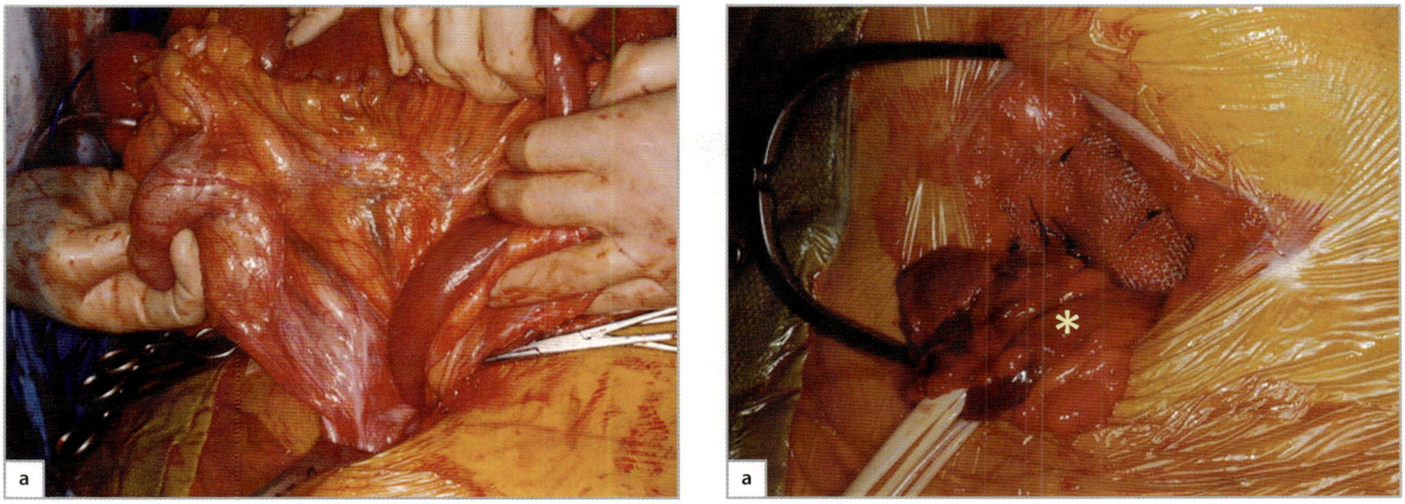

Figure 12.1 (a) Massive recurrent right-sided scrotal hernia with reduced contents (small bowel and colon) prior to placing within the abdomen. (b) Open Lichtenstein repair in same patient (*spermatic cord).

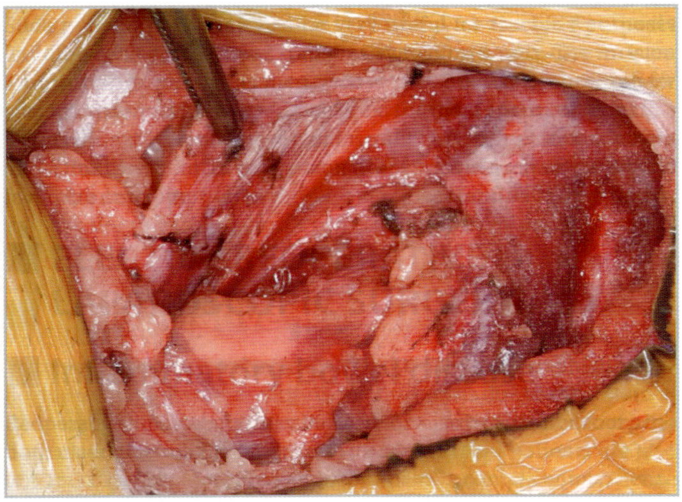

Figure 12.2 Scarred and disrupted anatomy when anterior approach is undertaken in a setting of previous anterior repair.

approach with a laparoscopic, preperitoneal approach. Conversely, in those patients with recurrent inguinal hernias who have undergone a previous laparoscopic approach, our preference is to perform an open, anterior mesh-based repair (**Figure 12.3**). For patients with multiple previous groin repairs with both anterior and posterior repairs, with or without mesh, the choice of repair is based on many considerations (use of anticoagulation, type of mesh present, the presence of groin pain, fitness and activity of patient, etc.).

TIMING OF REOPERATION

Most hernia repairs do not break down (Bay-Nielsen et al. 2001, Haapaniemi et al. 2001, Nilsson et al. 1998). As hernia surgeons become more skilled at repairing larger and more difficult defects, our recurrence rates have decreased over time. When recurrences do occur, they typically appear more than a year after surgery and sometimes many decades later. This is ideal, because reoperating in a surgical field several weeks to a few months later is fraught with hazard. In our practice, we prefer that 12 months have elapsed since the prior operation. If symptoms dictate otherwise or aggressive surgical reintervention is necessary, then reoperation may be performed sooner if it can be done so in a virgin field (laparoscopy for a previous anterior repair or vice versa: an open anterior repair following a laparoscopic attempt).

PREOPERATIVE IMAGING

While our radiology colleagues have offered a myriad of imaging techniques to survey groin hernias [computed tomography (CT), magnetic resonance imaging (MRI), ultrasonography (US), etc.), a thorough history and physical examination still remains the most important preoperative evaluation. Assuming the general surgeon identifies a recurrence on physical examination and the history corroborates this finding, then doing any further imaging is usually unnecessary. However, in those instances where patients verbalize chronic groin pain and/or an intermittent bulge, but the physical examination is unremarkable, imaging may be of some benefit. Imaging is of low yield in most cases as the patient is placed supine and both CT and MRI studies may fail to show tissue caught within the inguinal or femoral canals. US is a dynamic study and is able to evaluate patients in real time. It, however, is a less objective or standardized examination and is highly dependent on the skill and performance of the operator. US is also contingent upon the patient's ability to perform a strong Valsalva maneuver, an adequate cough, or strain effectively. We have not found US to be very helpful in our practice.

If given a choice of imaging studies to use on someone we are considering operating on for a potential recurrent inguinal hernia, a CT with intravenous and enteric contrast would be our preference (**Figure 12.4**). While we rarely do this, even in reoperative settings, sometimes it is useful. It heightens our concern and awareness for incarcerated colon, small bowel, or bladder, and CT is very accurate when tissue is incarcerated. If the concern relates more to chronic pain, and consideration for athletic pubalgia or musculoskeletal troubles, then MRI with gadolinium infusion is the imaging modality of choice (Amid 2004, Aasvang et al. 2009, van den Berg 2002).

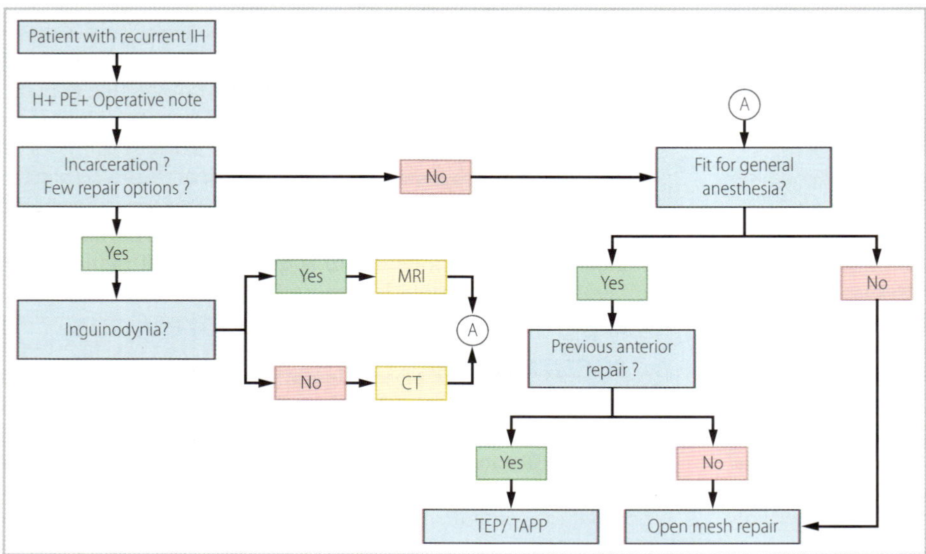

Figure 12.3 Basic algorithm for evaluation and treatment of patients with a recurrent inguinal hernia. H, history; PE, physical examination.

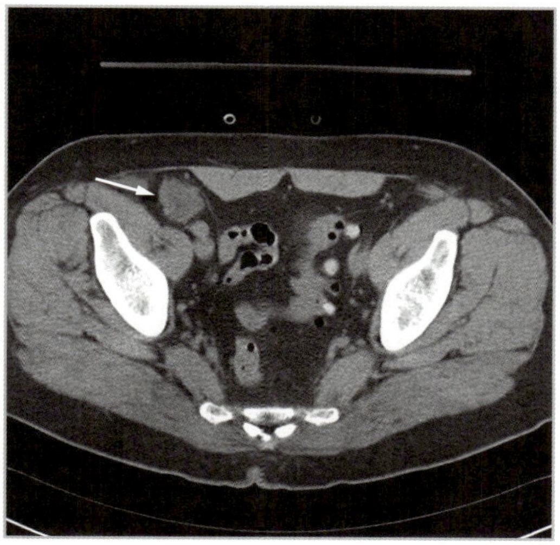

Figure 12.4 Computed tomography image of a mesh plug (arrow) residing in the right groin: 'meshoma.'

In summary, imaging is rarely necessary for patients undergoing re-do inguinal hernia surgery.

ADDITIONAL PREOPERATIVE CONCERNS

For patients undergoing reoperative hernia surgery, the operation is typically performed under general anesthesia; thus, careful evaluation of the patient's medical history, fitness, and medications is important. Assuming the patient is fit to undergo general anesthesia, then careful analysis of the use of anticoagulation (Plavix, Coumadin, aspirin, etc.) as well as insulin or steroid usage is important. In an ideal setting none of these medications would be required during surgical intervention. If possible, a month or two of rehabilitation and concerted effort improving physical fitness will benefit both patient and surgeon. Optimally, our patients should avoid tobacco usage for several months prior to surgery; cirrhotic patients will have ascites controlled, diabetic patients have improved compliance and better glucose control; morbidly obese patients begin losing weight and begin an exercise program; and patients with myocardial ischemia undergo therapy to enhance blood flow. Wound complications will be minimized if the preoperative health of the patient is maximized.

SURGICAL CONSIDERATIONS

Armed with a thorough history and physical examination and the previous operative reports in a fit patient undergoing general anesthesia, other pertinent considerations should surface in the surgeon's mind. Previous operations that suggest massive scarring, lax tissue, and difficult dissections should prompt concerns over a longer operation. Prophylactic intravenous antibiotics should be given and subcutaneous heparin or surgical compressive devices considered in patients with a greater risk of venous thromboembolism. Enlisting the support of another skilled or experienced surgeon may be of benefit in the most complex recurrent inguinal hernias. The possibility of needing a plastic surgeon is rare, but there have been times that our patients (and the general surgeon) have benefitted from such preoperative and intraoperative assistance. After careful induction of anesthesia, all patients are prepared and draped while supine on the operating table with arms tucked (or brought out to 90° if morbidly obese). If there is any concern about bladder injury or involvement of the bladder in a recurrent hernia, then urinary catheterization is prudent.

THE OPERATION

Previous open inguinal hernia recurrence

In a patient who has undergone an open inguinal hernia repair and now has a recurrence, our preference would be to perform laparoscopic surgery. However, the laparoscopic approach is typically abandoned if the patient has had a previous open prostatectomy [scarring makes totally extraperitoneal (TEP) and transabdominal preperitoneal (TAPP) hernia repairs more difficult). If there is a suggestion that the patient requires an urgent or emergent procedure with incarcerated bowel, we would favor initial laparoscopy as a viable option to immediately assess the intraoperative difficulties and then consider repair via TAPP or TEP or anterior approach.

With a straightforward recurrence from a previous open repair, whether with mesh (plug, hernia system, Lichtenstein) or a primary tissue based repair (Shouldice, Bassini, McVay), the preperitoneal placement of mesh is an excellent repair with a low risk of recurrence (Bisgaard et al. 2008, Sevonius et al. 2011). Caveats to laparoscopy in previous anterior repairs would be the importance of knowing that the patient has had a mesh plug, Kugel patch, or mesh hernia 'system' placed. This implies the previous operation violated the preperitoneal space and dissection may be a bit more difficult. While our experience has not found this to be overly problematic, the surgeon needs to recognize that mesh adherence to the epigastric vessels, the iliac vessels, and the spermatic cord may at times be troublesome and challenging. Unless the operation is for inguinodynia, most previously placed mesh is left in place. Patience, persistence, and finesse rather than brute strength in regions of scarring and mesh adherence will invariably serve the general surgeon well. Exposing widely the preperitoneal space and laying a panel of mesh at least 10 cm × 15 cm in size will allow for a dependable, outpatient hernia repair.

Previous laparoscopic recurrence

Whether the patient has had a TAPP or a TEP laparoscopic procedure, our usual strategy would be a subsequent open inguinal hernia repair. Prolene mesh is typically placed via a Lichtenstein technique in a tension free manner. Intraoperative findings will usually identify a direct defect and the previous mesh may not be visible or palpable. In such a case, the Lichtenstein repair is relatively straightforward; scarring to pelvic organs is uncommon but carefully assessed and meticulously released. In larger defects, omentum, bowel, and sometimes bladder may inhibit visualization of the inguinal floor and make repair difficult; placing several interrupted sutures in the shelving edge of the inguinal ligament and the conjoined tendon offers a pseudoclosure and facilitates later meticulous and tension-free mesh placement.

Open and laparoscopic previous recurrences: re-recurrences

We have had patients referred to see us with as many as a dozen inguinal hernia recurrences. Patients such as this often have had multiple open and one or two laparoscopic attempts at inguinal hernia repair. Clearly these patients are at extraordinarily high risk of a further hernia recurrence and potential complications postoperatively. First and foremost, these patients must be assessed on whether indeed another attempt at surgery is warranted. Often times the answer to that question is no, and use of a truss or bicycle shorts or even going without support is likely in the patient's best interest. If indeed an attempt at additional repair is made, then consultation with other physicians would be mandatory: plastic or bariatric surgeons, internists or the family practice physician. Many patients benefit greatly from weight loss, smoking cessation, and better diabetic control prior to attempting reoperative surgery for the second, third or fourth time.

Based on the individual, if the preperitoneal space is impossible to develop, there have been times in a multiply recurrent setting that we perform a laparoscopic hernia repair similar to mesh or Gore-Tex onlay seen with ventral hernia repairs. Advanced laparoscopic skills in attaching the mesh to the pubis, the abdominal wall, and potentially the anterior superior iliac spine are necessary. Anchoring devices including titanium tacks, intracorporeal suturing, as well as preformed tacks harboring sutures have been helpful. The larger the panel of mesh, the less likely hernias recur, but even in this setting many patients, due to their morbid obesity and poor tissue healing with increased intra-abdominal pressure, will develop recurrence. We freely admit that not all complex recurrent hernia repairs have been curative for our patients. Repairing multiply recurrent defects from the anterior aspect hoping that a larger panel of mesh with bigger purchases of scarred muscle and fascia is not a guarantee of success; placing these patients in a supportive garment postoperatively for several weeks will help fixate and scar in this region in a better manner and, more importantly, remind patients to avoid overexertion. Lifting >10 pounds is precluded for a full 90 days.

POSTOPERATIVE CARE

Most of these patients are repaired as an outpatient and are advised to avoid exertion for at least 4 weeks. Heavy exertion should be avoided at all costs. Aggressive management to assure regular bowel movements is started preoperatively and narcotic use is discouraged. Adequate hydration combined with the use of anti-inflammatory agents is preferred. Ice is a mainstay of therapy. Re-evaluating the patient in 1 month typically shows the resolution of edema and swollen genitalia and a satisfied patient. Patients should be counseled to minimize intra-abdominal pressure (avoid heavy exertion, smoking, and constipation) as much as is possible.

INGUINODYNIA

Patients undergoing reoperative groin surgery will typically do so for one of two problems: (1) symptomatic recurrent hernia or (2) inguinodynia. In the senior author's experience of evaluating approximately 3000 people with inguinal hernias, those patients, who are complaining preoperatively of a symptomatic recurrent inguinal hernia, have rarely, if ever, complained of inguinodynia postoperatively. They are first and foremost set on the repair of their hernia and do not seem to be troubled with pain and discomfort postoperatively. While we are meticulous about preserving nerves and carefully placing mesh and sutures, over 20 years of practice, several ilioinguinal, genitofemoral, and iliohypogastric nerves have surely been traumatized by the senior author. Nonetheless, patients with recurrent hernias seem to be very satisfied and minimize or diminish the importance of the pain that many have surely had. Hopefully careful placement of mesh and avoiding trauma to these important sensory nerves is part of our success.

The opposite idea of the previous paragraph is not true: patients who return with groin pain following hernia surgery *without* a recurrence are a very difficult lot to treat. Invariably these patients will be young men who previously had an asymptomatic hernia repaired. It is for this reason we try to avoid repairing inguinal hernias in young men who are asymptomatic. Only a handful of asymptomatic inguinal hernia patients have been offered an immediate repair in our experience: those being deployed overseas for military combat or those who are involved in wilderness exploration, or some patient who will be away from medical care for years at a time. If this is indeed the case, then we counsel them very carefully that they may have discomfort postoperatively, and we go to great lengths to avoid intraoperative trauma to any nerves.

With this in mind, from a laparoscopic standpoint, the important concept is to avoid tacks or sutures into the lateral femoral cutaneous nerve or the genitofemoral nerve. Placing tacks deep into muscle (using the tacker as an 'impaler') puts both the iliohypogastric and ilioinguinal nerves at risk. Laparoscopic repairs should never place tacks or sutures posteriorly, and all tacks used are lightly placed through the mesh to just 'tack' the mesh in place.

Mesh may cause inguinodynia, especially when wrapped circumferentially around the spermatic cord via TAPP or TEP procedures. We never wrap the cord with mesh for endoscopic inguinal hernia procedures. Removing mesh is difficult – whether anteriorly (**Figure 12.5**) or posteriorly (**Figure 12.6**) – but has alleviated groin pain in many patients referred to us.

From an anterior standpoint, careful evaluation and knowing where the iliohypogastric and ilioinguinal nerves reside are important. We prefer not to dissect them free from the surrounding tissues and only allow the mesh to lay safely under no tension. Sutures are kept well away from any of the visualized nerves (**Figure 12.7**). If indeed a nerve is identified and is in harm's way, the choices are two: (1) dissect it freely and place the nerve away from the mesh, or (2) if the mesh or sutures will abut, abrade, or bother the nerve in question, then the nerve is transected as lateral as possible and removed. Additionally, whenever inguinodynia and mesh exist together, if the previously placed mesh is removed, we avoid hernia repair at that operation. Prioritization of pain versus hernia recurrence is important to clarify preoperatively in all patients.

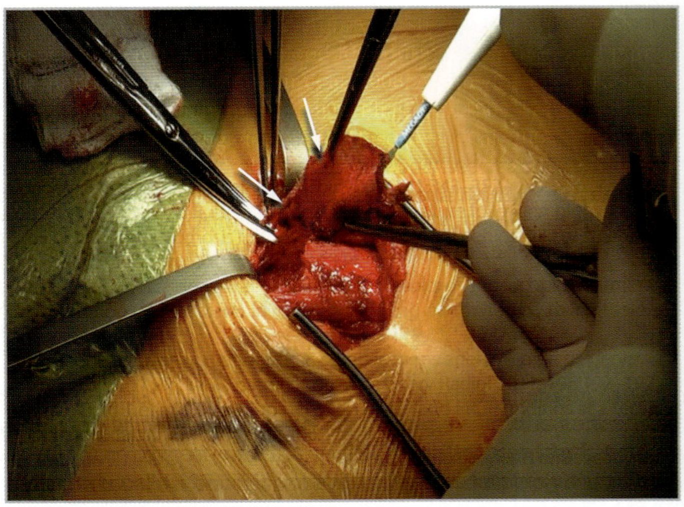

Figure 12.5 Explantation of mesh (arrows) from an anterior approach.

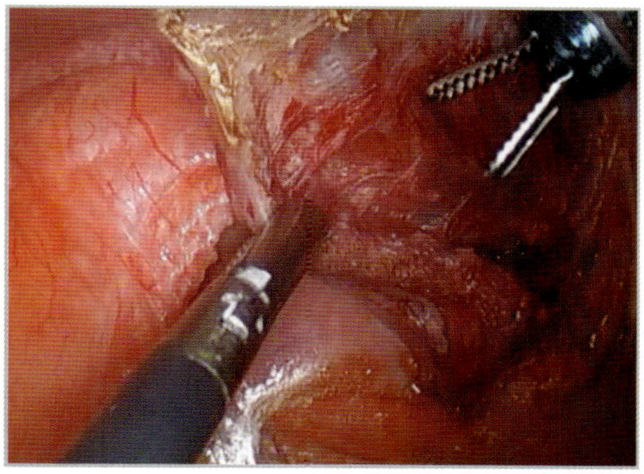

Figure 12.6 Intraoperative laparoscopic view for a previous totally extraperitoneal, demonstrating tenacious adhesions that obliterated the space of Bogros. Mesh explantation was performed for inguinodynia. Dissection can potentially increase the risk of injury to the lateral femoral cutaneous nerve.

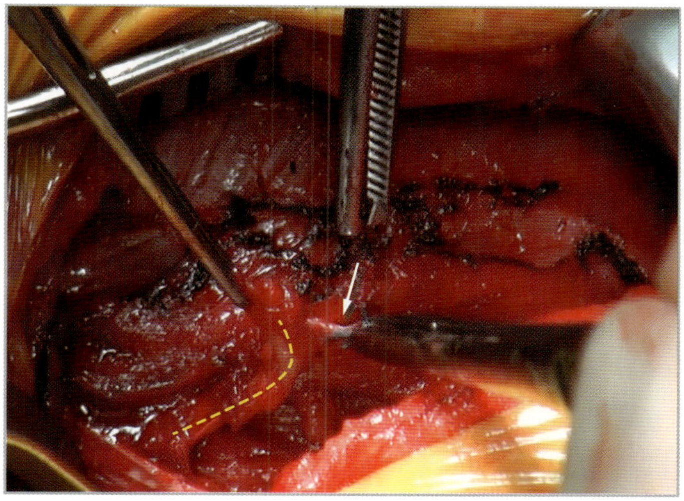

Figure 12.7 A blue 2-0 Prolene suture (arrow) found tied around the ilioinguinal nerve.

SUMMARY

Reoperative groin surgery may be complex with large defects, poor tissues, incarcerated bowel or bladder, and inguinodynia. The experienced general surgeon can tackle this problem and alleviate recurrence in well over 95% of patients in long-term follow-up. Invariably this will be done with a tension-free repair either done laparoscopically for previous open anterior approaches or vice versa through an anterior approach with mesh for those patients who have previously undergone laparoscopic surgery.

REFERENCES

Aasvang EK, Jensen KE, Fiirgaard B, Kehlet H. MRI and pathology in persistent postherniotomy pain. J Am Coll Surg 2009; 208:1023–1028, discussion 1028–1029.

Amid PK. Radiologic images of meshoma: a new phenomenon causing chronic pain after prosthetic repair of abdominal wall hernias. Arch Surg 2004; 139:1297–1298.

Bay-Nielsen M, Kehlet H, Strand L, Danish Hernia Database Collaboration. Quality assessment of 26,304 herniorrhaphies in Denmark: a prospective nationwide study. Lancet 2001; 358:1124–1128.

Bemdsen F, Sevonius D. Changing the path of inguinal hernia surgery decreased the recurrence rate ten-fold. Report from a county hospital. Eur J Surg 2002; 168:592–596.

Bisgaard T, Bay-Nielsen M, Kehlet H. Re-recurrence after operation for recurrent inguinal hernia. A nationwide 8-year follow-up study on the role of type of repair. Ann Surg 2008; 247:707–711.

Haapaniemi S, Gunnarsson U, Nordin P, Nilsson E. Reoperation after recurrent groin hernia repair. Ann Surg 2001; 234:122–126.

Lau WY. History of treatment of groin hernia. World J Surg 2002; 26:748–759.

McVay CB. Inguinal and femoral hernioplasty; anatomic repair. Arch Surg 1948; 57:524–530.

Nilsson E, Haapaniemi S, Gruber G, Sandblom G. Methods of repair and risk for reoperation in Swedish hernia surgery from 1992 to 1996. Br J Surg 1998; 85:1686–1691.

Rutkow IM. Demographic and socioeconomic aspects of hernia repair in the United States in 2003. Surg Clin North Am 2003; 83:1045–1051, v-vi.

Sevonius D, Gunnarsson U, Nordin P, Nilsson E, Sandblom G. Recurrent groin hernia surgery. Br J Surg 2011; 98:1489–1494.

Shouldice EB. The Shouldice natural tissue repair for inguinal hernia. BJU Int 2010; 105:428–439.

van den Berg JC. Inguinal hernias: MRI and ultrasound. Semin Ultrasound CT MR 2002; 23:156–173.

Chapter 13 Repair of the recurrent ventral hernia

Alla Zemlyak, Paul D. Colavita, B. Todd Heniford

If we could artificially produce tissues of the density and toughness of fascia and tendon the secret of the radical cure of hernia would be discovered.

Billroth, 1878 (From Beitrage zur Chirurgie by Vincenz Czerny, cited in Halsted, 1924)

HISTORICAL PERSPECTIVE

Hippocrates used the Greek *hernios* for 'bulge' to describe abdominal hernias. The Ebers papyrus, from approximately 1550 BC, described the use of a truss. Celsius advocated gradual pressure (taxis) in the management of incarcerated hernia. The earliest recorded surgical effort was the reduction in inguinal hernia through a scrotal incision, while the earliest prosthetic repair of hernia was performed by Phelps with silver coils in 1894 (Read 2004). Abdominal stiffness and patient discomfort have eventually resulted in the replacement of metal meshes with plastic ones. Repair of incisional hernias with Marlex (polypropylene) was first reported in 1958 (Read 2004). Mersilene and polytetrafluoroethylene (PTFE) meshes were first used for hernia repair in 1967 and 1980, respectively. Laparoscopic hernia repairs were first attempted in late 1980s and now play a competitive role in prosthetic hernia repair. So-called biologic meshes opened a new chapter in the history of hernia prosthetics, and their use for ventral hernias in contaminated wounds began in the first decade of this millennium. The search for the ideal hernia prosthetic continues today.

WHY DO HERNIA OPERATIONS FAIL?

Recurrence is the principal problem in ventral and incisional hernia repair. Recurrence rates of 25–50% have been reported after primary (suture) repairs and complicated abdominal hernia repairs (Hesse et al. 1993, Novitsky et al. 2006). Such high failure rates mandate investigation. It is said that the recurrence rate for incisional hernias nearly doubles without prosthetic mesh reinforcement (Hesselink et al. 1993, Luijendijk et al. 2000, Novitsky et al. 2006). The use of mesh reinforcement is based on the principle of tension-free repair and significantly reduces recurrence after hernia surgery (Luijendijk et al. 2000). This principle applies even to smaller abdominal wall defects that have often been repaired primarily. As has been shown by studies on umbilical hernias, even small hernias (<3 cm) have significantly higher (up to 11 times) recurrence rates when repaired primarily as opposed to mesh repair (Arroyo et al. 2001, , Farrow et al. 2008, Halm et al. 2005). Placing synthetic mesh has significantly improved the long-term success of ventral hernia operations in our opinion. In some studies, the recurrence rate after open ventral hernia repair with mesh was reported below 2% (Abdollahi et al. 2010), but these low numbers are rarely noted in other studies. However, the use of a synthetic mesh has introduced the problem of mesh infection. The overall rate of mesh infections is estimated at 1–5% in most studies (Collage & Rosengart 2010, Mavros et al. 2011). Mesh and subcutaneous tissue infection is a strong predictor of failure of hernia repair. Severe mesh infection may lead to systemic sepsis and necessitate mesh removal, although successful nonoperative treatment has been reported. Mesh harboring chronic low-grade infection does not become well incorporated with the tissues compromising the strength of the repair and eventually results in recurrence.

The advancement of laparoscopic techniques was an important milestone in the history of hernia surgery. The recurrence rate associated with laparoscopic repairs has been reported to be up to 12%, but in most series it does not exceed 5% (Asencio et al. 2009, Berger et al. 2002, Bingener et al. 2007, Heniford et al. 2000, 2003, LeBlanc 2007, Rudmik et al. 2006). The major advantages of laparoscopic technique are enhanced visualization of the ventral defect, the surrounding fascial integrity, reducing wound complications by minimizing soft tissue dissection and mesh exposure to potential sources of contamination, and possibly reducing incisional pain, although this is disputed in more recent studies. The studies that have analyzed the recurrence patterns after laparoscopic hernia repairs show that inadequate mesh overlap (mesh-to-defect area ratio <2) and failure to bridge the entire length of the fascial incision with mesh (in the case of incisional hernias) were the major factors associated with recurrence (LeBlanc et al. 2003, Wassenaar et al. 2009).

Among patient-related factors, the history of previous recurrence has been most strongly associated with hernia recurrence(Hesselink et al. 1993, Manninen et al. 1991, Novitsky et al. 2006, Varkarakis et al. 2010). Obesity has been shown by some studies, but not others to contribute to herniorrhaphy failure (Anthony et al. 2000, Hesselink et al. 1993,Manninen et al. 1991). Other factors, such as smoking, diabetes, cardiopulmonary disease, and steroid use, have been found to be associated with hernia recurrence by some studies, but these results have not been consistent across the board (Anthony et al. 2000, Bencini et al. 2009, Chang et al. 2011, Heartsill et al. 2005, Hesselink et al. 1993, Ko et al. 2009, Varkarakis et al. 2010). Based on current evidence, we believe that the best way to prevent hernia recurrence at the time of operation is to reinforce the repair with a mesh and have adequate overlap of the defect edges.

CHOOSING MESH FOR RECURRENT HERNIA REPAIR

As mentioned above, repair with prosthetic material significantly reduces the rate of hernia recurrence, and therefore it should be used whenever possible to reinforce a recurrent hernia regardless of how the original repair was performed. Synthetic materials are preferred for their durability and lower cost compared with the biologic meshes. In cases of active infection, contamination, or exposure of intestinal contents, bioprosthetics, such as human dermis, porcine dermis/submucosa, or bovine dermis/pericardium, should be considered.

There are a variety of synthetic meshes available today; these can consist of polypropylene, polyester, or expanded polytetrafluoroethylene (ePTFE). Composite meshes consist of multiple material types, typically polypropylene and ePTFE. Polypropylene promotes tissue ingrowth and integration into the abdominal wall but is fraught with adhesion formation when exposed to bowel, while ePTFE is more inert to the abdominal viscera. Composite meshes were popularized by laparoscopic repair techniques with intraperitoneal mesh placement, in order to provide integration on the fascial side and reduce adhesion formation on the visceral side (Balique et al. 2005). Unfortunately, the combination of meshes in these products has been shown to have a high infection rate and, secondly, to become very stiff with a resultant reduction in patient quality of life. Alternatively, dissolving antiadhesive coatings composed of hyaluronic acid, carboxymethyl cellulose, and omega-3 fatty acids are commonly used to minimize bowel adhesions. When planning a reoperative abdominal hernia repair, it is important to set proper expectations and safe exposure strategy based on the anticipated degree of visceral adhesions to the previously implanted materials, keeping in mind that none are exempted from adhesion formation.

Recently, laboratory and human experiments have shown that the traditional 'heavyweight' polypropylene mesh strength far exceeds the physiological range (Klinge et al. 1998, Schumpelick & Klinge 2003, Schmidbauer et al. 2005). Although the burst strength of a lightweight mesh is significantly lower than that of a heavyweight one, it is still more than double than that of the native fascia (Cobb et al. 2006). Lightweight mesh is also less prone to adhesions than heavyweight (Schug-Pass et al. 2008). Heavyweight polypropylene mesh without an adhesion barrier provides durable hernia repair, but may lead to erosion into the bowel and fistulization if placed in direct contact with intraperitoneal organs, especially in the face of infection or when multiple operations are required (Basoglu et al. 2004, Halm et al. 2007, Schug-Pass et al. 2008). Multifiber meshes show more propensity to infection than monofilament meshes based on some in vitro and animal studies, but the clinical significance of these observations is yet to be established (Harrell et al. 2006, Klinge et al. 2002).

A grading system for ventral incisional hernias was developed by Ventral Hernia Working Group (VHWG), which provides a relatively straightforward guide for decision making in regard to the use of synthetic versus biologic mesh (Breuing et al. 2010). Hernias are assigned to grades 1 through 4 based on the risk factors of the patient and their operative wound (**Table 13.1**). In general, based on available evidence and the consensus opinion of hernia experts, permanent synthetic material is not recommended for grades 3 and 4 hernias (Choi et al. 2012). In the context of recurrent hernias, this issue often arises when a patient has an active ongoing mesh infection (grade 4) or has had a prior excision of infected mesh (grade 3). If a synthetic mesh is used under such circumstances, there is greater than normal risk of developing postoperative infection or persistent draining sinus. The synthetic mesh can harbor bacteria and prevent the host immune defenses from eradicating the infection even with therapeutic levels of antibiotics in the bloodstream (Szczerba & Dumanian 2003). Traditionally, mesh excision was performed (Cavallaro et al. 2010), but, more recently, many of these cases can be managed without mesh removal. In this situation, consideration should be given to the use of biologic or newer bioabsorbable meshes. When used as a bridge, biologic meshes have a high rate of eventration or recurrence. In a clean, noncontaminated field, recurrent hernias should be repaired with a synthetic mesh in order to achieve the best, long-lasting, and cost-effective outcomes.

Table 13.1 Ventral Hernia Working Group classification (Bencini et al. 2009)

Grade 1	Healthy patient with no history of surgical site infections
Grade 2	Smoker, obese, diabetic, immunosuppressed, chronic obstructive pulmonary disease
Grade 3	Previous wound infection, stoma, violation of gastrointestinal tract
Grade 4	Infected mesh, septic dehiscence

Biologic mesh is made of an acellular collagen matrix derived from human or animal dermal, fascial, pericardial, or other tissues. Biologic meshes allow the body to eradicate small amounts of bacterial contamination (up to 10^4 CFU/ml) by promoting tissue ingrowth and allowing host immune cells into the mesh collagen matrix. The data available on the use of human acellular dermal matrix (HADM) show that it can be incorporated into contaminated tissue without becoming infected (Candage et al. 2008). Postoperative wound complications in the setting of HADM are often successfully treated with drainage (Kim et al. 2006). Compared with synthetic meshes, biologic meshes require explantation much less frequently (Shah et al. 2011). To date, there has not been a clinical trial comparing different biologic implants, and all available evidence comes from animal studies and small retrospective human reviews. Non-cross-linked collagen meshes demonstrate better ability to clear infections compared with cross-linked meshes (Harth et al. 2011), but eventration (thinning) of the mesh is more pronounced with non-cross-linked meshes as well as a tendency for a higher recurrence rate (Mulier et al. 2011, Shah et al. 2011).

PREOPERATIVE CARE AND IMAGING

Most often, a recurrent hernia is palpable, presents with patient symptoms, and is a straightforward clinical diagnosis. At times, however, confirmation of a recurrent hernia is more difficult because of the previous laparotomy scar, previously placed mesh, and/or obesity, which frequently accompanies a recurrent hernia. Computed tomography (CT) most often accurately identifies clinically occult abdominal wall hernias (Ianora et al. 2000). CT also reliably distinguishes hernias from hematomas, abscesses, and postoperative fluid collections (Ianora et al. 2000, Gossios et al. 2003, Wagenblast et al. 2004). Intestines within the hernia sac are easily identified with CT imaging, as well as incarceration and ischemia (Ianora et al. 2000, Gossios et al. 2003). Previously placed mesh and its boundaries, as well as the site of recurrence, are demonstrated very accurately with CT (Gossios et al. 2003).

Routine CT use when a recurrent hernia is suspected often aids with diagnosis and surgical planning. Reoperative hernia surgery is often difficult; simply accessing the postoperative abdomen can be problematic. Of particular concern with access is the presence of adhesions to both the mesh and the abdominal wall. Preoperative imaging, while certainly not required, can often reveal a plane of fat between the abdominal wall or mesh and the viscera, which may permit safe entry into the abdomen. Preoperative imaging will delineate the extent of the fascial defect, which is often obscured on the physical examination by the presence of previous, partially attached mesh or hernia incarceration. CT may also illustrate many undetected conditions that could impact the operative technique, such as inflammation from infection in the abdominal wall. The authors routinely attempt to acquire the most recent CT imaging, if available; while not mandatory, again, it may be helpful.

During operative planning, we often attempt to obtain the most recent surgical records, especially operative reports. A great deal of information can be gained from careful review of prior records: initial hernia defect, repair technique, mesh type, mesh placement (intraperitoneal, preperitoneal, posterior rectus, etc.), and fixation method, intraoperative complications, postoperative complications, and similar details from any repeated surgeries. All of these details can impact a surgeon's operative decisions for creating the best and final repair. In patients with multiple failed hernia repairs, the prior surgeons' descriptions of what has likely become an increasingly hostile abdomen will be of great assistance. Knowing which potential spaces have been previously used for mesh placement, and whether or not any extent of a component separation was performed will aid decision making; while these things can be sorted out intraoperatively, this knowledge is helpful preoperatively. Indeed, knowing the presence of prior metal fixation tacks can increase surgeon safety, as they can cause puncture through surgical gloves quite easily.

Understanding where and how the previous repair failed may influence the choice of mesh or fixation constructs and permit additional reinforcement in the area that is at highest risk of recurrence. Combining operative reports with preoperative imaging may illuminate the contributing factors to the failure of prior repairs, as well as the evolving recurrent hernia defect in patients with multiple failed operations.

OPERATIVE APPROACH: LAPAROSCOPIC REPAIR

Based on multiple reviews of ventral hernia repair, many of the patients with recurrent ventral hernias can undergo a laparoscopic repair (Cobb et al. 2006, Heniford & Ramshaw 2000, Heniford et al. 2000, Heniford et al. 2003, Hope et al. 2008, Novitsky et al. 2006, Tsereteli et al. 2008, Zerey & Heniford 2006). This operation can be performed in obese patients, with multiple previous hernia repairs or other operations, and a conversion rate of 5% or less has been seen in some experienced hands (Novitsky et al. 2006). The operation begins by establishing pneumoperitoneum with either Veress needle or cut-down approach. Preoperative imaging can help determine the safest point of entry; this is often between the costal margin and iliac crest on either side, even with the multiply recurrent hernia.

After access is achieved and additional laparoscopic ports are safely inserted under direct vision, adhesiolysis begins (**Figure 13.1a**). All adhesions to the mesh and abdominal wall must be taken down. The authors recommend a combination of blunt and sharp dissection. For the sharp dissection, laparoscopic scissors are most often used and electrosurgery is limited. In cases where extensive adhesions are present, the risk of intestinal injury is approximately 0.5–1.5% even in experienced hands and can yield additional complications postoperatively (Heniford et al. 2003, Novitsky et al. 2006).

An enterotomy does not preclude the use of synthetic mesh if it is recognized promptly without gross intestinal spillage. However, if spillage occurs, a staged herniorrhaphy or closure without mesh can be performed, or biologic mesh could be used. Some surgeons now believe that lightweight, widepore, monofilament meshes can be used in an at-risk field. Studies are ongoing to sort this out.

The complete resection of all previously placed mesh is not mandatory, but any loose or bridging material as well as any foreign material suspicious for having an active or past infection should be resected. Normal-appearing, well-incorporated mesh does not require removal. We strive for a mesh overlap on to normal fascia on all sides of the defect. However, for a small recurrence isolated at the edge of a previous repair, a patch repair can be undertaken. A new piece of mesh could be sutured intracorporeally or transcutaneously to the old mesh with a permanent suture. Dissolvable sutures or silk should never be used to sew mesh together. Transfascial suture fixation of mesh in addition to tacks alone has been disputed in the literature in terms of lowering recurrence rates (LeBlanc 2007). We routinely place transfascial sutures for added security in our laparoscopic ventral hernia repairs. Transfascial fixation provides a full-thickness anchor, which adds a layer of security to tack fixation (**Figure 13.1b**).

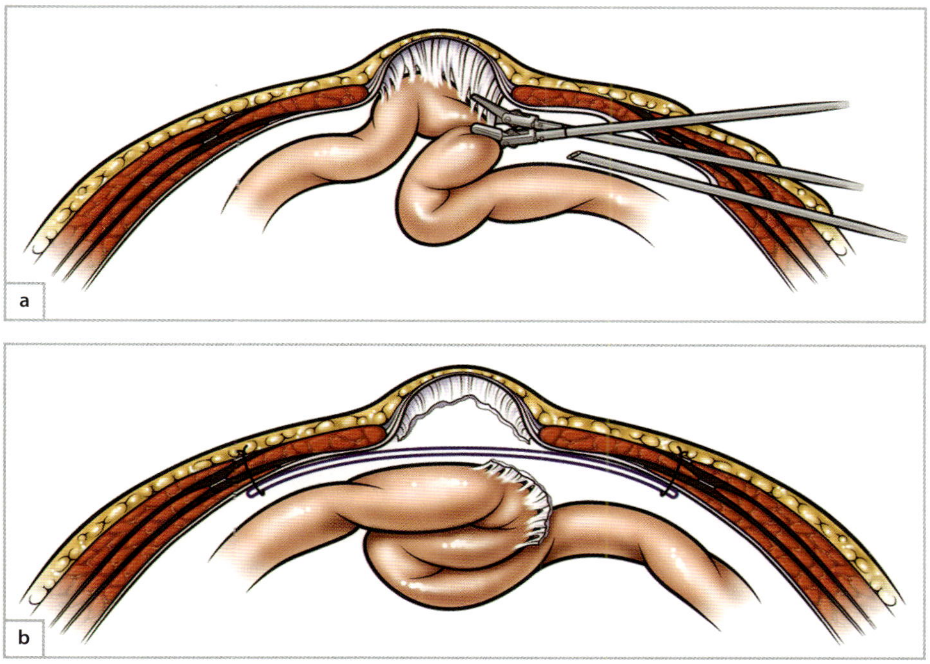

Figure 13.1 Laparoscopic hernia repair. (a) Enterolysis. (b) Completed repair with transfascial sutures. From Carolinas Healthcare System, with permission.

OPERATIVE APPROACH: OPEN REPAIR

Despite its inherent advantages, laparoscopy is not feasible in all patients. Patients with loss of abdominal domain, large pieces of mesh requiring resection, or complex and unusual hernias may not be good candidates for laparoscopy. Patients with thin or compromised abdominal skin, multiple scars, or a large pannus may benefit from concomitant panniculectomy, and these patients may be offered an open approach. Patients often express preference for an open repair, especially if they had a previous failed laparoscopic repair. The Rives--Stoppa technique, introduced in 1989 with reported recurrence rates of 1–14%, is popular among many surgeons and has been embraced as a standard for open ventral hernia repair (Awad et al. 2005, Bauer et al. 2002, Le & Bender 2005, Petersen et al. 2004, Stoppa 1989, Temudom et al. 1996). In this technique, a retrorectus plane (posterior to the rectus abdominis muscle and anterior to the posterior lamina of its sheath) is developed and a large piece of prosthetic mesh is placed in this plane (Stoppa 1989). An anterior rectus fascia is then closed on top of the mesh repair. According to Pascal's law of hydrostatics, the intra-abdominal pressures are uniformly distributed to the entire abdominal wall. With extensive mesh overlap, the same forces that are pushing on the mesh through the hernia defect are also pushing it against the adjacent abdominal wall thus holding it in place (Novitsky et al. 2006).

Our modification of this technique is the preperitoneal placement of the mesh (Novitsky et al. 2006). The peritoneum is carefully dissected from the transversalis fascia starting at the suprapubic space and extending cephalad to above the costal margin. Despite seeming difficulty, this can be successfully accomplished in cases with significant peritoneal scarring from previous hernia surgeries. The peritoneum is closed in the midline, the mesh secured in the preperitoneal plane, and the fascia reapproximated over the mesh (**Figure 13.2b**). There are three major advantages of our technique over the Rives–Stoppa. First, it allows much greater mesh overlap: the preperitoneal space can be dissected laterally and posteriorly and extended to the psoas muscle, while the retrorectus space is limited by the lateral borders of the rectus sheath. This permits fascial overlap of 8–10 cm or more. The use of mesh over 30 cm wide is not uncommon and affords lateral reinforcement of external oblique muscles release if a component separation is performed. Second, preperitoneal dissection can be easily carried down bluntly deep into the pelvis, in the space of Retzius, to the pubis. Lastly, the preperitoneal plane is usually bloodless and there is no risk of devascularizing the rectus muscle, which is especially important in the case of a compromised abdominal wall. With preperitoneal dissection, we can usually secure the mesh to the Cooper's ligaments inferiorly, as far as the psoas muscle laterally and beyond the costal margins superiorly. In our series, there have been few recurrences, and most are secondary to infection (Novitsky et al. 2006).

The open technique is often begun by excising the old scar (usually midline). We enter peritoneal cavity through the hernia sac or linea alba. Old mesh is routinely excised. We then perform lysis of adhesions. If serosal injuries or small enterotomies without spillage are inadvertently created, they are repaired with silk sutures and we proceed with the originally planned repair. Development of the preperitoneal plane may be challenging if the patient had multiple previous abdominal surgeries. We typically start this dissection by entering the space of Retzius at the lower midline level. Then using a blunt dissection technique, the plane is developed down to pubis, laterally, and cephalad toward the ribcage and then to the upper midline. Once the dissection is complete, the peritoneum is reapproximated with a running absorbable suture to cover the exposed visceral organs. If the peritoneum cannot be completely closed, we often secure omentum to edge of the peritoneum as a bridge to completely isolate the viscera from the space where the mesh will be placed.

Prior to mesh placement, the fascia is examined to determine whether or not primary closure will be possible. We use Kocher clamps to grasp the fascia on each side and pull toward the midline, gauging the amount of tension required to reapproximate the edges. If the fascia cannot be reapproximated, we consider other options, including component separation (see below). Once the mesh is placed in the preperitoneal space, it is secured to the abdominal wall with transfascial Prolene sutures. The sutures are placed 1–2 cm off the edge of the mesh and measured out at the corresponding position on the abdominal wall. Sutures are placed percutaneously using a transfascial suture passer, except where subcutaneous dissection is wide enough to permit transfascial sutures to be placed directly through the thickness of the abdominal wall. Sutures are placed superiorly on both sides of the xiphoid process and inferiorly just above the pubis and Cooper's ligament. The number of lateral fixation points depends on the extent of mesh-fascial overlap and ranges from 1 suture on each side to sutures spaced 3–5 cm apart. We routinely place closed suction drains over the mesh. The anterior fascia is closed over the mesh using a running permanent or slowly absorbing monofilament suture (**Figure 13.2c, d**).

COMPONENT SEPARATION

Reapproximation of the anterior fascia over the prosthetic mesh is ideal in open repair. Studies suggest that leaving anterior fascia open may lead to increased recurrence and higher rate of mesh infections (, Byrnes et al. 2011, Petersen et al. 2004). It is suggested that closure of anterior fascia results in better abdominal wall function and even pulmonary performance. Closed native tissue coverage over the mesh provides an additional antimicrobial barrier that prevents potential wound infections from extending onto the mesh. Fascial reapproximation may require excessive tension in cases of wide fascial defects. In such cases, a technique of abdominal components separation, first described by Ramirez, is used to create myofascial advancement flaps and reduce the tension on the reapproximated fascia (Ghazi et al. 2011, Nasajpour et al. 2011). Component separation may be performed on one or both sides of the abdominal wall by releasing the posterior rectus sheath, the external oblique muscle, or both. We chose to perform this prior to mesh placement.

The posterior rectus release is typically the first step of component separation. A longitudinal incision is made along the length of the posterior rectus fascia parallel to the hernia defect; it is often performed 1–2 cm lateral to the medial border of the rectus sheath, on one or both sides as necessary. This typically produces 2–3 cm of medial myofascial advancement on each side, which is frequently sufficient to approximate it without excessive tension. Otherwise, external oblique release can be performed on one or both sides. The external abdominal oblique fascia and muscle are incised lateral to the lateral border of rectus muscles from the iliac crest to the lower border of the ribcage, but the extent of the release can be taken to the inguinal ligament and well up onto the costal margin as needed. The external oblique release provides up to 10 cm of advancement on each side and is sufficient to reapproximate the anterior rectus fascia in most operations. We attempt to secure the mesh at a point lateral to the external oblique release for reinforcement of the potential abdominal wall weakness created by the release. In a patient with a large defect where a components separation will not result in closure

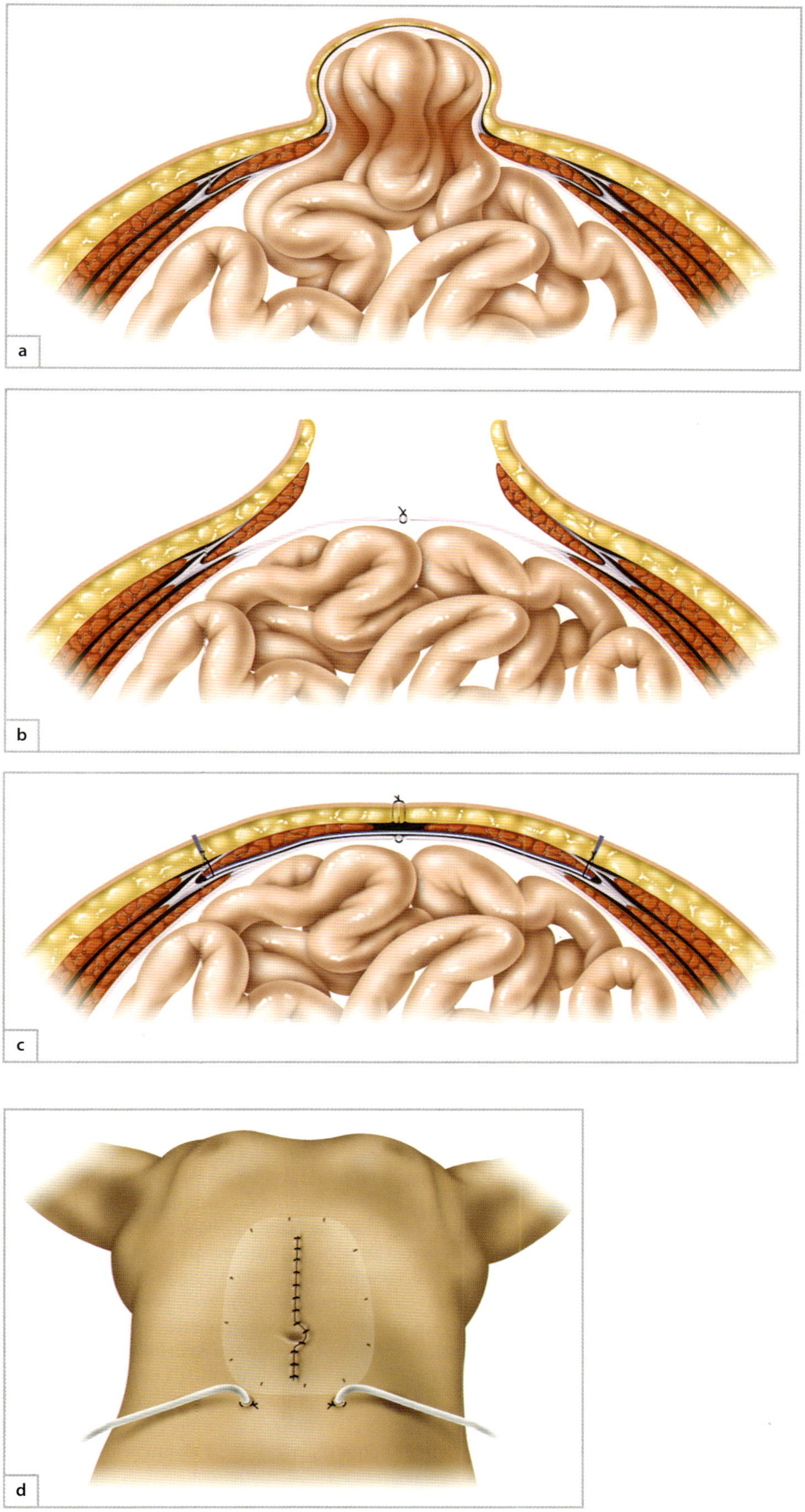

Figure 13.2 Open ventral hernia repair. (a) Ventral hernia. (b) Preperitoneal mesh placement. (c) Fascial closure after transfascial fixation of mesh. (d) Skin closure with prior drain placement. From Carolinas Healthcare System, with permission.

of the hernia or the oblique muscles are very thin, the anterior rectus fascia is left open.

PANNICULECTOMY

A concomitant panniculectomy can be offered to patients with recurrent ventral hernias who have thin or compromised skin, multiple scars, poorly vascularized tissue or to obese patients with a large pannus. Combining panniculectomy with ventral hernia repair allows one stage reconstruction of abdominal wall with results that are cosmetically and functionally pleasing to the patients (Berry et al. 2007, Hughes et al. 1996). Panniculectomy as an access procedure for ventral herniorrhaphy results in extensive exposure to the abdominal wall defect, which may facilitate repair (Downey et al. 2005). It has been shown that combining abdominoplasty with hernia repair is safe and has modest wound-related morbidity (Geffen & Simmermacher 2005, Hughes et al. 1996, Robertson et al. 2003). A plastic surgeon may perform the abdominoplasty or a general surgeon with such experience.

DRAINS

With extensive tissue dissection that is usually required for large recurrent hernias, there is great potential for seroma formation. During the extensive subcutaneous dissection, microscopic blood and lymphatic vessels are disrupted across a large area of soft tissue, which leads to accumulation of serous fluid (Beacon et al. 1980, Sarmah & Holl-Allen 1984). Closed suction drains should be placed above the prosthetic and in the subcutaneous tissues if abdominoplasty was performed. We recommend leaving them in place until a daily output is approximately 30 mL or less. It has been shown that drains decrease the seroma formation where extensive subcutaneous dissection was performed (Divino et al. 2000, Pearl et al. 1998, Somers et al. 1992). Closed suction drains are often quite simple for the patients to manage, and patients can be safely discharged home with them (Reid & Dumanian 2003).

SUBCUTANEOUS TALC TO PREVENT SEROMA FORMATION

Reducing the incidence of postoperative seromas in large recurrent hernia repairs, especially after panniculectomy and/or wide subcutaneous dissection, is a challenge for surgeons. Seromas can be chronic and occur despite drain placement during surgery. They can be unremitting and require multiple drainage procedures. Various agents have been used in an attempt to prevent subcutaneous seromas. Fibrin glue has been used in hernia operations and lymph node dissections with varying degrees of success (Moore et al. 2001, Mortenson et al. 2008, Santoro et al. 2007). We have published significant improvement in the rates of postoperative seroma and required interventions, as well as a decrease in the drain duration, with the use of subcutaneous talc (Klima et al. 2011). Talc (magnesium silicate hydroxide) is a sclerosing agent that has been used for pleurodesis of malignant pleural effusions with high degree of success (Kilic et al. 2005, Shaw & Agarwal 2004). It has been found to be effective in the treatment of chronic seromas (Holthouse & Chleboun 2001, Lehr & Schuricht 2001). We have demonstrated that it is also an effective prophylactic agent (Klima et al. 2011).

POSTOPERATIVE COMPLICATIONS AND THEIR TREATMENT AND PREVENTION

The incidence of postoperative complications after a laparoscopic repair demonstrates its overall safety (Heniford & Ramshaw 2000, Heniford et al. 2003). In our series of 850 patients, the overall complication rate was 13.2%, with the most common complications being prolonged ileus (3%) and seroma requiring intervention (2.6%) (Heniford et al. 2003). In our series of open preperitoneal repair, the overall incidence of complications was 18.8%, with 12.5% of patients developing surgical site infection and half of those eventually requiring operative debridement (Novitsky et al. 2006). From this experience, the most significant patient factor affecting wound morbidity is smoking (Novitsky et al. 2006). We, therefore, strongly encourage patients to quit smoking before the surgery.

Surgical site infections can have devastating consequences in hernia patients. Infections of the implanted mesh prosthetics are difficult to treat and can lead to mesh resection and hernia recurrence. Therefore, preventative strategies are important. Antibiotic prophylaxis should be administered at least 30 minutes before the incision. If a procedure lasts longer than 2–3 hours, we usually redose antibiotics intraoperatively depending on the half-life.

If a wound or mesh becomes infected, conservative management strategies are used first. Antibiotics and percutaneous drain placement for intra-abdominal or deep subcutaneous collections are the standard first step. Local wound explorations can also be performed. We have found that areas of exposed, lightweight polypropylene may be treated effectively with local wound care and vacuum-assisted devices in up to 75% of patients (Novitsky et al. 2006). Failure of mesh salvage is common in smokers.

CONCLUSIONS

Recurrent ventral hernias are a challenging problem. The approach to each patient should be individualized according to the number and types of previous hernia repairs, the patient's state of health and activity level, body habitus, and presence of infection or abdominal wounds. However, several general guidelines may facilitate a successful repair of recurrent ventral hernias. The principles of tension-free repair must be respected. Synthetic mesh under most circumstances should not be placed in infected or contaminated fields. At least 5 cm of mesh overlap should ideally be created on each side of the defect whether repair is performed in an open fashion or laparoscopically. Component separation is a useful technique to help achieve a tension-free closure of abdominal wall. Panniculectomy in certain patients may provide better surgical access to the ventral hernia. Intraoperative drain placement and subcutaneous talc help decrease the rates of seroma formation and wound breakdown. Controlling patient comorbidities (i.e. obesity and smoking) and preventive strategies for decreasing surgical site infections improve the surgical outcomes.

REFERENCES

Abdollahi A, Maddah GH, Mehrabi BM, et al. Prosthetic incisional hernioplasty: clinical experience with 354 cases. Hernia 2010; 14:569–573.

Anthony T, Bergen PC, Kim LT, et al. Factors affecting recurrence following incisional herniorrhaphy. World J Surg 2000; 24:95–100;discussion 101.

Arroyo A, Garcia P, Perez F, et al. Randomized clinical trial comparing suture and mesh repair of umbilical hernia in adults. Br J Surg 2001; 88:1321–1323.

Asencio F, Aguilo J, Peiro S, et al. Open randomized clinical trial of laparoscopic versus open incisional hernia repair. Surg Endosc 2009; 23:1441–1448.

Awad ZT, Puri V, LeBlanc K, et al. Mechanisms of ventral hernia recurrence after mesh repair and a new proposed classification. J Am Coll Surg 2005; 201:132–140.

Balique JG, Benchetrit S, Bouillot JL, et al. Intraperitoneal treatment of incisional and umbilical hernias using an innovative composite mesh: four-year results of a prospective multicenter clinical trial. Hernia. 2005; 9:68–74.

Basoglu M, Yildirgan MI, Yilmaz I, et al. Late complications of incisional hernias following prosthetic mesh repair. Acta Chir Belg 2004; 104:425–428.

Bauer JJ, Harris MT, Gorfine SR, Kreel I. Rives-Stoppa procedure for repair of large incisional hernias: experience with 57 patients. Hernia 2002; 6:120–123.

Beacon J, Hoile RW, Ellis H. A trial of suction drainage in inguinal hernia repair. Br J Surg 1980; 67:554–555.

Bencini L, Sanchez LJ, Bernini M, et al. Predictors of recurrence after laparoscopic ventral hernia repair. Surg Laparosc Endosc Percutan Tech 2009; 19:128–132.

Berger D, Bientzle M, Muller A. Postoperative complications after laparoscopic incisional hernia repair. Incidence and treatment. Surg Endosc 2002; 16:1720–1723.

Berry MF, Paisley S, Low DW, Rosato EF. Repair of large complex recurrent incisional hernias with retromuscular mesh and panniculectomy. Am J Surg 2007; 194:199–204.

Bingener J, Buck L, Richards M, et al. Long-term outcomes in laparoscopic vs open ventral hernia repair. Arch Surg 2007; 142:562–567.

Breuing K, Butler CE, Ferzoco S, et al. Incisional ventral hernias: review of the literature and recommendations regarding the grading and technique of repair. Surgery 2010; 148:544–558.

Byrnes MC, Irwin E, Carlson D, et al. Repair of high-risk incisional hernias and traumatic abdominal wall defects with porcine mesh. Am Surg 2011; 77:144–150.

Candage R, Jones K, Luchette FA, et al. Use of human acellular dermal matrix for hernia repair: friend or foe? Surgery 2008; 144:703–709; discussion 709–711.

Cavallaro A, Lo Menzo E, Di Vita M, et al. Use of biological meshes for abdominal wall reconstruction in highly contaminated fields. World J Gastroenterol 2010; 16:1928–1933.

Chang EI, Galvez MG, Padilla BE, et al. Ten-year retrospective analysis of incisional herniorrhaphy following renal transplantation. Arch Surg 2011; 146:21–25.

Choi JJ, Palaniappa NC, Dallas KB, et al. Use of mesh during ventral hernia repair in clean-contaminated and contaminated cases: outcomes of 33,832 cases. Ann Surg 2012; 255:176–180.

Cobb WS, Burns JM, Peindl RD, et al. Textile analysis of heavy weight, mid-weight, and light weight polypropylene mesh in a porcine ventral hernia model. J Surg Res 2006; 136:1–7.

Cobb WS, Kercher KW, Matthews BD, et al. Laparoscopic ventral hernia repair: a single center experience. Hernia 2006; 10:236–242.

Collage RD, Rosengart MR. Abdominal wall infections with in situ mesh. Surg Infect (Larchmt) 2010; 11:311–318.

Divino CM, Kuerer HM, Tartter PI. Drains prevent seromas following lumpectomy with axillary dissection. Breast J 2000; 6:31–33.

Downey SE, Morales C, Kelso RL, Anthone G. Review of technique for combined closed incisional hernia repair and panniculectomy status post-open bariatric surgery. Surg Obes Relat Dis 2005; 1:458–461.

Farrow B, Awad S, Berger DH, et al. More than 150 consecutive open umbilical hernia repairs in a major Veterans Administration Medical Center. Am J Surg 2008; 196:647–651.

Van Geffen HJ, Simmermacher RK. Incisional hernia repair: abdominoplasty, tissue expansion, and methods of augmentation. World J Surg 2005; 29:1080–1085.

Ghazi B, Deigni O, Yezhelyev M, Losken A. Current options in the management of complex abdominal wall defects. Ann Plast Surg 2011; 66:488–492.

Gossios K, Zikou A, Vazakas P, et al. Value of CT after laparoscopic repair of postsurgical ventral hernia. Abdom Imaging 2003; 28:99–102.

Halm JA, de Wall LL, Steyerberg EW, Jeekel J, Lange JF. Intraperitoneal polypropylene mesh hernia repair complicates subsequent abdominal surgery. World J Surg 2007; 31:423–429; discussion 430.

Halm JA, Heisterkamp J, Veen HF, Weidema WF. Long-term follow-up after umbilical hernia repair: are there risk factors for recurrence after simple and mesh repair. Hernia 2005; 9:334–337.

Halsted WS. Surgical Papers by William Stewart Halstead. Baltimore, MD: The Johns Hopkins Press, 1924; 1:271.

Harrell AG, Novitsky YW, Kercher KW, et al. In vitro infectability of prosthetic mesh by methicillin-resistant Staphylococcus aureus. Hernia 2006; 10:120–124.

Harth KC, Broome AM, Jacobs MR, et al. Bacterial clearance of biologic grafts used in hernia repair: an experimental study. Surg Endosc 2011; 25:2224–2229.

Heartsill L, Richards ML, Arfai N, et al. Open Rives-Stoppa ventral hernia repair made simple and successful but not for everyone. Hernia 2005; 9:162–166.

Heniford BT, Park A, Ramshaw BJ, Voeller G. Laparoscopic ventral and incisional hernia repair in 407 patients. J Am Coll Surg 2000; 190:645–650.

Heniford BT, Park A, Ramshaw BJ, Voeller G. Laparoscopic repair of ventral hernias: nine years' experience with 850 consecutive hernias. Ann Surg 2003; 238:391–399; discussion 399–400.

Heniford BT, Ramshaw BJ. Laparoscopic ventral hernia repair: a report of 100 consecutive cases. Surg Endosc 2000; 14:419–423.

Hesselink VJ, Luijendijk RW, de Wilt JH, Heide R, Jeekel J. An evaluation of risk factors in incisional hernia recurrence. Surg Gynecol Obstet 1993; 176:228–234.

Holthouse DJ, Chleboun JO. Talc serodesis – report of four cases. J R Coll Surg Edinb 2001; 46:244–245.

Hope WW, Lincourt AE, Newcomb WL, et al. Comparing quality-of-life outcomes in symptomatic patients undergoing laparoscopic or open ventral hernia repair. J Laparoendosc Adv Surg Tech A 2008; 18:567–571.

Hughes KC, Weider L, Fischer J, et al. Ventral hernia repair with simultaneous panniculectomy. Am Surg 1996; 62:678–681.

Ianora AA, Midiri M, Vinci R, Rotondo A, Angelelli G. Abdominal wall hernias: imaging with spiral CT. Eur Radiol 2000; 10:914–919.

Kilic D, Akay H, Kavukcu S, et al. Management of recurrent malignant pleural effusion with chemical pleurodesis. Surg Today 2005; 35:634–638.

Kim H, Bruen K, Vargo D. Acellular dermal matrix in the management of high-risk abdominal wall defects. Am J Surg 2006; 192:705–709.

Klima DA, Brintzenhoff RA, Tsirline VB, et al. Application of subcutaneous talc in hernia repair and wide subcutaneous dissection dramatically reduces seroma formation and postoperative wound complications. Am Surg 2011; 77:888–894.

Klinge U, Junge K, Spellerberg B, et al. Do multifilament alloplastic meshes increase the infection rate? Analysis of the polymeric surface, the bacteria adherence, and the in vivo consequences in a rat model. J Biomed Mater Res 2002; 63:765–771.

Klinge U, Klosterhalfen B, Conze J, et al. Modified mesh for hernia repair that is adapted to the physiology of the abdominal wall. Eur J Surg 1998; 164:951–960.

Ko JH, Wang EC, Salvay DM, Paul BC, Dumanian GA. Abdominal wall reconstruction: lessons learned from 200 "components separation" procedures. Arch Surg 2009; 144:1047–1055.

Le H, Bender JS. Retrofascial mesh repair of ventral incisional hernias. Am J Surg 2005; 189:373–375.

LeBlanc KA. Laparoscopic incisional hernia repair: are transfascial sutures necessary? A review of the literature. Surg Endosc 2007; 21:508–513.

LeBlanc KA, Whitaker JM, Bellanger DE, Rhynes VK. Laparoscopic incisional and ventral hernioplasty: lessons learned from 200 patients. Hernia 2003; 7:118–124.

Lehr SC, Schuricht AL. A minimally invasive approach for treating postoperative seromas after incisional hernia repair. JSLS 2001; 5:267–271.

Luijendijk RW, Hop WC, van den Tol MP, et al. A comparison of suture repair with mesh repair for incisional hernia. N Engl J Med 2000; 343:392–398.

Manninen MJ, Lavonius M, Perhoniemi VJ. Results of incisional hernia repair. A retrospective study of 172 unselected hernioplasties. Eur J Surg 1991; 157:29–31.

Mavros MN, Athanasiou S, Alexiou VG, et al. Risk factors for mesh-related infections after hernia repair surgery: a meta-analysis of cohort studies. World J Surg 2011; 35:2389–2398.

Moore M, Burak WE, Jr., Nelson E, et al. Fibrin sealant reduces the duration and amount of fluid drainage after axillary dissection: a randomized prospective clinical trial. J Am Coll Surg 2001; 192:591–599.

Mortenson MM, Xing Y, Weaver S, et al. Fibrin sealant does not decrease seroma output or time to drain removal following inguinofemoral lymph node dissection in melanoma patients: a randomized controlled trial (NCT00506311). World J Surg Oncol 2008; 6:63.

Mulier KE, Nguyen AH, Delaney JP, Marquez S. Comparison of Permacol and Strattice for the repair of abdominal wall defects. Hernia 2011; 15:315–319.

Nasajpour H, LeBlanc KA, Steele MH. Complex hernia repair using component separation technique paired with intraperitoneal acellular porcine dermis and synthetic mesh overlay. Ann Plast Surg 2011; 66:280–284.

Novitsky YW, Cobb WS, Kercher KW, et al. Laparoscopic ventral hernia repair in obese patients: a new standard of care. Arch Surg 2006; 141:57–61.

Novitsky YW, Porter JR, Rucho ZC, et al. Open preperitoneal retrofascial mesh repair for multiply recurrent ventral incisional hernias. J Am Coll Surg 2006; 203:283–289.

Pearl ML, Valea FA, Chalas E. Panniculectomy and supraumbilical vertical midline incisions in morbidly obese gynecologic oncology patients. J Am Coll Surg 1998; 186:649–653.

Petersen S, Henke G, Zimmermann L, et al. Ventral rectus fascia closure on top of mesh hernia repair in the sublay technique. Plast Reconstr Surg 2004; 114:1754–1760.

Read RC. Milestones in the history of hernia surgery: prosthetic repair. Hernia 2004; 8:8–14.

Reid RR, Dumanian GA. A minimalist approach to the care of the indwelling closed suction drain: a prospective analysis of local wound complications. Ann Plast Surg 2003; 51:575–578.

Robertson JD, de la Torre JI, Gardner PM, et al. Abdominoplasty repair for abdominal wall hernias. Ann Plast Surg 2003; 51:10–16.

Rudmik LR, Schieman C, Dixon E, Debru E. Laparoscopic incisional hernia repair: a review of the literature. Hernia 2006; 10:110–119.

Santoro E, Agresta F, Buscaglia F, et al. Preliminary experience using fibrin glue for mesh fixation in 250 patients undergoing minilaparoscopic transabdominal preperitoneal hernia repair. J Laparoendosc Adv Surg Tech A 2007; 17:12–15.

Sarmah BD, Holl-Allen RT. Porcine dermal collagen repair of incisional herniae. Br J Surg 1984; 71:524–525.

Schmidbauer S, Ladurner R, Hallfeldt KK, Mussack T. Heavy-weight versus low-weight polypropylene meshes for open sublay mesh repair of incisional hernia. Eur J Med Res 2005; 10:247–253.

Schug-Pass C, Sommerer F, Tannapfel A, Lippert H, Kockerling F. Does the additional application of a polylactide film (SurgiWrap) to a lightweight mesh (TiMesh) reduce adhesions after laparoscopic intraperitoneal implantation procedures? Experimental results obtained with the laparoscopic porcine model. Surg Endosc 2008; 22:2433–2439.

Schumpelick V, Klinge U. Prosthetic implants for hernia repair. Br J Surg 2003; 90:1457–1458.

Shah BC, Tiwari MM, Goede MR, et al. Not all biologics are equal! Hernia 2011; 15:165–171.

Shaw P, Agarwal R. Pleurodesis for malignant pleural effusions. Cochrane Database Syst Rev 2004:CD002916.

Somers RG, Jablon LK, Kaplan MJ, Sandler GL, Rosenblatt NK. The use of closed suction drainage after lumpectomy and axillary node dissection for breast cancer. A prospective randomized trial. Ann Surg 1992; 215:146–149.

Stoppa RE. The treatment of complicated groin and incisional hernias. World J Surg 1989; 13:545–554.

Szczerba SR, Dumanian GA. Definitive surgical treatment of infected or exposed ventral hernia mesh. Ann Surg 2003; 237:437–441.

Temudom T, Siadati M, Sarr MG. Repair of complex giant or recurrent ventral hernias by using tension-free intraparietal prosthetic mesh (Stoppa technique): lessons learned from our initial experience (fifty patients). Surgery 1996; 120:738–743; discussion 743–734.

Tsereteli Z, Pryor BA, Heniford BT, et al. Laparoscopic ventral hernia repair (LVHR) in morbidly obese patients. Hernia 2008; 12:233–238.

Varkarakis G, Daniels J, Coker K, et al. Effects of comorbidities and implant reinforcement on outcomes after component reconstruction of the abdominal wall. Ann Plast Surg 2010; 64:595–597.

Wagenblast AL, Kristiansen VB, Fallentin E, Schulze S. Computed tomography scanning and recurrence after laparoscopic ventral hernia repair. Surg Laparosc Endosc Percutan Tech 2004; 14:254–256.

Wassenaar EB, Schoenmaeckers EJ, Raymakers JT, Rakic S. Recurrences after laparoscopic repair of ventral and incisional hernia: lessons learned from 505 repairs. Surg Endosc 2009; 23:825–832.

Zerey M, Heniford BT. Laparoscopic versus open surgery for ventral hernia repair – which is best? Nat Clin Pract Gastroenterol Hepatol 2006; 3:372–373.

Chapter 14 Reoperative bariatric surgery

Yaniv Cozacov, Raul Rosenthal

INTRODUCTION

In the morbidly obese, surgery has in recent years been declared the most effective approach in achieving long-term weight loss with resolution of comorbidities (Demaria & Jamal 2005, National Institutes of Health 1991), and as such, there has been a surge of cases performed over the last decade.

Bariatric procedures, and their technical aspects, have gone through many modifications and evolved over the past few decades into today's standard procedures, mainly laparoscopic adjustable gastric banding (LAGB), Roux-en-Y gastric bypass (RYGB), laparoscopic sleeve gastrectomy (LSG), and biliopancreatic diversion and duodenal switch (BPD-DS) (Gumbs et al. 2007, Ikramuddin et al. 2007). As improvements made operations safer and more efficient, at the same time there are many patients with procedures that are less utilized, or even abandoned, that the bariatric surgeon must anticipate when taking into consideration reoperation on such individuals. This is an age where reoperative bariatric procedures are increasingly and rapidly becoming a daily presence in the bariatric surgeon's practice (Patel et al. 2011).

Bariatric surgeons are left to manage these patients on a case-by-case basis. We hope to provide some insight into not only the preoperative indications that lead to reoperations, but also to the postoperative complications that may appear. Whether it's due to procedure failure or complication, up to 25% of bariatric patients will undergo a reoperative procedure (Gagner et al. 2002). The indications and variety of these operations will be discussed in this chapter.

INDICATIONS AND TYPES OF REOPERATIONS

Reoperation of a patient after a bariatric procedure can fall into the following three main nonexclusive categories (**Table 41.1**). (1) Is it band related or nonband related? (2) Is it due to a complication or failure of the procedure?; and (3) the nature of the procedure to be performed - emergency, conversion, revision, or reversal. Using this classification system, it is easier to grasp and understand reoperative bariatric procedures. For example, while emergencies and reversals are exclusively related to complications, revisions and conversions can be the result of both complications and, more frequently, failures. Conversions utilize a variety of bariatric procedures, while revisions are mainly related to RYGB (Patel et al. 2011).

Table 14.1 Nonexclusive main categories of reoperative bariatric surgery. Conversions are more commonly performed due to failures, whereas revisions are due to complications (Patel et al. 2011)

	I	II	III
Bariatric reoperation	Band related	Complication	Emergency
			Revision
	Nonband related	Failure	Conversion
			Reversal

The term revision is used to designate a case in which the reoperation does not change the primary surgery's principal anatomy and mechanism. A conversion denotes when the primary surgery is transformed into another class within the bariatric procedure armamentarium.

Failure describes lack of postoperative weight loss, weight gain, or loss of restriction, and in such presentation, the operation is done electively. The definition of weight loss surgery failure is yet to be carefully designed. Failure is regarded as either weight gain or lack of weight loss, where the latter varies from patient to patient, depending on the preoperative outcome assessment and comorbidities resolution. Some complications, though, can be a cause for a procedure to fail, as in the case of a gastrogastric (GG) fistula. Failure can also pertain to loss of restriction, which is based on patients' subjective reports of being able to eat larger quantities of food.

Complications are classified either into early or 'acute' and late or 'chronic.' *Early* complications occur early (within 30 days) in the postoperative period and can include leaks, bleeding, gastrojejunostomy or jejunojejunostomy obstruction, and acute gastric remnant dilation. Late complications (>30 days) of a chronic nature are those in which pathological processes slowly take form and these result in strictures, ulcers, GG fistulas, internal hernias, intussusception, etc. (Patel et al. 2011) (**Table 14.2**).

The initial approach to reoperation has to evolve from the aforementioned indications and proceed into a conversion, revision, or reversal. Without exception, all of the aforementioned procedures should be approached with the laparoscopic technique, if possible.

Table 14.2 Early and late complications of bariatric surgery

Early complications:		
Bleeding		
Wound infection		
Leaks		
Obstruction		
Pulmonary		
Acute gastric remnant distension		
Cardiovascular/pulmonary embolism and deep venous thrombosis.		
Late complications:		
Roux-en-Y gastric bypass	**Gastric banding**	**Sleeve gastrectomy**
Gastrogastric fistula	Stomal obstruction	Bleeding
Stomal stenosis	Port infection	Stenosis
Marginal ulcers/strictures	Band erosion	Gastric leaks
Cholelithiasis	Band slippage and gastric prolapsed	
Internal/ventral incisional hernias	Port malfunction	
Functional syndromes	Esophageal dilatation	
Intussusception	Hiatal hernia	

Complications could impose an elective or urgent operation, depending on their nature. Chronic cases could and should be treated in optimized conditions. Acute operations relate to patients having perforation, bleeding, leaks, small bowl obstruction due to internal hernia, incarcerated trocar site hernia, or adhesions. Reoperations of acute emergencies will not be part of our discussion.

NON-LAGB-RELATED REOPERATIONS

Non-LAGB-related reoperations, otherwise known as stapling procedures, have a much wider variety of outcomes due to the use of different anatomical modifications in the primary procedures. Some outdated and outcasted procedures, such as the minidistal bypass, are converted to RYGB in most instances. In other cases, a BPD is converted to LSG, as well as jejunoileal bypasses. In non-LAGB reoperations, above 90% of cases can be performed in a totally laparoscopic technique, and the feasibility of laparoscopic reoperative procedures has been well documented (Gagner et al. 2002, Khaitan et al. 2005, McCormick et al. 2003, Nesset et al. 2007). Still, surgeons are urged not to underestimate the challenging nature of laparoscopic revisional surgery and should be performed by surgeons who are well trained in both bariatric surgery and minimally invasive surgery (**Table 14.3**).

Reversal and conversion

Reversal or conversional reoperations involve patients who required that their primary procedure be undone with restoration of their original anatomy or change into another bariatric subtype. These procedures are performed due to either failures or complications of a primary bariatric procedure. Reversal procedures simply due to failure are rarely ever performed.

Reversals of RYGB and jejunoileal bypasses are most commonly performed (Patel et al. 2011). The standard treatment of malabsorptive symptoms in patients with jejunoileal bypass is to reverse (Owens et al. 1996, Requarth et al. 1995), and in patients with RYGB either reversal or the Roux limb is shortened. The most common indication includes dumping syndrome and/or nonrefractory diarrhea along with signs and symptoms of malnutrition. Reversal of a procedure should only be considered an option if the aforementioned side effects of the operation cannot be resolved with medical intervention. Patients should be made aware that regardless of the time that transpired since the primary operation or the amount of weight loss achieved, reversing the procedure will result in weight regain and recurrence of comorbid illnesses in up to 98% of this patient population.

Another example is the minigastric bypass procedures that have been reported to have extremely high rates of bile reflux gastritis and marginal ulceration up to 53%, 3 months postoperatively (Johnson et al. 2007, Owens et al. 1996). These ulcers and the continuous mucosal injury may precipitate malnutrition. Conversion to RYGB is the recommended revisional procedure (Johnson et al. 2007).

In selected cases of severe diarrhea and weight loss, a step approach is warranted by the initial placement of a gastrostomy tube, in order to improve protein balance (for a period up to 3 months) due to severe malnutrition, followed by the conversion procedure once protein levels have normalized (Dang et al. 2009).

Revisional

Revisional procedures should not be taken lightly. Mortality rates in this group of patients range from 0% to 2.5% (Acholonu et al. 2009, Behrns et al. 1993, Ikramuddin et al. 2007, Nesset et al. 2007, Sugerman & Wolper 1984). Many times the patient has been in the OR repeatedly, once for the primary bariatric procedure, and then following that, for complications or revision. It is strongly suggested that the surgeon possesses a vast experience and understanding of the impending challenge. The most common indication for a revision is removal of the gastric remnant due to a variety of causes following RYGB procedures.

Loss of restriction in patients with prior RYGB can occur due to dilation of the gastric pouch, dilation of the GJ anastomosis, or a combination of both. Strictures at the GJ anastomosis and maladaptive eating habits can stress and dilate the gastric pouch (Mller et al. 2005). Patients presenting with a dilated pouch and/or anastomosis present on average 4 years after the primary operation (Patel et al. 2011).

Table 14.3 Complications following reoperative bariatric procedure (Patel et al. 2011)

	Conversions (N = 35)	Reversal (N = 7)	Revisions (N = 109)	Total (N = 151)
Leaks	7	0	13	20 (13.2%)
Gastrojejunal leak*	4	0	10	14 (9.3%)
Lateral pouch leak	2	0	3	5 (3.3%)
Leak jejunojejunostomy.†	1	0	0	1 (0.7%)
Wound infection	2	0	3	5 (3.3%)
Intra-abdominal abscess*	0	0	4	4 (2.6%)
Trocar site hernia†	1	0	2	3 (2.0%)
Gastrointestinal bleeding†	0	0	1	1 (0.7%)
Mortality	0	1	2	3 (2.0%)
Procedure performed by laparotomy	5	0	9	14 (9.3%)

*One patient required operative intervention.

†All patients required immediate operative intervention.

Once detailed with an imaging modality, a revision by either trimming of the pouch or redoing of the gastrojejunostomy is performed. Less commonly, revision of jejunojejunostomies is sought due to strictures, ulcers, irritable bowel disease (IBD), or other pathological processes taking place. In addition to these, the challenge increases simply due to the fact that in more than a third of cases, the revisional surgery requires multiple modifications (i.e. redoing the gastrojejunostomy, performing remnant gastrectomy, and pouch trimming) all done in the same, already lengthy by nature operation.

Marginal ulceration

Marginal ulceration is a concerning complication of RYGB, with incidence ranging from 0.6% to 16% (Gumbs et al. 2006, Siilin et al. 2005). The association between GG fistula and ulcer formation is well known and the incidence increases to 53.3% in such cases where a GG fistula is concomitantly present (Capella & Capella 1999, Carrodeguas et al. 2005, MacLean et al. 1997). Fistulas are most often associated with stapled and nondivided gastric pouches (Carrodeguas et al. 2005, Capella & Capella 1999, Cucchi et al. 1995). Treatment algorithm for patients with GG fistula is discussed below. Ulcer disease as a cause of GG fistula or vice versa leading to weight gain demonstrates the multifactorial nature of postoperative complications after primary RYGB surgery.

Ulcer disease, reflux, and bleeding will almost always present with additional symptoms, such as stricture, GG fistula, eroded silastic rings, or dilated gastric pouch. These patients may require a revision, conversion, or even reversal, according to patient request and surrounding determining factors. Ulcers are also an important cause for the formation of strictures, among other factors, such as operative technique, tension, and ischemia at the anastomosis site (Nguyen et al. 2003).

The mainstay of therapy is similar to that of gastroesophageal reflux disease (GERD) and GG fistulas, making use of proton pump inhibitors and cytoprotective agents such as sucralfate. These medications can be given for prolonged periods, but if they fail, revisional surgery via redoing the gastrojejunal (GJ) anastomosis may be required, and remnant gastrectomy if a GG fistula is present.

Treatment of intractable GERD or acute gastric outlet obstruction (**Figure 14.1**) in patients after having LSG has also been shown to be successfully treated only with the conversion to RYGB. Thus, one may conclude that LSG can be performed as a sole and definitive bariatric intervention, with conversion to RYGB as an exit strategy (Abdemur et al. 2012, Bellorin et al. 2010).

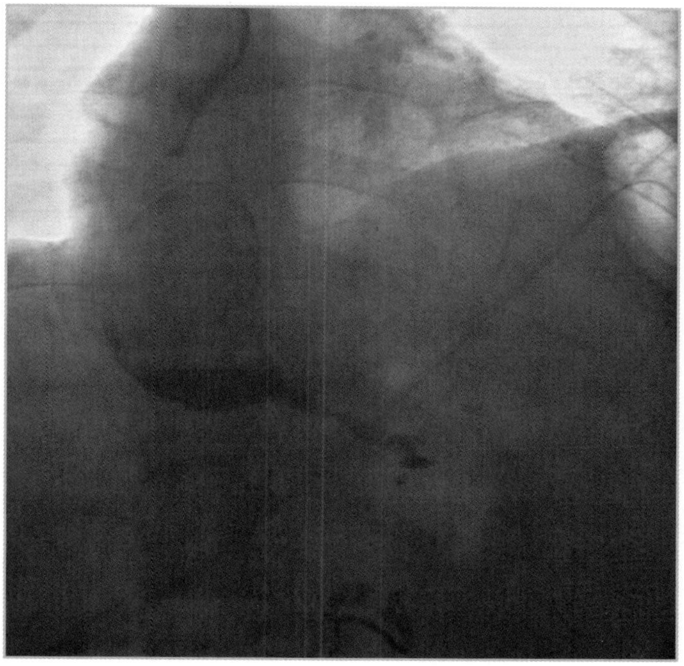

Figure 14.1 Gastric outlet obstruction. The patient is status post laparoscopic sleeve gastrectomy showing distention of the esophagus with air, and trace Gastrografin extending into the duodenum.

Gastrogastric fistula (Figure 14.2)

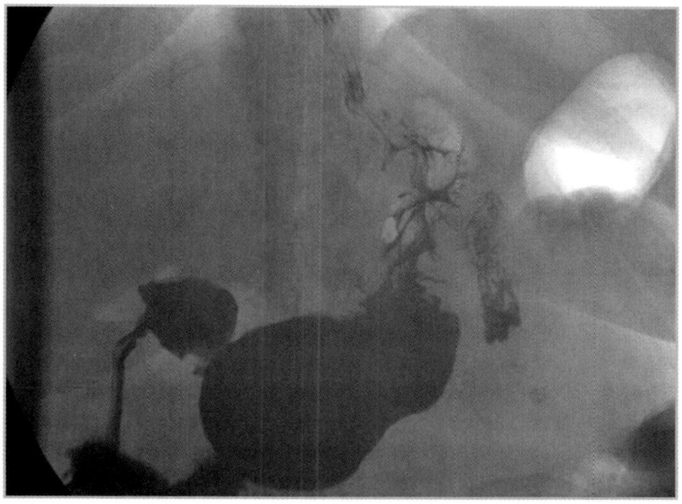

Figure 14.2 Gastrogastric fistula. Contrast preferentially extends into the 'bypassed' native stomach and duodenum, which appear to demonstrate the relatively normal native gastric and duodenal anatomy. Only a small amount of contrast extends from the gastric fundus directly into the jejunum.

GG fistula incidence can be as high as 49% in patients who undergo nondivided or partially divided RYGB, and a rate of 1.5–6% after divided RYGB (Acholonu et al. 2009, Capella & Capella 1999, Cucchi et al. 1995, Gustavsson & Sundbom 2003, Sapala et al. 1998). The exact etiology of GG fistula is unknown; various causes have been postulated, such as operative technique (nondivided gastric pouch), inadvertent failure to divide the stomach, anastomotic leak, gastric wall tissue migration, marginal ulceration, perforation of pouch or remnant, and erosions from a foreign body (Acholonu et al. 2009). The most common symptom of GG fistula is epigastric abdominal pain, along with nausea, vomiting, hematemesis, hematochezia, and weight regain.

Once diagnosed endoscopically, the majority of patients can be managed conservatively (MacLean et al. 1997) with the use of proton pump inhibitors to reduce acid production and sucralfate to provide protective coating to the pouch and ulcer, relieving pain and decreasing exposure to acids. This regimen is usually prescribed for 6–8 weeks (Carrodeguas et al. 2005, MacLean et al. 1997). Surgical options include fistulectomy and remnant gastrectomy. The latter is most useful and feasible. Division of the GG fistula alone can be done, or resection of the fistula along with redo of the GJ anastomosis and/ or pouch trimming. It is noteworthy that a third of patients with a GG fistula also present with active ulcer disease, of which 25% could have active bleeding from the ulcer bed at time of presentation (Patel et al. 2011).

The operative technique involves mobilizing the gastric remnant from the short gastric vessels proximally to the level of the gastroesophageal junction. A window is established between the pouch and the gastric remnant, and dissection is performed on both the anterior and posterior walls of the stomach. An endoscope is intraoperatively used to identify the location of the fistulous tract. The stomach should be transected at the level of antrum, and then transverse remnant gastrectomy is to be performed. This assures the complete mobilization of the stomach. An Ewald tube can be placed for marking the gastroesophageal junction and the anastomosis level. Finally, the pouch, if warranted, is then trimmed by resecting the fistulous tract. If the pouch is not enlarged or too small, the gastric remnant is excised, and a margin of the remnant tissue attached to the GG fistula side can be left behind. The practice of oversewing staple lines has many advocates and should also be performed. Endoscopy and a leak test using both air and/or methylene blue confirm the closure of the fistulous tract and assure the staple lines' integrity.

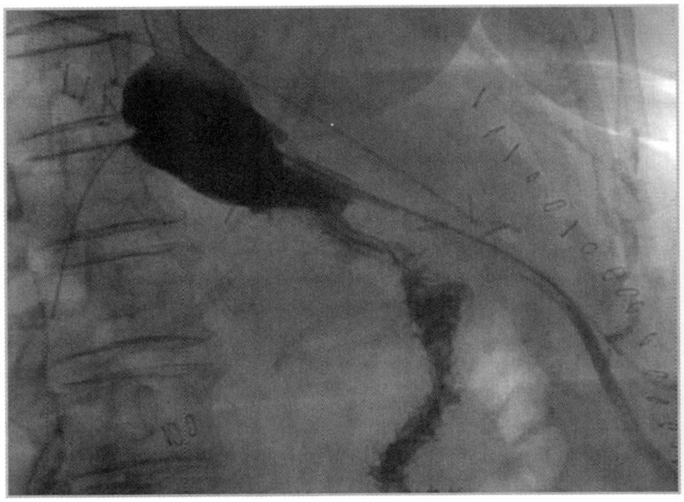

Figure 14.3 Roux-en-Y gastric bypass leak. The gastric pouch and gastrojejunostomy appeared unremarkable in the erect projection. When the patient drank contrast in the prone oblique projection, contrast extended from the base of the pouch into one of the drainage catheters adjacent to the anastomosis.

Strictures

Stricture formation at the GJ anastomosis is a relatively common complication following laparoscopic Roux-en-Y gastric bypass (LRYGB) that is reported in 3–27% of patients (Rosenthal 2009). Furthermore, strictures can be classified according to acute or chronic, and into membranous (due to prolonged fasting), cicatricial (ulcer or foreign body), or granular (tissue ischemia and tension) strictures. Acute cases are rare and are the result of technical errors. Chronic strictures are more commonly seen, and present on an average of 2 months range (Ahmad et al. 2003, Barba et al. 2003, Go et al. 2004). Nausea and vomiting are the first symptoms to appear, but they could be more severe, such as extreme belching and sialorrhea. The former symptoms are very unspecific, and thus a more common underlying cause should be ruled out – usually metabolic or dehydration in nature. Diagnosis is made by Gastrografin UGI series, along with a lateral decubitus film in order to rule out the presence of a GG fistula.

Treatment options of this complication can vary and include observation, endoscopic dilatation, or surgical revision depending on the time of onset and nature of the stricture (Ahmad et al. 2003, Gonzalez et al. 2003, Rosenthal 2009). In cases of acute stricture, endoscopic dilatation after RYGB should be considered 7 days postoperatively to be a safe option, and the indication should be intolerance to liquids or inability to meet daily nutrient requirements. Endoscopic dilatation should be performed according to the institute's standard and experience, keeping in mind that multiple attempts may be needed for the same patient. Surgical or laparoscopic revision of strictures is relatively uncommon and should be performed after several attempts of the above had failed. Incidence of the latter is close to 0.5% of all cases in need of dilatation, and patients usually had at least four prior attempts (Rosenthal 2009). Corkscrew stomach due to nonparallel stapling or kinking at the trimmed incisura could also present as a stricture, as well as local hematoma or edema. The former two might also require revisional surgery, whereas the latter two need conservative treatment and observation alone initially.

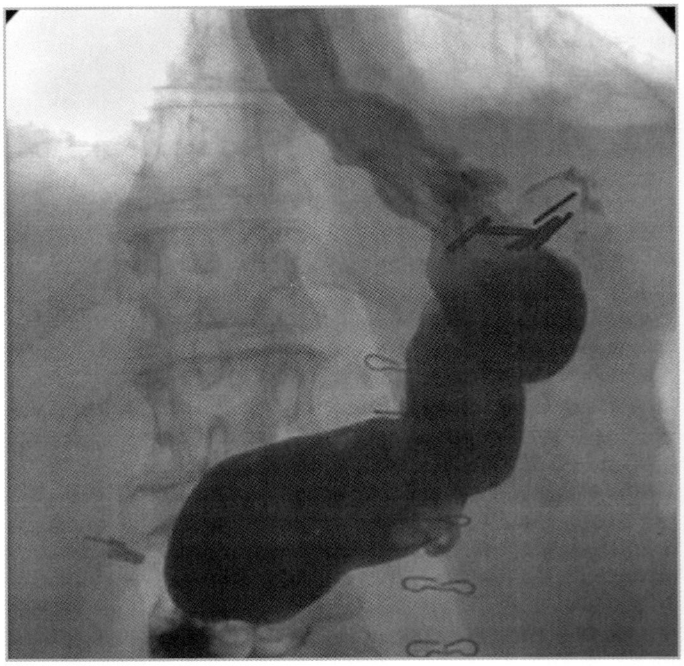

Figure 14.4 Laparoscopic sleeve gastrectomy leak. From a suture line in the upper aspect of the stomach, there is a small 2–3 cm fistulous or sinus tract extending superior and to the left that does not communicate with any other structure.

Leaks (Figures 14.3 and 14.4)

Leak rates are known to be higher in revisional procedures than in primary bariatric surgery (Roller & Provost 2006). They usually present during the postoperative stay, or by the time of the first postoperative office visit. They are recognized initially by drain outputs and later should be confirmed with either an upper gastrointestinal (UGI) series or a computed tomography (CT) scan. In over 90% of cases, leaks can be treated nonsurgically with broad-spectrum antibiotics, drainage, nil per os (NPO), total parenteral nutrition (TPN), or a gastrostomy tube feeding. Drains can be placed either through pre-existing drain tracts, percutaneous placement, or with the help of interventional radiology. Once a leak is detected, the primary goal is to obtain adequate drainage (thereby creating a controlled fistula), and prevent sepsis. Due to the lengthy nature of the leak's resolution, a feeding jejunostomy for nutritional support is advised, allowing recovery to take place (Fuks et al. 2009, Han-Geurts et al. 2005, Lee et al. 2007).

There are several different treatment modalities currently in use, once conservative treatment fails. Proximal leaks can be treated by the additional use of endoscopic procedures, such as fibrin sealing in combination with somatostatin and placement of endoluminal stents (Court et al. 2010, Papavramidis et al. 2008, Serra et al. 2007). If the latter fails in LSG, the use of a Roux limb can be done (Baltasar et al. 2007). The treatment of distal leaks is more complex and has been less described. The author of this chapter has described the use of a T-tube in conjunction with laparoscopy successfully performed with positive outcomes (Court et al. 2010). There is always a fear that a distal leak may develop into a stricture; in that case, if LSG was performed, the conversion to RYGB would be the recommended definite solution.

Internal herniation and small bowel obstruction

Internal herniation (IH) and small bowel obstruction (SBO) are complications of the gastric bypass procedure that can have devastating consequences. SBO could be the result of IH or from a myriad of other causes. To improve communication, study, and analysis of SBO, a simplified classification system has been devised (Tucker et al. 2007). The first part of the latter relates to the site of obstruction. It is at the level of the alimentary limb (type A), the biliopancreatic limb (type B), or at the level of the common channel (type C) (**Figure 14.5**). The second part of the classification pertains to the time of onset – acute early (30 days or less), acute late (>30 days and <12 months), or chronic (>12 months).

Obstruction at the jejunojejunostomy usually occurs when the anastomosis is closed using a stapler. Hemobezoars develop as a result of bleeding in the gastric remnant and can cause obstruction in the biliopancreatic limb, leading to the dreaded complication of closed loop obstruction. Intussusception often occurs at or in the vicinity of the jejunojejunostomy, while adhesions can form at any site along the GI tract. When patients present with symptoms of SBO, a diagnostic evaluation is warranted. However, with unstable vital signs and high clinical suspicion, resuscitation and immediate exploration should be performed without diagnostic tests. In the stable patient, appropriate blood tests should be drawn. Abnormal liver function indicates type B SBO. The most sensitive radiologic examination in the case of SBO is a CT scan with oral contrast (Deitel 2010), although that may be normal in 20% of cases. If enough clinical suspicion exists, a diagnostic exploration is warranted even in the face of normal radiographic evaluations.

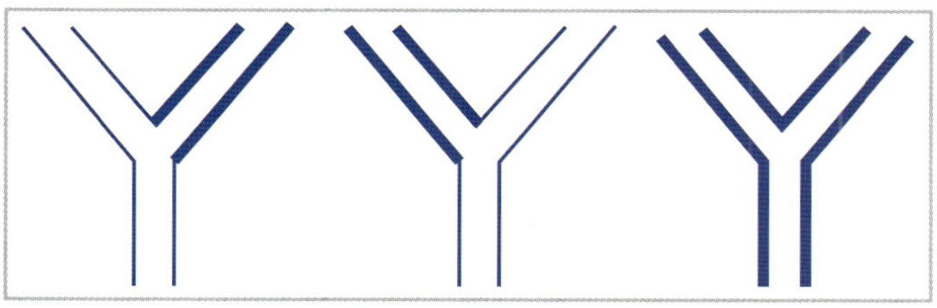

Figure 14.5 Schematic representation of the ABC system of classification of small bowel obstruction after laparoscopic Roux-en-Y gastric bypass. (a) Alimentary limb, (b) biliopancreatic limb, and (c) common channel. With permission from Tucker et al. (2007).

LAGB RELATED

LAGB is one of the most common bariatric procedures performed worldwide and has many perceived advantages, such as 50% excess weight loss at 2 years, low operative morbidity, and reversibility (OBrien & Dixon 2002, Patel et al. 2010, Rosenthal et al. 2006, Wittgrove & Clark 2000). It has also been shown by some advocates, mainly in Europe and Australia, to be more effective among the bariatric procedures, but at the same time, a significant number of patients and surgeons experience lack of satisfaction, mainly related to poor outcomes, such as a high rate of band removals. As a result, the number of cases performed is declining (Tucker et al. 2008). In experienced centers, LAGB has an acceptable safety profile with a short-term mortality rate of 0.05% and low perioperative morbidity (Favretti et al. 2007, OBrien et al. 2006, Ren et al. 2004, Te Riele et al. 2007) (**Table 14.4**). However, complications vary vastly, with reported morbidity rates as great as 30% in some series (Holczy et al. 2001, Ponce et al. 2005, Stroh et al. 2005, Zehetner et al. 2005). Reoperation rates for LAGB range widely from 1.7% to 66.7% due to several factors, including learning curves and various adjustable gastric banding systems. All revisions on LAGB patients should be set out to be performed laparoscopically, as this has been clearly shown by many to be advantageous, safe, and feasible (Patel et al. 2010).

The most significant morbidity in some series with band-related complications includes slippage (0.9–13%), pouch dilation (1.3–5%), band erosion, esophageal dilation, and port-related morbidity, including infection, leaks, and hardware-related problems (4.5–7%) (Brown et al. 2003, Chevallier et al. 2004, Dargent 2005, DeMaria et al. 2001, Te Riele et al. 2007, Tucker et al. 2008). As a result of the above, band removal rates have been reported from 0.5% to 20% by Patel et al. (Favretti et al. 2007, Doldi et al. 2000, Lattuada et al. 2007, Patel et al. 2010, Suter et al. 2004). The reported failure and complication rates increase with time and the annual reoperation rates typically range between 3% and 4.7%, but may be as high as 9.4% (Biertho et al. 2005, Suter et al. 2006, Vella & Galloway 2003).

Among all reoperations in LAGB patients, 85% of cases involve a band-related revision and the remaining 15% are port-related revisions (Patel et al. 2010). In 85% of LAGB patients undergoing a revisional operation, the band is removed, whether as a sole procedure or in association with another (Tucker et al. 2008). When examining the band-related causes of revision, indications are as follows: 45% weight loss failure, 32% band prolapse, 9% band erosion, 5% revision secondary to megaesophagus, and 4% for patients presenting with severe reflux/ulcer disease (Patel et al. 2010). The most common cause for port-related revisions is disconnection of the tubing system from the port, at a frequency of 46% among these type cases.

In cases of reoperating on LAGB patients, the most common end point is solely band removal. Repositioning of the band occurs frequently as well, and in a few cases the band is to be replaced and repositioned as in the primary procedure. In approximately a third of the cases, failed LAGB is converted to either LSG or RYGB, with similar frequency for either. In a few selected cases, a band could be placed over an enlarged pouch of a RYGB failure. Patients may require a two-step approach, as in cases presenting with megaesophagus causing the failures of LAGB, where the band is removed first and the conversion is performed at a later date (Patel et al. 2010).

In selected cases, and according to patients' wishes and circumstances, conversion to LSG can be performed. This group of

Table 14.4 Reported complications of LAGB by different institutions

Investigator	(n)	Postoperative complication rate (%)	Reoperation rate (%)	Prolapsed band and dilated pouch (%)	Erosion/ migration (%)	Portrelated complications (%)	Removal secondary to weight loss failure (%)
O'Brien and Dixon (2002)	1120	NR	NR	4.7–25	3	5.4	1
Silecchia et al. (2004)	313	8.3	13.7	3.2	5.1	2.2	3.2
Martikainen et al. (2004)	123	54	52	21	9	19	NR
Zinzindohoue et al. (2003)	500	18.8	10.4	8	1	7.2	NR
Chevallier et al. (2004)	1000	19.2	11.1	2.0–24	0.1	5.7	NR
Belachew et al. (2002)	763	13.4	11.1	8	0.9	2.5	NR
Favretti et al. (2007)	830	NR	3.9*	10	0.5	11	0.4
Furbetta and Coli (2003)	540	9.6	9.6	2.6	0.5	6.5	NR
Sarker et al. (2004)	154	14.8	9	3.2	0.6	4.5	NR
Weiner et al. (2003)	984	4.7	NR	3.7–17	NR	4	NR
Susmallian et al. (2003)	333	25.8	23.1	9	NR	13.5	NR
Angrisani et al. (2001)	1265	11.3	6.6	5.2	1.9	4.2	NR
Weiner et al. (1999)	184	9	6.4	2.2	1.1	3.2	NR
Vertruyen (2002)	543	NR	8.7	4.6	1	2.9	NR
Lyass et al. (2005)	270	NR	13	6	NR	5	3

*Included only 'major' postoperative complications.

LAGB, laparoscopic adjustable gastric banding.

patients, where conversion to LSG after failed LAGB might be regarded as superior to RYGB, includes cases of morbidly obese adolescents, patients on lifelong anticoagulation, endangering bleeding from marginal ulcers (more commonly associated with RYGB), and other high-risk patients who are poor candidates to withstand serious complications (leaks) as seen after RYGB. LSG may also be appropriate in cases of body mass index (BMI) between 35 and 40 with no or relatively insignificant comorbidity, low BMI patients requiring a second surgical procedure (such as kidney or liver transplantation, joint replacement, or recurrent incisional hernia repair), those without metabolic syndrome, and for patients with small bowel diseases and other contraindications for malabsorptive procedures, such as Crohn's disease, where one would rather not manipulate the small bowel (Acholonu et al. 2009). The end point of re-operating electively has to take into consideration case-by-case presentation, whether it is to be converted, reversed, or revised.

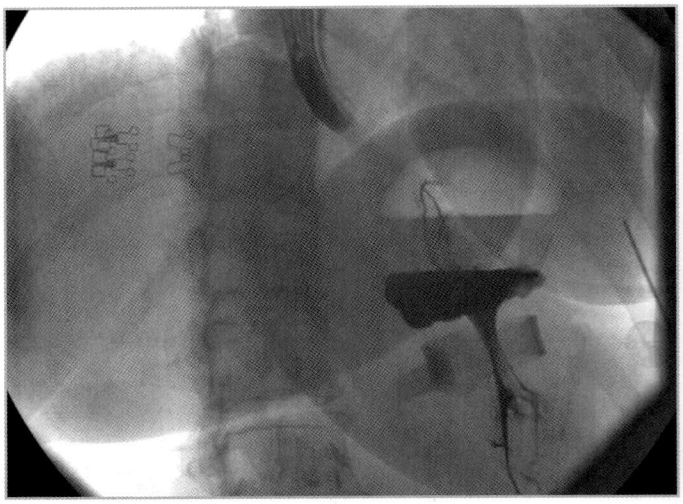

Figure 14.6 Band slippage. The gastric band in place has slipped distal to the gastroesophageal junction. The fundus of the stomach is herniated through the gastric band. There is moderate obstruction and hold up of contrast at the level of the gastric band.

Band prolapse (Figure 14.6)

Reoperation rates due to prolapse of the band are reported at 5–6% (Belachew et al. 2002, Martikainen et al. 2004). The latter figure has been achieved largely by abandoning the perigastric approach to band placement, having a 25% incidence of band prolapse (Patel et al. 2010). The nature of reoperation of band prolapse largely depends on presenting signs. Nausea, vomiting, dysphagia, reflux, and abdominal pain are indications that reoperation can be done electively. Clinical signs and symptoms of incarceration, such as elevated white blood count, fever, and epigastric tenderness, require an emergency surgery, within 24 hours of presentation. Rebanding or repositioning of a prolapsed band, although debatable, is not effective and results show disappointing outcomes for two-thirds of patients, including repeat prolapse, erosion, and weight loss failure (Suter 2001, Van Gemert et al. 1998, Weber et al. 2003). Close to half of reoperations on patients with a prolapsed band result with the removal of the entire band system. Second most common result is repositioning of the band. The replacement of the band or correction of placement for initially failed bands is questionable at best, and it has been reported that a failed restrictive procedure, if repeated, is rarely successful (Van Gemert et al. 1998, Weber et al. 2003), and thus other options should be sought after (Dargent 2004, Schouten et al. 2006). Several authors have shown that laparoscopic revision to RYGB is feasible and effective for failed LAGB (Spivak et al. 2007, Van Wageningen et al. 2006).

Band erosion

For band erosion, there is a bimodal presentation of early, at a period of 2–7 months, and late, between 52 and 54 months after band placement (Patel et al. 2010). Early erosions are attributed to technical errors such as tension from the wrap, a missed gastric perforation or injury, or pressure necrosis from a tight band. Delayed erosions are unexpected and might result from undiagnosed prolapse that eventually manifests itself as an eroded band.

Signs and symptoms are composed of upper abdominal pain and dysphagia, or more severe fever and sepsis, and may also concomitantly present with an infected port site in association with signs of systemic sepsis (Tucker et al. 2008). Numerous studies have shown that LRYGB as a primary bariatric procedure provides better weight loss and a reduced failure rate compared with LAGB (Weiner et al. 2003), and conversion of the purely restrictive procedure to a combined restrictive and malabsorptive procedure such as RYGB is becoming the preferred strategy for many surgeons, as it has been regarded as a rescue procedure after failed LAGB (Weber et al. 2003).

Short-term results have shown LSG to be a more effective restrictive procedure than LAGB, with an average excess weight loss of 33–83% and an average weight loss of 60–85% at the end of 1 year. In addition, LSG results in decreased hunger sensations and decreased incidence of GERD after 1 year compared with LAGB (Himpens et al. 2006, Van Gemert et al. 1998). LSG too has been found to be an effective revisional procedure after failed LAGB (Bernante et al. 2006, Gagner & Gumbs 2007).

PORT-RELATED

Port-related complications unjustly tend to be underestimated (Launay-Savary et al. 2008). Port-related morbidity accounts for 15% of LAGB cases needed for reoperation, and interventions have been reported in 1–8% of patients undergoing LAGB procedure (OBrien & Dixon 2002, Fen et al. 2002, Sarker et al. 2004) (**Table 14.5**).

Port tubing disconnections and rupture appear to predominate (Launay-Savary et al. 2008). A 7.1% reoperation rate has been reported for port complications, of which two thirds are disconnections and one out of five were infections (Keidar et al. 2005). Symptoms of intractable lower abdominal pain often bring the patient back for evaluation, later to find the port tubing disconnection. Pressure from leaking fluid from the tube into the abdomen and the motion of the catheter itself can result in lower abdominal pain, keeping in mind the latter could also mimic acute appendicitis (Kirshtein et al. 2009).

Port system revisions require port relocation, reconnection, replacement, or complete removal. If any of the latter occurred due to infection, the whole band-port system has to be thoroughly inspected and band erosion or infection ruled out endoscopically for fear of severe deterioration of the patient. Infection of the band is an uncommon complication, but if occurs, once conservative management fails to improve, it is necessary to remove the entire band-port system. A ruptured band is also uncommon, and it must be removed. Tube disconnection could be reconnected by retrieving the tubing laparoscopically. Relocation of the ports due to either pain or discomfort, or due to port rotation, occurs at a smaller frequency. The port could also be replaced due to malfunction with a leak.

Megaesophagus (Figure 14.7)

Megaesophagus is a complication occurring in approximately 5% of cases indicated for reoperation in LAGB patients. Esophageal dilation is defined as a 100% increase in the baseline diameter or >5 cm diameter (Lew et al. 2006), secondary and tertiary peristaltic contractions, and insufficient emptying of the distal esophagus (Wiesner et al. 2001). Development of megaesophagus takes 2–3 years (Arias et al. 2009). In addition to being a complication, megaesophagus can also lead to failure by providing additional space for food reservoir and patients preferring liquid diets high in carbohydrates over solid, protein-rich foods. The latter also results in delayed esophageal emptying, impaired motility, or lower esophageal sphincter relaxation dysfunction (Dargent 2005, DeMaria et al. 2001, Suter et al. 2005, Weiss et al. 2000). Patients diagnosed with megaesophagus have a %EWL less than half of patients without it (Arias et al. 2009). It is believed by some that preoperative esophageal manometry may decrease the incidence for developing the disorder by excluding patients with

Table 14.5 Reported port-related complications by different institutions (Patel et al. 2010)

Investigator	Patients (port complications) (n)	Overall port-related complication rate (%)	Band-port disconnection or rupture rate (%)	Infection rate (%)	Reservoir leak or perforation rate (%)	Port rotation or dislodgement rate (%)
Sarker et al. (2004)	154 (7)	4.5	2.6	NR	1.3	0.6
Launay-Savary et al. (2008)	286 (43)	15	8.4	1.4	5.2	NR
Keidar et al. (2005)	1272 (103)	7.1	4.9	1.5	NR	0.5
Susmallian et al. (2003)	333 (45)	13.5	2.4	6.9	1.5	2.1
Lyass et al. (2005)	270 (13)	5	2.2	1.9	NR	0.7
Yoffe et al. (2003)	58 (6)	10.3	10.3	NR	NR	NR
Patel et al. (2010)	88 (13)	13.8	6.8	2.3	2.3	1.1

NR, not reported.

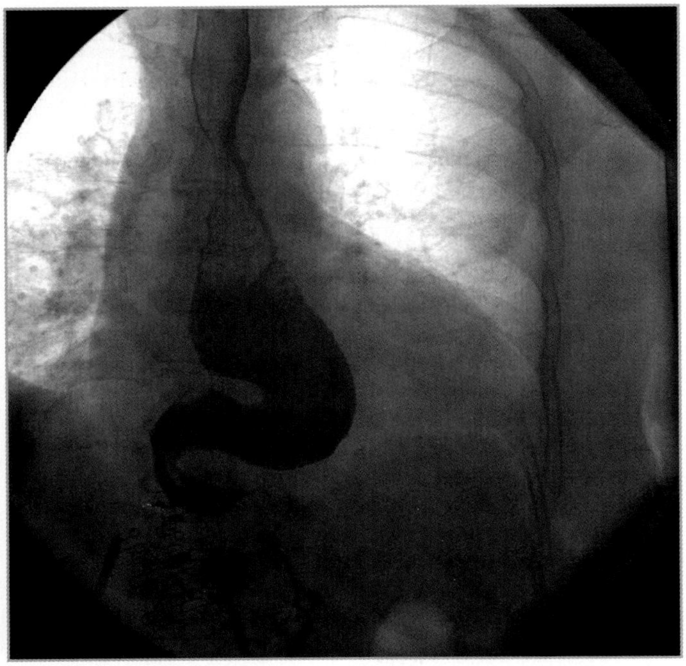

Figure 14.7 Megaesophagus. The esophagus is markedly dilated and tortuous, demonstrating numerous tertiary contractions. Also, there is a small hiatal hernia with a herniation of a small portion of the stomach above the level of the gastric band, and above the diaphragm. The gastric band does appear in normal position and orientation.

abnormal motility from undergoing the procedure. This has not been the experience of the author, and similar results were published by others (Arias et al. 2009, Lew et al. 2006).

Once megaesophagus is diagnosed, deflation of the band and re-evaluation of the patient in 3–12 weeks is recommended (Patel et al. 2010). The latter results in some improvement in all patients, but does not always resolve entirely; thus, if clinical signs and symptoms of outlet obstruction persist despite deflation, the band must be removed (Arias et al. 2009).

Preoperative imaging

Regardless of the indication, whether mechanical, anatomical, or metabolic abnormality, a thorough medical and surgical history is needed.

Prior to going into surgery, we must have all the available knowledge at hand:

- When the first surgery was performed
- Who was the surgeon (and call that surgeon for more information if necessary)
- Details of the surgery from reading the operative report of the first surgery
- Length of the alimentary and biliary limbs of the RYGB
- Whether the alimentary limb was passed in an antecolic, antegastric, or retrocolic retrogastric fashion.

This information will help us understand the nature of the complication or mechanism of failure and guide us in our strategy of reoperation.

Performing a bariatric reoperation requires much more than just anatomical knowledge. Details regarding the type of band in the case of a primary LAGB, such as the locking mechanism and port system, are needed. If RYGB is revised, then the type of bypass performed should be in one's mind – distal, proximal, divided versus nondivided, presence of preanastomotic ring, was a gastrostomy performed, route of retro-retro, ante-ante, etc. Whether cholecystectomy was performed should also be discovered.

Esophagogastroduodenoscopy (EGD), UGI series, or a CT scan can all provide an important road map to our approach. The UGI should be done in supine, erect, and lateral decubitus positions, in order to delineate all the existing channels and identify the presence of fistulas. Visualization of any dilation of a hollow organ, such as the esophagus (due to a band), the stomach pouch or remnant, or small bowel is critical. A large anastomosis or a GG fistula is best viewed with an UGI in left lateral decubitus. The presence of a preanastomotic ring can be used as an anatomic landmark to identify the site of the GJ. The CT scan is far superior to any imaging modality in identifying internal hernias, intussusception, an eroded band, and presence of nephrolithiasis and cholelithiasis, which are also part of the preoperative workup. The EGD is useful in assessing the size of the pouch, the size of the anastomosis, and the presence of a GG fistula. It is also the most accurate examination in visualizing foreign bodies such as staples, sutures, eroded bands, or rings. Last, it is the only method to truly assess a marginal ulceration. It is strongly suggested that the surgeon performs or is present during the EGD, so the surgeon must have a clear view and understanding of the anatomy.

PREOPERATIVE AND POSTOPERATIVE CARE

Preoperative

As for any primary bariatric procedure, reoperation for failure or complications call again for perioperative management, which includes a nutritional consult to assess the patient's eating habits, protein intake, and alcohol consumption, which is the culprit of ulcers. Psychological evaluation is a must in reoperative surgery, both in support and in maintenance, thus it is imperative to have in surgery due to weight gain or failure of weight loss.

A thorough medical examination is required prior to any operation. It is essential to rule out incisional hernias (presence of mesh) and lower extremity edema or anasarca, indicating malnutrition or low albumin, respectively, as well as hair loss. A full neurological examination is required in cases where malnutrition is suspected, due to vitamins B1 and B12 deficiency. The medical examination should be followed by relevant laboratory tests, of which albumin and prealbumin levels are of particular interest.

The standard lab tests (according to the institute's preference when performing surgery) are done, including complete blood count, basic metabolic panel, coagulation factors, vitamin B12 levels, serum thiamine and folic acid levels, iron levels, chest X-ray, electrocardiogram (ECG), and either an upper endoscopy, UGI series with Gastrografin, or both. Prior to surgery, all patients are to be evaluated by an anesthesiologist and preoperative clearance must be obtained from the patient's primary physician. Patients with prior abnormal cardiac or pulmonary history should be evaluated by a cardiologist and/or pulmonologist preoperatively.

Prior to any bariatric procedure, a clear liquid diet for diabetic with low sugar, low carbohydrate, and high protein shakes for 2 weeks is recommended. Deep venous thrombosis prophylaxis should be given as well, taking into consideration the possibility of a prolonged stay and immobility, and utilizing pneumatic compression devices and anticoagulation.

Postoperative

Postoperatively, patients should be admitted to an intermediate care unit. NPO along with intravenous hydration and pain medications (patient-controlled analgesia is suggested) should be administered. Proton pump inhibitors given for ulcer prophylaxis and deep breathing exercises with the use of an incentive spirometer are encouraged, along with early ambulation, with assistance if needed.

An UGI series using water-soluble contrast should be done prior to oral feedings, excluding the possibility of a hidden leak, and vital signs should be monitored, as they could be the only presenting signs. Patients having a contraindication for undergoing an UGI could be given methylene blue dissolved in water and drains be monitored for extraction. Patients are usually able to be discharged by postoperative Day 3 or 4 (Patel et al. 2011). Once discharged, patients should be asked to record the nature and amount of the drains' daily output. They are to be removed at the first postoperative outpatient visit.

ANTICIPATED LONG CASE AND NEED FOR CONSULTS

Due to the nature of the procedure, prolonged surgery is inevitable, and thus subjects the patient to a greater risk of complications. Routine medical clearance is a cornerstone for a successful and smooth perioperative field. Patients should be cleared through cardiology and pulmonology, and should undergo a routine ECG and chest X-ray, as well as routine laboratory tests to rule out any metabolic or blood abnormalities that would subject them to greater unnecessary risk.

Performing a reoperation

When converting an LAGB to a LRYGB, the most common approach, regardless of the selected end point, is to first take down the capsule that surrounds the band (leaving the band in place), and identify the right and left crus of the diaphragm. Next step is to remove the band, dissect the capsule from the stomach, and identify the first gastric pedicle (vessel pedicle) on the lesser curvature of the stomach. Going under the left gastric artery, dividing the stomach and creating the pouch would be the next step. These are the highlights of any LAGB conversion. The reconstruction that follows in a Roux-en-Y fashion is the same as the standard one used in primary RYGB.

When converting a vertical banded gastroplasty (VBG), dissecting through the short gastric vessels on the greater curvature, reaching under the ring and dividing the stomach distally is done first. Once under the left gastric artery, a pouch is created by stapling superior and medial from the vertical banded area. Knowing the stomach is to be removed, a Hasson technique should be used due to the standardized larger port in which the specimen would later be obtained.

When we convert a VBG to a bypass, there are two techniques: one incorporates removing the stomach remnant and the other does not. Removing the remnant is advantageous since the feasibility of the technique presumably prevents potential complications. So once the right and left crus and the left gastric artery are identified, a window is created behind the stomach. Next step is to take down all the short gastric vessels and staple superior and medial, resecting the stomach distally. The procedure should then be completed into a RYGB in the standard approach.

A pitfall to remember is that at the fundus in the area of the gastric band, the tissue is thick with more difficult apposition. It is strongly recommend to use the tallest staples (green cartridges) when transecting that portion of the gastric wall (Acholonu et al. 2009).

CONCLUSION

It has well been established that revisional procedures have a higher morbidity and mortality rate than primary operations (Behrns et al. 1993, De Csepel et al. 2001, Ikramuddin et al. 2007, Patel et al. 2011, Schwartz et al. 1988, Sugerman & Wolper 1984). Complication rates as high as 33–62% have been reported (Ikramuddin et al. 2007, Khaitan et al. 2005).

Reoperative emergencies after the secondary procedure (the revisional operations) are uncommon, but one should always be prepared and foresee these types of cases as those with an increased risk for further complications. It is the authors' experience to be confronted with approximately 22% of postoperative complications, most commonly leaks that can reach in experienced hands up to 12%, though they can be treated in over 90% of cases conservatively (NPO, antibiotics, TPN, and drainage).

Certain principles should be applied to the primary procedure to prevent and avoid the unwanted need for reoperation, or to make for a smoother reoperative procedure if one is necessary. Choosing the right patient has been a tough call for all, but a growing amount of data suggests and supports a more specific subpopulation that is suitable for and that will benefit from different bariatric procedures, and selecting the best approach for the right patient is critical.

A solid technique in the primary procedure makes for an easier reoperative procedure when one is necessary. Creating a small pouch, narrow stoma, and proper limb length and having a rigorous patient follow-up, along with support, are the main technical key points for success. In regard to a reoperative procedure, have experienced help available (gray hair), make use of the 'one centimeter rule,' test the anastomosis (both air and methylene blue, as well as intraoperative endoscopy), treat thin or ischemic tissue properly, and familiarize yourself with the proper use of G-tubes and drains.

REFERENCES

Abdemur A, Fendrich I, Rosenthal R. Laparoscopic conversion of laparoscopic sleeve gastrectomy to gastric bypass for intractable gastroesophageal reflux disease. Surg Obes Relat Dis 2012; 8:654.

Acholonu E, McBean E, Court I, et al. Safety and short-term outcomes of laparoscopic sleeve gastrectomy as a revisional approach for failed laparoscopic adjustable gastric banding in the treatment of morbid obesity. Obes Surg 2009; 19:1612–1616.

Ahmad J, Martin J, Ikramuddin S, Schauer P, Slivka A. Endoscopic balloon dilation of gastroenteric anastomotic stricture after laparoscopic gastric bypass. Endoscopy 2003; 35:725–728.

Angrisani L, Alkilani M, Basso N, et al. Laparoscopic Italian experience with the Lap-Band. Obes Surg 2001; 11:307–310.

Arias IE, Radulescu M, Stiegeler R, et al. Diagnosis and treatment of megaesophagus after adjustable gastric banding for morbid obesity. Surg Obes Relat Dis 2009; 5:156–159.

Baltasar A, Bou R, Bengochea M, Serra C, Cipagauta L. Use of a Roux limb to correct esophagogastric junction fistulas after sleeve gastrectomy. Obes Surg 2007; 17:1408–1410.

Barba CA, Butensky MS, Lorenzo M, Newman R. Endoscopic dilation of gastroesophageal anastomosis stricture after gastric bypass. Surg Endosc 2003; 17:416–420.

Behrns KE, Smith CD, Kelly KA, Sarr MG. Reoperative bariatric surgery. Lessons learned to improve patient selection and results. Ann Surg 1993; 218:646–653.

Belachew M, Belva PH, Desaive C. Long-term results of laparoscopic adjustable gastric banding for the treatment of morbid obesity. Obes Surg 2002; 12:564–568.

Bellorin O, Lieb J, Szomstein S, Rosenthal RJ. Laparoscopic conversion of sleeve gastrectomy to Roux-en-Y gastric bypass for acute gastric outlet obstruction after laparoscopic sleeve gastrectomy for morbid obesity. Surg Obes Relat Dis 2010; 6:566–568.

Bernante P, Foletto M, Busetto L, et al. Feasibility of laparoscopic sleeve gastrectomy as a revision procedure for prior laparoscopic gastric banding. Obes Surg 2006; 16:1327–1330.

Biertho L, Steffen R, Branson R, et al. Management of failed adjustable gastric banding. Surgery 2005; 137:33–41.

Brown SL, Reid MH, Duggirala HJ. Adjustable silicone gastric banding adverse events reported to the Food and Drug Administration. J Long Term Eff Med Implants 2003; 13:509–517.

Capella JF, Capella RF. Gastro-gastric fistulas and marginal ulcers in gastric bypass procedures for weight reduction. Obes Surg 1999; 9:22–27; discussion 28.

Carrodeguas L, Szomstein S, Soto F, et al. Management of gastrogastric fistulas after divided Roux-en-Y gastric bypass surgery for morbid obesity: analysis of 1,292 consecutive patients and review of literature. Surg Obes Relat Dis 2005; 1:467–474.

Chevallier J-M, Zinzindohoué F, Douard R, et al. Complications after laparoscopic adjustable gastric banding for morbid obesity: experience with 1,000 patients over 7 years. Obes Surg 2004; 14:407–414.

Court I, Wilson A, Benotti P, Szomstein S, Rosenthal RJ. T-tube gastrostomy as a novel approach for distal staple line disruption after sleeve gastrectomy for morbid obesity: case report and review of the literature. Obes Surg 2010; 20:519–522.

Cucchi SG, Pories WJ, MacDonald KG, Morgan EJ. Gastrogastric fistulas. A complication of divided gastric bypass surgery. Ann Surg 1995; 221:387–391.

Dang H, Arias E, Szomstein S, Rosenthal R. Laparoscopic conversion of distal mini-gastric bypass to proximal Roux-en-Y gastric bypass for malnutrition: case report and review of the literature. Surg Obes Relat Dis 2009; 5:383–386.

Dargent J. Surgical treatment of morbid obesity by adjustable gastric band: the case for a conservative strategy in the case of failure - a 9-year series. Obes Surg 2004; 14:986–990.

Dargent J. Esophageal dilatation after laparoscopic adjustable gastric banding: definition and strategy. Obes Surg 2005; 15:843–848.

De Csepel J, Nahouraii R, Gagner M. Laparoscopic gastric bypass as a reoperative bariatric surgery for failed open restrictive procedures. Surg Endosc 2001; 15:393–397.

Deitel M. Handbook of obesity surgery : current concepts and therapy of morbid obesity and related disease. Toronto: FD-Communications, 2010.

Demaria EJ, Jamal MK. Surgical options for obesity. Gastroenterol Clin North Am 2005; 34:127–142.

DeMaria EJ, Sugerman HJ, Meador JG, et al. High failure rate after laparoscopic adjustable silicone gastric banding for treatment of morbid obesity. Ann Surg 2001; 233:809–818.

Doldi SB, Micheletto G, Lattuada E, et al. Adjustable gastric banding: 5-year experience. Obes Surg 2000; 10:171–173.

Favretti F, Segato G, Ashton D, et al. Laparoscopic adjustable gastric banding in 1,791 consecutive obese patients: 12-year results. Obes Surg 2007; 17:168–175.

Fuks D, Verhaeghe P, Brehant O, et al. Results of laparoscopic sleeve gastrectomy: a prospective study in 135 patients with morbid obesity. Surgery 2009; 145:106–113.

Furbetta F, Coli E. Codification of techniques for reoperation after Lap-Band. Obes Surg 2003; 13:289–293.

Gagner M, Gentileschi P, De Csepel J, et al. Laparoscopic reoperative bariatric surgery: experience from 27 consecutive patients. Obes Surg 2002; 12:254–260.

Gagner M, Gumbs AA. Gastric banding: conversion to sleeve, bypass, or DS. Surg Endosc 2007; 21:1931–1935.

Go MR, Muscarella P 2nd, Needleman BJ, Cook CH, Melvin WS. Endoscopic management of stomal stenosis after Roux-en-Y gastric bypass. Surg Endosc 2004; 18:56–59.

Gonzalez R, Lin E, Venkatesh KR, Bowers SP, Smith CD. Gastrojejunostomy during laparoscopic gastric bypass: analysis of 3 techniques. Arch Surg 2003; 138:181–184.

Gumbs AA, Duffy AJ, Bell RL. Incidence and management of marginal ulceration after laparoscopic Roux-Y gastric bypass. Surg Obes Relat Dis 2006; 2:460–463.

Gumbs AA, Pomp A, Gagner M. Revisional bariatric surgery for inadequate weight loss. Obes Surg 2007; 17:1137–1145.

Gustavsson S, Sundbom M. Excellent weight result after Roux-en-Y gastric bypass in spite of gastro-gastric fistula. Obes Surg 2003; 13:457–459.

Han-Geurts IJM, Lim A, Stijnen T, Bonjer HJ. Laparoscopic feeding jejunostomy: a systematic review. Surg Endosc 2005; 19:951–957.

Himpens J, Dapri G, Cadière GB. A prospective randomized study between laparoscopic gastric banding and laparoscopic isolated sleeve gastrectomy: results after 1 and 3 years. Obes Surg 2006; 16:1450–1456.

Holéczy P, Novák P, Králová A. 30% complications with adjustable gastric banding: what did we do wrong? Obes Surg 2001; 11:748–751.

Ikramuddin S, Kellogg TA, Leslie DB. Laparoscopic conversion of vertical banded gastroplasty to a Roux-en-Y gastric bypass. Surg Endosc 2007; 21:1927–1930.

Johnson WH, Fernanadez AZ, Farrell TM, et al. Surgical revision of loop ("mini") gastric bypass procedure: multicenter review of complications and conversions to Roux-en-Y gastric bypass. Surg Obes Relat Dis 2007; 3:37–41.

Keidar A, Carmon E, Szold A, Abu-Abeid S. Port complications following laparoscopic adjustable gastric banding for morbid obesity. Obes Surg 2005; 15:361–365.

Khaitan L, Van Sickle K, Gonzalez R, et al. Laparoscopic revision of bariatric procedures: is it feasible? Am Surg 2005; 71:6–10; discussion 10–12.

Kirshtein B, Avinoach E, Mizrahi S, Lantsberg L. Presentation and management of port disconnection after laparoscopic adjustable gastric banding. Surg Endosc 2009; 23:272–275.

Lattuada E, Zappa MA, Mozzi E, et al. Band erosion following gastric banding: how to treat it. Obes Surg 2007; 17:329–333.

Launay-Savary MV, Slim K, Brugère C, et al. Band and port-related morbidity after bariatric surgery: an underestimated problem. Obes Surg 2008; 18:1406–1410.

Lee S, Carmody B, Wolfe L, et al. Effect of location and speed of diagnosis on anastomotic leak outcomes in 3828 gastric bypass cases. J Gastrointest Surg 2007; 11:708–713.

Lew JI, Daud A, DiGorgi MF, et al. Preoperative esophageal manometry and outcome of laparoscopic adjustable silicone gastric banding. Surg Endosc 2006; 20:1242–1247.

Lyass S, Cunneen SA, Hagiike M, et al. Device-related reoperations after laparoscopic adjustable gastric banding. Am Surg 2005; 71:738–743.

MacLean LD, Rhode BM, Nohr C, Katz S, McLean AP. Stomal ulcer after gastric bypass. J Am Coll Surg 1997; 185:1–7.

Martikainen T, Pirinen E, Alhava E, et al. Long-term results, late complications and quality of life in a series of adjustable gastric banding. Obes Surg 2004; 14:648–654.

McCormick JT, Papasavas PK, Caushaj PF, Gagné DJ. Laparoscopic revision of failed open bariatric procedures. Surg Endosc 2003; 17:413–415.

Müller MK, Wildi S, Scholz T, Clavien P-A, Weber M. Laparoscopic pouch resizing and redo of gastro-jejunal anastomosis for pouch dilatation following gastric bypass. Obes Surg 2005; 15:1089–1095.

National Institutes of Health. Gastrointestinal surgery for severe obesity. Consens Statement 1991; 9:1–20.

Nesset EM, Kendrick ML, Houghton SG, et al. A two-decade spectrum of revisional bariatric surgery at a tertiary referral center. Surg Obes Relat Dis 2007; 3:25–30; discussion 30.

Nguyen NT, Stevens CM, Wolfe BM. Incidence and outcome of anastomotic stricture after laparoscopic gastric bypass. J Gastrointest Surg 2003; 7:997–1003; discussion 1003.

Owens BM, Owens ML, Hill CW. Effect of revisional bariatric surgery on weight loss and frequency of complications. Obes Surg 1996; 6:479–484.

O'Brien PE, Dixon JB. Weight loss and early and late complications – the international experience. Am J Surg 2002; 184:42S–45S.

O'Brien PE, McPhail T, Chaston TB, Dixon JB. Systematic review of medium-term weight loss after bariatric operations. Obes Surg 2006; 16:1032–1040.
Papavramidis TS, Kotzampassi K, Kotidis E, Eleftheriadis EE, Papavramidis ST. Endoscopic fibrin sealing of gastrocutaneous fistulas after sleeve gastrectomy and biliopancreatic diversion with duodenal switch. J Gastroenterol Hepatol 2008; 23:1802–1805.
Patel S, Eckstein J, Acholonu E, Abu-Jaish W, Szomstein S, Rosenthal RJ. Reasons and outcomes of laparoscopic revisional surgery after laparoscopic adjustable gastric banding for morbid obesity. Surg Obes Relat Dis 2010; 6:391–398.
Patel S, Szomstein S, Rosenthal RJ. Reasons and outcomes of reoperative bariatric surgery for failed and complicated procedures (excluding adjustable gastric banding). Obes Surg 2011; 21:1209–1219.
Ponce J, Paynter S, Fromm R. Laparoscopic adjustable gastric banding: 1,014 consecutive cases. J Am Coll Surg 2005; 201:529–535.
Ren CJ, Horgan S, Ponce J. US experience with the LAP-BAND system. Am J Surg 2002; 184:46S–50S.
Ren CJ, Weiner M, Allen JW. Favorable early results of gastric banding for morbid obesity: the American experience. Surg Endosc 2004; 18:543–546.
Requarth JA, Burchard KW, Colacchio TA, et al. Long-term morbidity following jejunoileal bypass. The continuing potential need for surgical reversal. Arch Surg 1995; 130:318–325.
Roller JE, Provost DA. Revision of failed gastric restrictive operations to Roux-en-Y gastric bypass: impact of multiple prior bariatric operations on outcome. Obes Surg 2006; 16:865–869.
Rosenthal RJ. Dilating the stenotic gastrojejunostomy after laparoscopic Roux-en-Y gastric bypass for morbid obesity: when things go wrong. J Gastrointest Surg 2009; 13:1561–1563
Rosenthal RJ, Szomstein S, Kennedy CI, Soto FC, Zundel N. Laparoscopic surgery for morbid obesity: 1,001 consecutive bariatric operations performed at The Bariatric Institute, Cleveland Clinic Florida. Obes Surg 2006; 16:119–124.
Sapala JA, Wood MH, Sapala MA, Flake TM Jr. Marginal ulcer after gastric bypass: a prospective 3-year study of 173 patients. Obes Surg 1998; 8:505–516.
Sarker S, Herold K, Creech S, Shayani V. Early and late complications following laparoscopic adjustable gastric banding. Am Surg 2004; 70:146–149; discussion 149–150.
Schouten R, Van Dielen FMH, Greve JWM. Re-operation after laparoscopic adjustable gastric banding leads to a further decrease in BMI and obesity-related co-morbidities: results in 33 patients. Obes Surg 2006; 16:821–828.
Schwartz RW, Strodel WE, Simpson WS, Griffen WO Jr. Gastric bypass revision: lessons learned from 920 cases. Surgery 1988; 104:806–812.
Serra C, Baltasar A, Andreo L, et al. Treatment of gastric leaks with coated self-expanding stents after sleeve gastrectomy. Obes Surg 2007; 17:866–872.
Siilin H, Wanders A, Gustavsson S, Sundbom M. The proximal gastric pouch invariably contains acid-producing parietal cells in Roux-en-Y gastric bypass. Obes Surg 2005; 15:771–777.
Silecchia G, Perrotta N, Boru C, et al. Role of a minimally invasive approach in the management of laparoscopic adjustable gastric banding postoperative complications. Arch Surg 2004; 139:1225–1230.
Spivak H, Beltran OR, Slavchev P, Wilson EB. Laparoscopic revision from LAP-BAND to gastric bypass. Surg Endosc 2007; 21:1388–1392.
Stroh C, Hohmann U, Schramm H, Manger T. [Long-term results after gastric banding]. Zentralbl Chir 2005; 130:410–418.
Sugerman HJ, Wolper JL. Failed gastroplasty for morbid obesity. Revised gastroplasty versus Roux-Y gastric bypass. Am J Surg 1984; 148:331–336.
Susmallian S, Ezri T, Elis M, Charuzi I. Access-port complications after laparoscopic gastric banding. Obes Surg 2003; 13:128–131.
Suter M. Laparoscopic band repositioning for pouch dilatation/slippage after gastric banding: disappointing results. Obes Surg 2001; 11:507–512.
Suter M, Calmes JM, Paroz A, Giusti V. A 10-year experience with laparoscopic gastric banding for morbid obesity: high long-term complication and failure rates. Obes Surg 2006; 16:829–835.
Suter M, Dorta G, Giusti V, Calmes J-M. Gastric banding interferes with esophageal motility and gastroesophageal reflux. Arch Surg 2005; 140:639–643.
Suter M, Giusti V, Héraief E, Calmes J-M. Band erosion after laparoscopic gastric banding: occurrence and results after conversion to Roux-en-Y gastric bypass. Obes Surg 2004; 14:381–386.
Te Riele WW, Dejong JR, Vogten JM, et al. [Sustained weight loss 2 years after laparoscopic adjustable gastric banding for morbid obesity]. Ned Tijdschr Geneeskd 2007; 151:1130–1135.
Tucker ON, Escalante-Tattersfield T, Szomstein S, Rosenthal RJ. The ABC system: a simplified classification system for small bowel obstruction after laparoscopic Roux-en-Y gastric bypass. Obes Surg 2007; 17:1549–1554.
Tucker O, Sucandy I, Szomstein S, Rosenthal RJ. Revisional surgery after failed laparoscopic adjustable gastric banding. Surg Obes Relat Dis 2008; 4:740–747.
Van Gemert WG, Van Wersch MM, Greve JW, Soeters PB. Revisional surgery after failed vertical banded gastroplasty: restoration of vertical banded gastroplasty or conversion to gastric bypass. Obes Surg 1998; 8:21–28.
Van Wageningen B, Berends FJ, Van Ramshorst B, Janssen IFM. Revision of failed laparoscopic adjustable gastric banding to Roux-en-Y gastric bypass. Obes Surg 2006; 16:137–141.
Vella M, Galloway DJ. Laparoscopic adjustable gastric banding for severe obesity. Obes Surg 2003; 13:642–648.
Vertruyen M. Experience with Lap-band system up to 7 years. Obes Surg 2002; 12:569–572.
Weber M, Müller MK, Michel J-M, et al. Laparoscopic Roux-en-Y gastric bypass, but not rebanding, should be proposed as rescue procedure for patients with failed laparoscopic gastric banding. Ann Surg 2003; 238:827–833; discussion 833–834.
Weiner R, Blanco-Engert R, Weiner S, et al. Outcome after laparoscopic adjustable gastric banding - 8 years experience. Obes Surg 2003; 13: 427–434.
Weiner R, Wagner D, Bockhorn H. Laparoscopic gastric banding for morbid obesity. J Laparoendosc Adv Surg Tech A 1999; 9:23–30.
Weiss HG, Nehoda H, Labeck B, et al. Treatment of morbid obesity with laparoscopic adjustable gastric banding affects esophageal motility. Am J Surg 2000; 180:479–482.
Wiesner W, Hauser M, Schöb O, Weber M, Hauser RS. Pseudoachalasia following laparoscopically placed adjustable gastric banding. Obes Surg 2001; 11:513–518.
Wittgrove AC, Clark GW. Laparoscopic gastric bypass, Roux-en-Y- 500 patients: technique and results, with 3-60 month follow-up. Obes Surg 2000; 10:233–239.
Yoffe B, Sapojnikov S, Lebedev V, Goldblum C. Disconnection of port after laparoscopic gastric banding: causes and solution. Obes Surg 2003; 13:784–787.
Zehetner J, Holzinger F, Triaca H, Klaiber C. A 6-year experience with the Swedish adjustable gastric band Prospective long-term audit of laparoscopic gastric banding. Surg Endosc 2005; 19:21–28.
Zinzindohoue F, Chevallier J-M, Douard R, et al. Laparoscopic gastric banding: a minimally invasive surgical treatment for morbid obesity: prospective study of 500 consecutive patients. Ann Surg 2003; 237:1–9.

Chapter 15 Reoperations for pancreatic surgery complications

Mitsugi Shimoda, Keiichi Kubota

HISTORICAL PERSPECTIVE

Over the past decade, the number of pancreatic resections have increased. Pancreatic cancer is a major cause of cancer-related mortality worldwide, ranking as the fifth leading cause of death. Over 26,000 people die from pancreatic cancer every year in Japan, and the survival rate in the last 5 years was 5.5% (Jemal et al. 2011, Matsuda et al. 2011). Surgery is historically associated with a high operative mortality rate, although technical advances and the centralization of care have both improved outcomes and reduced the mortality rate of patients with pancreatic cancer. Surgical morbidity remains high, with patients commonly suffering one or more complications. Furthermore, advancements in diagnostic imaging may now detect atypical, small early neoplasms thus allowing earlier intervention. Although the exact nature of such tumors may be difficult to diagnose by preoperative imaging only, resection is still required due to the suspected malignancy. Formal pancreatic resection like pancreatoduodenectomy (PD), distal pancreatectomy (DP), or total pancreatectomy (TP) is the only way to treat these patients.

Although mortality after pancreatic surgery in several high-volume centers has decreased to <3%, morbidity still remains high at about 18–52% (Adam et al. 2004, Buchler et al. 2003, DeOliveira et al. 2006, Gouma et al. 2000, Sohn et al. 2003, Trede & Schwall 1988, Winter et al. 2006). Frequent complications are anastomoses related [pancreatojejunostomy (PJ), pancreaticogastrostomy (PG), gastrojejunostomy (GJ), duodenojejunostomy (DJ), hepaticojejunostomy (HJ)] and include: bleeding complications, pancreatic fistulas (PFs), biliary stricture (BS), delayed gastric empting, and intra-abdominal infection. Most importantly, hemorrhage after pancreatic surgery is the most frequently reported complication and the incidence of hemorrhage after pancreatic surgery is found to be about 4% (Limongelli et al. 2008, Roulin et al. 2011). However, one-third of patients with bleeding died even if they received interventional radiology (IR) or an endoscopic procedure. Limongelli et al (2008) and Roulin at al (2011) demonstrated the optimal treatment for postpancreatectomy hemorrhage (PPH). As the management of this life-threatening situation is very difficult, the outcome of PPH is dependent on the clinical status of the patient and the performance of the medical center and physicians. BS is another major complication following PD, and is present in about 2.6% of cases (Limongelli et al. 2008). Patients with BS need interventional treatment, endoscopic procedures, or reoperation.

This chapter outlines the surgical approach for treatment of PPH and BS.

POSTPANCREATECTOMY HEMORRHAGE

Cause of PPH

1. Gastrointestinal tract hemorrhage (intraluminal) was reported in one-third of patients after pancreatic surgery (Wente et al. 2007). Gastrointestinal tract hemorrhage is sometimes related to the ulcer at the anastomosis or at the suture lines of gastrojejunostomy (GJ). Pancreatic anastomosis (PJ or PG) is also a potential site for intraluminal hemorrhage after PD. Some patients suffered a stress ulcer in the remnant stomach, which was one of the causes of intraluminal bleeding
2. Approximately two-thirds of patients with postpancreatic surgery hemorrhage had extraluminal bleeding. This was detected, in most patients, by bleeding in abdominal drains, most of which was associated with a leak of the PJ or PG. In pancreatic surgery, regional lymphadenectomy and extensive vascular skeletonization (celiac trunk and around supramesenteric artery, SMA and splenic vessels) must be performed for curative resection. If pancreatic juice leakage occurs, stepwise erosion of the celiac trunk, SMA, and especially the stump of the gastroduodenal artery (GDA), may cause pseudoaneurysm formation that subsequently ruptures
3. Technical failure with inadequate hemostasis in the operative field or excess bleeding is related to reconstruction of the portal vein, hepatic artery (HA), common hepatic artery (CHA), and SMA

Site of PPH

1. The main potential bleeding sites after PD are, as shown in **Figure 15.1a,** (1) stump of GDA, (2) portal vain or HA, (3) superior mesenteric vein, (4) branch of SMA including jejunal mesenteric arterial branch and inferior pancreaticoduodenal artery, (5) cut line and suture line at PJ or PG, (6) liver bed after cholecystectomy, (7) suture line of the DJ or GJ, and (8) surgical field (retroperitonium). Bleeding arising from GDA is most frequently encountered in PPH (Standop et al. 2005, Wente et al. 2007)
2. The main bleeding points after DP are, as shown in **Figure 15.1b,** (1) stump of pancreas, (2) stump of splenic artery or vein, (3) splenic hilus or small-ligated vessels (in cases of splenic preservation), and (4) surgical field (Wente et al. 2007)

Definition of PPH

The International Study Group of Pancreatic Surgery (ISGPS) classified PPH into early and delayed onset and Roulin et al. described a systemic review of delayed PPH (Roulin et al. 2011, Wente et al. 2007). They defined PPH as follows:

1. Early PPH: This mostly occurs within 24 hours of surgery; this type of PPH is mostly due to technical failure of appropriate hemostasis during the operation or an underlying perioperative coagulopathy. It is easily found in the area of the surgical fields and is discovered by abdominal drain bleeding in most cases
2. Delayed PPH: The definition of delayed PPH is 'bleeding observed after 24 hours postoperatively.' It is related to gastrointestinal anastomosis bleeding, leakage of venous or arterial anastomosis after vessel resection, or erosion after PF. Occasionally, delayed PPH may be observed several days or even months after the patient's

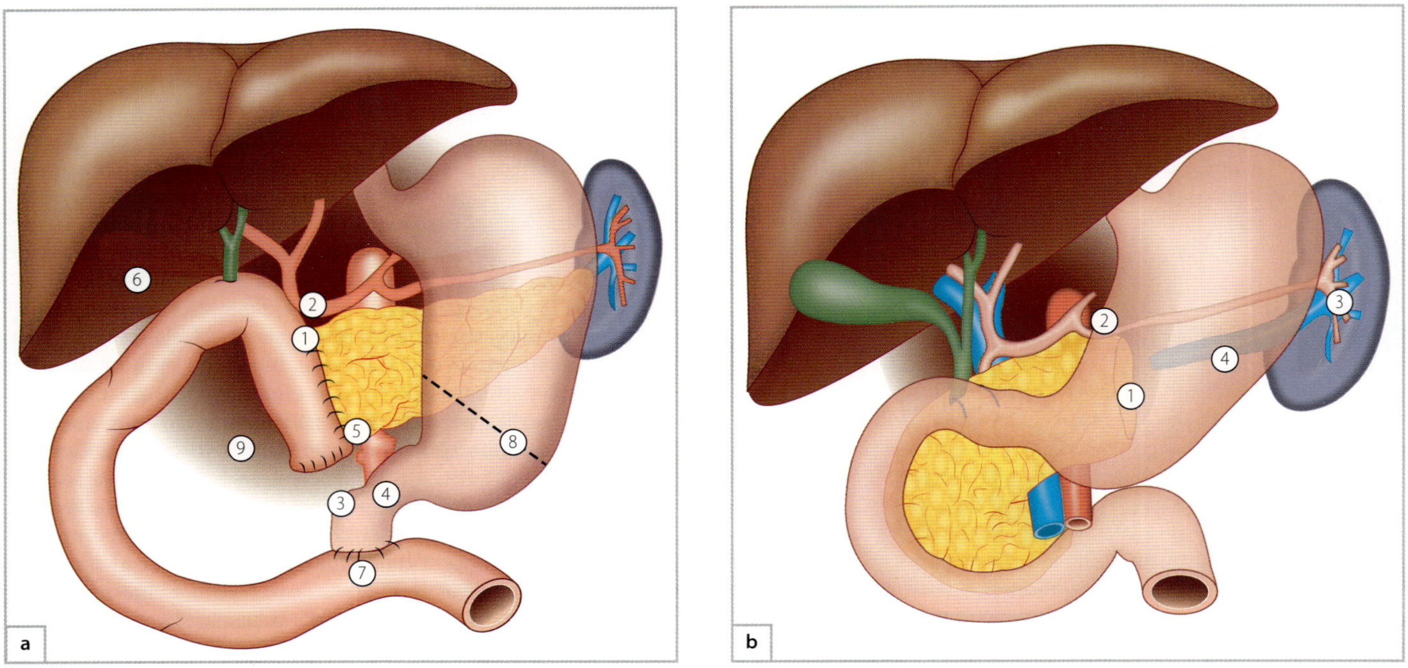

Figure 15.1 (a) Common sites of hemorrhage post pancreatico-duodenectomy: (1) stump of gastro-duodenal artery, (2) portal vain or hepatic artery, (3) superior mesenteric vein, (4) branch of superior mesenteric artery including jejunal mesenteric arterial branch and inferior pancreaticoduodenal artery, (5) cut line and suture line at pancreatico-jejunostomy or pancreatico-gastrostomy, (6) liver bed after cholecystectomy, (7) suture line of the duodeno-jejunostomy or gastro-jejunostomy, and (8) surgical field (retroperitonium). (b) Common sites of hemorrhage post distal pancreatectomy: (1) stump of pancreas, (2) stump of splenic artery or vein, (3) splenic hilus or small-ligated vessels (in cases of splenic reservation), and (4) surgical field.

discharge. Delayed PPH occurs in only 3.3% of patients, but is associated with a mortality rate as high as 35% (Roulin et al. 2011)

Timing of reoperation and preoperative imaging for PPH

Several major reports and systemic reviews described the timing of reoperation for PPH (Limongelli et al. 2008, Makowiec et al. 2005, Roulin et al. 2011, Yekebas et al. 2007). Indications for reoperation were, as indicated below, a life-threatening unstable hemodynamic status, with a decrease in hemoglobin (3 g/dL/h), or bleeding from the surgical field (extraluminal) or hematemesis and melena (intraluminal):

1. Early PPH in stable patients requires thorough investigation to detect intraluminal or extraluminal bleeding sites using endoscopy or helical computed tomography (CT). For intraluminal bleeding, endoscopic examination is performed first. If the bleeding source is detected, endoscopic treatment provides the optimal management. When endoscopic hemostasis is not technically feasible, reoperation is indicated. For extraluminal bleeding, IR should be performed first. If IR cannot demonstrate an active bleeding source or accomplish hemostasis, reoperation must be performed. If the diagnostic modalities are not promptly available or there is no time for examinations, immediate reoperation is required without diagnostic delay. Early PPH is associated with the surgeon's skill and has often been attributed to technical failure (**Figure 15.2**)
2. In delayed PPH, when patients are bleeding through an abdominal drain or nasogastric tube with a stable or unstable hemodynamic status, abdominal angiography, abdominal helical CT or endoscopic examinations should first be performed to locate the bleeding source. In most cases, delayed PPH is related to PF.

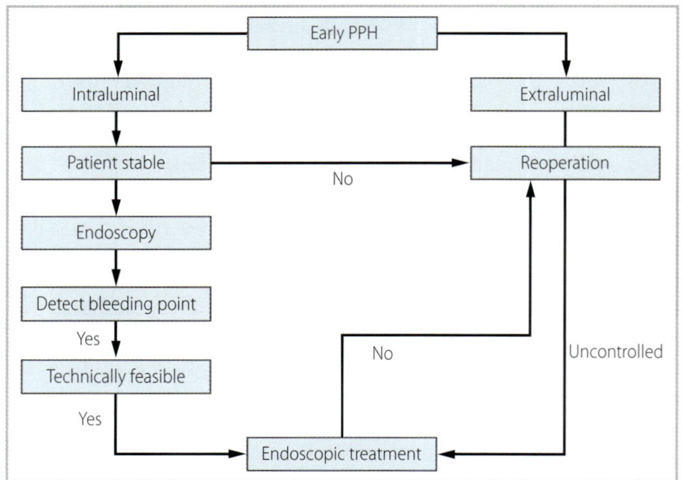

Figure 15.2 Algorithm for early PPH.

Therefore, if bleeding points or pseudoaneurysms are identified by the above examinations, endoscopic hemostasis or transarterial embolization (TAE) should be employed to control the hemorrhage. Recently, interventional techniques have shown remarkable results, and when extraluminal PPH is suspected to be associated with PF, an interventional technique is chosen first in most institutions. In the authors' institution, if the bleeding point or pseudoaneurysm cannot be identified at the time of angiogram, two choices remain: observation or TAE of a potential bleeding point (stump of GDA, splenic artery, HA or CHA).

In most cases, after bleeding, the exact bleeding sites can be identified and TAE therefore becomes feasible. When observation is selected, re-bleeding within 7 days occurs in most cases and TAE then becomes necessary. After failure of repeated TAE treatment due to technical unfeasibility, reoperation must be considered (**Figure 15.3**). As mentioned above, the operation serves as a final cure for PPH. However, surgical access to the bleeding point is always difficult due to the overlying pancreaticoenteric and bilioenteric anastomosis, peripancreatic inflammation, as well as the presence of intra-abdominal adhesion. Even if the bleeding point is exposed, it is often difficult to repair or ligate it due to peripancreatic inflammation and vessel wall fragility

Type of operation for PPH

After failure of an endoscopic technique to control the bleeding of intraluminal early and delayed PPH, reoperation should be immediately performed by opening the anterior wall of the stomach and suturing the bleeding site. When PF is significant, completion pancreatectomy is performed to control the bleeding at the PJ anastomosis.

When TAE is unsuccessful for extraluminal delayed PPH associated with PF, the surgical techniques for delayed PPH comprise the following steps:

1. Identify the bleeding point and encircle the proximal and distal part of the artery, compressing the bleeding point using a finger.
2. If possible, suture the pore using 6-0 Proline (Ethicon Inc. Somerville, NJ). Even if hemostasis is obtained, this is not sufficient in most patients. In such cases, take a small part of the fascia of the abdominal rectal muscle and cover the sutured part using the fascia patch.
3. When PF is significant, extirpate the remnant pancreas leaving behind the spleen. This procedure, however, may be technically difficult to perform.

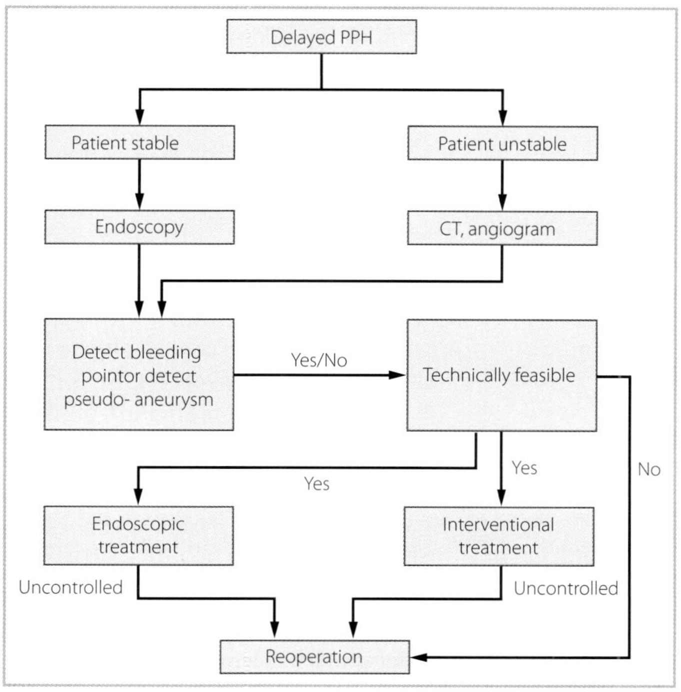

Figure 15.3 Algorithm for delayed PPH.

4. Place two large sump drains and wash the surgical field continuously using saline (1200–2400 mL/day). When suturing of the pore is technically difficult due to the fragility of the vessel wall, the proximal and distal sites of the artery should be ligated.

Anticipated PPH

Protection of major vessels from PF

The falciform or greater omentum graft patch method

The greater omentum graft is used to separate and cover the stump of GDA from the PJ anastomosis. When the greater omentum graft is not available, the falciform ligament is used. The greater omentum is divided at the center (**Figure 15.4a**), the right-side omentum graft is brought behind the PJ anastomosis (**Figure 15.4b**), and then covers the stump of GDA (**Figure 15.4c**). Kapoor et al. (2006) described no deaths due to PJ leak. This procedure is one of the options for preventing PPH caused by PF.

Two-stage PD with external drainage of pancreatic juice method

Generally, patients with soft pancreatic parenchyma, massive amounts of intraoperative bleeding, a high BMI, extensive previous surgery, and liver cirrhosis are known to be at risk of PF (Reid-Lombardo et al. 2007, Shimoda et al. 2012). This two-stage technique has been used in these high-risk patients.A pancreatic tube is inserted into the main pancreatic duct, a posterior row of sutures is placed between the seromuscular layer of jejunum and pancreatic parenchyma and an incomplete anterior row of sutures is also inserted (**Figure 15.5a**). The pancreatic tube is brought out of the abdominal cavity. A 16 Fr tube is placed in the jejunum to reduce the intraluminal pressure. Three months later, at reoperation, the incomplete anterior row of sutures between the pancreas and jejunum is exposed. At this stage, the fibrous tissue covering the tube must be preserved. A new pancreatic tube is inserted into the main pancreatic duct and the other end is inserted into the jejunal lumen and then brought out of the jejunum using a jejunostomy tube route. The PJ is achieved with an additional anterior row of sutures between the anterior wall of the pancreas (with the fibrous tissue) and the jejunum (**Figure 15.5b** and **c**) (Kubota et al. 2000, Seyama et al. 1998).

Placement of endoscopic nasopancreatic drainage

Endoscopic nasopancreatic drainage (ENPD) is often used for pancreatic duct injury, acute pancreatitis, and cytological diagnosis (Iiboshi et al. 2012, Ito et al. 2012, Kimura et al. 2011, Quan et al. 2003). ENPD is one of the treatment options for PF after DP. However, only one report has described the utility of ENPD for the treatment of PF (Nagatsu et al. 2011). Reduction of the pancreatic ductal pressure using ENPD may improve the PF. In six patients, ENPD was used for grade C PF after DP. None of the six patients developed PPH after ENPD tube placement. However, this procedure has not become a standard treatment for PF due to the small number of patients in this study.

Continuous peritoneal irrigation for infected cavity after PF

When PF is significant, the surgical field is lavaged continuously using saline. This procedure may reduce the infectious complications after PD and subsequently prevent the occurrence of PPH (Nakano et al. 2008). Horiuchi et al. (2010) reported that irrigation using saline solution containing gabexate mesilate was also effective for resolving PF in 27 patients with PF after PD. Eight of the 27 patients had grade A or B PF. There were no cases of PPH in this series.

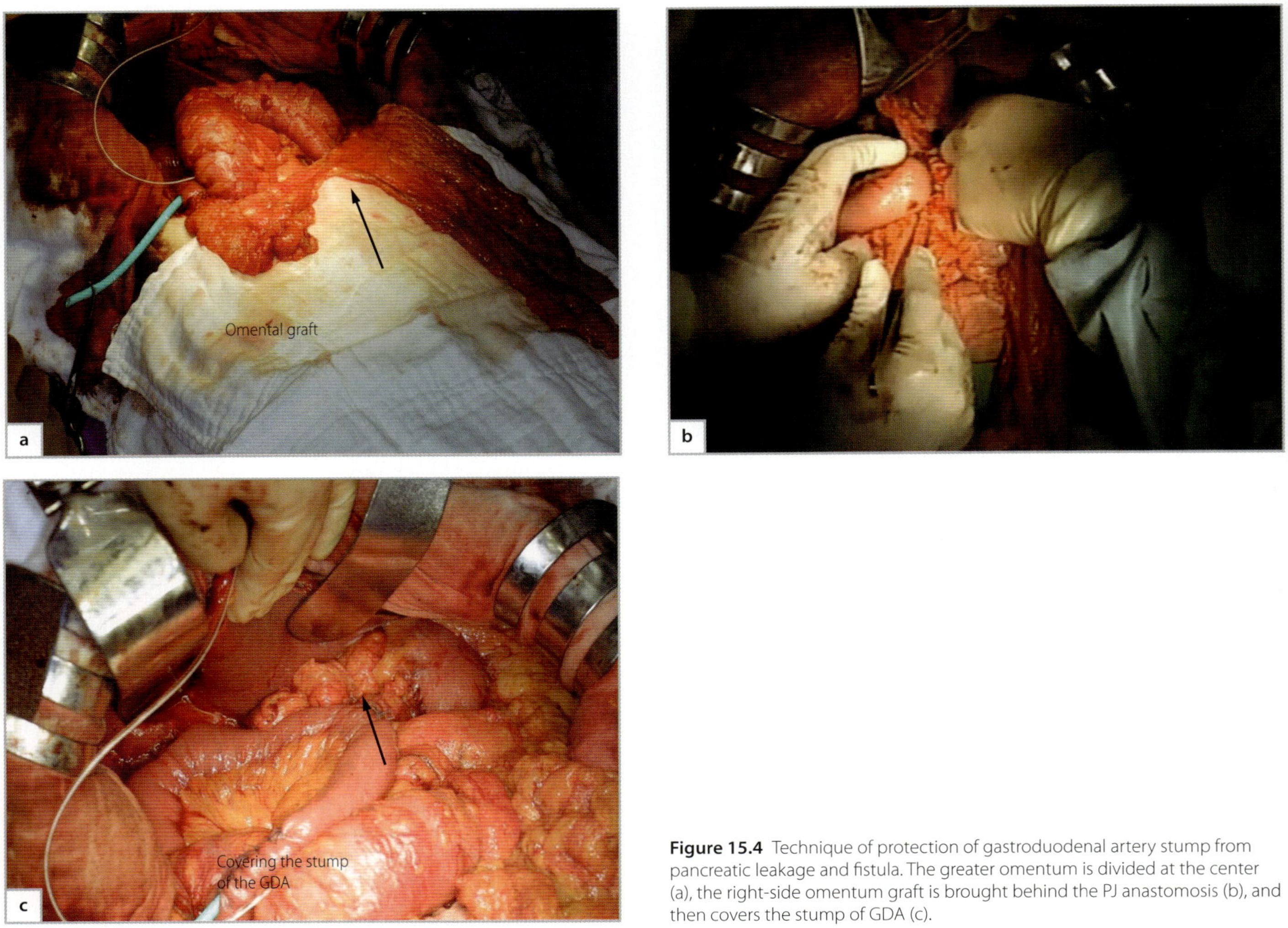

Figure 15.4 Technique of protection of gastroduodenal artery stump from pancreatic leakage and fistula. The greater omentum is divided at the center (a), the right-side omentum graft is brought behind the PJ anastomosis (b), and then covers the stump of GDA (c).

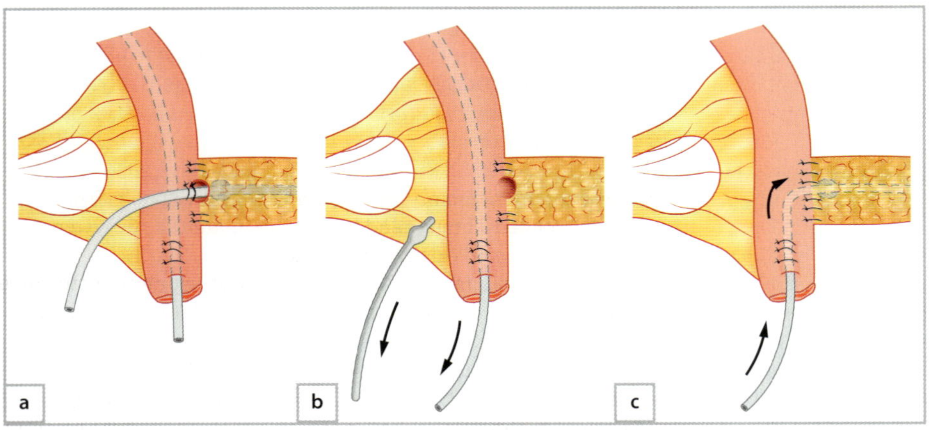

Figure 15.5 A pancreatic tube is inserted into the main pancreatic duct; a posterior row of sutures is placed between the seromuscular layer of jejunum and pancreatic parenchyma and an incomplete anterior row of sutures is also inserted (a). The pancreatic tube is brought out of the abdominal cavity. A 16 Fr tube is placed in the jejunum to reduce the intraluminal pressure (b), three months later, at reoperation, the incomplete anterior row of sutures between the pancreas and jejunum is exposed. At this stage, the fibrous tissue covering the tube must be preserved. A new pancreatic tube is inserted into the main pancreatic duct and the other end is inserted into the jejunal lumen and then brought out of the jejunum using a jejunostomy tube route. The PJ is achieved with an additional anterior row of sutures between the anterior wall of the pancreas (with the fibrous tissue) and the jejunum (c).

Continuous irrigation methods

When patients are diagnosed as having grade B or C PF, continuous irrigation using saline solution only should be started immediately. The drainage tubes are placed at the upper and lower sides of the PJ (**Figure 15.6a**), 24-hour continuous irrigation is started using saline (1200–2400 mL/day) through one tube, and then a stoma pouch is attached to drain the discharge fluid (**Figure 15.6b** and **c**). The other tube is sucked for 30 minutes continuously with a 5-minute release. Octreotide is simultaneously injected subcutaneously. The authors usually make a jejunostomy at the site of the jejunal stump to reduce intraluminal pressure. Reducing pressure is important for protecting PJ and HJ anastomosis.

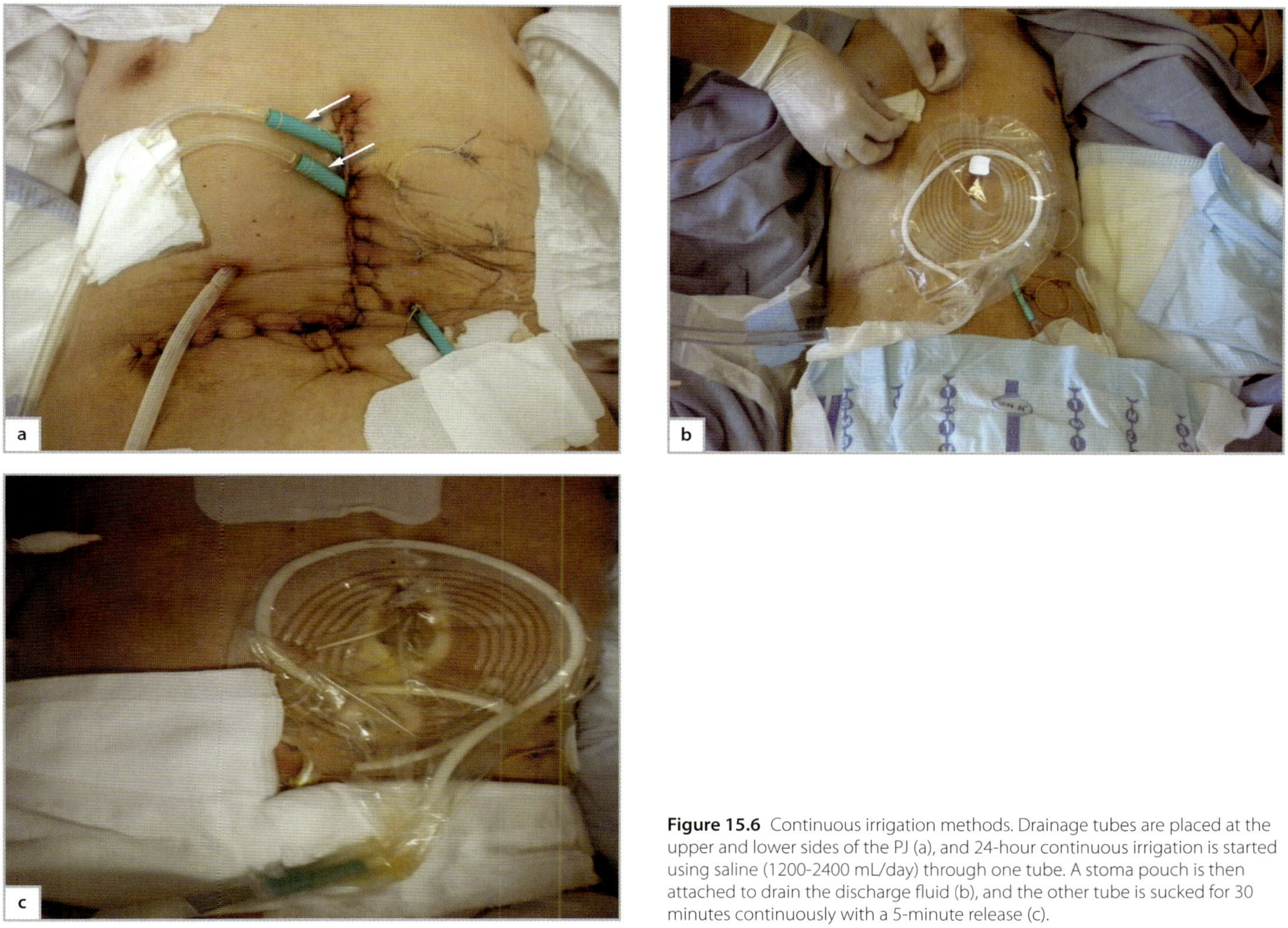

Figure 15.6 Continuous irrigation methods. Drainage tubes are placed at the upper and lower sides of the PJ (a), and 24-hour continuous irrigation is started using saline (1200-2400 mL/day) through one tube. A stoma pouch is then attached to drain the discharge fluid (b), and the other tube is sucked for 30 minutes continuously with a 5-minute release (c).

Postoperative principles to maximize results

After PPH treatment, parenteral nutrition is important for maintaining the patient's condition. If the patient's oral intake is poor, the authors recommend making a jejunostomy or placing a nasojejunostomy tube at the time of reoperation, or after TAE or endoscopic hemostasis. Starting nutrition will prevent PF and infection and also protect against rebleeding.

Major complications after reoperations are bleeding shock, septic shock, disseminated intravascular coagulation (DIC), and multiple organ failure. Ligations of the proper HA or CHA can induce cholangitis, hepatic abscess, or fatal hepatic failure. Previous reports have described the death of several patients from liver failure after ligation of the HA or CHA (Brodsky & Turnbull 1991). For recurrent bleeding after operation, the authors recommend IR initially, followed by TAE for the bleeding site.

BILIARY STRICTURE

BS formation after PD is a frequently encountered complication. House et al. (2006) reported that 42 of 1595 (2.6%) patients who had undergone PD between 1995 and 2003 developed BS. Ten patients had a benign tumor and the remaining 32 patients had a malignant tumor at the periampullary region. The median time to BS formation resulting in jaundice was 13 months.

Cause of BS

There are three risk factors for BS after PD as described below:

1. Patient-related factors: gender, age, race, comorbidities, preoperative jaundice, and origin of malignancy.
2. Disease-related factors: this type of BS was usually a recurrence of a malignant neoplasm at the site of a biliary enteric anastomosis.
3. Procedure-related factors: risk factors included bile duct issues (size, hardness and thickness, preoperative biliary drainage etc.), surgical technique issues, operative factors (operating time, amount of bleeding, dissection of lymph nodes around biliary tree etc.), and postoperative factors (bile leakage, PF etc.).

Otherwise, BS formation is uncommon after PD. House et al. (2006) suggested that preoperative biliary drainage was associated with BS. Previous reports have suggested that bile duct ischemia has been one of the risk factors for BS (Mueller et al. 1986, Pitt et al. 1989).

Treatment of BS

House et al. (2006) described and evaluated the incidence and outcome of 42 patients with BS. Forty of the 42 patients received percutaneous biliary drainage (PBD) initially and were then treated with balloon dilatation or Wallstent placement. Only two patients had undergone reanastomosis of HJ after failure of repeated dilations. After failure of repeated IR treatment, surgical repair was the only way to recover the BS patients. Reanastomosis is technically difficult: isolate the right, middle, and left HAs carefully; identify the portal vein; and then isolate and encircle the bilioenteric anastomosis (**Figure 15.7a**). Divide the anterior wall of the anastomosis (**Figure 15.7b**) and then confirm the severity of the stricture by inserting a surgical sonde (**Figure 15.7c**). The narrow orifice is widened by dividing the bile duct wall (**Figure 15.7d**). After a sufficient orifice is obtained, bilioenteric reanastomosis is performed in a standard manner (**Figure 15.7e**).

Example case

A 57-year-old male patient was admitted to our medical center with a diagnosis of pancreatic body cancer. The patient underwent DP with splenectomy in November 2009. He was doing well and discharged on 21st POD (postoperative day).

He was readmitted to our department as an emergency with hematemesis and shock signs. Endoscopy demonstrated a deep ulcer with massive hemorrhage at the posterior wall of the duodenum (**Figure 15.8a**). As an endoscopic procedure was considered to be ineffective, we decided to perform an emergency laparotomy. At laparotomy, a huge amount of clotted blood was present behind the stomach and at the pancreatic stump. The main bleeding points were the splenic artery and a branch of the SMA, and hemostasis by suture and ligation with aortal clamping was performed. After controlling the bleeding, several drainage tubes were placed at the surgical fields. We considered this hemorrhage to be due to PF, because amylase-rich fluid collection was confirmed in the abdominal cavity. After operation, we immediately started continuous irrigation with gabex-

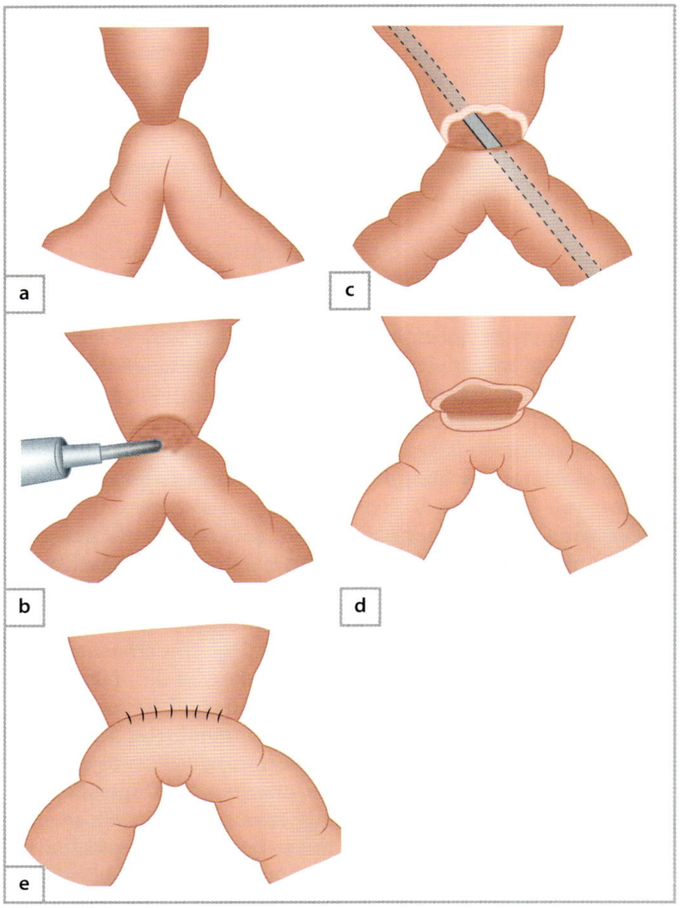

Figure 15.7 Technique of re-anastomosis for BS. The bilioenteric anastomosis is isolated and encircled (a), the anterior wall of the anastomosis is divided (b), then the severity of the stricture is confirmed by inserting a surgical sonde (c), the narrow orifice is widened by dividing the bile duct wall (d), after a sufficient orifice is obtained, bilioenteric reanastomosis is performed in a standard manner (e).

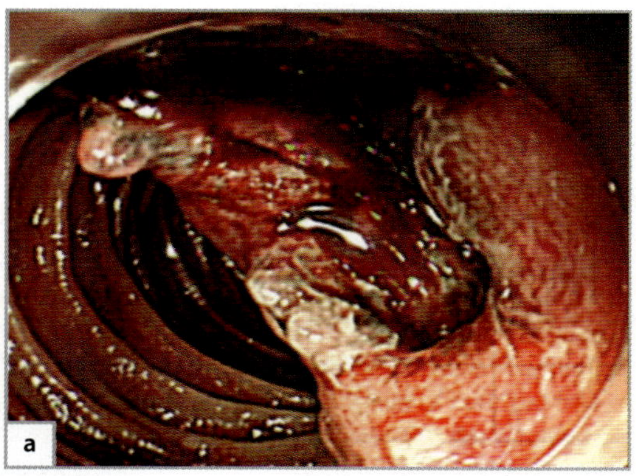

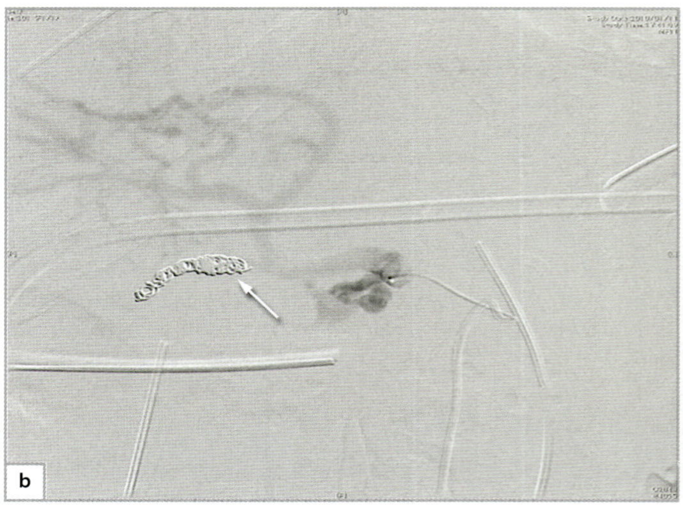

Figure 15.8 *See opposite page for details.*

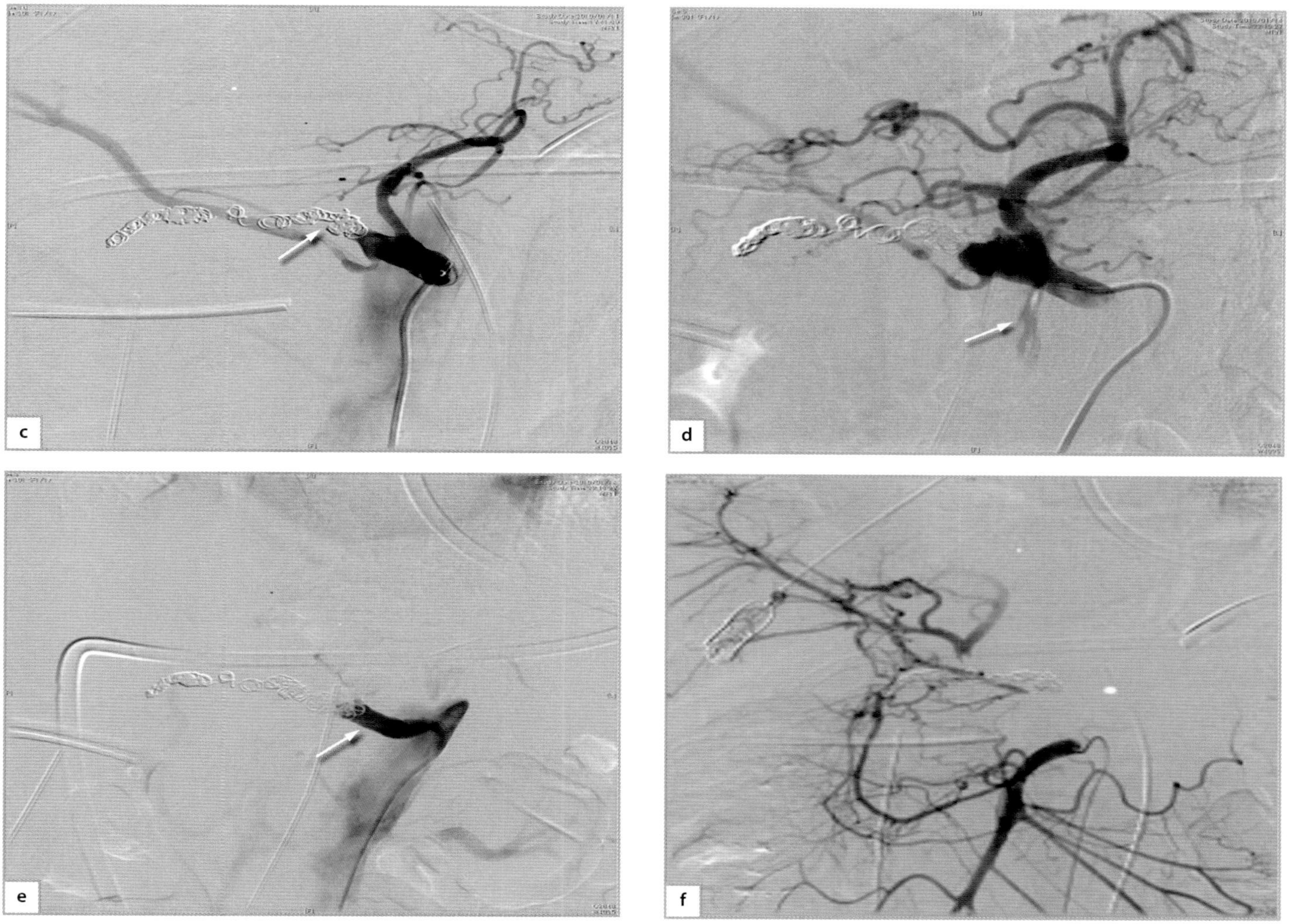

Figure 15.8 Post pancreatectomy hemorrhage case presentation (see case description in text) hemorrhage from erosion at the posterior duodenal wall (a), due to re-bleeding, angiography with coiling (arrow) of a GDA pseudoaneurysm was performed (b), recurrent bleeding required second angiography with embolization of the common hepatic artery (arrow) (c),third bleeding from celiac trunk required another embolization (arrows) (d, e), angiography showing replaced right hepatic artery from SMA (f).

ate mesilate in the abdominal cavity. On the 10th POD, the patient had some re-bleeding from the abdominal drain. At this time, since he was stable, we performed angiography first, which revealed a pseudoaneurysm at the GDA. TAE using coiling was then performed (**Figure 15.8b**). Five days after the first IR, the patient had recurrent bleeding at the CHA. We performed TAE again (**Figure 15.8c**). Three days after the second TAE, the patient had re-bleeding, this time from the celiac trunk. The third TAE was performed for the celiac trunk (**Figure 15.8d, e**). Fortunately, this patient had a replaced right HA coming from the SMA (**Figure 15.8f**). He never presented with any complications of liver failure or abscess. We placed a nasoduodenal tube and nutrition was initiated (**Figure 15.9**). He recovered, was discharged on 174 th POD and is now without any evidence of recurrence of his pancreatic cancer.
Comment: In this case, a combination treatment of operation and IR was very effective in controlling PPH. Postoperative nutrition was also a very important factor in the improvement of the general condition of the patient.

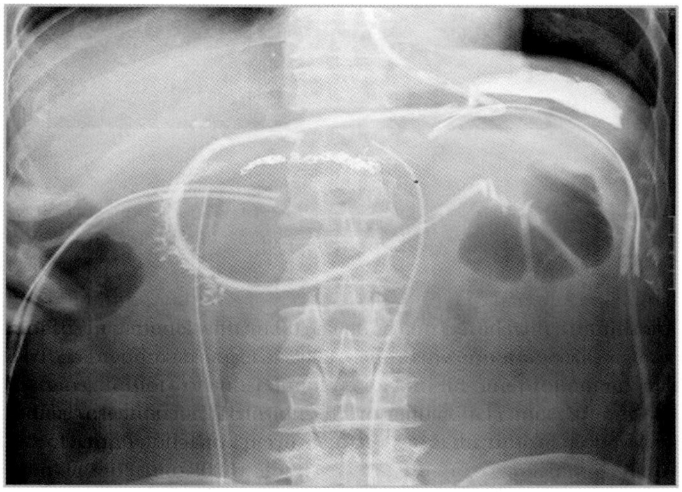

Figure 15.9 Placement of a nasoduodenal tube.

REFERENCES

Adam U, Makowiec F, Riediger H, et al. Risk factors for complications after pancreatic head resection. Am J Surg 2004; 187:201–208.

Brodsky JT, Turnbull AD. Arterial hemorrhage after pancreatoduodenectomy. The 'sentinel bleed'. Arch Surg 1991; 126:1037–1040.

Buchler MW, Wagner M, Schmied BM, et al. Changes in morbidity after pancreatic resection: toward the end of completion pancreatectomy. Arch Surg 2003; 138:1310–1314; discussion 1315.

DeOliveira ML, Winter JM, Schafer M, et al. Assessment of complications after pancreatic surgery: a novel grading system applied to 633 patients undergoing pancreaticoduodenectomy. Ann Surg 2006; 244:931–917; discussion 937–939.

Gouma DJ, van Geenen RC, van Gulik TM, et al. Rates of complications and death after pancreaticoduodenectomy: risk factors and the impact of hospital volume. Ann Surg 2000; 232:786–795.

Horiuchi A, Watanabe Y, Sato K, et al. Continuous irrigation with gabexate mesilate around pancreaticojejunostomy after pancreaticoduodenectomy. Hepatogastroenterology 2010; 57:1291–1294.

House MG, Cameron JL, Schulick RD, et al. Incidence and outcome of biliary strictures after pancreaticoduodenectomy. Ann Surg 2006; 243:571–576; discussion 576–578.

Iiboshi T, Hanada K, Fukuda T, et al. Value of cytodiagnosis using endoscopic nasopancreatic drainage for early diagnosis of pancreatic cancer: establishing a new method for the early detection of pancreatic carcinoma in situ. Pancreas 2012; 41:523–529.

Ito Y, Kenmochi T, Irino T, et al. Endoscopic management of pancreatic duct injury by endoscopic stent placement: a case report and literature review. World J Emerg Surg: WJES 2012; 7:21.

Jemal A, Bray F, Center MM, et al. Global cancer statistics. CA Cancer J Clin 2011; 61:69–90.

Kapoor VK, Sharma A, Behari A, Singh RK. Omental flaps in pancreaticoduodenectomy. JOP: Journal of the Pancreas 2006; 7:608–615.

Kimura H, Furukawa Y, Yamasaki S, et al. A study of the usefulness of pancreatic juice cytology obtained via an endoscopic nasal pancreatic drainage (ENPD) tube. Nihon Shokakibyo Gakkai zasshi: The Japanese Journal of Gastroenterology 2011; 108:928–936.

Kubota K, Makuuchi M, Takayama T, et al. Appraisal of two-staged pancreatoduodenectomy: its technical aspects and outcome. Hepatogastroenterology 2000; 47:269–274.

Limongelli P, Khorsandi SE, Pai M, et al. Management of delayed postoperative hemorrhage after pancreaticoduodenectomy: a meta-analysis. Arch Surg 2008; 143:1001–1007; discussion 1007.

Makowiec F, Riediger H, Euringer W, et al. Management of delayed visceral arterial bleeding after pancreatic head resection. J Gastrointest Surg: Official Journal of the Society for Surgery of the Alimentary Tract 2005; 9:1293–1299.

Matsuda T, Marugame T, Kamo K, et al. Cancer incidence and incidence rates in Japan in 2005: based on data from 12 population-based cancer registries in the Monitoring of Cancer Incidence in Japan (MCIJ) project. Jpn J Clin Oncol 2011; 41:139–147.

Mueller PR, van Sonnenberg E, Ferrucci JT, Jr., et al. Biliary stricture dilatation: multicenter review of clinical management in 73 patients. Radiology 1986; 160:17–22.

Nagatsu A, Taniguchi M, Shimamura T, et al. Endoscopic naso-pancreatic drainage for the treatment of pancreatic fistula occurring after LDLT. World J Gastroenterol: WJG 2011; 17:3560–3564.

Nakano H, Asakura T, Sakurai J, et al. Prophylactic irrigation around a pancreaticojejunostomy for the treatment of a pancreatic fistula after a pancreaticoduodenectomy in patients with a risky pancreatic remnant. Hepatogastroenterology 2008; 55:717–721.

Pitt HA, Kaufman SL, Coleman J, et al. Benign postoperative biliary strictures. Operate or dilate? Ann Surg 1989; 210:417–425; discussion 426–427.

Quan ZF, Wang ZM, Li WQ, Li JS. Use of endoscopic naso-pancreatic drainage in the treatment of severe acute pancreatitis. World J Gastroenterol: WJG 2003; 9:868–870.

Reid-Lombardo KM, Farnell MB, Crippa S, et al. Pancreatic anastomotic leakage after pancreaticoduodenectomy in 1,507 patients: a report from the Pancreatic Anastomotic Leak Study Group. J Gastrointest Surg: Official Journal of the Society for Surgery of the Alimentary Tract 2007; 11:1451–1458; discussion 1459.

Roulin D, Cerantola Y, Demartines N, Schafer M. Systematic review of delayed postoperative hemorrhage after pancreatic resection. J Gastrointest Surg: Official Journal of the Society for Surgery of the Alimentary Tract 2011; 15:1055–1062.

Seyama Y, Kubota K, Kobayashi T, et al. Two-staged pancreatoduodenectomy with external drainage of pancreatic juice and omental graft technique. J Am Coll Surg 1998; 187:103–105.

Shimoda M, Katoh M, Yukihiro I, et al. Body mass index is a risk factor of pancreatic fistula after pancreaticoduodenectomy. The Am Surg 2012; 78:190–194.

Sohn TA, Yeo CJ, Cameron JL, et al. Pancreaticoduodenectomy: role of interventional radiologists in managing patients and complications. J Gastrointest Surg: Official Journal of the Society for Surgery of the Alimentary Tract 2003; 7:209–219.

Standop J, Overhaus M, Schaefer N, et al. Pancreatogastrostomy after pancreatoduodenectomy: a safe, feasible reconstruction method? World J Surg 2005; 29:505–512.

Trede M, Schwall G. The complications of pancreatectomy. Ann Surg 1988; 207:39–47.

Wente MN, Veit JA, Bassi C, et al. Postpancreatectomy hemorrhage (PPH): an International Study Group of Pancreatic Surgery (ISGPS) definition. Surgery 2007; 142:20–25.

Winter JM, Cameron JL, Campbell KA, et al. 1423 pancreaticoduodenectomies for pancreatic cancer: a single-institution experience. J Gastrointest Surg 2006; 10:1199–1210; discussion 1210–1211.

Yekebas EF, Wolfram L, Cataldegirmen G, et al. Postpancreatectomy hemorrhage: diagnosis and treatment: an analysis in 1669 consecutive pancreatic resections. Ann Surg 2007; 246:269–280.

Chapter 16 Reoperative liver surgery

Myron E. Schwartz, Parissa Tabrizian, Sasan Roayaie

INTRODUCTION

The transformation of liver surgery from a prohibitive and risky endeavor to a standardized treatment modality has been remarkable in the last 30 years (Tanabe 2008). The safety and effectiveness of liver surgery has not only improved largely due to the segmental approach but also due to increased experience with techniques for vascular control and exclusion used in liver transplantation (Fortner et al. 1974, Heaney et al. 1966) Techniques such as portal vein embolization (PVE), percutaneous local tumor destruction, and more effective chemotherapy agents have increased the number of curative resections. However, despite recent advances, major challenges remain, among which is reoperative liver surgery. Since the mid-1980s, a number of reports have demonstrated the safety and improved long-term results of repeat resection in recurrent malignancies (Fong et al. 1999, Fong et al. 2005, Morris et al. 2006, Weitz et al. 2005). The outcomes reported following repeat hepatectomy for metastatic colorectal cancer and hepatocellular carcinoma (HCC) are comparable with those described after initial resection (Adam et al. 1997, Fong et al. 1994, Kobayashi et al. 2006, Lee et al. 1995, Petrowsky et al. 2002, Roayaie et al. 2011). Extended survival has been demonstrated, and in select cases, survival is equivalent to that observed after primary hepatectomy (Adam et al. 1997, Fong et al. 1994, Kobayashi et al. 2006, Lee et al. 1995, Petrowsky et al. 2002, Roayaie et al. 2011). In this chapter, we focus on the key technical aspects of reoperative liver surgery, discussing the indications, patient selection, operative planning, and outcome.

ANATOMICAL CHALLENGES

Repeat liver resection carries certain technical difficulties that are not commonly encountered during the initial resection. A thorough knowledge of liver anatomy and a clear understanding of the nature of the prior resection are prerequisites (**Figure 16.1**).

Adhesions at the prior parenchymal transection line can make reexposure of the liver difficult. The previously resected edge adheres intimately to nearby organs. This is particularly likely after a right hepatectomy or bisegmentectomy VI–VII, where the liver has rotated through 90° and the resected edge adheres to the diaphragm. It is not unusual for reoperative dissection of the liver to be subcapsular or include the diaphragm. Remobilization of the liver off of the vena cava and exposure of the hepatic veins and porta hepatis can be particularly risky. Steatosis due to systemic chemotherapy can further increase friability, leading to capsular tearing and hemorrhage (Adam et al. 1997, Elias et al. 1993). After extensive hepatectomy and resultant

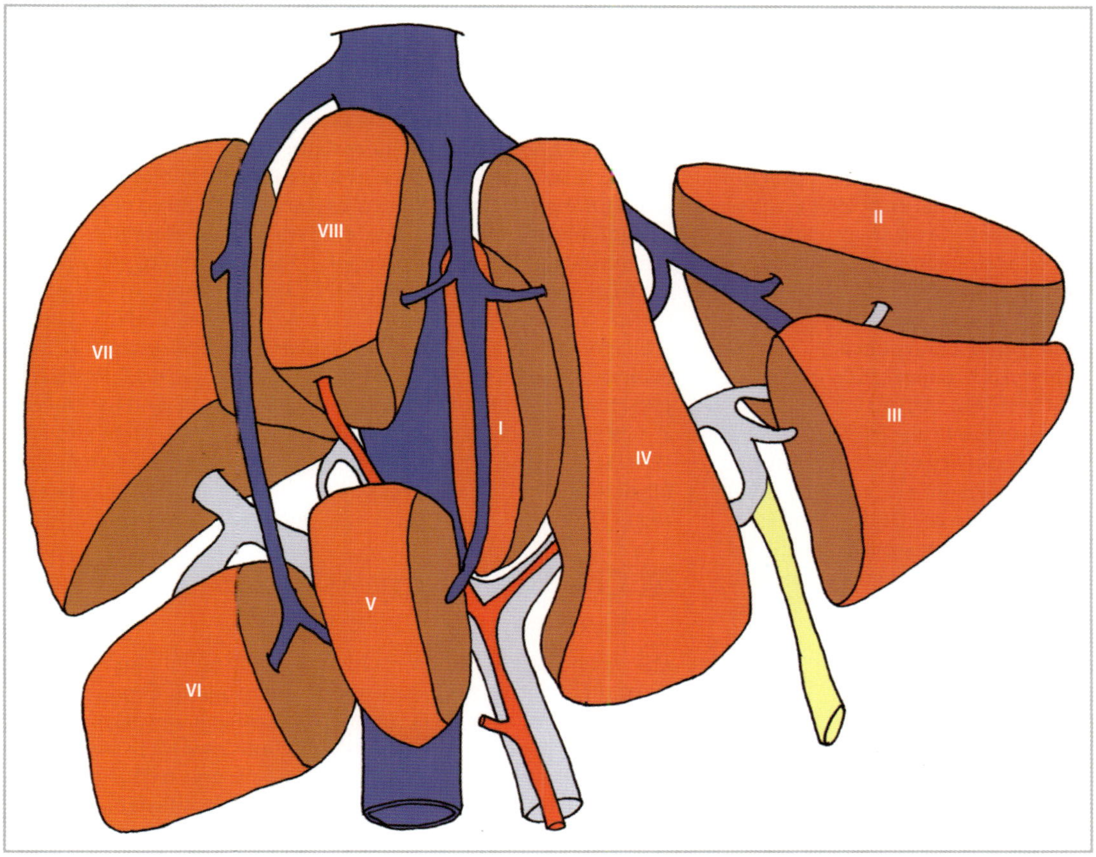

Figure 16.1 Segmental liver anatomy. Courtesy of Dr Parissa Tabrizian.

regeneration, the liver parenchyma is commonly more friable than in the normal state. Lastly, distortion of anatomy should be considered. This change is infinitely variable and depends both on the type of previous resection and on pre-existing anatomic variations. This is seen, e.g. after right liver resections where the three-dimensional orientation and classic anatomical landmarks disappear. The porta hepatis is rotated posteriorly and to the right, thereby displacing the bile duct posteriorly and the portal vein anteriorly.

The difficulty of reoperative surgery can often be estimated by noting the operative duration, hepatic clamping, blood loss, and reported difficulties during the primary resection, but it is not unusual for reoperative surgery to be either easier or considerably more difficult than anticipated. Defining external landmarks within the liver remnant helps in identifying the anatomic structures. In a repeat resection after a previous right hepatectomy, care should first be taken to identify the remnant of the ligamentum teres, also known as the round ligament of the liver, which demarcates segments 2–3 from segment 4. Following this structure to the base of the umbilical fissure helps to identify the location of the left hepatic artery. The second step should aim to define the porta hepatis. This may be facilitated by identifying the caudate lobe, opening the lesser omentum, and creating a plane anterior to the caudate lobe toward the obliterated foramen of Winslow.

The third step is identifying the portocaval plane, which can be achieved by kocherization of the duodenum. This enables isolation of the hepatoduodenal ligament for dissection of the inflow vessels and application of the Pringle maneuver. In a repeat resection after a previous left hepatectomy, anterior displacement of the portal vein due to hepatic regeneration is common. It is therefore recommended to mobilize the right liver remnant and duodenum in order to follow the vena cava and identify the portal vein from the right side. Excellent visualization is key to avoiding iatrogenic injury of important structures, and this is best achieved by maintaining a dry operative field; the authors use cautery extensively even when mobilizing adherent stomach and colon. Care must be taken to avoid injury of the middle hepatic vein, which may be a source of hemorrhage during the dissection.

Blood loss and transfusion requirements are major determinants of morbidity and mortality following liver resection, and intraoperative blood loss is of particular concern in reoperative cases (Cunningham et al. 1994, Katz et al. 2009, Melendez et al. 2001). Low central venous pressure is important (Jones et al. 1998, Melendez et al. 1998); inflow and/or outflow vascular control may be difficult due to scarring as a result of the previous operation. In situations where extensive extrahepatic dissection was previously performed to control inflow vasculature, control of these vessels may be more safely accomplished via intraparenchymal pedicle ligation. Intraoperative ultrasonography greatly facilitates resection by enabling visualization of major intrahepatic vessels (Castaing et al. 1985, Sietses et al. 2010).

In general, anatomic resection is theoretically preferable over nonanatomic resection because of the tendency of vascular invasion into segmental portal venous branches, the reported association with decreased blood loss, and higher rate of negative margins (Hasegawa et al. 2005, Weber et al. 2000). However, the technical challenges posed by reoperative surgery and the need to spare parenchyma often make nonanatomic resection preferable in the reoperative setting (Sarpel et al. 2009).

OPERATIVE PLANNING

Both tumor stage and hepatic reserve must be considered when selecting the optimal treatment strategy. The indications for repeat hepatectomy should be the same as for primary resection with respect to patient characteristics (general condition, age, liver function) and tumor parameters (number, size, site, predicted resection margin). The same operative techniques and planning should be considered.

Extent of resection and preoperative portal vein embolization

Because the liver returns nearly to its original volume after primary resection, the risk of hepatic failure is not necessarily increased in repeat liver surgery (Shirabe et al. 1999). There is nevertheless a tendency in reoperative surgery to perform nonanatomic resections and to accept limited margins in order to maximally spare parenchyma (Sarpel et al. 2009). While major resection is less common in the reoperative than in the primary setting, preoperative PVE may be used to induce growth of the future liver remnant when hepatic reserve is borderline, and major resection is anticipated. In patients with normal liver parenchyma and function, a future liver remnant volume of 25–30% is considered adequate (Abulkhir et al. 2008, Makuuchi et al. 1990, Ribero et al. 2007). In patients with chronic liver disease, cirrhosis, or documented hepatic steatosis, a future liver remnant volume of 40–50% is desired (Abulkhir et al. 2008, Makuuchi et al. 1990, Ribero et al. 2007).

Liver cirrhosis

One of the greatest challenges in hepatic surgery, reoperative or otherwise, is the presence of cirrhosis. Cirrhotic patients have by definition reduced hepatic functional reserve. Therefore, these patients are at a higher risk of repeat hepatectomy and require careful assessment of liver function. While a variety of tests have been used to assess hepatic reserve, none have been proven more useful than the Child – Pugh classification; resection should be limited to patients with Child – Pugh A cirrhosis, ideally with a serum bilirubin level <1 (Okamoto et al. 1984). In addition to Child – Pugh class, portal hypertension (as judged by absence of varices on imaging, platelet count >100,000/mm^3, and/or hepatic venous pressure gradient <10 mm Hg) seems to be an independent factor in determining postresection outcome (Llovet et al. 1999).

Reoperative liver resection in cirrhotic patients is also associated with specific technical difficulties that increase the complexity of the operation. Mobilization of the liver may be difficult due to the firmness of the parenchyma. Care must be taken to avoid vessel injury. In addition, the anatomic landmarks may be distorted secondary to fibrosis and atrophy/hypertrophy. Lastly, portal hypertension is associated with increased blood loss during dissection and parenchymal transection (Abulkhir et al. 2008, Adam et al. 1997, Castaing et al. 1985, Cunningham et al. 1994, Elias et al. 1993, Fong et al. 2005, Fong et al. 1999, Fong et al. 1994, Hasegawa et al. 2005, Jones et al. 1998, Katz et al. 2009, Kobayashi et al. 2006, Lee et al. 1995, Llovet et al. 1999, Makuuchi et al. 1990, Melendez et al. 2001, Melendez et al. 1998, Morris et al. 2006, Okamoto et al. 1984, Petrowsky et al. 2002, Ribero et al. 2007, Roayaie et al. 2011, Sarpel et al. 2009, Shirabe et al. 1999, Sietses et al. 2010, Weber et al. 2000).

Chemotherapy-associated liver injury

The development of newer chemotherapy agents increased the feasibility of curative resection by downstaging hepatic tumors (Kornprat et al. 2007). It is common for patients to receive multiple chemotherapeutic agents before being considered for liver resection. Chemotherapy-associated liver injury is common; oxaliplatin-based regimens can cause a veno-occlusive type of injury resulting in portal hypertension with splenomegaly and thrombocytopenia. Irinotecan-based regimens commonly induce steatohepatitis (Fernandez et al. 2005, Fong & Bentrem 2006). Such patients should be handled similar to patients with early cirrhosis, and preoperative PVE should be considered if liver reserve is marginal.

PREOPERATIVE IMAGING

Preoperative imaging is even more essential for repeat liver resections than for primary resections. Modern high-resolution imaging with contrast-enhanced CT or MR enables accurate preoperative assessment, sparing unresectable patients unnecessary morbidity and defining the locations of tumors relative to adjacent structures (Murakami et al. 2011, Parikh & Taouli 2013, Strasberg & Siegal 2002). With access to the liver limited by scarring, intraoperative assessment via palpation or even ultrasound can be difficult; a clear picture of the exact number and locations of the lesions allow a targeted approach in many cases without the need for full mobilization of the liver. Positron emission tomography (PET) imaging has particular applicability when considering second resection for metastatic liver tumors since recurrence in the liver may be accompanied by extrahepatic recurrence, and PET facilitates the identification of inconspicuous sites of extrahepatic disease (Strasberg & Siegal 2002).

ANESTHESIA AND PATIENT POSITIONING

Reoperative liver surgery is among the complex surgical procedures for which results are directly linked to experience, with shorter lengths of stay and a reported fourfold difference in mortality between the lowest- and highest-volume centers (Choti et al. 1998, Dimick et al. 2003, Glasgow et al. 1999). The experience of the anesthesia team is as important as that of the operating surgeon. As in all liver surgery, the possibility of significant intraoperative bleeding should be anticipated. Careful monitoring and sufficient vascular access to permit rapid transfusion should be in place. Inflow occlusion by the operating team is useful to limit bleeding during parenchymal transection, but does not prevent bleeding from hepatic venous tributaries; maintenance of low central venous pressure (< 5 mmHg) by the anesthesiologist is the best way to limit bleeding from hepatic veins during the division of the liver (Chen et al. 2000, Jones et al. 1998, Rees et al. 1996).

The patient is placed in supine position; lateral position is not necessary even for the largest tumors. Preparation and draping should allow exposure of the lower chest and the abdomen down to the pubis. In open hepatectomy, the choice of incision is critical to exposure and efficiency (**Figure 16.2**). Increasingly, we have come to perform hepatic resection, including second resection, via a midline incision. A right- or bilateral subcostal incision with upper midline extension is preferred when a large tumor or the patient's body habitus makes exposure of the suprahepatic vena cava difficult. While not usually necessary, in repeat resection after previous right hepatectomy, it is wise to anticipate the possibility that dense adherence of the prior resection margin to the diaphragm may make a thoracoabdominal incision the easiest approach.

ANTICIPATED HEMORRHAGE

Operative blood loss and need for perioperative transfusion have repeatedly been identified as predictors of poor outcome after liver surgery (Katz et al. 2009). Experience, knowledge of the anatomy, and a commitment to limited blood loss are important to limit bleeding.

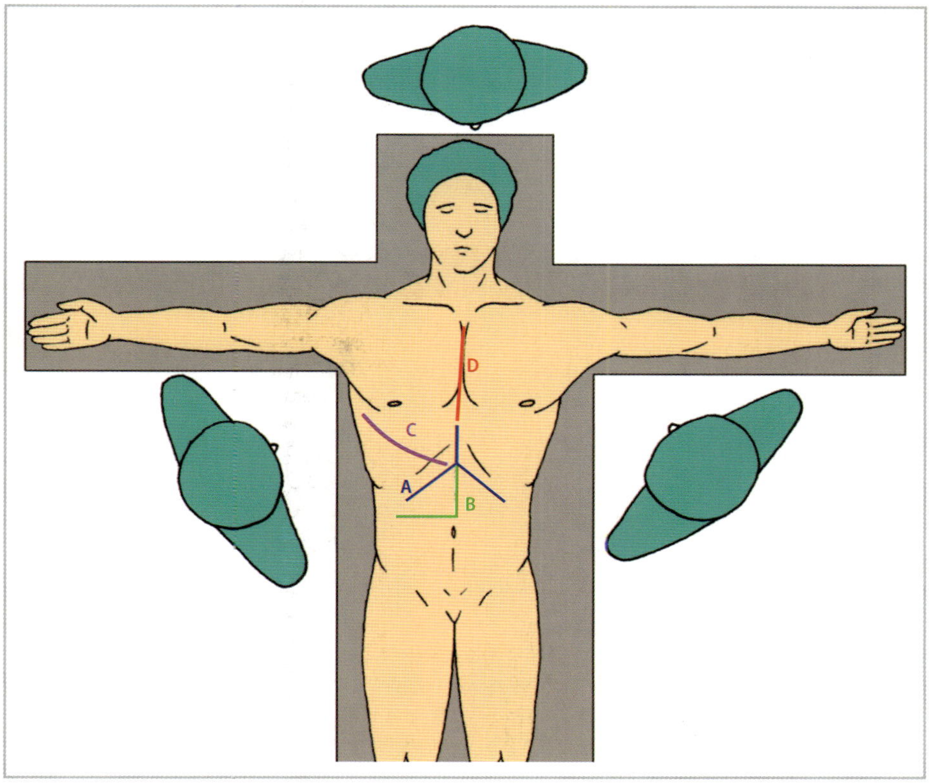

Figure 16.2 Patient positioning and recommended incisions. Courtesy of Dr Parissa Tabrizian.

Optimal exposure through an appropriate incision with suitable retraction is critical to minimizing blood loss. The most common source of massive intraoperative bleeding is from the hepatic veins. Special care should therefore be exercised when approaching the region of the hepatic veins and their confluence with the vena cava; in the reoperative setting there may be dense scars adjacent to these vessels, making dissection and control extremely difficult. Avoidance of excessive traction or torsion on the venous structures is necessary to avoid tearing. If a tear develops in the vena cava, or a clamp slips off of a large tributary after its division, finger occlusion and then serial placement of Allis clamps on the vessel across the opening can usually re-establish control.

Good operative technique and tissue handling, the liberal use of diathermy for dissection, and ligation of larger vessels all contribute toward a 'dry' operative field. As in any liver resection, there is an array of techniques for dividing liver parenchyma that will not be discussed here; since no one method is suitable for all situations, it is good to master a few techniques and to have a flexible approach.

Occlusion of hepatic vascular inflow (Pringle maneuver) is an effective way to limit blood loss during hepatic resection (Belghiti et al. 1999, Figueras et al. 2005, Petrowsky et al. 2006). Intermittent occlusion (cycles of approximately 15 minutes on and 5 minutes off) as compared with continuous occlusion has been shown to decrease ischemia/reperfusion injury with less elevation of postoperative liver enzyme levels, and is the method most commonly employed; however, a randomized trial comparing resection using ischemic preconditioning and subsequent continuous occlusion versus intermittent occlusion alone in noncirrhotic patients demonstrated markedly reduced blood loss and resection time in the ischemic preconditioning group (Petrowsky et al. 2006). Total hepatic vascular isolation, wherein the hepatic veins/vena cava is clamped along with the portal pedicle, is a useful technique when either tumor or previous surgery renders dissection of the hepatic veins hazardous (Belghiti et al. 1996).

OUTCOME OF REOPERATIVE LIVER RESECTION

The role of repeat hepatectomy in the management of patients with recurrent malignancy after primary resection remains somewhat controversial, despite the fact that numerous studies have described the short- and long-term outcomes in both HCC and metastatic colorectal cancer recurrence (Adam et al. 1997, Elias et al. 1993, Fong et al. 1994, Kobayashi et al. 2006, Katz et al. 2009, Lee et al. 1995, Petrowsky et al. 2002, Roayaie et al. 2011). With refinements in surgical technique, improvements in perioperative care, and better criteria for patient selection, repeat hepatectomy can be performed with a mortality rate comparable with that of primary resection (Adam et al. 1997, Elias et al. 1993, Fong et al. 1994, Katz et al. 2009, Kobayashi et al. 2006, Lee et al. 1995, Petrowsky et al. 2002, Roayaie et al. 2011).

Repeat hepatectomy for recurrent hepatocellular carcinoma

Recurrence after resection of HCC remains a significant problem with many series reporting rates of 60–70% at 5 years (Lizuka et al. 2003, Mazzaferro et al. 2006, Roayaie et al. 2011). The optimal treatment of patients who develop intrahepatic recurrence after hepatic resection and have maintained normal liver function remains unclear. Roayaie et al. present their large Western experience and confirm that second hepatectomy for recurrent HCC is a safe procedure (Roayaie et al. 2011) (see **Figure 16.3**). Repeat hepatectomy was applicable in only

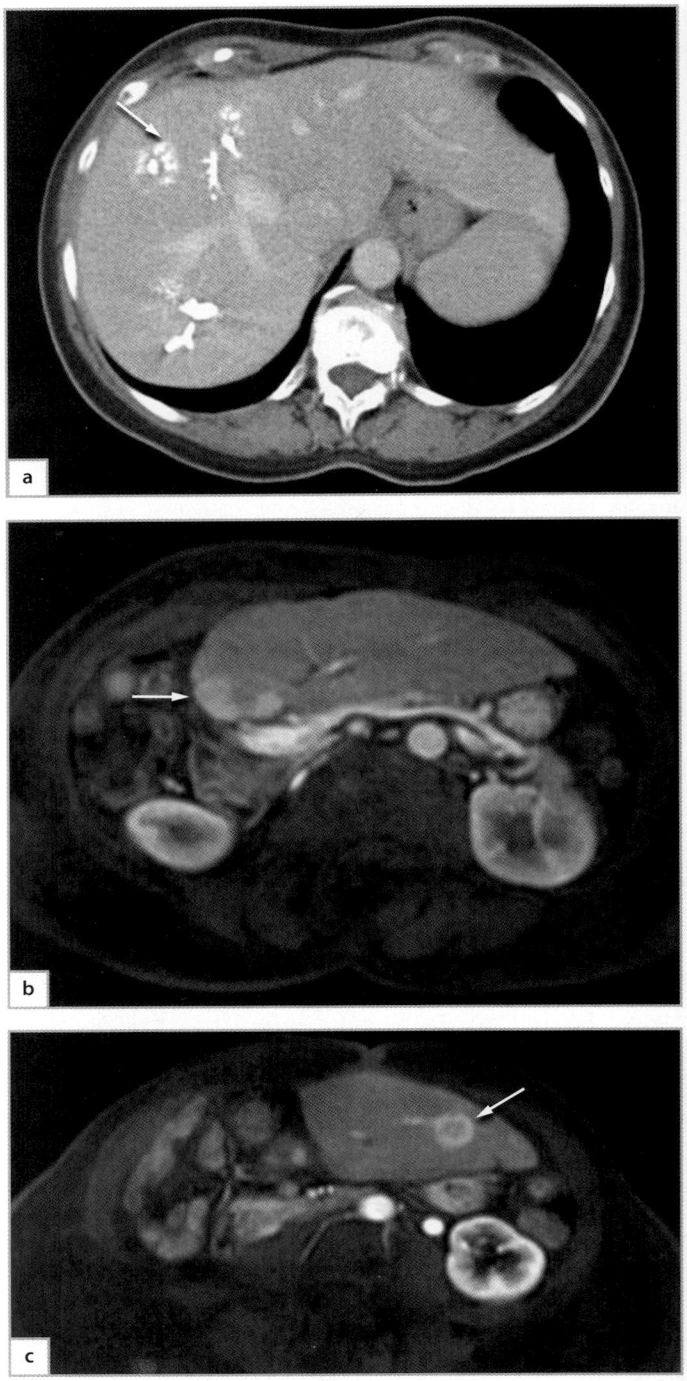

Figure 16.3 Repeat hepatectomy: hepatocellular cancer case (a) 9 cm right lobe hepatocellular carcinoma. (b) Second hepatectomy – segment 4. (c) Third hepatectomy – segment 3.

15% of patients with HCC recurrence (20% in patients with recurrence limited to the liver). The 5-year survival after second hepatectomy (67%) compared favorably with the 5-year intention-to-treat survival reported for liver transplantation for HCC in the United States (61%). The time from primary resection to recurrence of HCC and presence of gross vascular invasion were significant predictors of both recurrence and survival after second resection. Other authors have also identified time to recurrence as an important prognostic variable; time to recurrence <1 year, along with multiple recurrent tumor nodules and interval hepatic decompensation, is a reason to avoid repeat resection (Minigawa et al. 2003, Sun et al. 2005).

Repeat hepatectomy for metastatic colorectal cancer

Resection of hepatic metastases of colorectal origin remains the only treatment that offers hope for long-term survival, but similar to HCC, most patients who undergo resection of metastatic colorectal cancer will recur (Adam et al. 1997, Fong et al. 1994). Second resection is feasible in 20–33% of these patients (Adam et al. 1997, Fong et al. 1994). Prior major resection limits the possibilities for second resection; this provides a rationale for parenchyma-sparing surgery during primary hepatectomy. Because patients are typically under surveillance, recurrent tumors are commonly small and few in number when discovered, facilitating limited resection. Repeat hepatectomy has been published in many series with reported risks and outcomes similar to those seen for primary liver resection, with perioperative morbidity seen in 7–40%, perioperative mortality ranging from 0% to 5%, and 5-year survival between 21% and 49% (Adam et al. 1997, Fong et al. 1994) (see **Figure 16.4**). Third hepatectomy has also been reported to provide survival benefit (Elias et al. 1993). In a multivariate analysis, the extent of liver resection (>2 segments) and tumor size (>3.5 cm) were independent predictors of poor outcome (Tanaka et al. 2007).

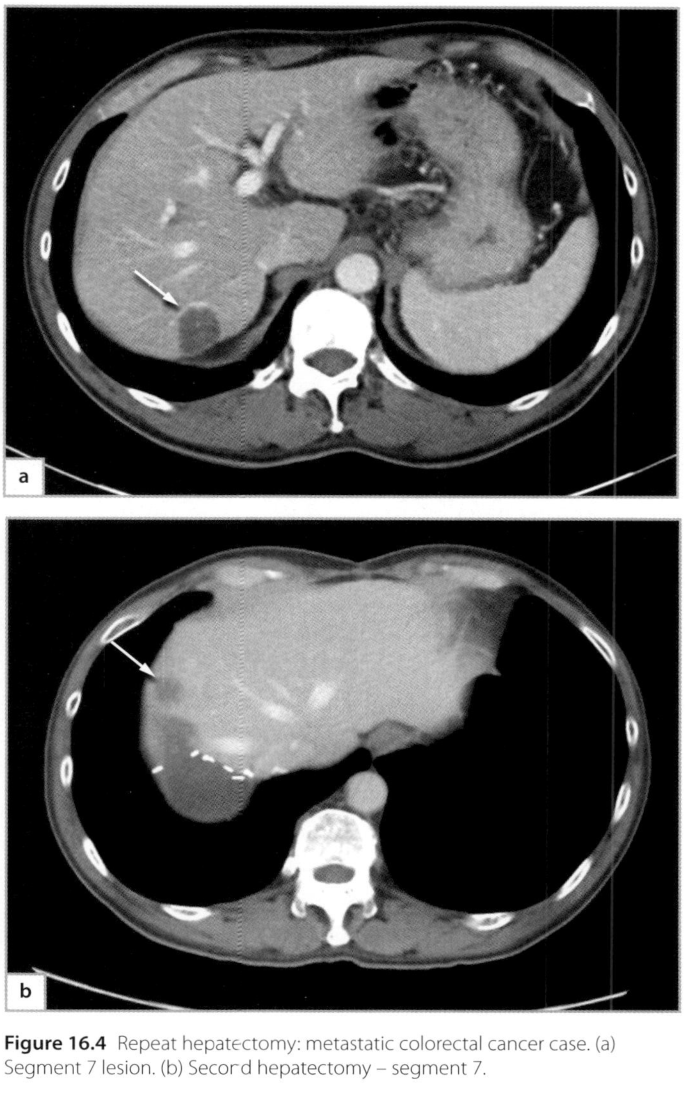

Figure 16.4 Repeat hepatectomy: metastatic colorectal cancer case. (a) Segment 7 lesion. (b) Second hepatectomy – segment 7.

ROLE OF LAPAROSCOPIC REPEAT HEPATIC RESECTION

Laparoscopic hepatectomy has expanded rapidly with growing experience and advances in technology and is safe and feasible for a selected group of patients with benign or malignant hepatic tumors (Asahara et al. 1998, Huscher et al. 1998). There is, however, a paucity of literature on laparoscopic repeat hepatic resection because even in centers where laparoscopic hepatectomy is commonly performed, the difficulties posed by right upper quadrant adhesions and altered anatomy have led most surgeons to choose an open approach. The greatest concern with laparoscopy is the limited ability to control bleeding; other issues include loss of tactile sensation that may lead to inadequate tumor clearance and, particularly in cirrhotic patients, difficulty mobilizing/moving the liver. The use of a hand access port can obviate many of these concerns, enabling ready manual compression of bleeding and the ability to feel the liver and the tumors within (Asahara et al. 1998). Recommended trocar and hand port placement are shown in **Figure 16.5**. Other technologic advances including laparoscopic staplers, ultrasonic dissectors, and electrosurgical devices that can seal and divide liver parenchyma further facilitate a laparoscopic approach for repeat resection (Buell et al. 2009, Koffron et al. 2006, Nguyen et al. 2009).

Studies have been performed to evaluate the safety, feasibility, and oncologic integrity of laparoscopic repeat hepatectomy (Belli et al. 2009, Shafaee et al. 2011). The most common indication for repeat hepatic resection was recurrence of colorectal liver metastasis. The criteria for application of the laparoscopic technique for repeat liver resection were the same as for the laparoscopic primary resections. The laparoscopic approach was typically preferred in patients who had undergone primary laparoscopic liver resection, but some repeat resections were performed laparoscopically after prior open resection. In a large study (n = 76) comparing group A (previous laparoscopic resection) and group B (previous open resection), reoperation after a previous laparoscopic procedure was associated with a lower blood loss and transfusion requirement (Shafaee et al. 2011). This may be explained by the extensive lysis of adhesions required after an open procedure. However, both groups reported similar postoperative outcomes (hospital stay, major complications, and mortality rates) (Shafaee et al. 2011). These findings were confirmed by another similar smaller study reviewing repeat laparoscopic resection in cirrhotic HCC patients after open resection (Belli et al. 2009).

Intraoperative ultrasonography and the selective use of hand ports were considered critical tools in reoperative laparoscopic liver resection. Although intraoperative bleeding has been a concern, intraoperative blood loss and transfusion requirements were comparable with reported primary laparoscopic resection series, and the postoperative morbidity rate of 32% and bile leakage rate of 6.6% fall within the range previously reported for laparoscopic primary liver resections (Belli et al. 2009, Kazaryan et al. 2010, Sarpel et al. 2009, Shafaee et al. 2011). With no perioperative deaths and a conversion rate of 11%, second laparoscopic resection appears to be a viable option in selected cases (Shafaee et al. 2011).

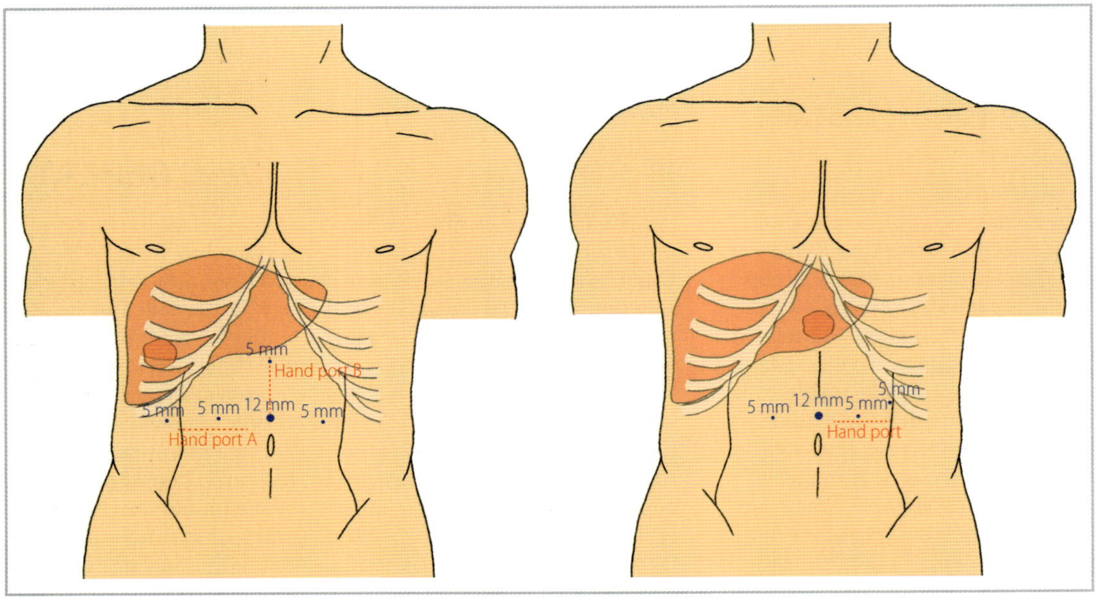

Figure 16.5 Laparoscopic trocar and hand port placement. Courtesy of Dr Parissa Tabrizian.

CONCLUSION

Due to its complexity and challenges, repeat hepatectomy remains a controversial topic. However, with appropriate patient selection, careful operative planning, and performance by an expert hepatobiliary surgeon, perioperative and long-term results largely comparable with those obtained after primary resection can be achieved.

REFERENCES

Abulkhir A, Limongelli P, Healey AJ, et al. Preoperative portal vein embolization for major liver resection: a meta-analysis. Ann Surg 2008; 247:49–57.

Adam R, Bismuth H, Castaing D, et al. Repeat hepatectomy for colorectal liver metastases. Ann Surg 1997; 225:51–60.

Asahara T, Dohi K, Nakahara H, et al. Laparoscopy-assisted hepatectomy for a large tumor of the liver. Hiroshima J Med Sci 1998; 47:163–166.

Belghiti J, Noun R, Malafosse R, et al. Continuous versus intermittent portal triad clamping for liver resection. A controlled study. Ann Surg 1999; 229:369–375.

Belghiti J, Noun R, Zante E, et al. Portal triad clamping or hepatic vascular exclusion for major liver resection: a controlled study. Ann Surg 1996; 224:155–161.

Belli G, Cioffi L, Fantini C, et al. Laparoscopic redo surgery for recurrent hepatocellular carcinoma in cirrhotic patients: feasibility,safety, and results. Surg Endosc 2009; 23:1807–1811.

Buell JF, Cherqui D, Geller DA, et al. The international position on laparoscopic liver surgery: The Louisville Statement, 2008. Ann Surg 2009; 250:825–833.

Castaing D, Kunstlinger F, Habib N. Intraoperative ultrasound study of the liver: methodology and anatomical results. Am J Surg 1985; 149:676–682.

Chen H, Merchant NB, Didolkar MS. Hepatic resection using intermittent vascular inflow occlusion and low central venous pressure anesthesia improves morbidity and mortality. J Gastrointest Surg 2000; 4:162–167.

Choti MA, Bowman HM, Pitt HA, et al. Should hepatic resections be performed at high-volume referral centers? J Gastrointest Surg 1998; 2:11–19.

Cunningham JD, Fong Y, Shriver C, et al. One hundred consecutive hepatic resections: blood loss, transfusion and operative technique. Arch Surg 1994; 129:1050–1056.

Dimick JB, Cowan JA, Jr, Knol JA, Upchurch GR, Jr. Hepatic resection in the United States: indications, outcomes, and hospital procedural volumes from a nationally representative database. Arch Surg 2003; 138:185–191.

Elias D, Lasser P, Hoang JM, et al. Repeat hepatectomy for cancer. Br J Surg 1993; 80:1557–1562.

Fernandez FG, Ritter J, Goodwin JW, et al. Effect of steatohepatitis associated with irinotecan or oxaliplatin pretreatment on resectability of hepatic colorectal metastases. J Am Coll Surgeons 2005; 200:845–853.

Figueras J, Llado L, Ruiz D, et al Complete versus selective portal triad clamping for minor liver resections: a prospective randomized trial. Ann Surg 2005; 241:582–590.

Fong Y, Bentrem DJ. CASH (Chemotherapy-Associated Steatohepatitis) costs. Ann Surg 2006; 243:8–9.

Fong Y, Blumgart LH, Cohen A, Fortner J, Brennan MF. Repeat hepatic resections for metastatic colorectal cancer. Ann Surg 1994; 220:657–662.

Fong Y, Gonen M, Rubin D, et al. Long-term survival is superior after resection N10CD6 for cancer in high-volume centers. Ann Surg 2005; 242:540–544.

Fong Y, Sun RL, Jarnagin W, et al. An analysis of 412 cases of hepatocellular carcinoma at a Western center. Ann Surg 1999; 229:790–799.

Fortner JG, Shiu MH, Kinne DW, et al. Major hepatic resection using vascular isolation and hypothermic perfusion. Ann Surg 1974; 180:644–652.

Glasgow RE, Showstack JA, Katz PP, et al. The relationship between hospital volume and outcomes of hepatic resection for hepatocellular carcinoma. Arch Surg 1999; 134:30–35.

Hasegawa K, Kokudo N, Imamura H, et al. Prognostic impact of anatomic resection for hepatocellular carcinoma. Ann Surg 2005; 242:252–259.

Heaney JP, Stanton WK, Halbert DS, et al. An improved technic for vascular isolation of the liver: experimental study and case reports. Ann Surg 1966; 163:237–241.

Huscher CGS, Lirici MM, Chiodini S. Laparoscopic liver resections. Semin Laparosc Surg 1998; 5:204–210.

Jones RM, Moulton CE, Hardy KJ. Central venous pressure and its effect on blood loss during liver resection. Br J Surg 1998; 85:1058–1060.

Jones RM, Moulton CE, Hardy KJ. Central venous pressure and its effect on blood loss during liver resection. Br J Surg 1998; 85:1058–1060.

Katz SC, Shia J, Liau KH, et al. Operative blood loss independently predicts recurrence and survival after resection of hepatocellular carcinoma. Ann Surg 2009; 249:617–623.

Kazaryan AM, Marangos IP, Rosseland AR, et al. Laparoscopic liver resection for malignant and benign lesions: 10 year Norwegian single centre experience. Arch Surg 2010; 145:34–40.

Kobayashi A, Kawasaki S, Miyagawa S, et al. Results of 404 hepatic resections including 80 repeat hepatectomies for hepatocellular carcinoma. Hepatogastroenterology 2006; 53:736–741.
Koffron A, Geller D, Gamblin TC, et al. Laparoscopic liver surgery: shifting the management of liver tumors. Hepatology 2006; 44:1694–1700.
Kornprat P, Jarnagin WR, Gonen M, et al. Outcome after hepatectomy for multiple (four or more) colorectal metastases in the era of effective chemotherapy. Ann Surg Oncol 2007; 14:1151–1160.
Lee PH, Lin WJ, Tsang YM, et al. Clinical management of recurrent hepatocellular carcinoma. Ann Surg 1995; 222:670–676.
Lizuka N, Oka M, Yamada-Okabe H, et al. Oligonucleotide microarray for prediction of early intrahepatic recurrence of hepatocellular carcinoma after curative resection. Lancet 2003; 361:923–929.
Llovet JM, Fuster J, Bruix J. Intention-to-treat analysis of surgical treatment for early hepatocellular carcinoma: resection versus transplantation. Hepatology 1999; 30:1434–1440.
Makuuchi M, Thai BL, Takayasu K, et al. Preoperative portal embolization to increase safety of major hepatectomy for hilar bile duct carcinoma: a preliminary report. Surgery 1990; 107:521–527.
Mazzaferro M, Romito R, Schiavo M, et al. Prevention of hepatocellular carcinoma recurrence with alpha-Interferon after liver resection in HCV cirrhosis. Hepatology 2006; 44:1543–1554.
Melendez JA, Arsian V, Fischer M, et al. Perioperative outcomes of major hepatic resections under low central venous pressure anaesthesia: blood loss, blood transfusion, and the risk of postoperative renal dysfunction. J Am Coll Surg 1998; 187:620–625.
Melendez J, Ferri E, Zwillman M, et al. Extended hepatic resection: a 6-year retrospective study of risk factors for perioperative mortality. J Am Coll Surg 2001; 192:47–53.
Minigawa M, Makuuchi M, Takayama T, et al. Selection criteria for repeat hepatectomy in patients with recurrent hepatocellular carcinoma. Ann Surg 2003; 238:703–710.
Morris KT, Song TJ, Fong Y. Recent advancements in diagnosis and treatment of metastatic colorectal cancer to the liver N10CC1. Surg Oncol 2006; 15:129–134.
Murakami T, Imai Y, Okada M et al. Ultrasonography, computed tomography and magnetic resonance imaging of hepatocellular carcinoma: toward improved treatment decisions. Oncology 2011; 81:86–99.
Nguyen KT, Laurent A, Dagher DA, et al. Minimally invasive liver resection for metastatic colorectal cancer: a multi-institutional, international report of safety, feasibility, and early outcomes. Ann Surg 2009; 250:842–848.
Okamoto E, Kyo A, Yamanaka N, et al. Prediction of the safe limits of hepatectomy by combined volumetric and functional measurements in patients with impaired hepatic function. Surgery 1984; 95:586–592.
Parikh A, Taouli B. Imaging of hepatocellular carcinoma: current concepts Recent Results. Cancer Res 2013; 190:33-55.
Petrowsky H, Gonen M, Jarnagin W, et al. Second liver resections are safe and effective treatment for recurrent hepatic metastases from colorectal cancer: a bi-institutional analysis. Ann Surg 2002; 235:863–871.
Petrowsky H, McCormack L, Trujillo M, et al. A prospective, randomized, controlled trial comparing intermittent portal triad clamping versus ischemic preconditioning with continuous clamping for major liver resection. Ann Surg 2006; 244:921–928.
Rees M, Plant G, Wells J, Bygrave S. One hundred and fifty hepatic resections: evolution of technique toward bloodless surgery. Br J Surg 1996; 83:1526–1529.
Ribero D, Abdalla EK, Madoff DC, et al. Portal vein embolization before major hepatectomy and its effects on regeneration, resectability and outcome. Br J Surg 2007; 94:1386–1394.
Roayaie S, Bassi D, Tarchi P et al. Second hepatic resection for recurrent hepatocellular cancer: a Western experience. J Hepatol 2011; 55:346–350.
Sarpel U, Bonavia AS, Grucela A, et al. Does anatomic versus nonanatomic resection affect recurrence and survival in patients undergoing surgery for colorectal liver metastasis? Ann Surg Oncol 2009; 16:379–384. Epub 2008 Nov 20.
Sarpel U, Hefti MM, Wisnievsky JP, et al. Outcome for patients treated with laparoscopic versus open resection of hepatocellular carcinoma: case-matched analysis. Ann Surg Oncol 2009; 16:1572–1577.
Shafaee Z, Kazaryan AM, Marvin MR, et al. Is laparoscopic repeat hepatectomy feasible? A tri-institutional analysis. J Am Coll Surg 2011; 212:171–179.
Shirabe K, Shimada M, Gion T, et al. Postoperative liver failure after major hepatic resection for hepatocellular carcinoma in the modern era with special reference to remnant liver volume. J Am Coll Surg 1999; 188:304–349.
Sietses C, Meijerink MR, Meijer S, et al. The impact of intraoperative ultrasonography on the surgical treatment of patients with colorectal liver metastases. Surg Endosc 2010; 24:1917–1922.
Strasberg SM, Siegal BA. Survival of patients staged by FDG-PET before resection of hepatic metastases from colorectal cancer. Ann Surg 2002; 235:308.
Sun HC, Tang ZY, Ma ZC, et al. The prognostic factors for outcome following second resection for intrahepatic recurrence of hepatocellular carcinoma with a hepatitis B virus infection background. J cancer Res Clin Oncol 2005; 131:284–288.
Tanabe KK. The past 60 years in liver surgery. Cancer 2008; 113:1888–1896.
Tanaka K, Shimada H, Matsuo K, et al. Intra-operative blood loss predicts complications after a second hepatectomy for malignant neoplasms. Ann Surg Oncol 2007; 14:2668–2677.
Weber SM, Jarnagin WR, DeMatteo RP, et al. Survival after resection of multiple hepatic colorectal metastases. Ann Surg Oncol 2000; 7:643–650.
Weitz J, Blumgart LH, Fong Y, et al. Partial hepatectomy for metastases from noncolorectal, non-neuroendocrine carcinoma. Ann Surg 2005; 241:269–276.

Chapter 17 Reoperations for complications of biliary tract surgery

Kristina V. Spate, Michael H. Bahr, Gary C. Vitale

INTRODUCTION

Diseases of the gallbladder have become increasingly more common in the United States and around the world making the cost a major health burden to society. Cholelithiasis is the most common biliary tract disease, which affects approximately 10–15% of the adult population (Shaffer 2006). Although the majority of gallstones will remain asymptomatic, the potential for major gallstone complications is reported to be 1–2% per year. Many factors are associated with gallstone formation such as ethnicity, obesity, rapid weight loss, particular drugs, or hemolytic disorders. While the majority of gallstones are asymptomatic, they have the propensity to cause biliary colic, cholangitis, pancreatitis, or acute cholecystitis with an annual risk varied from 0.2% to 1.5% (Gracie & Ransohoff 1982, Frieman 1993, McSherry et al. 1985).

Since the advent of laparoscopic cholecystectomy in the 1990s, the cholecystectomy rate has increased with approximately 700,000 operations performed annually and has now become the most common elective abdominal operation performed (National Institutes of Health 1993). With this increase in the number of procedures, there has also been an increase in common bile duct (CBD) injuries with a quoted incidence of 0.4–0.6% (Adamsen et al. 1997, Wherry et al. 1996). This is a considerable problem for the surgeon and patient who must undergo a reoperation for a bile duct injury. Patients who sustain a bile duct injury have the potential to have an impaired quality of life due to the psychological, social, and medical impact of requiring reoperation when compared with the patients who experience an uncomplicated cholecystectomy (Melton et al. 2002). Not only is the medical impact of great significance in this setting, but large legal compensation is often awarded to patients who have to undergo reoperation due to an inadvertent injury (Kern 1997).

Additional complications following cholecystectomy that may also require reoperation include primary biliary stones, biliary leaks, subhepatic abscesses, and biliary strictures. The management of these different complications varies from patient to patient with regard to a conservative approach or reoperation. The options of placing biliary stents with the use of endoscopic retrograde cholangiopancreatography (ERCP) or percutaneous drainage for drainage of abscesses amenable to nonoperative drainage are useful adjuncts in therapy, given that the reoperative field in these settings can pose a great technical challenge.

PREVENTIVE OPERATIVE TECHNIQUES

Risk factors for a bile duct injury during a cholecystectomy have been described as acute cholecystitis or pancreatitis, obesity, cirrhosis, bleeding in Calot's triangle, a scarred contracted gallbladder, short cystic duct, or a large stone in Hartmann's pouch. In addition, a prolonged operation of >120 minutes and male sex are also risk factors, but it is also common to have an unidentified injury during what is perceived by the surgeon as a technically easy operation if there is an anatomic variation that is unappreciated (Giger et al. 2006, Nuzzo & Giuliante 2004, Zdichavsky et al. 2012). In a study of 2184 patients who underwent a laparoscopic cholecystectomy with an overall CBD injury incidence of 0.69%, the risk of CBD injury was 3.5 times higher in patients with inflammation than noninflamed cholecystectomies (Georgidades et al. 2008).

With regard to the potential injuries that can occur during the laparoscopic cholecystectomy, the most important aspect is identifying anatomy correctly and using safe techniques during the operation. The use of clips and electrocautery should be minimized particularly in the setting where the cystic duct and artery have not been accurately identified (Strasberg 2002). The identification of Calot's triangle and attaining the 'critical view' as described by Strasberg et al. in 1995 is also important in the prevention of an intraoperative complication (Strasberg et al. 1995). Using the above-described technique, with a clear dissection between the gallbladder and the liver bed leaving only the cystic duct and artery visible, there is a lower incidence of bile duct injury and has now become the gold standard technique with regard to biliary dissection during a cholecystectomy.

When faced with a question of variable biliary anatomy secondary to dense adhesions or if excessive bleeding is encountered making the anatomy difficult to visualize with certainty, conversion to an open procedure is recommended. An intraoperative consult to a senior partner with more experience is one way to have a fresh perspective and added technical assistance when biliary anatomy is in question. Prior studies have reported a lower rate of CBD injury with 1.7 per 1000 laparoscopic cholecystectomies in more experienced surgeons versus 3.2 per 1000 in younger surgeons in practice (Flum et al. 2001).

The importance of knowing when to 'bail out,' perform a subtotal cholecystectomy, leave a drain, or simply leave a cholecystostomy tube in place with the expectation of a definitive delayed operation is also a critical skill in surgical judgment. This has been proven to provide a safe and successful bridge to an operation in an acutely ill patient who is at higher risk of presenting with acute cholecystitis with success rates of 80–85% (Berber et al. 2000, Cherng et al. 2012). One study comparing the postoperative outcome in patients who underwent a subtotal versus total cholecystectomy for complicated cholecystitis demonstrated twice the number of postoperative complications in the total cholecystectomy group with 12% versus 6% in the subtotal cholecystectomy group. No CBD injuries occurred in the subtotal cholecystectomy group, while there were two CBD injuries in the total cholecystectomy group in this study (Davis et al. 2012).

The debate as to whether routine intraoperative cholangiography (IOC) actually prevents inadvertent injury to the bile duct still remains a topic of debate among surgeons (Buddingh et al. 2011, Hamad et al. 2011, Sanjay et al. 2010). One study compared 421 patients who underwent a selective IOC versus 435 patients who underwent a routine IOC during cholecystectomy. This study reported fewer CBD injuries in the routine IOC group with 0%, while the selective IOC group had CBD injury rate of 1.9% with choledocholithiasis leading to intraoperative management also higher in the routine IOC group (4.8% vs. 1.0%) (Buddingh et al. 2011). Conversely, several studies and systematic reviews have failed to demonstrate compelling evidence to support the practice of routine IOC; however, cholangiography has been reported to add an average of 16 minutes of operative time during the cholecystectomy (Ford et al. 2012). At our institution, we advocate the use of routine IOC unless the cystic duct is unusually short or brittle making the risk of obtaining the cholangiogram too high to proceed.

PREOPERATIVE IMAGING

Delineating biliary anatomy is essential in preparing an operative strategy for repair once a CBD injury is identified. The use of ERCP and percutaneous transhepatic cholangiography (PTC) accommodates both the need for diagnostic evaluation and provides a therapeutic modality. The use of PTC is useful in defining the proximal biliary tree anatomy and placing catheters across injuries located in the biliary system with a quoted success rate of 85% (Fidelman et al. 2011) (**Figure 17.1a** and **b**). It can also be utilized to alleviate proximal biliary strictures that are difficult to stent across via the endoscopic route such as in metastatic gastric cancer with technical success rates approaching 90% (Gwon et al. 2012). This technique can be easily performed if the intrahepatic ductal system is dilated but can be unsuccessful if the biliary system is decompressed. PTC is associated with a 2% complication rate that is mainly attributed to bleeding and occasionally cholangitis (Ginat et al. 2011). The bleeding can occur at the tract site, into the gastrointestinal tract, or into the hepatic parenchyma with subsequent hemobilia that can usually be managed with maneuvers such as coil embolization in the radiological suite.

ERCP is another diagnostic imaging tool that provides imaging and a mode of therapeutic intervention with regard to the biliary system. It provides similar imaging to PTC; however, a method of internal drainage into the gastrointestinal tract versus an external mode of biliary drainage is possible with ERCP. A biliary stent may be used to treat a biliary leak, sequentially dilate a biliary stricture of malignant or benign origin with the use of either metallic or plastic stents (**Figure 17.2** and **17.3a** and **b**). The complications of an ERCP include gastrointestinal perforation (<1%), pancreatitis (3%), cholangitis (3%), and bleeding (2%) (Glomsaker et al. 2012).

The use of abdominal MR cholangiopancreatography is a noninvasive diagnostic tool that can also be utilized to demonstrate biliary anatomy and delineate ductal injuries. This can be a useful diagnostic tool if a patient has a contrast allergy or has renal insufficiency making contrast use detrimental. It has been demonstrated to have similar diagnostic results in identifying ductal pathology and the proximal biliary system. It can also be useful in identifying biliary anatomical variants that may not be appreciated on ERCP or PTC (Rahman et al. 2010).

Hepatobiliary scintigraphy has limited use in the diagnosis of biliary anatomy and the preoperative evaluation of a biliary tract injury. This test can demonstrate a biliary leak but does not demonstrate which bile duct the leak originates from and will require further imaging with ERCP if simple computed tomography (CT)-guided drainage does not improve symptoms or there is evidence of biliary obstruction.

BILE DUCT INJURIES

The type and location of a bile duct injury will dictate which type of repair is necessary and what type of preoperative preparation will be needed in order to perform a successful repair with a good postoperative outcome. The Strasberg classification is a system that describes the various bile duct injuries most commonly encountered following a complicated laparoscopic cholecystectomy (Strasberg et al. 1996). This system has five types of described injuries A–E with subset types for the E type of injury. Type A describes a bile leak that originates from the cystic duct or a small accessory duct originating from the liver bed such as a duct of Luschka. Type B injuries are described as injuries to an aberrant right hepatic duct, and type C injuries are the same injury but with concomitant bile leak. Type D injury is a partial transection of the CBD located along the lateral aspect of the duct. The type E injury can be the most complex of these injuries necessitating

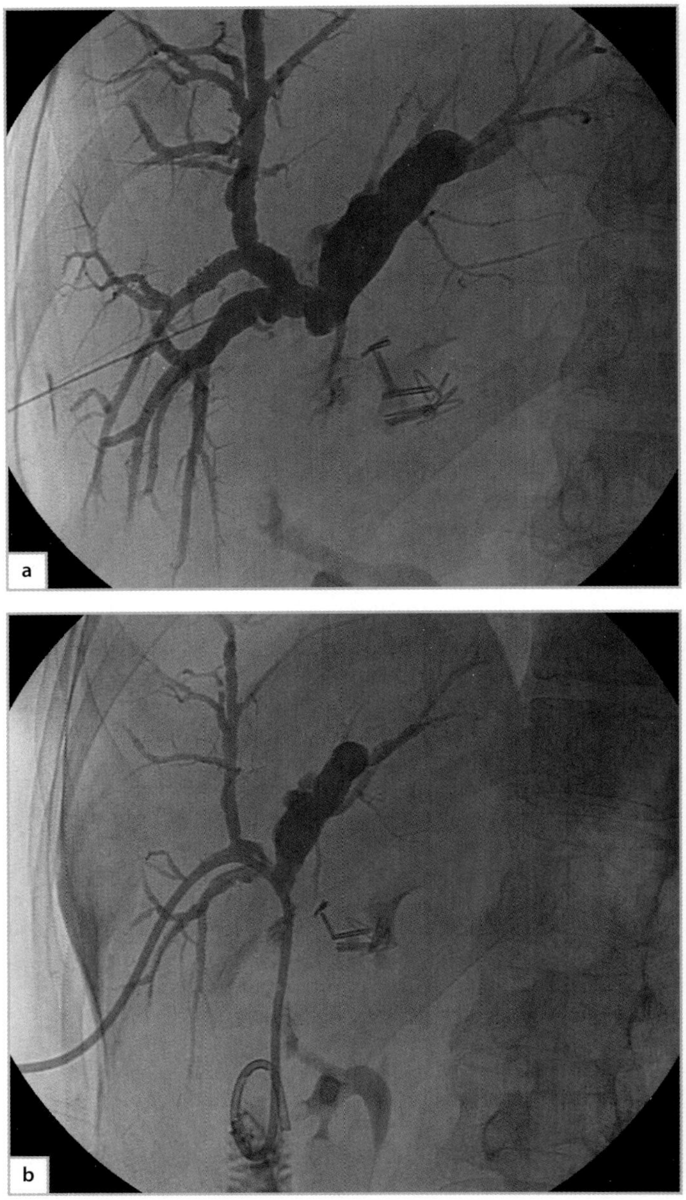

Figure 17.1 (a) Excision of segment of common hepatic duct and common bile duct as evidenced by percutaneous transhepatic cholangiography. (b) Placement of internal–external percutaneous cholangiocatheter into the duodenum.

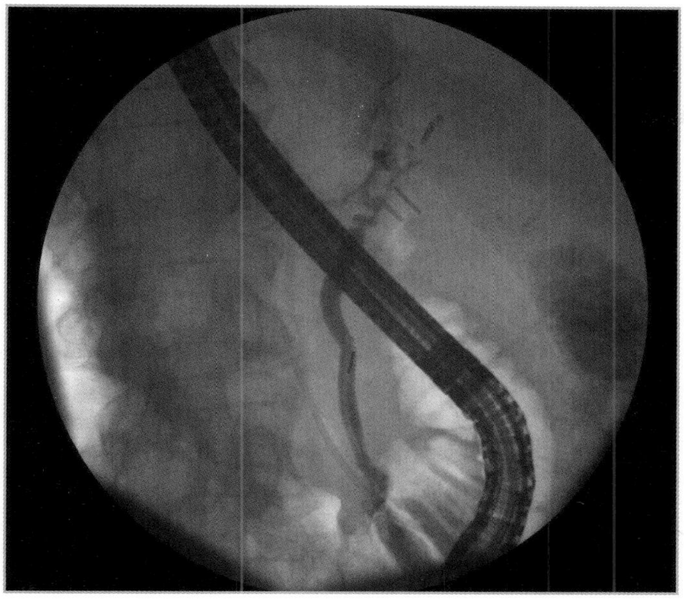

Figure 17.2 Common bile duct, obstructed by transversely placed metallic clips. When associated with contrast leak (as pictured here), one must be concerned about excisional loss of the common duct tissue above the clips.

biliary reconstruction or possible hepatic segmentectomy depending on which subtype of injury exists (Mercado & Dominguez 2011).

The majority of bile duct injuries present in a delayed fashion with only 25–32% of the injuries identified during the operation (Lau et al. 2010). In the setting of a recognized injury that is identified during the initial operation, it is certainly feasible for an experienced surgeon to primarily repair a bile duct injury. Results from studies looking at these outcomes have suggested this is not the ideal method and prompt referral to a tertiary referral center is associated with improved outcomes (Sicklick & Camp 2005, Stewart & Way 1995). Flum et al. (2001) reported an increase in risk of death by 11% in Medicare beneficiaries who underwent repair by the injuring surgeon.

After a bile duct injury is identified, controlling bile peritonitis is important and can be accomplished by simply placing a t-tube or a bulb suction drain to divert and control the bile outflow away from the abdominal cavity. Further manipulation or persistence in handling the tissues should be avoided as this may potentially devascularize the bile duct making the future definitive operation more challenging. In the absence of intra-abdominal sepsis and if the injury is identified within 7 days of the initial operation, repair of the injury is feasible with a postoperative complication rate of 7–21% and a mortality rate of 2% (Fischer et al. 2009).

Depending on the type of injury, there are several options for repair ranging from endoscopic therapy to hepatic resection. The Strasburg type A injury with a cystic duct or accessory duct leak may resolve with simple drainage if the output decreases over the course of time during the postoperative period. If the output remains high, an attempt at repair with ERCP and placement of a biliary stent across the leak after performing a sphincterotomy to preferentially drain the bile into the duodenum is also a reasonable option (**Figure 17.4a–c**). The success rate of ERCP in the management of bile leaks in the absence of transection has been quoted to be as high as 90–100% and has been described to resolve over a shorter period of time with placement of a stent versus sphincterotomy alone (Vitale & Davis 2011).

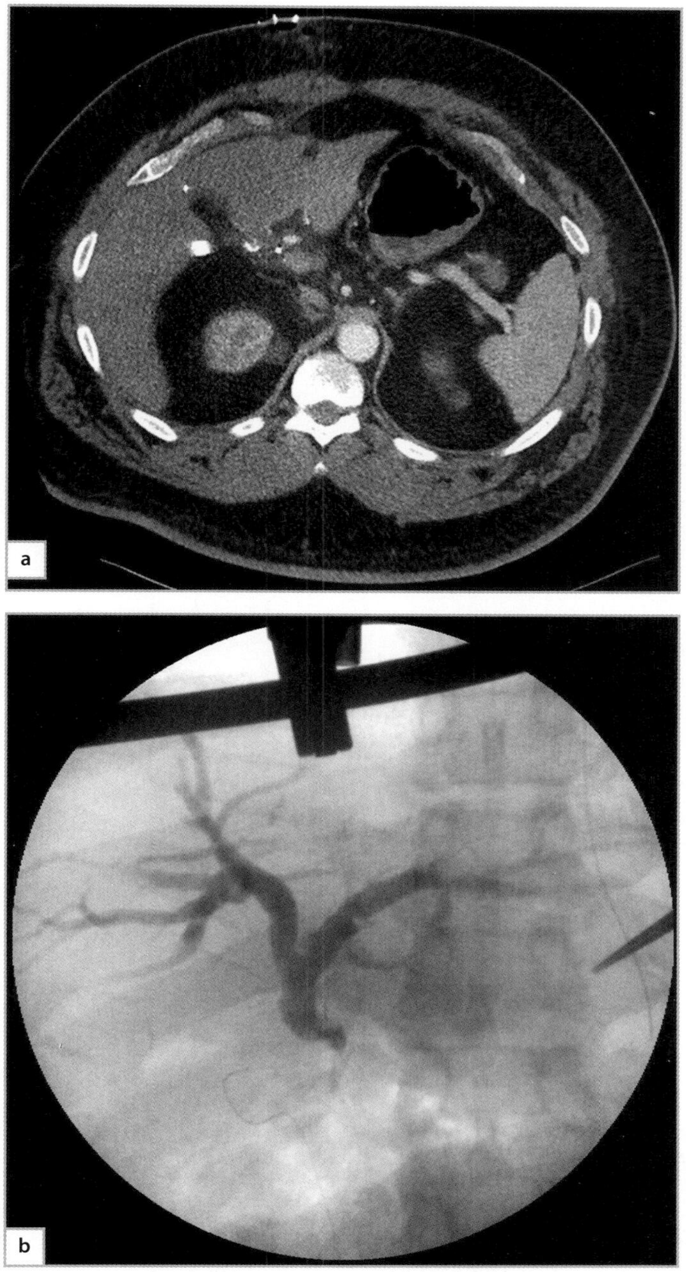

Figure 17.3 (a) Postoperative computed tomography scan showing radiodense vascular load stapling device placed across common bile duct. (b) The segment of common bile duct that was transected with the stapling device was excised intraoperatively and the subsequent cholangiogram is shown above.

In the setting of a small isolated partial transection located on the lateral aspect of the CBD, a simple repair can be performed with a 4-0 or 5-0 monofilament absorbable suture and placement of a t-tube. The two key principles to a successful outcome in reconstruction of the biliary system are a well-vascularized bile duct and a tension-free anastomosis. If the injury is located in the proximal portion of the CBD or at the bifurcation, the best operation for this location is a Roux-en-Y hepaticojejunostomy.(**Figure 17.5a–e**) Several studies have reported their postoperative outcomes with regard to the rate of anastomotic stricture of 5–67%, cholangitis 13–63%, reoperation 11–45%, and a mortality rate of 1–9% (Fischer et al. 2009, , Mercado & Dominguez 2011, Pottakkat et al. 2010).

The most morbid of injuries is an injury located above the confluence necessitating a portoenteral anastomosis. Occasionally, these injuries require removing hepatic segments IV and V to provide exposure of the left hepatic duct, which can be difficult to access for reconstruction at that level. These repairs are complicated by a higher rate of biliary fistulas and biliary strictures and are generally associated with a higher overall mortality rate (Mercado & Dominguez 2011). The routine use of anastomotic stents has been found unnecessary, can compromise the quality of the anastomosis, and has fallen out of favor over recent years. Other technical considerations include the creation of a neoconfluence of the hepatic bifurcation versus performing two separate anastomoses to the roux limb. If necessary, lowering the hilar plate may also be performed to augment visualization and operative exposure to both right and left hepatic ducts when high ductal injuries are identified.

It is rare that an injury is located in the distal CBD during a cholecystectomy, but in the event that this does occur, a choledochoduodenostomy is a safe option if the bile duct has adequate blood supply. This is performed with a Kocher maneuver to freely mobilize the duodenum followed by a large oblique choledochotomy

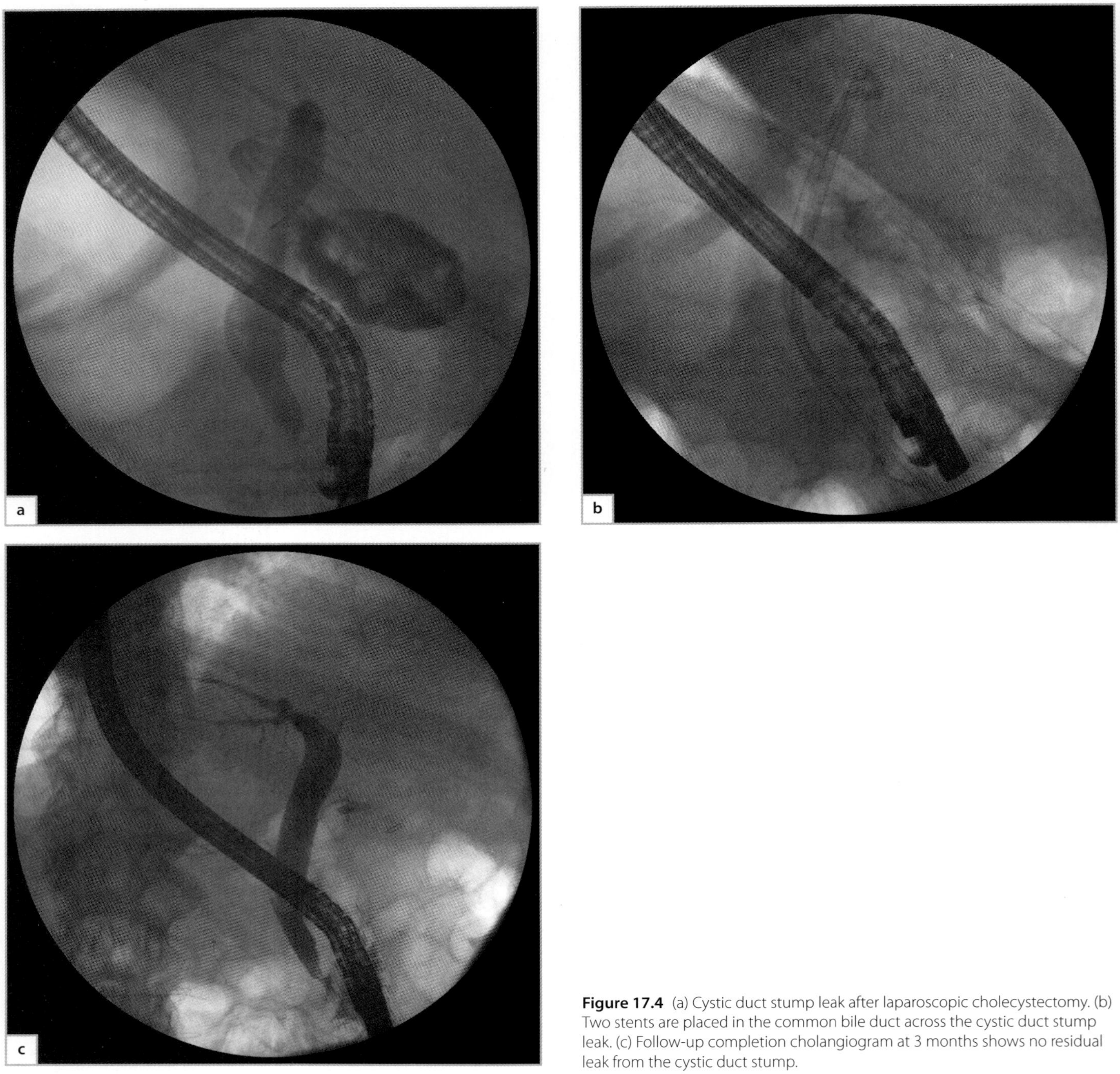

Figure 17.4 (a) Cystic duct stump leak after laparoscopic cholecystectomy. (b) Two stents are placed in the common bile duct across the cystic duct stump leak. (c) Follow-up completion cholangiogram at 3 months shows no residual leak from the cystic duct stump.

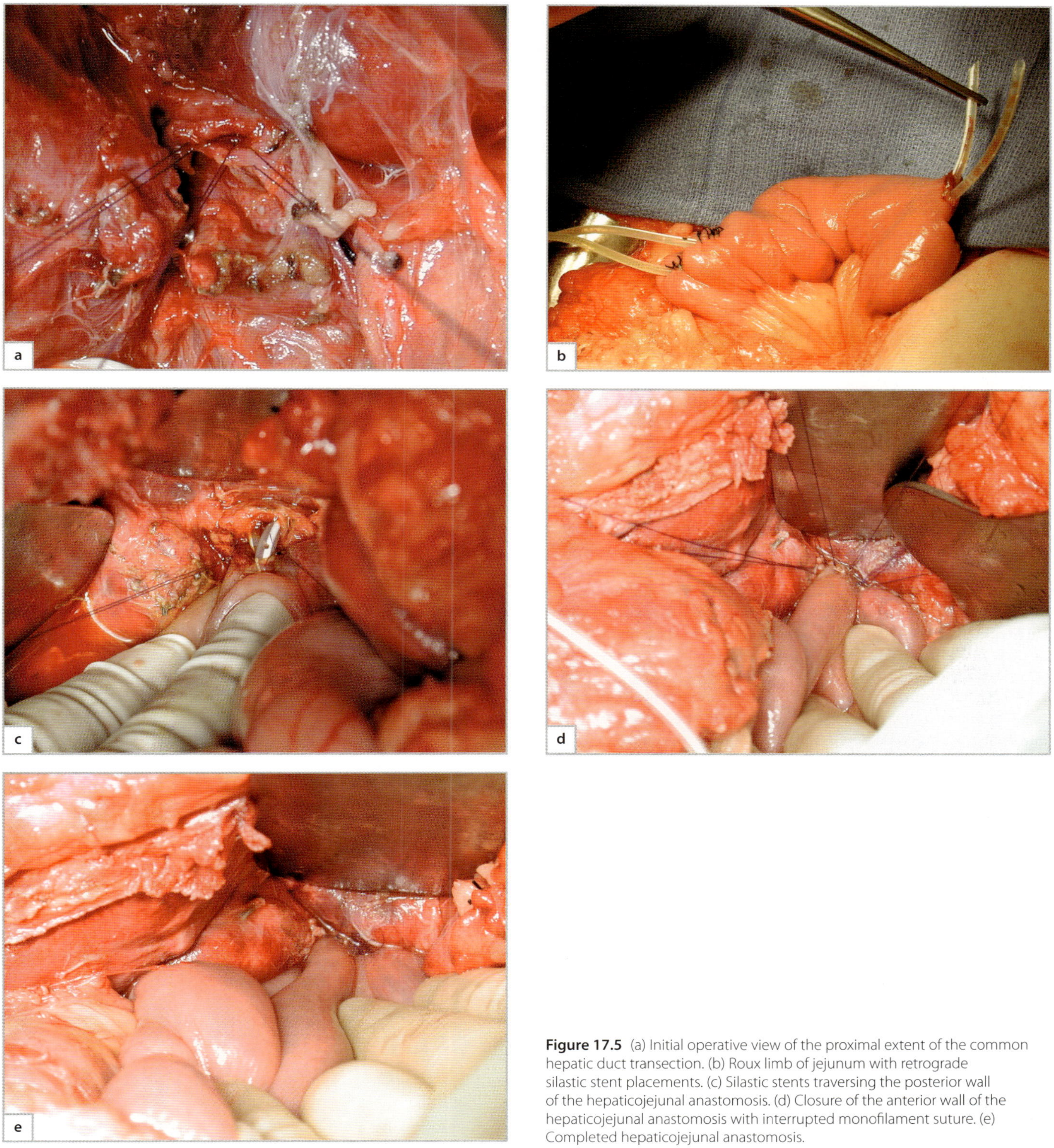

Figure 17.5 (a) Initial operative view of the proximal extent of the common hepatic duct transection. (b) Roux limb of jejunum with retrograde silastic stent placements. (c) Silastic stents traversing the posterior wall of the hepaticojejunal anastomosis. (d) Closure of the anterior wall of the hepaticojejunal anastomosis with interrupted monofilament suture. (e) Completed hepaticojejunal anastomosis.

where the bile duct injury is located. A posterior layer of 3-0 silk in a Lambert fashion is placed to keep the duodenum in place, and a running layer of 4-0 absorbable monofilament suture is then used to reapproximate the posterior row of the anastomosis followed by interrupted 4-0 monofilament suture for the anterior layer. Although there is a reported 1% complication of sump syndrome described with choledochoduodenostomy with the reflux of enteric contents into the biliary system, we routinely perform this procedure at our institution and have not observed this complication in the postoperative period.

BILIARY STRICTURES

Biliary strictures are a known complication that can present as many as 20 years after the initial operation. Determining the etiology and ruling out a malignancy is an important part of the initial evaluation. This can be difficult to discern at times, particularly with the accuracy of bile duct brushings on pathology having a low sensitivity of 37–56% (Glassbrenner et al. 1999, Lee et al. 1995). Benign biliary strictures can result after a cholecystectomy or from a CBD exploration, necrotizing, or gallstone pancreatitis. It will generally present as jaundice and can be accompanied by recurrent episodes of cholangitis. These strictures are generally caused by inadvertent thermal injury or stripping of the blood supply to the bile duct at the location of the resulting stricture.

There are several studies describing the results of endoscopic therapy for bile duct strictures (Costamagna et al. 2010, Pozsar et al. 2004, Regimbeau et al. 2012, Tuvignon et al. 2011). Endoscopic treatment is performed at the time of ERCP with placement of single to multiple biliary stents over recommended treatment duration of at least 12 months. This requires a stent exchange every 3–4 months over this time period. Multiple side-by-side stents should be placed or can be exchanged for a retrievable expanding metallic stent to help progress dilatation of the stricture over time with subsequent cholangiogram demonstrating resolution of the stricture. A persistent stricture seen on subsequent cholangiograms is one quoted predictor of recurrence or failure, but success following endoscopic therapy is quoted to be 60–82% for benign biliary strictures (Pozsar et al. 2004, Tuvignon et al. 2011) (**Figure 17.6a–d**) The incidence of associated cholangitis has been reported to occur in 20% of patients, and surgical treatment of these patients who have recurrent cholangitis should be considered in addition to patients who have a persistent stricture (Costamagna et al. 2010).

If surgical treatment is necessary, then operative repair with a hepaticojejunostomy, choledochojejunostomy, or choledochoduodenostomy is indicated depending on the extent and location of the stricture. These surgical procedures for benign biliary strictures can be performed successfully but are accompanied by a complication rate up to 49% (Zafar et al. 2011). These rates include various complications ranging from a local wound infection, recurrent cholangitis, and pancreatic fistulas to many other systemic disorders such as venous thromboembolism, postoperative pulmonary, or cardiac complications. Recurrent anastomotic strictures have been quoted to occur at a low rate of 8% and can be treated successfully with percutaneous transhepatic balloon dilatation with long-term success in 90% of patients with minimal risk to patients (Bonnel & Fingerhut 2012, Pottakkat et al. 2010).

POSTOPERATIVE CARE

The early postoperative period is mainly focused on the postoperative recovery of bowel function and monitoring for evidence of anastomotic breakdown and resultant leak. Depending on the health and age of the patient, a short stay in the intensive care unit may be necessary with emphasis on early ambulation and adequate pulmonary toilet to minimize the risk of postoperative pneumonias. After the patient is having bowel function and there is no evidence of residual bile in the postoperative drain left near the anastomosis, this drain is usually removed prior to discharge home if the output is <30 mL/day. Patients can generally return to their normal daily activities approximately 2–3 weeks following the operation.

The late postoperative follow-up should include annual visits and labwork to evaluate for evidence of anastomotic strictures following biliary enteric bypass procedures. If the patient is having symptoms of jaundice, abdominal pain, or a notable increase in their hepatic function panel, further imaging with a CT scan to evaluate for intrahepatic ductal dilatation and further evidence of stricture is needed.

POSTOPERATIVE HEMORRHAGE

The management of postoperative hemorrhage is approached differently depending on whether this presents early or delayed in the postoperative period. Early postoperative hemorrhage occurs within 24 hours of the operation and is oftentimes apparent by the presence of blood in a drain and hemodynamic instability in the patient (Wente et al. 2006). This requires surgical re-exploration with the goal of identifying the source of blood loss. Early postoperative hemorrhage is usually accompanied by coagulopathy in the affected patient and should be treated concomitantly, while the surgeon prepares and proceeds with reoperation. Following a pancreaticoduodenectomy, one of the most common locations for early postoperative bleeding is the gastroduodenal artery stump or small vessels associated with dissection of the pancreatic uncinate near the portal vein and superior mesenteric vessels. This type of hemorrhage can be stopped with ligation of the bleeding vessels or temporarily packing the abdominal cavity if the bleeding appears to be confounded by coagulopathy.

Delayed postoperative hemorrhage clinically manifests itself differently than early postoperative hemorrhage. It can present as a subtle change in hemodynamics that resolves or a sentinel bleed that manifests with drifting hemoglobins. In this scenario, the bleeding can be either extraluminal or intraluminal. The source of extraluminal bleeding can originate from a pseudoaneurysm of an artery or arterial erosion. The gastroduodenal artery is a described source of pseudoaneurysm and can be treated with coil embolization, while arterial erosion can occur anywhere from the common or proper hepatic artery to the splenic artery. This can also be treated by interventional radiology with either placement of stents or embolization depending on its location (Puppala et al. 2011). If the bleeding is coming from an intraluminal source, the source of blood loss can be identified with the presence of melenic stools or bloody output into a nasogastric tube. Treatment of this process with endoscopy can be performed effectively and hemostasis can be achieved on a mucosal vessel or bleeding site with endoscopic clipping or coagulation.

The incidence of postoperative hemorrhage is reported to be 3.5% and associated with a 30–40% mortality rate (Yeo et al. 1997). Most often these are associated with pancreatic fistulas, sepsis, or intra-abdominal abscesses. The mortality rate is significant and can be improved with early intervention.

GALLBLADDER CARCINOMA

Gallbladder carcinoma is a rare cancer with an overall incidence in the United States of 1.2/100,000 (Duffy et al. 2008). This incidental finding following a cholecystectomy is not uncommon and is a large percentage of how this diagnosis is found at initial presentation. Regardless of whether the initial procedure is performed by a laparoscopic or an open approach, it is common that a subsequent operation is required for curative intent. There has been some debate regarding the topic of worse outcomes in patients who initially undergo a laparoscopic cholecystectomy prior to their diagnosis but further studies have proven this to have no effect in the overall

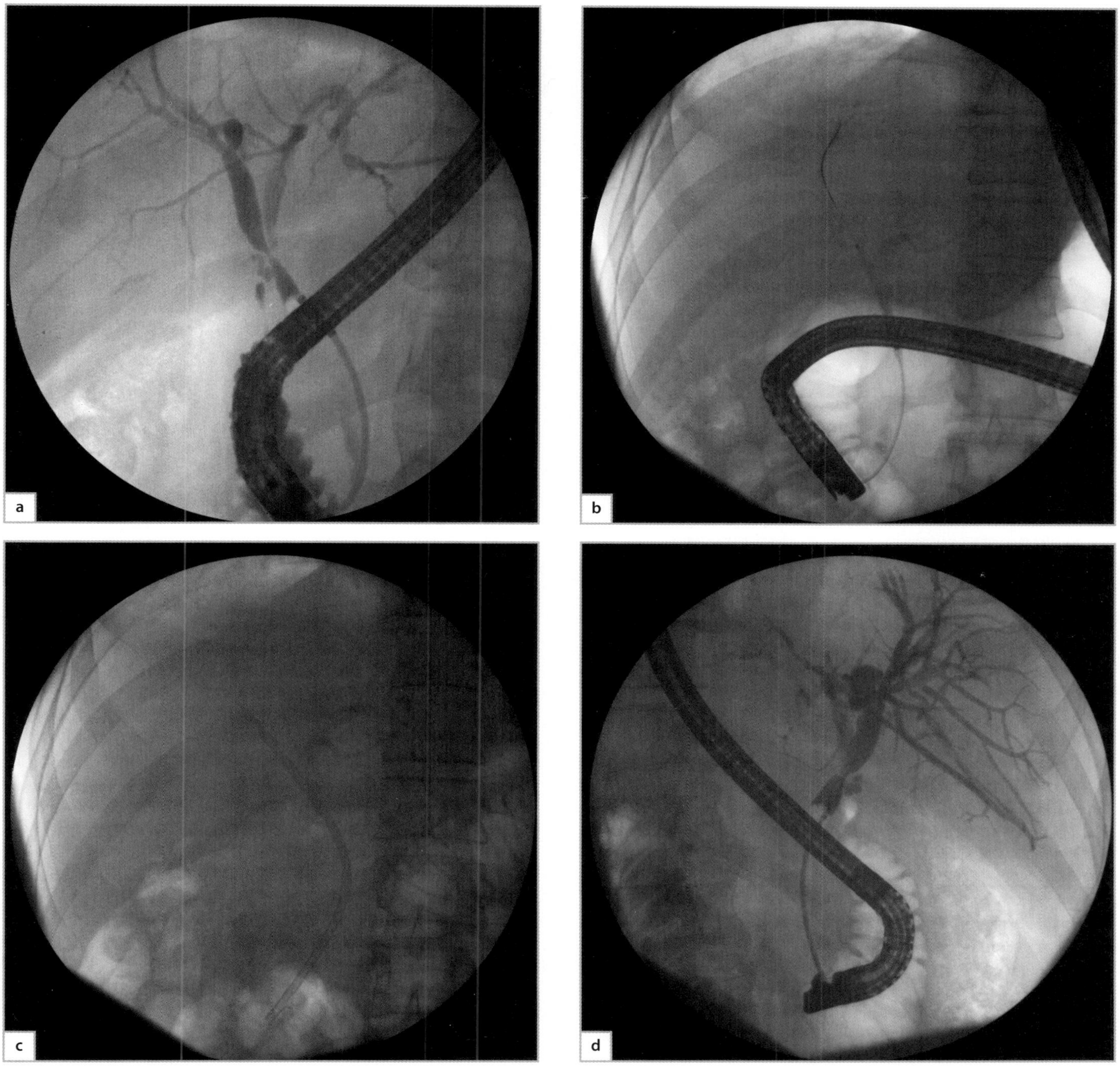

Figure 17.6 (a) Initial endoscopic retrograde cholangiopancreatography (ERCP) after cholecystectomy exhibits a significant stricture at the bifurcation of the common hepatic duct, near the insertion of the cystic duct stump. This was believed to be consistent with an ischemic stricture. (b,c) The stricture at the bifurcation of the common hepatic duct was balloon dilated and a single stent was placed initially. (d) Follow-up ERCP failed to demonstrate improvement in the degree of ductal stenosis with endoscopic techniques. This patent ultimately went on to have a Roux-en-Y hepaticojejunostomy.

prognosis in these patients. Important prognostic factors that are associated with improved survival are the complete excision of tumor with an R0 resection, negative tumor margins, and the absence of perineural or vascular invasion. The overall 5-year survival rate for patients who undergo surgery for gallbladder cancer has been quoted in a recent study to be 26.2% with a longer median survival of 97 months in patients with an R0 resection compared with 8 months for R1/R2 resections (Liang et al. 2008). Due to the importance of negative margins, authors of subsequent recent studies are proponents of a radical resection for T1b lesions due to gallbladder cancer's increased risk of lymph nodal and peritoneal disease at the time of reoperation (Shukla & Barreto 2008).

POSTCHOLECYSTECTOMY SYNDROME

Postcholecystectomy syndrome is a disorder composed of recurrent right upper quadrant abdominal pain following a cholecystectomy. The diagnosis can be attributed to a multitude of various disorders such as reflux, esophagitis or gastritis, peptic ulcer disease, choledocholithiasis, or sphincter of Oddi dysfunction. These patients will benefit from endoscopy, esophageal manometry, and further imaging to aid in establishing these diagnoses. The treatments can span from medical therapy for peptic ulcer disease to ERCP for the treatment of sphincter of Oddi dysfunction and choledocholithiasis with various degrees of success.

Occasionally this disorder can be attributed to a retained gallbladder remnant from a partial cholecystectomy performed during the initial operation (**Figure 17.7a** and **b**). There have been reports of this procedure not having symptomatic sequelae, and proponents of this procedure encourage this strategy as a bailout technique to safely avoid a bile duct injury. This is a reasonable option in the difficult case of acute or chronic cholecystitis; however, there have been published case reports describing patients who had to undergo a reoperation for recurrent symptoms from a retained gallbladder segment and associated cholelithiasis (Demetriades et al. 2008). The diagnosis was generally made by the patient's history and the demonstration of a gallbladder remnant on abdominal ultrasound or magentic resonance cholangiopancreatography (MRCP). These studies all reported excellent results with a reoperation performed primarily utilizing a laparoscopic approach.

POSTOPERATIVE BILE LEAK

The event of a postoperative bile leak is a common complication postcholecystectomy (**Figure 17.4a–c**). The diagnosis should be suspected in any patient postcholecystectomy with abdominal pain, fevers, or occasionally an elevated bilirubin level. The diagnosis can be made with a CT if there is a large fluid collection and accompanied by a positive hepatobiliary iminodiacetic acid scan (HIDA). If the potential for a postoperative bile leak is highly probable as determined during intraoperative findings, a drain can simply be placed at the time of the operation and kept in place until the bile leak resolves. In the event of an undrained biloma, a percutaneous drain can simply be placed by either CT or ultrasound guidance. An ERCP and sphincterotomy can also be performed in the setting of a persistent bile leak. With a high-output biliary fistula, placement of a biliary stent is recommended with quoted 90–95% resolution (Tzovaras et al. 2001, Vitale & Davis 2011).

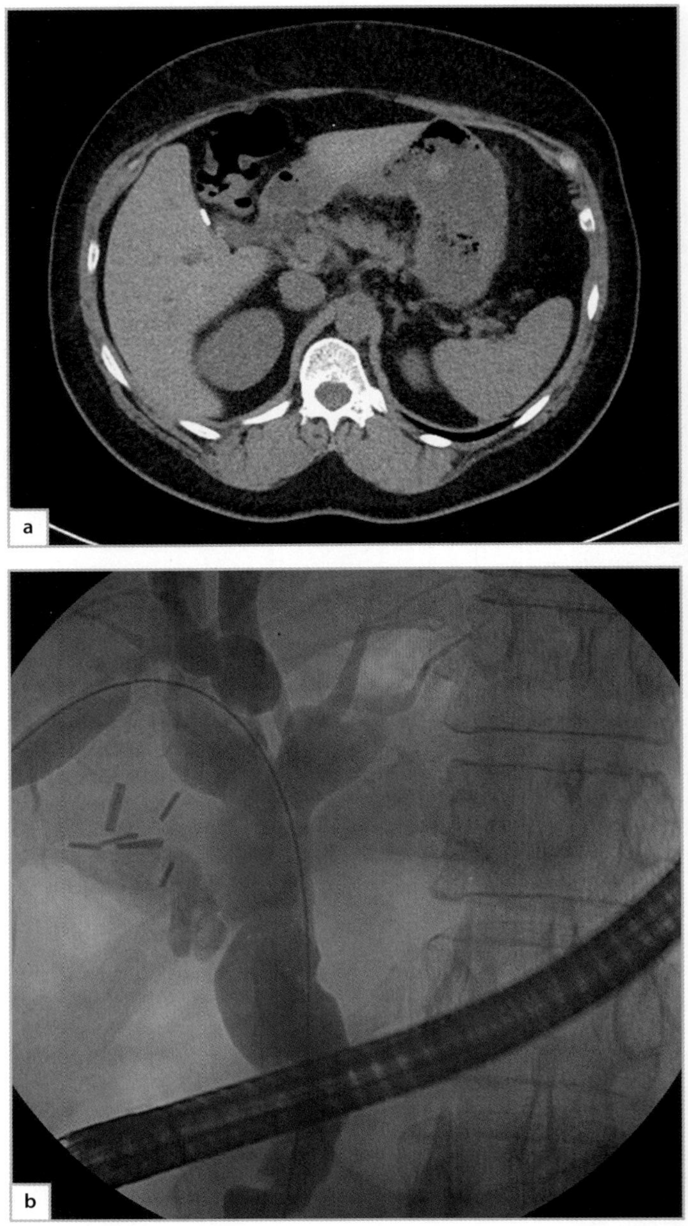

Figure 17.7 (a) Postcholecystectomy computed tomography exhibiting a retained gallbladder segment with stones (arrow). (b) endoscopic retrograde cholangiopancreatography with retained gallbladder and stones.

PRIMARY CHOLEDOCHOLITHIASIS

Bile duct stones recur in approximately 4–24% of patients postcholecystectomy (Attasaranya et al. 2008). The diagnosis can be established with noninvasive imaging with abdominal ultrasound or MRCP; however, ERCP is the gold standard in providing both a diagnosis and therapeutic intervention. Treatment consists of endoscopic sphincterotomy to aid in the passage of bile and subsequent stones as well as stone extraction (**Figure 17.8a–e**). The stone extraction is performed using balloon or basket extraction techniques with a success rate of 85–95% (Shaw et al. 1993). If the stone is a large size, i.e. >1.5 cm, complete extraction during the first endoscopy may prove to be difficult. Partially fragmenting the stone with mechanical lithotripsy can be performed, and a biliary stent placed for aid in passage of bile with a repeat endoscopy for further attempt at stone fragmentation and extraction is a reasonable option.

Regarding an operative approach to choledocholithiasis, a laparoscopic or open CBD exploration can be performed with success rates of 83–96% (Martin et al. 2006). Laparoscopic CBD explorations, when performed by an experienced laparoscopic surgeon, can be performed with a morbidity rate as low as 6% compared with 12% with the open technique (Grubnik et al. 2012). The laparoscopic approach is a technically difficult procedure and can be challeng-

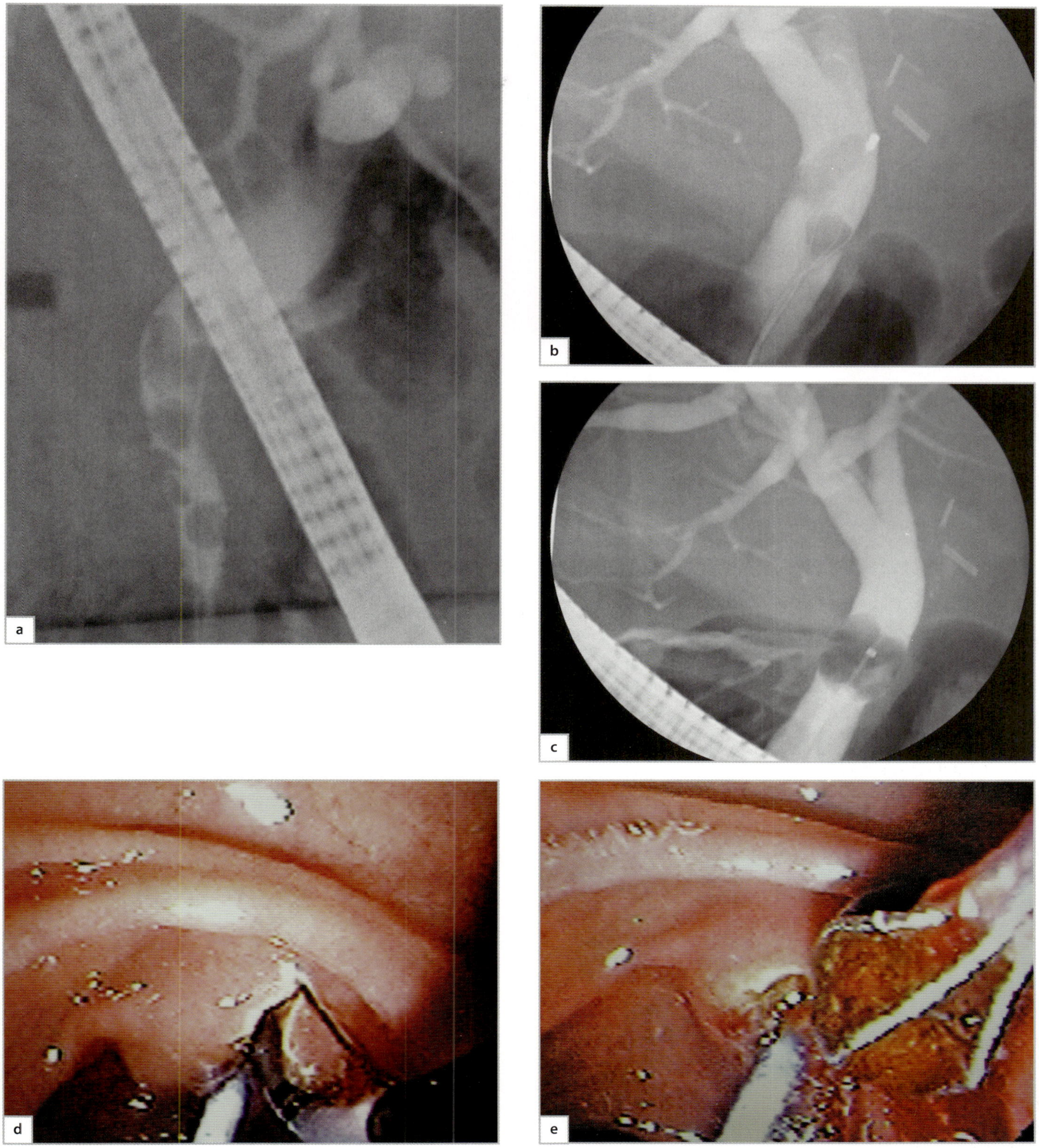

Figure 17.8 (a) Retained common bile duct stones after cholecystectomy. (b) Wire-guided basket extraction of common bile duct stone. (c) Balloon sweep of common bile duct after stone extraction. (d) Endoscopic sphincterotomy and (e) stone extraction.

ing if the size of the stone is >8–10 mm in size, particularly through a transcystic approach. If the stone cannot be removed through a transcystic approach, a choledochotomy can be performed laparoscopically or via an open technique and stone extraction can be attempted with a wire basket or Fogarty catheter. Placement of a t-tube after this procedure is beneficial to help decompress the biliary system but must be left in place at least 2 weeks prior to removal to ensure the development of a well-formed sinus tract prior to removal. This will avoid complications of biliary peritonitis after the t-tube is removed.

CONCLUSION

Performing a reoperation in the biliary tract can be a successful yet challenging task for a surgeon. The anatomy of the biliary system can be complex and highly variable making the identification of vital structures a critical component of this process. While there are many therapeutic options ranging from endoscopy to a reoperation to treat these various biliary pathologies, the key principles for a successful outcome are preoperative preparation and prudent decision making during and after the operation.

REFERENCES

Adamsen S, Hansen O, Funch-Jensen P, et al. Bile duct injury during laparoscopic cholecystectomy: a prospective nationwide series. J Am Coll Surg 1997; 184:571.

Attasaranya S, Fogel E, et al. Choledocholithiasis, ascending cholangitis and gallstone pancreatitis. Med Clin North Am 2008; 92:925–960.

Berber E, Engle K, et al. Selective use of tube cholecystostomy with interval laparoscopic cholecystectomy in acute cholecystitis. Arch Surg 2000; 135:341–346.

Bonnel DH, Fingerhut A. Percutaneous transhepatic balloon dilatation of benign bilioenteric stricture: long-term results in 110 patients. Am J Surg 2012; 203:675–683.

Buddingh K, Nieuwenhuijs V, et al. Intraoperative assessment of biliary anatomy for prevention of bile duct injury: a review of current and future patient safety interventions. Surg Endosc 2011; 25:2449–2461.

Buddingh K, Weersma RK, Savenije RA, et al. Lower rate of major bile duct injury and increased intraoperative management of common bile duct stones after implementation of routine intraoperative cholangiography. J Am Coll Surg 2011; 213:267–274.

Cherng N, Witkowski E, et al. Use of cholecystostomy tubes in the management of patients with primary diagnosis of acute cholecystitis. J Am Coll Surg 2012; 214:196–201.

Costamagna G, Tringali A, Mutgnani M, et al. Endotherapy of postoperative biliary strictures with multiple stents: results after more than 10 years of follow-up. Gastrointest Endosc 2010; 72:551–557.

Davis B, Castaneda G, Lopez J. Subtotal cholecystectomy versus total cholecystectomy in complicated cholecystitis. Am Surg 2012; 78:814–817.

Demetriades H, Pramateftakis M, et al. Retained gallbladder remnant after laparoscopic cholecystectomy. J Laparoendosc Adv Surg Tech 2008; 18:276–279.

Duffy A, Capanu M, et al. Gallbladder cancer: 10 year experience at Memorial Sloan-Kettering Cancer Centre. J Surg Oncol 2008; 1:485–489.

Fidelman N, Kerlan R, Laberge JM, et al. Accuracy of percutaneous transhepatic cholangiography in predicting the location and nature of major bile duct injuries. J Vasc Interv Radiol 2011; 22:884–892.

Fischer CP, Fahy BN, Aloia TA, et al. Timing of referral impacts surgical outcomes in patients undergoing repair of bile duct injuries. HPB 2009; 11:32–37.

Flum DR, Koepsell T, et al. Common bile duct injury during laparoscopic cholecystectomy and the use of intraoperative cholangiography: adverse outcome of preventable error? Arch Surg 2001; 136:1287–1292.

Ford JA, Soop M, Du J, et al. Systematic review of intraoperative cholangiography in cholecystectomy. Br J Surg 2012; 99:160–167.

Frieman G. Natural history of asymptomatic and symptomatic gallstones. Am J Surg 1993; 165:399–404.

Georgidades CP, Mavromatis T, Kourlaba GC, et al. Is inflammation a significant predictor of bile duct injury during laparoscopic cholecystectomy? Surg Endosc 2008; 22:1959–1964.

Giger U, Michel J, et al. Risk factors for perioperative complications in patients undergoing laparoscopic cholecystectomy: analysis of 22,953 consecutive cases from the Swiss Association of Laparoscopic and Thoracoscopic Surgery database. J Am Coll Surg 2006; 203:723–728.

Ginat D, Saad W, et al. Incidence of cholangitis and sepsis associated with percutaneous transhepatic biliary drain cholangiography and exchange: a comparison between liver transplant and native liver patients. Am J Roentgenol 2011; 196:73–77.

Glassbrenner B, Ardan M, Boeck W, et al. Prospective evaluation of brush cytology of biliary strictures during endoscopic retrograde cholangiopancreatography. Endoscopy 1999; 31:712–717.

Glomsaker T, Hoff G, Kvaloy JT, et al. Patterns and predictive factors of complications after endoscopic retrograde cholangiopancreatography. Br J Surg 2012; 100:373–380.

Gracie W, Ransohoff D. The natural history of silent gallstones: the innocent gallstone is not a myth. N Engl J Med 1982; 307:798–800.

Grubnik W, Tkachenko A, Ilyashenko W, et al. Laparoscopic common bile duct exploration versus open surgery: comparative prospective randomized trial. Surg Endosc 2012; 26:2165–2171.

Gwon DI, Ko G, Sung KB, et al. Clinical outcomes after percutaneous biliary interventions in patients with malignant biliary obstruction by metastatic gastric cancer. Acta Radiol 2012; 53:422–429.

Hamad M, Nada A, et al. Major biliary complications in 2714 cases of laparoscopic cholecystectomy without intraoperative cholangiography: a multicenter retrospective study. Surg Endosc 2011; 25:3747–3751.

Kern K. Malpractice litigation involving laparoscopic cholecystectomy. Cost, cause and consequences. Arch Surg 1997; 132:392–397.

Lau WY, Lai E, Laus SH. Management of bile duct injury after laparoscopic cholecystectomy: a review. ANZ J Surg 2010; 80:75–81.

Lee JG, Leung J, Baillie J, et al. Benign, dysplastic or malignant – making sense of endoscopic bile duct brush cytology: results in 149 consecutive patients. Am J Gastroenterol 1995; 90:722–726.

Liang JW, Dong S, Zhou ZX. Surgical management for carcinoma of the gallbladder: a single-institution experience for 25 years. Chin Med J 2008; 121:1900–1905.

Martin DJ, Vernon D, Toouli J. Surgical versus endoscopic treatment of bile duct stones. Cochrane Database Syst Rev 2006; 19(2):CD003327.

McSherry C, et al. The natural history of diagnosed gallstone disease in symptomatic and asymptomatic patients. Ann Surg 1985; 202:59–63.

Melton G, Lillemoe K, et al. Major bile duct injuries associated with laparoscopic cholecystectomy. Ann Surg 2002; 235:888–895.

Mercado M, Dominguez I. Classification and management of bile duct injuries. World J Gastrointest Surg 2011; 3:4348.

National Institutes of Health Concensus Development Conference statement on gallstones and laparoscopic cholecystectomy. Am J Surg 1993; 165:390–398.

Nuzzo G, Giuliante F, Persiani R. The risk of biliary ductal injury during laparoscopic cholecystectomy. J Chir 2004; 141:343–353.

Pottakkat B, Vijayahari R, et al. Factors predicting failure following high bilioenteric anastomosis for post-cholecystectomy benign biliary strictures. J Gastrointest Surg 2010; 14:1389–1394.

Pozsar J, Sahin P, Laszlo F, et al. Medium term results of endoscopic treatment of common bile strictures in chronic calcifying pancreatitis with increasing number of stents. J Clin Gastroenterol 2004; 38:118–123.

Puppala S, Patel J, et al. Hemorrhagic complications after Whipple surgery: imaging and radiologic intervention. Vasc Interv Radiol 2011; 196:192–197.

Rahman R, Ju J, et al. Correlation between MRCP and ERCP findings at a tertiary care hospital. W V Med J 2010; 106:14–29.

Regimbeau J, Fuks D, et al. A comparative study of surgery and endoscopy for the treatment of bile duct stricture in patients with chronic pancreatitis. Surg Endosc 2012; 26:2902–2908.

Sanjay P, Fulke J, et al. 'Critical view of Safety' as an alternative to routine

intraoperative cholangiography during laparoscopic cholecystectomy for acute biliary pathology. J Gastrointest Surg 2010; 14:1280–1284.
Shaffer EA. Gallstone disease: epidemiology of gallstone disease. Best Pract Res Clin Gastroenterol 2006; 20:981–996.
Shaw M, Mackie R, et al. Results of a multicenter trial using a mechanical lithotripter for the treatment of large bile duct stones. Am J Gastroenterol 1993; 88:730–733.
Shukla, P, Barreto G. Revision surgery for incidental gallbladder cancer: factors influencing operability and further evidence for T1b tumours. HPB 2008; 10:43–47.
Sicklick J, Camp M. Surgical management of bile duct injuries sustained during laparoscopic cholecystectomy: perioperative results in 200 patients. Ann Surg 2005; 241:786–792.
Stewart L, Way L. Bile duct injuries during laparoscopic cholecystectomy. Factors that influence the results of treatment. Arch Surg 1995; 130:1123–1128.
Strasberg S. Avoidance of biliary injury during laparoscopic cholecystectomy. J Hepatobiliary Pancreat Surg 2002;9:543-7.
Strasberg S., Callery MP, Soper NJ. Laparoscopic surgery of the bile ducts. Gastrointest Endosc Clin North Am 1996; 6:81–105.
Strasberg S, Hertl M, et al. An analysis of the problem of biliary injury during laparoscopic cholecystectomy. J Am Coll Surg 1995; 180:101–125.
Tuvignon N, Liguory C, et al. Long-term follow-up after biliary stent placement for postcholecystectomy bile duct strictures: a multicenter study. Endoscopy 2011; 43:208–216.
Tzovaras G, Peyser P, et al. Minimally invasive management of bile leak after laparoscopic cholecystectomy. HPB 2001; 3:165–168.
Vitale G, Davis B. Evaluation and treatment of biliary leaks after gastrointestinal surgery. J Gastrointest Surg 2011; 15:1323–1324.
Wente M, Shrikhande S, et al. Management of early hemorrhage from pancreatic anastomoses after pancreaticoduodenectomy. Dig Surg 2006; 23:203–208.
Wherry D, Marohn M, et al. An external audit for laparoscopic cholecystectomy in the steady state performed in medical treatment facilities of the Department of Defense. Ann Surg 1996; 224:145–154.
Yeo C, Cameron J, et al. Six hundred fifty consecutive pancreaticoduodenectomies in the 1990s: pathology, complications and outcomes. Ann Surg 1997; 226:248–260.
Zafar S, Khan M, et al. Early complications after biliary enteric anastomosis for benign disease: a retrospective analysis. BMC Surg 2011; 11:11–19.
Zdichavsky M, Bashin Y, et al. Impact of risk factors for prolonged operative time in laparoscopic cholecystectomy. Eur J Gastoenterol Hepatol 2012; 24:1033–1038.

Chapter 18 Reoperations after abdominal organ transplants

Christoph E. Broelsch, G. Felix Broelsch

INTRODUCTION

Abdominal organ transplants encompass a variety of organs including liver, kidney, pancreas, small bowel, and multivisceral transplants such as en bloc transplants of liver and small bowel, liver and pancreas plus small bowel, as well as combined transplants like kidney and pancreas. Virtually, any abdominal organ can be surgically removed to substitute a failing or missing one.

Consequently, each organ or organ system presents its own set of complications that require immediate diagnosis and treatment. While organ transplants have increased dramatically and long-term survival has reached an unthinkable level of success since the early days, one event has not changed since then: 'Most severe complications and death occur within the first 3 months following operation' (Koneru et al. 1988).

Any postoperative phase is marked by disturbances of graft function, pre-existing morbidities and anomalies, and potential technical difficulties. Not every early complication necessarily requires reintervention, but does require clarification for its cause. Advances in imaging, interventional procedures, endoscopies, and laboratory screening frequently allow for prompt diagnosis without the need for reoperation. The latter needs to be weighed up against any surgical trauma presenting additional morbidity and stress to the patient – as well as to their relatives – and, thus, has to provide substantial benefit for the recovery and overall prognosis of the patient.

Reoperations in the later postoperative phase depend on the cause and severity of dysfunctions. Threat to graft survival challenges the surgical experience if a graft can be salvaged or needs to be replaced. Often, retransplantation presents the only viable option to rescue the patient.

The most common causes for reoperations in transplantation are related to primary graft quality, vascular or drainage disturbances, circulatory or respiratory collapse, and potential infections under immunosuppression. Several complications may occur simultaneously and, thus, require continuous monitoring in any phase of postoperative care. Timing of reoperation presents a key factor, while watchful waiting may result in graft loss or patient death.

ANATOMICAL AND PHYSIOLOGICAL ISSUES

As the largest cavity of the human body, the abdomen presents a unique conglomerate of intrinsically connected organs sustaining life through digestion, absorption, metabolism, secretion and excretion, hematopoiesis, and circulation. Particularly, its enteric circulation from the intestines to the liver allows the utilization of nutrition, hormonal metabolism, detoxification, and biliary excretion to yield optimal digestive and regulatory effects.

Each organ in this cavity can be replaced by transplantation, most frequently being kidney, liver, and pancreas. Subsequently combined transplants consist of kidney and pancreas, liver and kidney, liver and pancreas, or liver and small bowel with or without pancreas. The small bowel alone presents a special entity, because of its gastrointestinal and immunological complications and has not yet received broad acceptance.

LIVER

The liver presents the largest organ within the abdomen. Its special subphrenic position requires an orthotopic position to maintain its circulatory relationship with the portal vein, the hepatic artery, and as a drainage channel with venous blood, returning from the lower portion of the body. The subphrenic drainage of the hepatic veins presents an anatomic prerequisite without which a long-term function cannot be preserved. The low (negative) pressure during inspiration and its relative increase during expiration (positive pressure) present a vital factor for sinusoidal drainage of portal venous blood, passing through the liver parenchyma. The pressure gradients are supported by the respiratory mechanics, i.e. expanding the chest during inspiration and compression of the diaphragm and abdominal wall during expiration. In comparison with a sponge, the normal liver receives circulatory support in lieu of its own effective contractile regulatory system. Therefore, heterotopic positioning of the liver or parts of it in the groin, the chest, or neck has failed in the long run (Maki & Slapak 1974).

PORTAL VENOUS REVASCULARIZATION

For liver transplantation, the portal venous circulation has to be re-established under almost any circumstance. The nutritional portal blood is essential for the maintenance of liver regeneration, as well as for splanchnic blood decompression. As a completely detached and denervated isolated organ, the microcirculation of this huge organ depends on intrinsic interaction between the portal and arterial blood supply. Thus, excessive portal hypertension maintains a risk factor for intrahepatic circulation and should be lessened pharmacologically or by technical flow-reducing measures. Today, the incidence of portal venous complications (e.g. thrombosis, kinking, and steal syndrome) is one of the rarest problems due to anatomical circumstances.

VENOUS OUTFLOW

While veno-vasomotor reactions are virtually absent in cirrhotic livers and the hyperdynamic vascular status allows for predominance of arterial blood supply, the transplanted, full-size normal liver requires circulatory adaptation maintaining a low venous outflow pressure and a rather proportional arterial (40%) and portal blood flow (60%) to keep a homogenous sinusoidal perfusion. In the present era of living-related partial liver transplants and/or segmental and/or reduced size and/or split livers, hemodynamic considerations have received vital attention because of too many graft failures and consequent loss due to hyperperfusion or venous outflow obstruction (Broelsch et al. 1990).

Today, few problems arise from venous outflow and obstruction of caval blood flow. With the frequently performed 'piggyback technique' (**Figure 18.1**), a large anastomosis allows for unhindered return of venous blood from the lower body as well as from the hepatic veins, provided that the anastomosis is well placed directly under the diaphragmatic hiatus (Audet et al. 2010, Calne & Williams 1968). However, local stenoses are extremely difficult to repair, even through stenting, and oftentimes require retransplantation.

Arterial revascularization

Arterial revascularization still remains as the focus of attention. Depending on the vascular pedicles obtained from the donor, the recipient´s anatomy requires subtle dissection and – particularly in small children – an anastomosis sufficient in size and diameter. Anomalies such as aberrant gastroduodenal or pancreaticoduodenal arteries (12–20% in normal individuals) have to be reconstructed to maintain adequate blood supply. Thus, integrity of the common hepatic artery for the viable liver organ takes precedence in cases of multiorgan retrieval. However, arrangements between the donor team and the transplant team have yielded excellent cooperation and result in a fair distribution of vascular pedicles whenever a liver is being retrieved together with a pancreas (Molmenti et al. 2004).

The subtlety of performing arterial anastomoses has been improved by applying microvascular methods and magnifications, as well as by involving plastic and reconstructive surgeons for this part, at the end of a sometimes long and tedious operation (Fan et al. 2002). Arterial thromboses can still occur in the early postoperative phase due to hypotension or increased vascular resistance of the graft due to swelling and postperfusion edema and require immediate medical attention. Reconstruction and interposition grafting need to be successful, or else, parenchymal necroses occur and render the graft nonfunctional that consequently would require a retransplantation. Also, the incidence of manifest arterial thrombosis qualifies for requesting another graft through a 'high urgency' listing.

PARTIAL LIVER GRAFTS

Anatomical issues related to segmental or partial liver grafts include the size of the organ, the cut surface, and the biliary drainage. Biliary anastomoses were long considered to be the Achilles heel of the operation. Studies on blood supply of this intra- and extrahepatic structure clearly point toward the arterial supply of the proper hepatic artery, mostly the right one. Limited collateral circulation to the duct in the hilum of the liver often leads to ductal necrosis and anastomotic leakage. Thus, dissection of the whole liver, a lobe or, a segment has to ascertain the intact vascular circulation! In particular, in cases of segmental transplants of the left lobe or lateral segment, the duct rarely lends itself to an end-to-end anastomosis. In children with biliary atresia a Roux-en-Y loop is required anyhow (Bismuth & Houssin, 1984, Broelsch et al. 1990).

The cut surface should represent an exact segmental/lobar anatomy to prevent bleeding or leakage from the soft parenchymal tissue (**Figure 18.2**). Unfortunately, hypoperfusion of small areas because of nonanatomical resections gives rise to severe infections and sepsis and, thus minimizes the functional parenchyma of the graft. In borderline cases, this can turn the balance of the graft into a nonfunctional one.

Dissection techniques guided by preoperative imaging of the organ have allowed easy, transparenchymal sparing of the organ tissue,

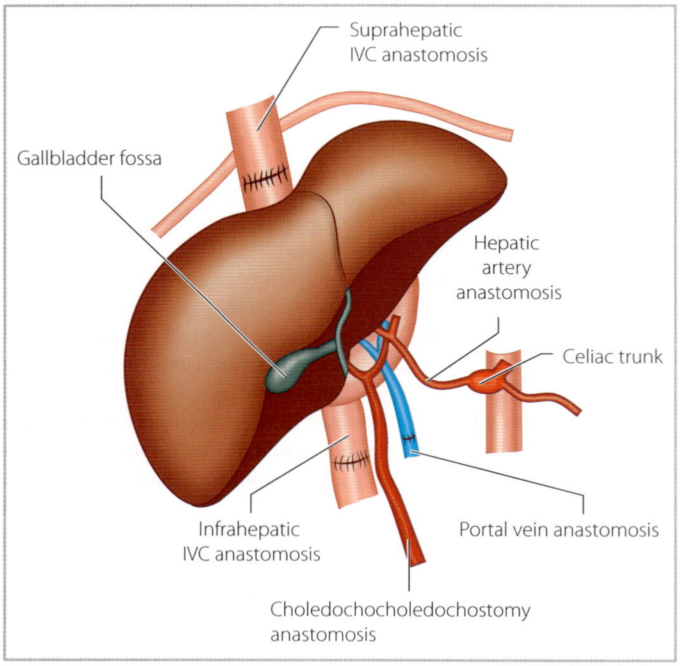

Figure 18.1 Orthotopic liver transplantation with preservation of the retrohepatic vena cava. 'Piggyback technique' to ascertain maximal venous outflow and avoid dissection of retroperitoneal collaterals. With permission from Savitsky et al. Evaluation of orthotopic liver transplant recipients presenting to the emergency department. Ann Emerg Med 1998; 31:507–517.

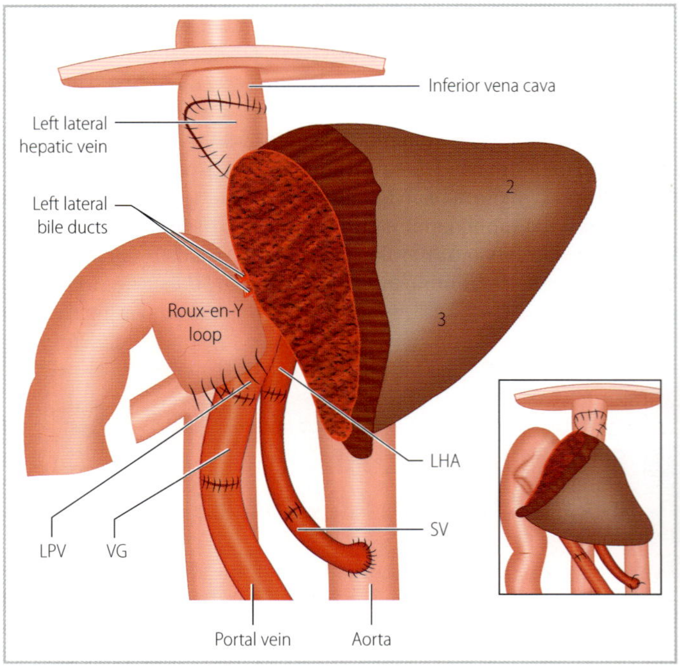

Figure 18.2 Completed recipient implantation of left lateral segment graft (segments 2 and 3) with two bile ducts. Interposition grafts [venous allograft (VG) and arterial interposition graft (AIG = SV)] were used for both hepatic artery (LHA) and portal vein (LPV) to assure adequate length. With permission from Broelsch et al. (1990).

while transparenchymal dissection during intact circulation of an organ yielded optimal grafts with few complications arising from the transplant itself (Fan et al. 2002, Nadalin et al. 2007, Rogiers et al. 1996) (**Table 18.1**).

In due consideration of a live donor or any partial hepatectomy, sufficient liver mass has to be maintained to sustain the life of an individual, while a compromise is unacceptable for both, donor and recipient. Graft size becomes relevant whenever a partial graft is used. Several studies have recommended a graft-to-body weight ratio (GBWR) of 0.8. Thus, a 50-kg individual should receive at least 400 mg liver parenchyma (Nadalin et al. 2007, Shehata et al. 2012). Interestingly, the GBWR required renders hepatic cell cultures to be ineffective in cases of needed liver support unless a critical mass can be substituted.

KIDNEY AND PANCREAS

Although thousands of kidney transplants have been performed worldwide since its inception in 1956 (Harrison et al. 1956), anatomical issues have rarely been discussed since the extraperitoneal approach was established using the vessels of the iliac fossa and its vicinity to the bladder. Arterial and venous anastomoses have been adapted to the anatomy of the donor organ, by end-to-side anastomoses either directly or by ex situ constructions of patches or joint orifices, observing a 10% incidence of polar arteries (Barba et al. 2013). Anastomoses between the transplant ureter and the bladder prevent antireflux by using established procedures like ureterocystostomies or pyeloureterostomies and prove to be reliable for primary anastomoses, as well as for diagnostic or reconstructive procedures (Saidi et al. 2012). Temporary stenting remains a matter of individual preference. In children, intra-abdominal placement of grafts is performed due to size differences using the vicinity of large iliac vessels or vena cava for anastomoses.

Implantation of the pancreas into the iliac fossa (intraperitoneally) and contralaterally to the implanted kidney allows for drainage into the bladder as well as through an enteric conduit (duodenum) into the small bowel. Both drainage procedures have their pros and cons in regard to early diagnosis of rejection by measuring amylase in the bladder versus destruction of the bladder wall and subsequent pain during urination. Today, enteric duct management is preferred, although there seems to be no difference in outcome as far as techniques are concerned in larger series (Humar et al. 2004, Gruessner & Sutherland 2005). However, improved results have led to an increase in solitary pancreas transplants. Also, pancreatic blood drainage into the portal vein instead of into a systemic vein has failed to provide a substantial survival benefit. Despite initial controversies, vascular reconstruction procedures often required in multiorgan harvesting to preserve the gastroduodenal artery as well as the pancreaticoduodenal artery have yielded favorable results (Molmenti et al. 2004).

Table 18.1 Accumulated indications for reintervention (%) following full-size liver transplants.

Complication	Incidence (%)
Biliary Surface leakage Anastomotic leakage Anastomotic stricture	13 69 23 8
Vascular	9
Hemorrhage	3
Nonspecific (e.g. peritonitis, ischemic parenchymal lesions, bowel obstruction, Roux-limb hemorrhage)	7

Modified from Taketomi et al. (2010).

Nevertheless, technical failures in pancreas and kidney transplants are still the highest in abdominal organ transplants, ranging from 12% to 33% depending on the sequence of operations, e.g. a simultaneous pancreas and kidney (SPK), a pancreas following the kidney (PAK), or an isolated pancreas transplant (PTA) (Banga et al. 2012, Sollinger et al. 2009). For SPK, relaparotomy rates range from 1 to 36 reoperations per patient with an enormous economic impact. PAK have a 25% probability of reoperation, while PTA account for 16%. In this context, organ quality is of paramount importance, because the use of older or marginal organs will definitely increase the rate of re-explorations. Recipients for pancreas transplants are severely diabetic, uremic, and immunocompromised. Intra-abdominally, two hollow viscera are involved in a multimorbid patient. Thus, morbidity and mortality are higher compared with other procedures in solid organ transplantation.

In terms of the need for reoperations, pancreas transplants require special expertise not only during implantation but even more so during the onset of complications, i.e. removing the graft, changing the drainage, extent of local damage, and chance of recovery. Kidney transplants have become such a routine that reoperation rate is below 5% in comparison with reoperation rates for general surgical patients such as with intra-abdominal infections.

Ureteral complications following simple leakages or necroses caused by lack of blood supply require reanastomosis and stenting or reconstructions using the recipient ureter (Saidi et al. 2012). However, malformations require the preparation of intestinal conduits (Barba et al. 2013).

TIMING OF REOPERATIONS

Any reoperation increases the length of hospital stay and health care costs aside from placing the patient to another risk! (Lock et al. 2010a, 2010b) Nevertheless, any failure to miss the point of reintervention can evolve into a life-threatening crisis for the immunosuppressed patient.

Early indications

Bleeding

In visceral transplants no abdomen is closed, while active bleeding still occurs. In the presence of coagulopathy due to liver failure or sepsis, correction of coagulation through platelets, clot factors, or plasma transfusions can be achieved, and toward the end of time-consuming operations, surgical bleeding is controlled. Occasionally, packing of the upper abdominal area around the liver and the retroperitoneum can be successful such as in severe liver trauma for staged reintervention, and removal of lap-pads and closure of the abdomen. In the intensive care unit (ICU), hemoglobin and hematocrit need to be measured hourly. Also, drainage output has to be measured. Dilution factors during fluid resuscitation should improve, while pulse rate, urine output, central venous pressure (CVP), and/or pulmonary artery pressure (PAP) indicate stability of the circulation. Slow, continuous drop of the hematocrit despite transfusion is indicative of ongoing intra-abdominal blood loss. Hence, examination of the abdominal circumference and the tenderness of the abdomen provide clues about the intra-abdominal situation. Percutaneous drainages placed around critical sites toward the end of an operation present a doubtful reliance when the efflux does not correspond to the clinical parameters!

Primary graft failure

Although a rare incidence since the established use of Euro-Collins solution (ECS) or histidine – tryptophan – ketoglutarate solution (HTK), primary graft failure (PGF) requires immediate attention and verification either by exploration and exclusion of correctable factors or other interventional measures, such as biopsy or angiography. Specific functional tests are employed by some centers most often representing cellular destruction, mitochondrial enzyme release, failure to correct coagulopathy, bile production, urine output, hyperglucosemia, and intestinal motility (Singer et al. 1989). Early removal of the graft (pancreas) or retransplantation (liver) presents the only treatment option, which obviously then depends on graft availability. Several days of monitoring are accredited to a center by the organ distribution agency to allow for an urgent request for another organ (high urgency). Nonvital organs (e.g. kidney, pancreas, and small bowel) can be left in situ but need to be removed quickly once they cause infectious, toxic, or circulatory problems (i.e. hyperacute rejection).

For a vital liver graft, a rescue graft can be awaited in an anhepatic state. Personal experience with a few cases (<5) over 30 years has not yielded any long-term survival (unpublished data). In cadaveric kidney transplants, grafts may require several weeks to resume reasonable function and do not need to be removed unless local reasons call for reintervention. PGF can almost be suspected once certain donor risk factors accumulate like age >65 years, prolonged ischemia time, circulatory instability, hypernatremia, and respiratory-intensive care treatment >7 days (Freeman 2013).

Initial graft dysfunction

Within 72 hours post-transplant, graft function should reveal itself according to its organ-specific parameters, e.g. bile secretion, correction of coagulopathy and encephalopathy after a liver transplant, urine output and creatinine clearance after a kidney transplant, and correction of serum glucose after a pancreas transplant. Delayed function can be temporarily compensated by support medication, dialysis, or plasmapheresis. Reintervention is definitely required whenever indefinable causes are suspected, i.e. vascular occlusion, partial necrosis of the graft, early leakages, and intestinal obstructions; delayed incidences of graft function are sometimes foreseeable and dependent on the various retrieval procedures (Lock et al. 2010a) but can usually be compensated.

Vascular stenosis occlusion

Arterial thrombosis has decreased to <5–7% (Cherqui et al. 2002, Sotiropoulos et al. 2011) in all transplants as causes of relaparotomy and graft failure, except for pancreas transplants. Detected <12 hours post-transplant by Doppler ultrasound or angiography, revascularization presents a valid option for organ rescue, though even partial graft necrosis can lead to sepsis and multiorgan failure (Broelsch et al. 1990). Removal of necrotic areas can be successful but often provides only a temporary solution with ultimate graft failure. In principle, any graft remains vital only with a homogenous circulation, while a defect graft resembles a 'timebomb' within a body. In particular, operative techniques using microscopes and appropriate adaptation of anastomotic sites have led to significant decrease in such complications (Fan et al. 2002, Lock et al. 2010a, Shehata et al. 2012, Wang et al. 2008).

In contrast, portal vein occlusion often remains compatible with sufficient graft function in liver transplantation, while in other transplants, venous drainage (pancreas, small bowel, and kidney) remains as essential as arterial inflow (Northup et al. 2009).

Hepatic venous outflow also needs to allow for unrestricted sinusoidal drainage into the low-pressure right atrium. An extremely rare intervention can be provided by stenting rather than operation! Appropriate adaptation of outflow sites by triangular incision of the vena cava in children (Millis et al. 2000) and the use of piggyback implantations of the graft have minimized the incidence of outflow problems, which were addressed already in the early years of transplantation (Calne & Williams 1968).

Drainage and leakage

Biliary drainage has long been the 'Achilles heel' in liver transplantation, but has lost its perils. Modifications of end-to-end or side-to-side anastomoses with or without T-Tubes performed under scrutiny with magnifiers have proven to be safe as well as Roux-en-Y anastomoses even with multiple ductules as required in reduced size or living-related transplants (Malago et al. 2003).

Bile, amylase or intestinal secretion, urinary leakage into the abdomen within the first days or week of transplantation requires reoperation, no matter how much! Most complications following kidney transplants are located in the iliac fossa around the ureterocystostomy. Fluid collections, lymphoceles, and perirenal hematomas, with or without wound infection, require local revisions and decompression.

In small bowel transplantation, anastomotic dehiscences, necroses, or infections require surgical repair by either reconstruction or exteriorization through fistulas or stomata. The immunocompromised status of the patient warrants particular consideration.

Late complications

Persistent graft dysfunction

Any graft eventually has to function normally to restore the patient's health and quality of life. Dysfunctions caused by reperfusion or rejection normally do not require reoperations; however, in small bowel, particularly in multivisceral transplants (small bowel plus liver plus kidney plus pancreas), various sites require reinspection, biopsies, partial removal of a single graft and, thus, present an ongoing alert to the transplant surgeon for monitoring and immediate re-exploration sometimes only because of anxiety!

Graft dysfunction can persist and deteriorate with or without obstruction of bile duct, pancreatic duct, or ureter. For the liver, obstruction through sludge or stenosis leads to irreversible intrahepatic dilatation of the biliary system and cholestasis; similarly for the kidney, obstruction through sludge or stenosis leads to hydronephrosis, and in the pancreas, depending on the drainage site, leads to necrotic inflammation. Parenchymal destruction can cause dysfunction as well through ischemia, rejection, or inflammation.

Within the first 3 months after liver transplantation, enzyme release, vanishing bile ducts, and progressive cholestasis unresponsive to antirejection therapy are indicative of chronic rejection or even early recurrence of a viral or an autoimmune disease of the liver. In the kidney, glomeruli and tubuli are affected by inflammation and/or necroses. Kidney function is monitored by measuring urine output and creatinine clearance. Pancreas function is measured by serum glucose and insulin dependency of the recipient. Through a pancreatocystostomy, amylase can be measured through the bladder. Excretory blockage of a graft still provides sufficient residual endocrine functions. Thus, for reoperation, a clear, mechanical, correctable or infectious cause of disturbance needs to be identified.

Source of infection

Despite ultrasound, magnetic resonance imaging, and refined computed tomography (CT) diagnostics, repeat infections or ongoing sepsis often require search for the focus by exploration, drainage, and abdominal lavages. Specimen for bacterial cultures is mandatory to permit appropriate adjustment for antibiotic therapy. Infections can occur at any time point during the course and require diagnosis by sampling from any external site, fluids, or feces as well as from the lung and abdomen. Locally confined infections surrounding any visceral transplant require open lavage treatment and eventually stepwise abdominal closure. Almost always, an abdominal wall hernia develops and may require later repair.

Intestinal obstructions

The clinical diagnosis is made by conventional measures and occurs as often as in any conventional laparotomy. However, motility problems in small bowel transplants repeatedly require re-exploration, decompression, and elimination of the cause. Ischemic intestines and perforations do not allow for reanastomosis but require exteriorization due to the immunocompromised status of the patient.

Graft loss and retransplantation

Any patient receiving a transplant will either leave the hospital with a satisfactory functioning graft or never. Thus, reoperations including comprehensive diagnostic workups of the treatment aiming at redeeming the potential threat also inevitably produce costs.

While the costs of post-transplant complications accumulate in the length of stay, or number of readmissions, various studies (Brown et al. 2003, Lock et al. 2010a) have found that vascular complications increase costs by 62% and renal failure, coinciding with graft failure, by 175%. Not surprisingly, biliary leakages, primary nonfunctioning grafts and sepsis, double the costs of transplantation. Early identification of intra-abdominal causes of graft dysfunction by relaparotomy is therefore an opportunity to reduce costs rather than to increase expenditures.

Transplant-associated complications requiring surgery are frequent and any patient undergoing a transplant for a visceral organ, with the exception of the kidney, may face at least two to three other procedures to be done before discharge. Once a complication occurs, the repair itself and the additional trauma could potentially give rise to other complications. Most reports of transplant centers do not reveal the actual number of reinterventions, instead refer to patient and graft survival as the significant parameter. However, in calculating costs for transplant procedures, transplant-associated reinterventions should be included in the calculations along with other factors, i.e. the number of reoperations, length of stay in the ICU, pulmonary and/or renal failure, and graft loss.

The issue of retransplantation cannot be discussed within this context of reoperations. However, for a vital organ, retransplantation presents a lifesaving reoperation with two different contexts: Timely removal and replacement of a primary nonfunctioning graft are overtly different from retransplantation after 6 months or beyond a year after the first transplant. The outcome is not simply related to techniques but to different stages of the underlying diseases. Early retransplant rates are similar to late ones (7–11%) (Brown et al. 2003, Northup et al. 2009) yielding survival rates beyond 80% for the first year. In contrast, the results for the latter group in view of donor organ scarcity may justify the use of a graft for recurrent organ failure due to infection, recurrent disease, or uncontrollable rejection. The desperate – though inevitable – attempt to rescue a failing graft with strong antirejection, antiviral, or antibiotic therapy leads to more sepsis and in some series leads to 60% death (Freeman 2013). This ethical issue is very challenging.

REOPERATIONS

Any reoperation following the primary transplant procedure has to target the obvious cause either originating from the graft itself or from the surrounding organs. The indication has to consider the immunocompromised status of the patient and thus, has to relieve any infectious source, any anastomotic leakages, and any potential source creating ischemia with subsequent necroses such as caused by vascular thromboses.

In liver transplantation, postoperative bleeding presented the most frequent indication for reintervention in the past. The patient with a severe coagulopathy can be successfully managed through the operation by substitution of plasma, factors, platelets, and red blood cells. Intraoperative monitoring of fibrinolysis and coagulopathy, rapid transfusions, prevention of loss of body temperature, and improved surgical techniques that shorten the operations usually below 6–8 hours have eliminated previous risk factors. Rarely, a patient expires on the operation table due to circulatory arrest despite the preoperative critical status. Thirty years ago, anesthesiologists rejected the institution of a liver transplant program by saying 'It is a hundred hour procedure, with a hundred units of blood and a hundred percent mortality.' Today, some patients leave the operating room extubated and spontaneously breathing.

The most frequent need for a reoperation in visceral organ transplantation occurs within the first 3–5 days! Depending on the type of transplant received, monitoring of arterial and venous (portal) flow by Doppler ultrasound presents the standard, while any minor changes of even failure of arterial flow require immediate reoperation. If in doubt, make sure that the transplant is well perfused and the first reoperation often presents a quasi 'second look,' whereby irrigation, control of anastomoses, and evacuation of minor hematomas can also be performed. Interruption of blood flow has to be detected immediately and restored, while graft examination per se prevents graft failure.

Any transplant connected to a part of intestines faces particular immunological responses and allows intra-abdominal infections including sepsis. Abdominal closure calls for multiple reinterventions under strong immunosuppression. Healing is delayed, endangering other intra-abdominal anastomoses. The reoperation rate for pancreas transplants ranges from 50% to 60%, frequently involving a sequence of reoperations attempting to return to an undisturbed healing process. In some Western countries, only 'standard' transplants like kidney or liver are covered by health insurances. The costs of any 'additional' organs like pancreas or small bowel have to be covered by the primary procedure. This economical imbalance causes the variable incidence of transplant procedures even throughout the Western world.

For liver transplantation, reoperation rates range between 15% and 60% depending on the graft received. Considering an identical outcome, however, recipients of split grafts have to face a significant higher chance of a necessary reoperation as compared with full-size grafts (Broering et al. 2004, Busuttil & Goss 1999, Renz et al. 2004, Taketomi et al. 2010). Reoperations of kidney recipients alone are <8% including high-risk obese patients, retransplant patients, and elderly patients receiving double kidney grafts from elderly donors presenting a high standard in surgical techniques.

PREOPERATIVE IMAGING

Particular imaging for transplantation of visceral organs is practically only required for segmental liver transplantation. Other organs, like kidneys or pancreas, not even require any more preharvesting angiography to detect aberrant arteries. However, retrieval teams have to carefully consider their responsibility to the transplant surgeons, to deliver intact, well-perfused grafts including intact vascular pedicles. Preparing liver grafts from live donors, today, noninvasive CT provides information about vascular anatomy, feeding or drainage of individual liver segments, and, specifically, the biliary anatomy. Primarily, live donors are subjected to imaging procedures detailing the lobar anatomy of livers and kidneys. The historical description of Couinaud fails to allow for safe separation of liver segments, although the principle of a segmental anatomy of the liver still prevails.

The need for small grafts for children, coinciding with advances in hepatic surgery for removing cancerous lesions, originated the idea of reducing the size of a transplant, to fit the need for space and function in the abdomens of small babies (Broering et al. 2004, Millis et al. 2000). However, there was no gain in organs, by simply reducing organs for children, leaving the major portion unused (Bismuth & Houssin 1984, Broering et al. 2004). The application of split livers in the eighties, initially, gave rise to additional complications at the site of dissection, but was eventually established for the use between donor and a child recipient (Busuttil & Goss 1999, Northup et al. 2009, Renz et al. 2004).

In 1989, individual transplants from live donors were performed until the Chicago Series was published presenting an ethical protocol for the selection and performance of 20 consecutive cases with equivalent results (Broelsch et al. 1988, Broering et al. 2004). The donors were subjected to celiac angiography and simple hepatic CT volumetry. The information obtained was helpful, but did not include biliary anatomy. Thus, initial obstacles in any segmental or lobar transplants evolved around biliary complications. Endoscopic retrograde cholangiography (ERC) became necessary to identify abnormalities at the cost of some few cases of pancreatitis. Thus, morbidity during semi-invasive donor examination was considerable and switching to appropriate, informative imaging procedures became mandatory. Innovative research cooperation with the MeVIS Institution yielded the nowadays widespread application of three-dimensional CT to identify the precise segmental/lobar anatomy of the donor organ, which is presently widely being used prior to hepatic resections for cancer removal as well.

In contrast to the simplified anatomy of the liver consisting of two lobes encompassing eight individual segments, the specifics are notoriously variable when a surgical approach is being planned. The problems start in the hilum and extend into the intrahepatic branching of the vessels and bile ducts. Each aberration can result in a complicated reoperation affecting donors and recipients equivalently. While on the donor side, there is no 'margin for error,' the recipient side needs to be well dissected.

For adult recipients, the right lobe is being used because of its size and its divisible structure, particularly its individual venous drainage, while the cut surface can be severed and secured with stitches. The biliary system gives rise to frequent reoperations because of its unpredictable branching within the hilum and the intraparenchymal distribution (Malago et al. 2002, Northup et al. 2009). Only in the last few decades, surgical approach into the hilum for the treatment of cancer was feasible. The operation of the donor has to extend far deeper into the recipient part of the liver because integrity on the donor side presents the primary necessity. Thus, the computer-assisted three-dimensional CT and color Doppler ultrasonography have allowed the evaluation of functional remnant volumes, decreasing the need for extended resections and vascular reconstructions. Several software packages are available for this purpose like HepaVision (MeVis Medical Solutions AG, Bremen, Germany) (**Figure 18.3**) (Malago et al. 2003, Radtke et al. 2010).

In essence, a three-dimensional virtual resection can be performed prior to surgery outlining the critical phases of dissection and even decide about risk or inoperability of the procedure. With these logistics, operations were performed to allow for reanastomoses of multiple bile ducts even in an end-to-side fashion and to reconstruct venous outflow by using autologous or allograft patches.

RECIPIENT REOPERATIONS

Initially, 30% of reoperations had to deal with biliary tract leakages or stenoses. Today, early complications rarely entail <10% of the indications for reoperation. Consequent monitoring of blood flow by Doppler ultrasound accounts for another 5–8% for detecting blood flow changes or even clotting of the nutrient vessel. The small graft is usually exposed to elevated portal blood flow in a cirrhotic recipient, and graft edema develops a higher parenchymal resistance to the arterial flow, while the arterial inflow presents the same condition. Thus, immediate response is required to investigate the cause. Sometimes pharmacological lowering of vascular resistance suffices. Sometimes reanastomosis or portal venous banding is required, maybe even shunting, when the flow exceeds an estimated limit of >1.5 L/min. The pattern of complications and reoperations resembles the findings in the split series, which definitely show that receiving a surgically cut down transplant presents a chance of >10% to undergo a reoperation, while the survival statistic is identical even at a higher MELD score (>31) (Nadalin et al. 2006, Sotiropoulos et al. 2011).

Complications in liver transplantation can be frequent and severe. However, 'The worst complication is to receive no transplant at all.' *(H. Bismuth)*

DONOR REOPERATIONS

The healthy donor, subjected to any reoperation following the primary procedure, requires utmost attention! For comparison of various complications, classifications have been established varying between I (= no complication) and VI (= death) (Dindo et al. 2004). For a live donor, surgical complications present only a somatic portion of the event, but equally severe, psychological traumata can develop and possibly persist for quite longer time. There are two classifications published describing minor, major, and severe complications. Our own classification includes psychiatric aspects accompanied by surgical complications and adds chronic abnormalities, which have rarely occurred (Nadalin et al. 2006, Nadalin et al. 2007).

Thus, indications for reoperation present grade lll and lV and account for <7% of all postoperative morbidities. Reports mostly include biliary leakages or bleeding from the cut surface of right hemihepatectomies. Left lateral segmentectomies can result in >90% of cases without any even minor complication and virtually no reoperation. A substantial part of reoperations results in pre-emptive laparotomies to explore and exclude potential threats. The application of minimal invasive techniques is expected to reduce regional complications because of less trauma to the abdomen (Buell et al. 2009, Cherqui et al. 2002), while hernia repairs were the most frequent reason for reoperation (<W3%).

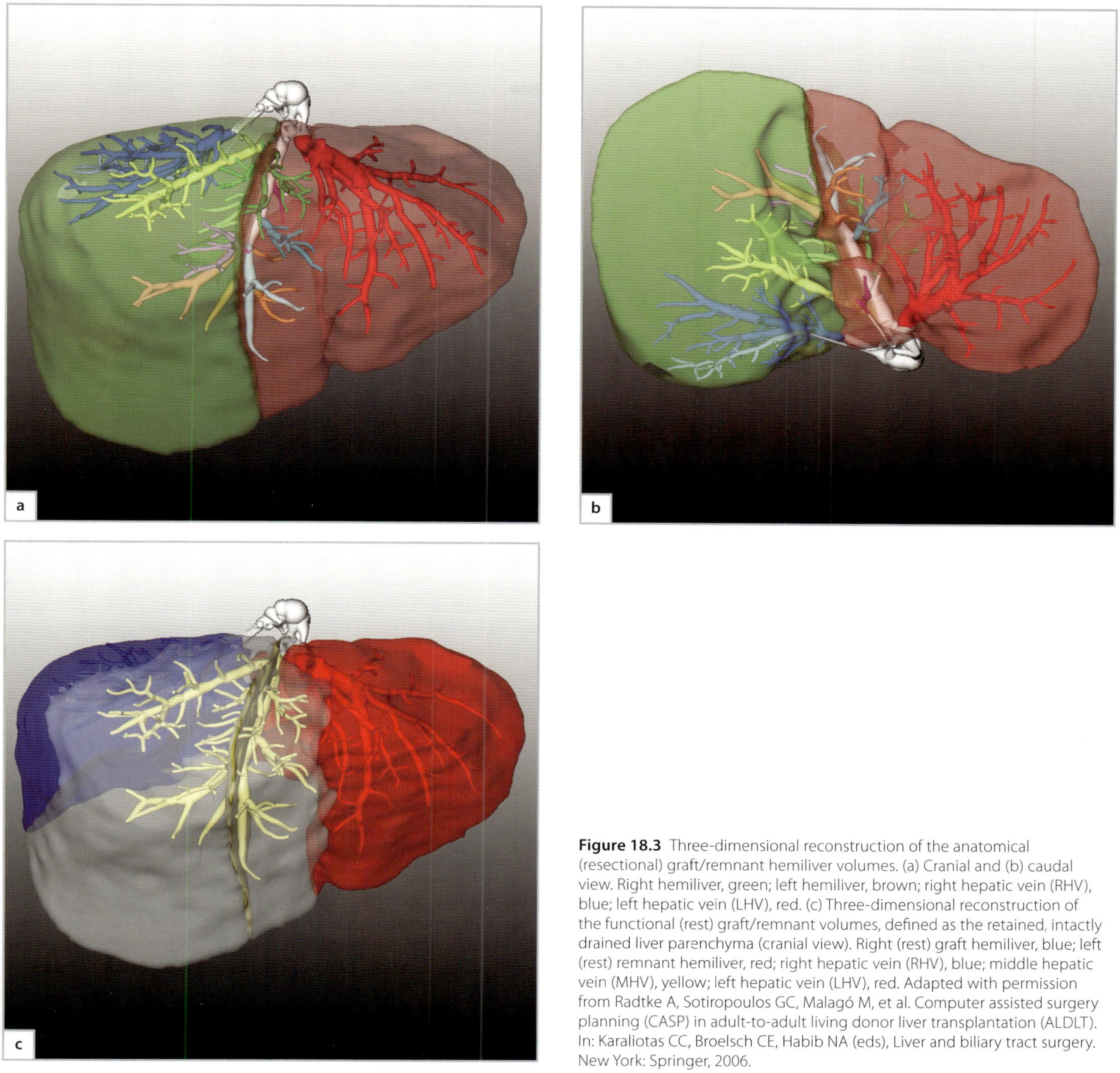

Figure 18.3 Three-dimensional reconstruction of the anatomical (resectional) graft/remnant hemiliver volumes. (a) Cranial and (b) caudal view. Right hemiliver, green; left hemiliver, brown; right hepatic vein (RHV), blue; left hepatic vein (LHV), red. (c) Three-dimensional reconstruction of the functional (rest) graft/remnant volumes, defined as the retained, intactly drained liver parenchyma (cranial view). Right (rest) graft hemiliver, blue; left (rest) remnant hemiliver, red; right hepatic vein (RHV), blue; middle hepatic vein (MHV), yellow; left hepatic vein (LHV), red. Adapted with permission from Radtke A, Sotiropoulos GC, Malagó M, et al. Computer assisted surgery planning (CASP) in adult-to-adult living donor liver transplantation (ALDLT). In: Karaliotas CC, Broelsch CE, Habib NA (eds), Liver and biliary tract surgery. New York: Springer, 2006.

Anticipated long case and need for consultants

Any organic disease eventually requiring a transplant is preceded by a lengthy course of suffering, treated by medical specialists such as hepatogastroenterologists, nephrologists, or pediatricians. Already in the pretransplant phase, they often present the decisive consultants as to the time of transplantation as well as thereafter. The surgeon's role is not of the 'technician' to retrieve and implant the graft, but to continue the treatment and to assure the vitality of the graft in the context of secondary recovery of other organ systems. Thus, a transplanted patient remains a 'surgical patient forever, but not any more a suffering individual.'

Following discharge, most expertise in the long run is required to monitor organ function, sustain effective immunosuppression, and prevent recurrence of the original disease. The basis of immunosuppression still is corticosteroids, although in minimal application, complemented by purin derivatives (mycophenolate mofetil), calcineurin inhibitors (e.g. cyclosporin, sirolimus, and tacrolimus), and/or m-Tor inhibitors (everolimus). Since its gradual introduction in 1981, results have skyrocketed and survival rates exceeded any expectation of earlier years. Pharmacological monitoring allows for effective immunosuppression by determining the appropriate trough level. The clinical follow-up requires both the medical specialist in clinical chemistry and consultant services, mainly pathologists and microbiologists.

The number of prospective studies to minimize side effects and simultaneously sustain efficacy of immunosuppression is legion! While in the immediate post-transplant period rejection has lost its perils, nephrotoxicity, beta cell toxicity, development of skin cancer, and lymphoma and recurrent diseases present new side effects in the long term.

At present patients with diseases of viral or immunological origin may experience recurrence of their diseases after years of survival at a high rate. Prevention seems only feasible in viral hepatitis infections, most effectively in hepatitis B virus by application of hyperimmunoglobulin (Hepatect) sustaining an antibody level >200 ng/mL. Viral monitoring (i.e. replication rates of DNA, RNA, and genotype determinations) through consultant specialists is a constituent for a transplant team as are pathologists for determining the differential diagnosis between rejection, recurrence, or persistent ischemic or structural damage through biopsy.

Treatment for hepatitis C virus consists of application of pegylated interferon and ribavirin with different response rates depending on genotype and dosage. However, the progression of the disease after transplantation can be accelerated with 25% of recipients, developing cirrhosis within 5 years requiring retransplantation.

CONDUCT OF OPERATION

Transplantation of visceral organs has evolved from various specializations in general surgery and urology. While a plastic surgeon (Joseph E. Murray) began with kidney transplants in identical twins to circumvent immunosuppression (Brown et al. 2003), the task was taken up by general, pediatric, and urological surgeons to serve their particular patients. Further specialization in hepatobiliary pancreatic surgery focused on the right upper quadrant to eventually combine physiological, immunological, and technical understanding of the specific need of transplanting isolated abdominal organs.

Professional requirements needed to conduct any transplant procedure depend on training and verification programs that differ worldwide. Transplantation depends on organ availability, which is contingent on individual preparedness to donate after death or as live donors. Willingness to donate depends on legislation and public opinion. Transplanters conduct their work under the public eye, definitely not intending to withhold criticism, deterring stories and, thus, always remaining within the scope of control and regulations.

The unusual 'material' transplantation requirements demand the highest degree of ethical and technical conduct. Ever since its inception and widespread application, organ transplantation has presented its problems, developments, and results in a transparent and organized fashion, i.e. data controlling, adaptation of allocation rules for scarce organs, and establishment of consulting and controlling committees. Nevertheless, the technical and scientific conduct of transplant procedures was guided by pioneers in the field, namely Thomas Starzl in the United States, Sir Roy Calne in the United Kingdom, Henry Bismuth in France and Rudolf Pichlmayr in Germany. Initially, heavily criticized by the medical community, these pioneers pushed the limits to improve techniques, immunosuppression, and selection criteria. In the course, they contributed massively to the development of new fields in medicine, in particular, hepatology.

Live donation has been part of transplantation from the start in kidney transplantation (Harrison et al. 1956). Since 1983, within the evolution of liver transplantation the need for organs became dramatic for pediatric recipients with biliary atresia. By size reduction and splitting of larger adult grafts, mortality of children on the waiting list declined (Millis et al. 2000). Initially inferior results had to be overcome, to establish the procedure in particular, when organs were split after harvesting (Broering et al. 2004, Rogiers et al. 1996).

The ethical guidelines for conducting live donor operations were established according to the following principles: need for the procedure, an alternative for the procedure, and an informed consent (Singer et al. 1989). Although cadaveric organ donation still remains the backbone of transplantation, live donation should be offered whenever a frame within ethical guidelines allows for responsible conduct.

In countries with limited or absent cadaveric organ donation (e.g. Korea and Japan), live donor procedures are being performed by thousands. The ethical conduct remains within the competence and responsible selection of candidates by the physicians and surgeons and it has convincingly been demonstrated that the responsibility is being seriously executed by surgeons as well as by their institutions. By contrast, in Western countries media and public consider the live donor procedure a disproportionate risk for the healthy donor converting it into a substantial risk for any surgeon or transplant center drawn under public critic. The pressure discourages surgeons to progress with this particular procedure, which is by now carried out mostly for children, where the donor operation is limited to the left lateral segment, easily being performed by laparoscopic approaches (Buell et al. 2009, Cherqui et al. 2002).

Postoperative principles and other treatments to maximize results do not differ from general surgical practices, except for keeping in mind that a transplant recipient remains extremely receptive for tissue healing and for viral infections like Epstein–Barr virus (EBV) or cytomegalovirus (CMV) and any bacterial seeding (Terrault 2012). Prevention of drug toxicity, disease recurrence and rejection are equally important factors as patient compliance and monitoring by competent and committed physicians.

REFERENCES

Audet M, Piardi T, Panaro F, et al. Four hundred and twenty-three consecutive adults piggy-back liver transplantations with the three suprahepatic veins: was the portal systemic shunt required? J Gastroenterol Hepatol 2010; 25:591–596.

Banga N, Hadjianastassiou VG, Mamode N, et al. Outcome of surgical complications following simultaneous pancreas-kidney transplantation. Nephrol Dial Transplant 2012; 27:1658–1663.

Barba J, Algarra R, Romero L, et al. Recipient and donor risk factors for surgical complications following kidney transplantation. Scand J Urol 2013; 47:63–71.

Bismuth H, Houssin D. Reduced-sized orthotopic liver graft in hepatic transplantation in children. Surgery 1984; 95:367–370.

Broelsch CE, Emond JC, Thistlethwaite JR, et al. Liver transplantation, including the concept of reduced-size liver transplants in children. Ann Surg 1988; 208:410–420.

Broelsch CE, Emond JC, Whitington PF, et al. Application of reduced-size liver transplants as split grafts, auxiliary orthotopic grafts, and living related segmental transplants. Ann Surg 1990; 212:368–375; discussion 375–377.

Broering DC, Wilms C, Bok P, et al. Evolution of donor morbidity in living related liver transplantation: a single-center analysis of 165 cases. Ann Surg 2004; 240:1013–1024; discussions 1024–1026.

Brown RS, Jr., Russo MW, Lai M, et al. A survey of liver transplantation from living adult donors in the United States. N Engl J Med 2003; 348:818–825.

Buell JF, Cherqui D, Geller DA, et al. The international position on laparoscopic liver surgery: The Louisville Statement, 2008. Ann Surg 2009; 250:825–830.

Busuttil RW, Goss JA. Split liver transplantation. Ann Surg 1999; 229:313–321.

Calne RY, Williams R. Liver transplantation in man. I. Observations on technique and organization in five cases. Br Med J 1968; 4:535–540.

Cherqui D, Soubrane O, Husson E, et al. Laparoscopic living donor hepatectomy for liver transplantation in children. Lancet 2002; 359:392–396.

Dindo D, Demartines N, Clavien PA. Classification of surgical complications: a new proposal with evaluation in a cohort of 6336 patients and results of a survey. Ann Surg 2004; 240:205–213.

Fan ST, Lo CM, Liu CL, Tso WK, Wong J. Biliary reconstruction and complications of right lobe live donor liver transplantation. Ann Surg 2002; 236:676–683.

Freeman RB. Deceased donor risk factors influencing liver transplant outcome. Transpl Int 2013; 5:463–470.

Gruessner AC, Sutherland DE. Pancreas transplant outcomes for United States (US) and non-US cases as reported to the United Network for Organ Sharing (UNOS) and the International Pancreas Transplant Registry (IPTR) as of June 2004. Clin Transplant 2005; 19:433–455.

Harrison JH, Merrill JP, Murray JE. Renal homotransplantation in identical twins. Surg Forum 1956; 6:432–436.

Humar A, Ramcharan T, Kandaswamy R, et al. Technical failures after pancreas transplants: why grafts fail and the risk factors – a multivariate analysis. Transplantation 2004; 78:1188–1192.

Koneru B, Tzakis AG, Bowman J, 3rd, et al. Postoperative surgical complications. Gastroenterol Clin North Am 1988; 17:71–91.

Lock J, Reinhold T, Bloch A, et al. The cost of graft failure and other severe complications after liver transplantation – experience from a German Transplant Center. Ann Transplant 2010a; 15:11–18.

Lock JF, Schwabauer E, Martus P, et al. Early diagnosis of primary nonfunction and indication for reoperation after liver transplantation. Liver Transpl 2010b; 16:172–180.

Maki T, Slapak M. Can a heterotopically placed segmental liver graft be life-supporting? An affirmative finding. Br J Surg 1974; 61:33–39.

Malago M, Testa G, Frilling A, et al. Right living donor liver transplantation: an option for adult patients: single institution experience with 74 patients. Ann Surg 2003; 238:853–862; discussion 853–862.

Malago M, Testa G, Hertl M, et al. Biliary reconstruction following right adult living donor liver transplantation end-to-end or end-to-side duct-to-duct anastomosis. Langenbecks Arch Surg 2002; 387:37–44.

Millis JM, Cronin DC, Brady LM, et al. Primary living-donor liver transplantation at the University of Chicago: technical aspects of the first 104 recipients. Ann Surg 2000; 232:104–111.

Molmenti EP, Klein AS, Henry ML. Procurement of liver and pancreas allografts in donors with replaced/accessory right hepatic arteries. Transplantation 2004; 78:770–771.

Nadalin S, Bockhorn M, Malago M, et al. Living donor liver transplantation. HPB (Oxford) 2006; 8:10–21.

Nadalin S, Malago M, Radtke A, et al. Current trends in live liver donation. Transpl Int 2007; 20:312–330.

Northup PG, Abecassis MM, Englesbe MJ, et al. Addition of adult-to-adult living donation to liver transplant programs improves survival but at an increased cost. Liver Transpl 2009; 15:148–162.

Radtke A, Sotiropoulos GC, Molmenti EP, et al. Computer-assisted surgery planning for complex liver resections: when is it helpful? A single-center experience over an 8-year period. Ann Surg 2010; 252:876–883.

Renz JF, Emond JC, Yersiz H, Ascher NL, Busuttil RW. Split-liver transplantation in the United States: outcomes of a national survey. Ann Surg 2004; 239:172–181.

Rogiers X, Malago M, Gawad K, et al. In situ splitting of cadaveric livers. The ultimate expansion of a limited donor pool. Ann Surg 1996; 224:331–339; discussion 339–341.

Saidi RF, Elias N, Hertl M, et al. Urinary reconstruction after kidney transplantation: pyeloureterostomy or ureteroneocystostomy. J Surg Res 2013; 181:156–159.

Shehata MR, Yagi S, Okamura Y, et al. Pediatric liver transplantation using reduced and hyper-reduced left lateral segment grafts: a 10-year single-center experience. Am J Transplant 2012; 12:3406–3413.

Singer PA, Siegler M, Whitington PF, et al. Ethics of liver transplantation with living donors. N Engl J Med 1989; 321:620–622.

Sollinger HW, Odorico JS, Becker YT, D'Alessandro AM, Pirsch JD. One thousand simultaneous pancreas-kidney transplants at a single center with 22-year follow-up. Ann Surg 2009; 250:618–630.

Sotiropoulos GC, Radtke A, Molmenti EP, et al. Long-term follow-up after right hepatectomy for adult living donation and attitudes toward the procedure. Ann Surg 2011; 254:694–700; discussion 691–700.

Taketomi A, Morita K, Toshima T, et al. Living donor hepatectomies with procedures to prevent biliary complications. J Am Coll Surg 2010; 211:456–464.

Terrault N. Liver transplantation in the setting of chronic HCV. Best Pract Res Clin Gastroenterol 2012; 26:531–548.

Wang SN, Sturdevant M, Kandaswamy R, et al. Technical failure of the pancreas after SPK transplant: are these patients good candidates for later pancreas retransplant? Clin Transplant 2008; 22:50–54.

Chapter 19 Reoperative surgery for chronic inflammatory bowel disease

Fabrizio Michelassi, Léon Maggiori

INTRODUCTION

Crohn's disease and ulcerative colitis represent the two main chronic inflammatory bowel diseases in the Western world. Their cause is unknown and there is no curative medical treatment; surgical treatment is not curative in Crohn's disease either, but it is curative in ulcerative colitis if the entire colorectal mucosa is removed.

Crohn's disease is characterized by transmural bowel inflammation, which can affect any segment of the gastrointestinal tract from mouth to anus. This chronic inflammation can give rise to complications, such as strictures, abscesses, fistulae, hemorrhage, or malignant transformation, which are the main indications for surgery: despite optimal medical treatment, over 70% of all Crohn's patients require surgical treatment within 10 years of diagnosis (Bernell et al. 2000).

Surgical procedures in Crohn's patients are often challenging due to the presence of severe complications and to changes in the consistency of the tissues secondary to the disease and the medical treatment. This translates into a high rate of postoperative morbidity and reoperation. In addition, Crohn's disease is a recurring disease: up to 60% of Crohn's patients develop clinical symptoms of recurrence after their index procedure and up to 30% of the patients require additional surgical procedures (Chardavoyne et al. 1986, Michelassi et al. 1991, Post et al. 1996).

Ulcerative colitis is characterized by inflammation generally limited to the mucosa, which may affect the entire rectum and colon. Despite optimal medical treatment, ulcerative colitis may develop preneoplastic or neoplastic changes, or may result in multiple loose bowel movements daily, occasionally bloody, with weight loss and cachexia. Occasionally patients need to be admitted to the hospital for frank hemorrhage or toxic megacolon. When premalignant or malignant lesions are found on surveillance colonoscopy or medical treatment fails, surgical treatment is indicated.

Many surgical procedures are available for ulcerative colitis: proctocolectomy with ileostomy, abdominal colectomy with ileorectal anastomosis, and proctocolectomy with Kock pouch. Yet, nowadays the preferred surgical procedure in the majority of patients is a restorative proctocolectomy with J-pouch ileoanal anastomosis. Due to its magnitude and complexity, this procedure is complicated by some postoperative morbidity and by long-term complications, both requiring surgical reinterventions (Sagar & Pemberton 2012).

This chapter reviews early and late postoperative complications in Crohn's disease and ulcerative colitis in need of reoperation. Complications that do not need surgical treatment (i.e. superficial site infections, prolonged postoperative ileus, and decreased fertility after a pelvic pouch procedure) or complications after rare procedures (i.e. proctocolectomy with Kock pouch) are not dealt within this chapter.

GENERAL CONSIDERATIONS

Preoperative

Optimal preoperative evaluation and planning are essential prior to reoperative surgery to formulate an appropriate interventional strategy that assures the highest likelihood of success and the lowest chance of complications and unsatisfactory results. In the absence of emergent surgical indications, such as profuse hemorrhage or severe sepsis, preoperative assessment of the general conditions of the patient and of the extent of the disease should be as complete as possible.

In the immediate postoperative period after a major intestinal procedure for Crohn's disease or ulcerative colitis, imaging often relies on abdominal and pelvic computed tomography (CT) scans with both intravenous and oral contrast to assess the presence of intra-abdominal or pelvic fluid collections and abscesses, intestinal obstruction, and anastomotic dehiscences. If a dehiscence of an ileoanal anastomosis is suspected, an examination under anesthesia of the anal canal and ileal pouch-anal anastomosis (IPAA) may be necessary in addition to a pelvic CT scan or magnetic resonance imaging (MRI) to better define the degree of dehiscence and to inform optimal drainage.

Upper and lower endoscopy, CT. and/or an MR enterography (MRE) are well suited to investigate new complications that have arisen long time after a previous procedure for Crohn's disease. MRE is the most sensitive and specific imaging procedure for Crohn's disease assessment (Rimola et al. 2009) and it allows distinction between active inflammatory strictures, which might be medically managed, and fibrotic strictures, which should be surgically treated (Zappa et al. 2011). Well-contained intra-abdominal abscesses should be drained percutaneously, under radiologic guidance, prior to a surgical procedure, when feasible. If a patient is found to have a hydroureter or significant inflammation in proximity of the pelvic brim, consideration should be given to preoperative ureteral stenting to facilitate the conduct of the surgical procedure. By the same token, use of advanced abdominal wall reconstruction procedures (component separation, use of biological material) to decrease tension on the closure of an hostile abdominal wall or to repair complex hernias should be entertained and planned preoperatively. When operating for septic pelvic and perineal complications in Crohn's disease, consideration should be given to the use of muscular or myocutaneous flaps in the filling of the resultant pelvic dead space and in the closure of the perineum after an abdominal-perineal resection.

Pouchoscopy, pouchograms, CT, and/or an MRI are all well suited to investigate complications that have arisen in a pouch years after a restorative proctocolectomy with IPAA. An examination under anesthesia of the perineum, the anal canal, and the ileal pouch may be required to better understand the extent of the complication.

Patients with chronic inflammatory bowel disease frequently have severe metabolic derangements. Fluid and electrolytes abnormalities, anemia, and coagulopathies need to be aggressively corrected prior to any surgical intervention. Finally, reoperative surgery for inflammatory bowel disease often includes a stoma formation. Selection of the optimal placement of such stoma should be determined preoperatively (Bass et al. 1997) and will be preferably set over the rectus abdominis muscles, away from skin fold, navel, scars, or bony prominence.

Perioperative

Patients with chronic inflammatory bowel diseases are at high risk of postoperative superficial surgical site infections due to the nature of the procedure. Perioperative antibiotics need to be administered prior to skin incision and redosed appropriately. These patients are also at high risk of postoperative thromboembolic complications; hence they should receive perioperative deep vein thrombosis prophylaxis.

Intraoperative

Crohn's disease patients may have endured several previous surgical procedures and may present with dense adhesions. Inflammatory and septic complications may make adhesions difficult to lyse. These adhesions must be completely lysed in order to perform a thorough examination of the bowel to assess the location and the extent of the complications (strictures, phlegmonous masses, abscesses, fistulae) and to quantify the length of the remaining small bowel. We call this phase of the procedure 'the design of a road map.' A strategic approach to the patient's specific disease is then developed by studying the 'road map' and includes the use of strictureplasties, intestinal resections, drainage of abscesses, repair of fistulous openings on target intestinal loops or hollow viscera, or a combination of the above.

CROHN'S DISEASE

Bowel resection has represented the mainstay of surgical treatment for Crohn's disease complications until strictureplasties techniques were described in the early 80s by Emmanuel Lee (Lee & Papaioannou 1982) after he became aware of a similar technique for tubercular strictures of the terminal ileum described by Katariya et al. (1977). Strictureplasty is the treatment of choice for patients with symptomatic nonphlegmonous jejunoileal Crohn's fibrotic strictures, as highlighted in both American (Lichtenstein et al. 2009) and European (Dignass et al. 2010) guidelines for Crohn's disease management, especially in the recurrent setting. However, strictureplasty techniques are contraindicated when the patient is nutritionally profoundly impaired and in the presence of generalized peritonitis, a phlegmon, a thickened and unyielding intestinal wall, preneoplastic transformation (dysplasia), or cancer (Dietz et al. 2001, Roy & Kumar 2004).

Strictureplasty techniques may be divided into three subgroups: short, including the commonly performed Heineke–Mikulicz strictureplasty (**Figure 19.1**); intermediate, including the Finney strictureplasty (**Figure 19.2**); and long, like the side-to-side isoperistaltic strictureplasty (**Figure 19.3**). A large number of publications have highlighted the safety of strictureplasties for Crohn's disease. A meta-analysis, including >3000 strictureplasties, has been published in 2007 (Yamamoto et al. 2007). Overall, mortality was nil and 13% of patients developed postoperative complications, including 3% postoperative hemorrhages and 4% septic complications (anastomotic dehiscence, fistula, and abscess).

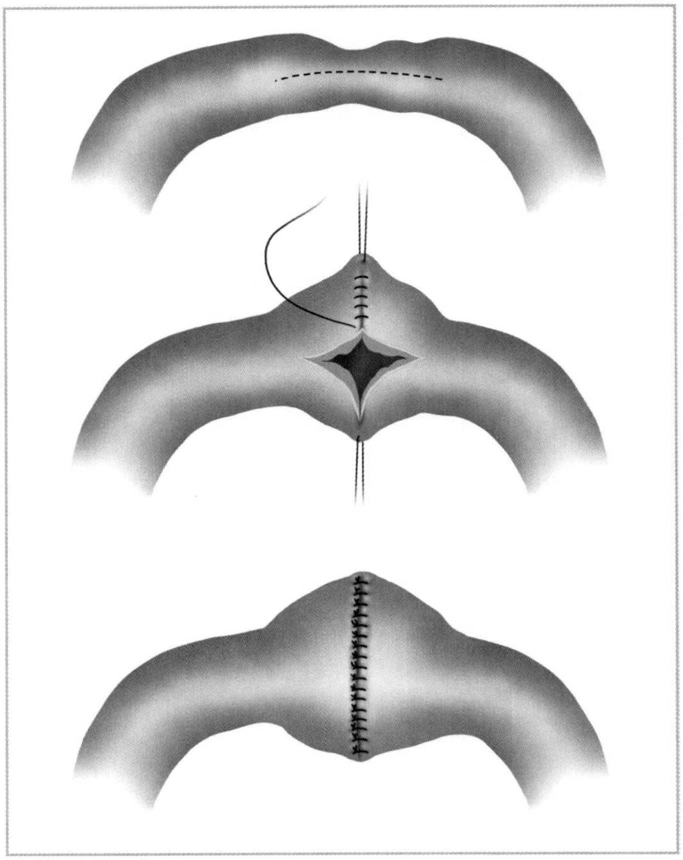

Figure 19.1 Heineke–Mikulicz strictureplasty. The most common strictureplasty technique is the Heineke–Mikulicz technique (Roy & Kumar 2004). Heineke–Mikulicz strictureplasties are optimal to address short strictures (≤7 cm). This technique is performed by making a longitudinal incision on the antimesenteric side of the bowel extending from 2 cm proximal to 2 cm distal to the stricture. The enterotomy is then closed in a transverse fashion in two layers using interrupted Lambert nonabsorbable 3-0 sutures for the outer layer and a running absorbable 3-0 suture for the inner layer.

Early postoperative complications

Hemorrhage

Hemorrhage can occur postoperatively after a bowel resection or after a strictureplasty, but the source of the hemorrhage differs after each one of the two procedures.

During a bowel resection, hemostatic control of the mesentery, which may be thickened and friable, can be quite challenging. In this situation, proximal control of the mesentery should be obtained with a large, noncrushing vascular clamp prior to transection of the mesentery. The cut edge of the mesentery is sequentially suture-ligated. The vascular clamp is then gradually released and additional suture ligatures are applied to the remaining bleeding vessels. Despite these maneuvers, postoperative hemoperitoneum requiring reoperation and control of the bleeding mesentery has been reported to occur in about 0.3–0.5% (Hurst et al. 1997).

After a bowel preserving procedure, the bleeding commonly originates from the strictureplasty site. Usually it is self-contained and does not require reoperation. If persistent, patients should undergo an angiogram to diagnose which strictureplasty is bleeding

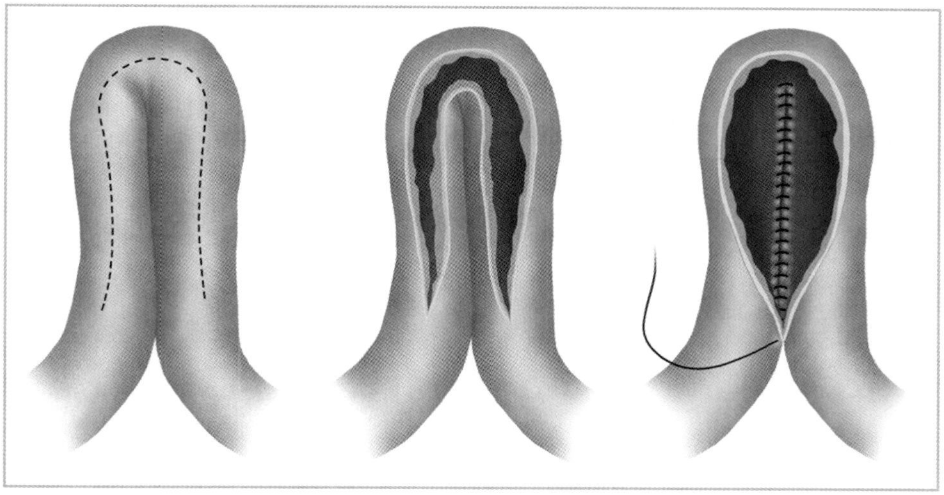

Figure 19.2 Finney strictureplasty. Intermediate length procedures, such as the Finney strictureplasty (Roy & Kumar 2004), are appropriate for longer strictures (> 7 cm and ≤15 cm). The strictured loop is folded over itself at its midpoint section, forming a 'U'-shaped configuration. An enterotomy is then performed half way between the mesenteric and the antimesenteric side on the folded loop. The opposed edges of the bowel are sutured together in a two-layer fashion to create a side-to-side isoperistaltic enteroenterostomy.

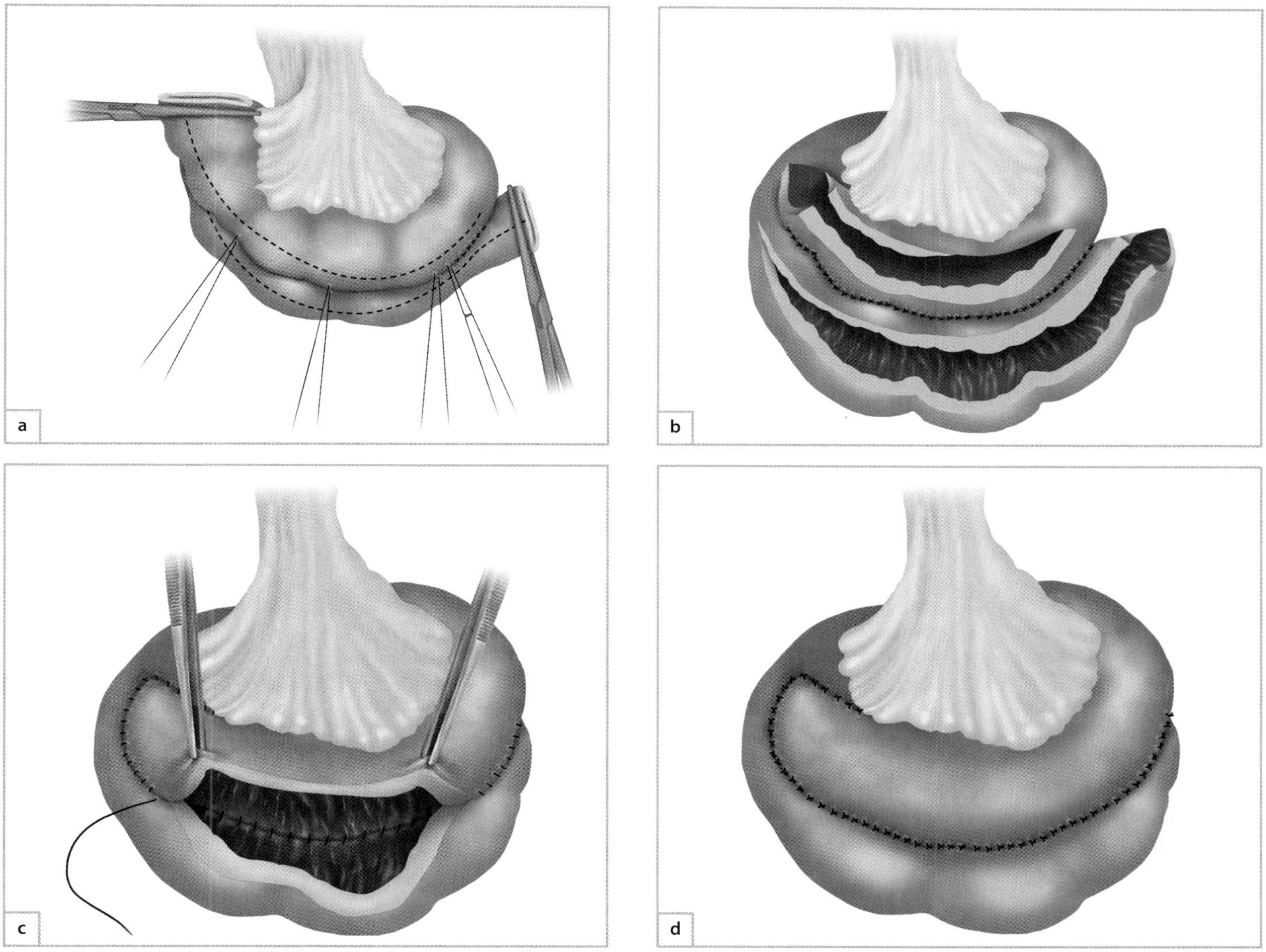

Figure 19.3 Side-to-side isoperistaltic strictureplasty. Finally, the side-to-side strictureplasty, first described in 1996 by the senior author (Michelassi 1996), is the technique of choice to address multiple short strictures closely clustered over a lengthy small bowel segment. In this technique, the mesentery of the small bowel loop to undergo the strictureplasty is first divided at its midpoint. The proximal intestinal loop is then moved over the distal one in a side-to-side fashion. Care is taken to ensure that stenotic areas of one loop are placed adjacent to the dilated areas of the other loop. The two loops are then approximated by a layer of interrupted seromuscular Lembert stitches, using nonabsorbable 3-0 sutures (a). A longitudinal enterotomy is performed on both loops, with the intestinal ends tapered to avoid blind stumps (b). Frozen-section biopsies of suspicious areas of disease are obtained in order to exclude occult malignancy. Hemostasis is obtained with suture ligatures or electrocautery. The outer suture line is reinforced with an internal row of running, full-thickness 3-0 absorbable sutures, continued anteriorly as a running Connell suture (c); this layer is reinforced by an outer layer of interrupted seromuscular Lembert stitches using non-absorbable 3-0 sutures (d).

in case of multiple strictureplasties and anastomoses. If the bleeding is identified, vasopressin can be infused into the feeding vessel in the hope of stopping the bleeding and avoiding surgery (Belaiche 1999). If the bleeding persists, the strictureplasty site needs to be explored and the bleeding controlled with topical measures or through a resection of the strictureplasty site.

Septic complications

The principles of treatment of postoperative septic complications and its timing after a resection and primary anastomosis or a strictureplasty in Crohn's disease do not differ from the principles followed after an intestinal resection for any other benign or malignant process and are based on the acuteness and severity of the presentation. In the presence of generalized peritonitis following a suture line dehiscence, appropriate antibiotics need to be started, resuscitation performed, and the patient needs to be explored promptly. The choice of a local repair of the dehiscence or a resection of the dehiscence with primary anastomosis or temporary stoma is based on the age and size of the dehiscence, the magnitude of the contamination, and the general conditions of the patient. Small abscesses (<2 cm in diameter) may be treated with antibiotics; larger abscesses need to be drained usually percutaneously, occasionally through a re-exploration. Enterocutaneous fistulae resulting from a dehiscence or a percutaneously drained abscess require initial control of sepsis with antibiotics and drainage, resuscitation, local care of the skin around the fistulous opening, possible parenteral nutrition, and surgical intervention 6–12 weeks later if the fistula does not heal.

Intestinal obstruction

Adhesive small bowel obstruction in Crohn's disease occurs in the early postoperative period with the same incidence after intestinal procedures for other benign and malignant intestinal disorders. Intestinal obstruction is a frequent postoperative complication after an abdominal colectomy with ileorectal anastomosis. The principles of treatment of early postoperative intestinal obstruction and the timing of possible surgical intervention in Crohn's disease do not differ from the principles followed after an intestinal resection for other benign or malignant intestinal processes.

Late postoperative complications

Recurrence

Crohn's disease is a recurrent disease (Bernell et al. 2000, Chardavoyne et al. 1986, Michelassi et al. 1991, Post et al. 1996). With the need for repeated intestinal resections, Crohn's patients may eventually develop short gut syndrome and intestinal insufficiency, leading to the need for total parenteral nutrition support. Recurrent surgery for Crohn's disease should therefore aim to address complications without jeopardizing bowel length and function.

Preoperative evaluation is mandatory to allow optimal surgical treatment of Crohn's disease recurrence (see General Consideration, *Preoperative*). A laparoscopic approach can be attempted in recurrent Crohn's disease. In 2010, Brouquet et al. compared the outcomes of 29 laparoscopic ileocolic resections for recurrent Crohn's disease to those of 33 open procedures for the same indication, suggesting that laparoscopic management of recurring Crohn's disease was feasible and safe, without an increase in postoperative morbidity as compared with the open approach, but was associated with a high-risk conversion (39%) (Brouquet et al. 2010). Two additional studies have compared results of primary and recurring Crohn's disease managed with laparoscopic approach, and did not observe any increased morbidity or conversion rate in patients with recurrent disease (Chaudhary et al. 2011, Hasegawa et al. 2003).

Crohn's recurrence in the rectum can be observed in 49–83% of patients at 10 years after abdominal colectomy with ileorectal anastomosis for Crohn's colitis (Cattan et al. 2002, Yamamoto & Keighley 2000). In medically refractory patients, this recurrent proctitis may lead to the necessity of a completion proctectomy, required in up to 20% of the cases (Cattan et al. 2002). The most commonly performed procedure in this setting is a completion proctectomy with end ileostomy. In the absence of suspected or demonstrated neoplastic transformation, the rectal dissection should be undertaken as close as possible to the rectal fascia, in order to avoid injury of the sympathetic and parasympathetic nerves. Postoperatively, the major complication is the occurrence of a pelvic sinus, observed in up to 25% of the patients (Yamamoto et al. 1999). To minimize this risk, and in the absence of severe perineal disease, the perineal dissection should be carried out along the intersphincteric plane, allowing preservation of the external sphincter for appropriate closure of the pelvic floor. Occasionally, however, septic complications of the anorectum and perineum may require an extensive resection of perineal skin and subcutaneous tissue. The resultant pelvic dead space needs to be filled with viable tissue (intestinal loops, omentum, muscle flaps) to avoid a postoperative pelvic abscess; similarly the resultant perineal defect may be too large for primary closure and its healing may therefore require muscular flaps or myocutaneous flaps (i.e. gluteal, gracilis, or myocutaneous rectus abdominis flaps) (Michelassi et al. 2000).

CANCER

Reports of development of small bowel adenocarcinoma arising at the site of strictureplasty have been documented. To date, four cases of such complication have been published (Jaskowiak & Michelassi 2001, Marchetti et al. 1996, Menon et al. 2007, Partridge & Hodin 2004), including one experienced by the senior author (Jaskowiak & Michelassi 2001). It is assumed that the risk of neoplastic transformation after strictureplasty is low and not sufficient to dissuade surgeons from performing those techniques. When occurring, an oncologically radical resection needs to be performed.

ULCERATIVE COLITIS

Since its initial description in 1978 (Parks & Nicholls 1978), the restorative proctocolectomy with IPAA has progressively become the standard procedure for surgical management of ulcerative colitis (Travis et al. 2008). This procedure is commonly performed with a protecting loop ileostomy that is then closed 2–3 months after the index procedure. The IPAA is technically demanding and associated with a high rate of postoperative morbidity (Lovegrove et al. 2007).

Early postoperative complications

Bowel obstruction

Bowel obstruction in the immediate postoperative period after an IPAA is treated as any postoperative bowel obstruction. To this extent, it may require reintervention. Before surgical reintervention is carried out, an obstructed loop ileostomy through a tight abdominal wall defect or the presence of intra-abdominal septic collections needs to be ruled out. In the former case, intubation of the ileostomy will resolve the obstructive picture; in the latter case, percutaneous drainage may resolve the associated paralytic ileus.

Anastomotic dehiscence and pelvic sepsis

Anastomotic dehiscence and pelvic sepsis after IPAA occur in 7–19% of cases (Fazio et al. 1995, Hueting et al. 2005, Meagher et al. 1998). Preoperative steroid therapy (Heuschen et al. 2002) and biological therapy administered within 2–3 months prior to surgery (Selvasekar et al. 2007) have been identified as independent risk factor of increased morbidity. However, neither azathioprine nor mercaptopurine has been shown to have any impact on postoperative dehiscence rate following IPAA (Aberra et al. 2003).

Clinical manifestations of acute anastomotic dehiscence after an IPAA are highly variable and include prolonged postoperative ileus, perineal tenderness, purulent exudate through the anus, low-grade fever, and leukocytosis.

Management of an anastomotic dehiscence is determined by the severity of local and systemic sepsis. In the absence of symptoms of peritonitis, continuous perineal pain and fever, patients may just need antibiotic treatment. An examination under anesthesia of the anal canal, ileoanal anastomosis, and pouch can be performed to assess the magnitude of the dehiscence and drain septic collections. If a diverting ileostomy is already in place, the stoma should be maintained until complete healing of the dehiscence has occurred. In the absence of a diverting ileostomy, a loop ileostomy should be performed (Heuschen et al. 2002) in most cases. A laparotomy may occasionally be required to address pelvic septic collections that cannot be treated with antibiotics or drained percutaneously.

The majority of anastomotic dehiscences heal spontaneously under fecal diversion by the loop ileostomy. Occasionally the healing process determines an anastomotic stricture (see below) or a chronic posterior presacral sinus. Healing of the presacral sinus can be accelerated by transanal curettage or by opening the pouch wall on top of the sinus facilitating healing by secondary intention.

Pouch-cutaneous fistula

After construction of a pouch, dehiscences can also occur from the pouch staple lines or the access enterotomies (Raval et al. 2007). These dehiscences may result in pelvic sepsis that spontaneously drains through the abdominal wound creating a pouch-cutaneous fistula. Alternatively, a pouch-cutaneous fistula is created when a pelvic abscess following a dehiscence of a pouch suture line or access enterotomies is drained percutaneously. Most of these fistulae heal spontaneously prior to closure of the loop ileostomy. If they do not, they are usually diagnosed through a pouchogram obtained prior to closure of the loop ileostomy or through a fistulogram in the presence of a nonhealing abdominal wound.

An abdominal approach is usually necessary to repair these dehiscences. After a complete lysis of intra-abdominal and pelvic adhesions, the pouch is mobilized completely, usually starting posteriorly. The dehiscence site is then identified and repaired according to its location. Anastomotic dehiscences originating from the proximal tip of the 'J' can be easily repaired, trimming and stapling the efferent limb (Kirat et al. 2011). Leaks arising from the antimesenteric pouch vertical staple lines can be directly sutured. Leaks from the distal third of the pouch or from the mesenteric vertical suture line require complete disconnection of the ileoanal anastomosis, revision or reconstruction of the pouch, and subsequent reconnection through a hand-sewn IPAA (Tekkis et al. 2006). Unless the repair is simple and technically satisfactory, the diverting ileostomy should be left in place.

Abdominal colectomy with ileostomy and closure of rectal stump

When patients come to surgery in poor nutritional conditions or on high doses of steroids or recent administration of biological therapy, or for emergent indications (hemorrhage, toxic, megacolon) or with severe acute colitis, the procedure of choice is an abdominal colectomy with ileostomy and closure of the rectal stump. A restorative proctectomy with IPAA is then carried out as a staged procedure when the patient has recovered from the original surgery and the devastating consequences of severe ulcerative colitis.

An abdominal colectomy with ileostomy and closure of the rectal stump may be complicated by ileostomy complications (necrosis, retraction) and by dehiscence of the rectal stump in the early postoperative period. In the former case, the patient requires to be reoperated promptly to fashion a new ileostomy, usually in the same location as the original one; in the latter case, antibiotic treatment and percutaneous drainage is frequently sufficient, although occasionally patient requires re-exploration and open drainage of the pelvic abscess if this is not approachable percutaneously.

Late postoperative complications

Bowel obstruction

Adhesive small bowel obstruction is one of the most common late postoperative complications after proctocolectomy with IPAA with an incidence reaching 30% in the 10 years following surgery, leading to reoperation in 25% of the cases (Meagher et al. 1998). Furthermore, for patients requiring relaparotomy for lysis of adhesions, the risk of recurring small bowel obstruction is high, up to 21%, leading to a 5% rate of patients requiring more than one surgical procedure for adhesive disease (MacLean et al. 2002).

Several strategies have been proposed to prevent the formation of intra-abdominal adhesions. Biologic membranes, such as Seprafilm, have been extensively studied after colorectal surgery. A meta-analysis by the Cochrane Foundation (Kumar et al. 2009) comprising seven randomized controlled trials showed a reduced incidence, extent, and severity of adhesions in patients treated with biological membranes. However, there was no significant reduction in the rates of clinical small bowel obstruction or required reoperation. Furthermore, the authors highlighted that there may be a higher risk of anastomotic leakage when those biologic membranes were wrapped around anastomoses. In light of these results, we do not advocate use of such membranes in routine practice.

However, the laparoscopic approach for IPAA is significantly associated with less severe intra-abdominal adhesions than the open approach (Indar et al. 2009), leading to a lower risk of long-term small bowel obstruction (Fichera et al. 2009).

Anastomotic stenosis

Stenosis of the IPAA occurs in 10–15% of patients (Fazio et al. 1995, Michelassi et al. 2003) and usually develops 6–9 months after the procedure. Moderate and soft strictures might be addressed by repeated digital dilatations in the office or using Hegar's dilatators under inhalation general anesthesia. A lumen that allows introduction of an index finger is adequate.

Long and narrow strictures, most of times occurring after a complete dehiscence following a complete mucosectomy and hand-sewn anastomosis, are likely to recur after simple dilatation. In an attempt to address these challenging situations, Fazio and Tjandra (1992) described use of the pouch advancement technique (**Figure 19.4**).

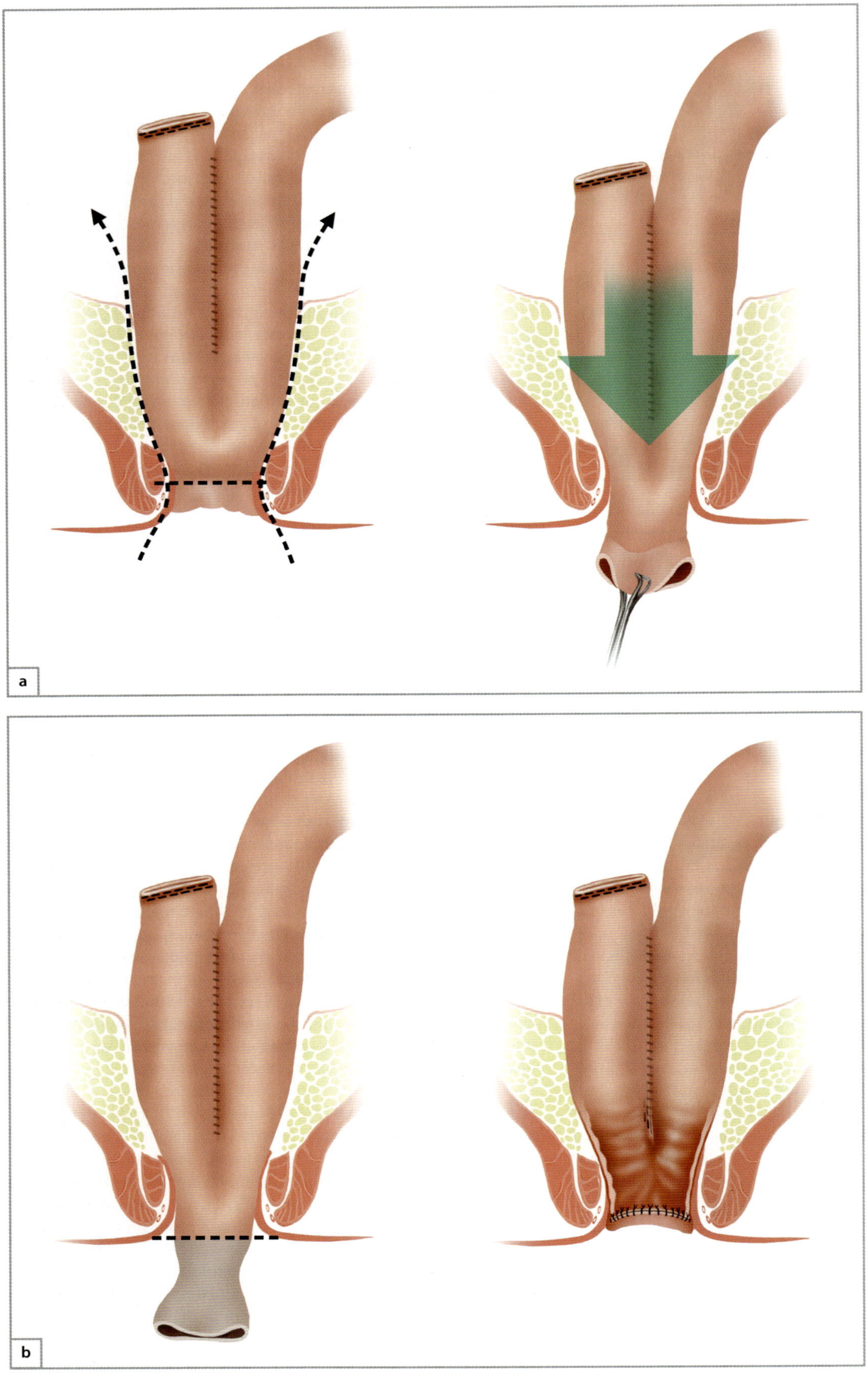

Figure 19.4 Ileal pouch advancement. (a) Under general anesthesia and using a perineal approach, a circumferential incision is performed at the dentate line, distally to the stenosis, and extended proximally in the sphincteric plane, until the ileal pouch serosa is reached. The pouch is then freed from its pelvic adhesions, in order to advance its distal third through the anal canal. (b) The fibrotic stricture is then excised and a new anastomosis is performed using the hand-sewn technique.

Pouch-vaginal fistula

Pouch-vaginal fistula occurs in approximately 6% of female patients undergoing IPAA (Lolohea et al. 2005) and is, most of the time, a result of postoperative pelvic sepsis (Groom et al. 1993). Once a pouch-fistula is suspected, the diagnosis can easily be confirmed by a simple clinical examination in 90% of the patients (Wexner et al. 1989). Its occurrence should always prompt questioning the original diagnosis of ulcerative colitis, especially if the fistula originates from a crypt of the dentate line after a stapled IPAA, and lead to pouch biopsies in order to eliminate Crohn's disease.

Surgical options for pouch-vaginal fistula include several perineal procedures. In the absence of a diverting stoma, fecal diversion should be discussed early with the patient. The Cleveland Clinic Foundation reported a 50% success rate after perineal repair of pouch-vaginal fistula, using a combination of direct suture, pouch mucosal advancement flap, and transvaginal repair (Lee et al. 1997). In case of multiple failures, the subsequent step should include an interposition muscle flap, performed with a bulbocavernous, a sartorius, or a gracilis muscle (Wexner et al. 2008, Zmora et al. 2006) with good reported results. If all fail and the fistulous drainage is voluminous and nonmanageable by the patient, a transabdominal removal of the pouch with construction of a new pouch or with a permanent ileostomy should be considered. Unfortunately the former approach is complicated by a high recurrence rate of the fistula, lower if an interposition gracilis graft is used at the time of the pouch construction.

Fistula-in-ano

Fistula-in-ano occurs in about 2–3% of patient (Fazio et al. 1995, Hueting et al. 2005, Meagher et al. 1998). Its occurrence, especially when the fistula originates from the crypts of the dentate line after a stapled IPAA, should always prompt questioning the original diagnosis of ulcerative colitis and lead to pouch biopsies in order to eliminate Crohn's disease. All operative procedure should start with a careful examination under general anesthesia, with the patient placed in a modified lithotomy position, to assess all fistula tracts and associated abscesses. If a superficial fistula, a rare occurrence, is diagnosed, a fistulotomy is all it is necessary; otherwise intervening abscesses need to be drained to obtain control of sepsis, and setons should be placed for better drainage of trans-sphincteric fistula tracts.

After complete control and abatement of the perineal sepsis, surgical options include simple suturing of the internal fistulous opening, fibrin glue sealing or pouch advancement (Dehni et al. 2005, Ahmed Ali et al. 2012, Akbari et al. 2009, Tulchinsky et al. 2003, Whitlow et al. 1997). Although minimally invasive, the first two options are rarely successful. The goal of the pouch advancement is to cover the internal opening of the fistula with viable tissue. The technique is similar to the one depicted in **Figure 19.4** but requires only refreshing of the opening of the pouch rather than a complete amputation.

Despite these procedures, a fistula-in-ano may persist or recur. In this situation, any intervening abscess should be drained and a seton should be placed to facilitate drainage. It will be up to the patient to decide whether the drainage of the fistula-in-ano is tolerable or whether removal of the pouch in favor of a permanent ileostomy is preferable.

Chronic pouchitis

Pouchitis is a nonspecific pouch inflammation of unknown origin that may occur in the absence of local complications. Its incidence increases with time, reaching 40% at 10 years after surgery and up to 70% at 20 years (Hahnloser et al. 2007). Its occurrence should lead to an endoscopy with biopsies to exclude a misdiagnosis of Crohn's disease. Pouchitis can be controlled with medical treatment in most of the cases: the first line of treatment includes ciprofloxacin (Gionchetti et al. 2000), followed by metronidazole in cases of no satisfactory response within 3–4 days. Third-line treatments, including steroids and/or immunosuppressive therapy, are only needed in 10% of the cases (Navaneethan & Shen 2010). In cases of resistant severe pouchitis, some authors advocate performing a fecal diversion with a loop ileostomy (Sandborn 1994); unfortunately, pouchitis usually relapses upon re-establishment of the intestinal continuity. When the symptoms of chronic pouchitis cannot be controlled satisfactorily, the pouch should be excised in favor of a permanent ileostomy.

Pouch with insufficient capacity

The pouch constructed during the IPAA procedure should have a length ranging from 15 to 18 cm. Shorter pouches have lesser capacity, resulting in impaired functional results with high stool frequency. Insufficient pouch volume should be suspected when medical treatment fails to provide a satisfactory daily stool frequency (six bowel movements per day). The diagnosis is then confirmed on pouchography with water-soluble contrast, highlighting a pouch length of <12 cm, and on pouch manometry to assess the maximum tolerable pouch volume (Oresland et al. 1990).

If insufficient pouch volume is confirmed, surgical correction can be entertained. Dehni et al. (2005) described three types of pouch enlargement procedures (**Figure 19.5**): type 1 includes integration of the blind end of the J into the pouch lumen, but can only be done when a long blind end was left in place during the initial procedure; type 2 and 3 are more complex and can only be performed in patients with sufficient mesenteric length. When performed, these procedures have satisfactory results as reported by Dehni et al. (2005) who successfully treated six cases of insufficient pouch volume and Fazio et al. (1998) who reported seven cases of successful pouch enlargement.

Pouch with large capacity

Occasionally, a normal-size pouch enlarges to very large dimensions (megapouch). Symptoms associated with this enlargement include constipation and abdominal distention. On initial examination, it is important to rule out a stricture at the ileoanal anastomosis as the cause of the dilatation. If this is the case, sequential mechanical dilatations of the anastomosis may take care of the cause of the pouch dilatation and of the symptoms. Otherwise, patients may require an abdominal approach with severance of the ileoanal anastomosis, tapering of the pouch with sequential applications of a linear GIA stapler ('sleeve pouchectomy'), a new hand-sewn ileoanal anastomosis and a temporary protecting ileostomy.

Development of Crohn's features in pouch

Three to seven percent of all patients operated with a firm diagnosis of ulcerative colitis develop Crohn's features in their pouches. The function of these pouches may deteriorate with high bowel movement frequency and incontinence or complications (obstructive: tight stenosis of the pouch outlet; septic: fistula-in-ano, pouch-vaginal fistula) may develop. If medical treatment fails to control symptoms or complications, the pouch may have to be excised in favor of a permanent ileostomy.

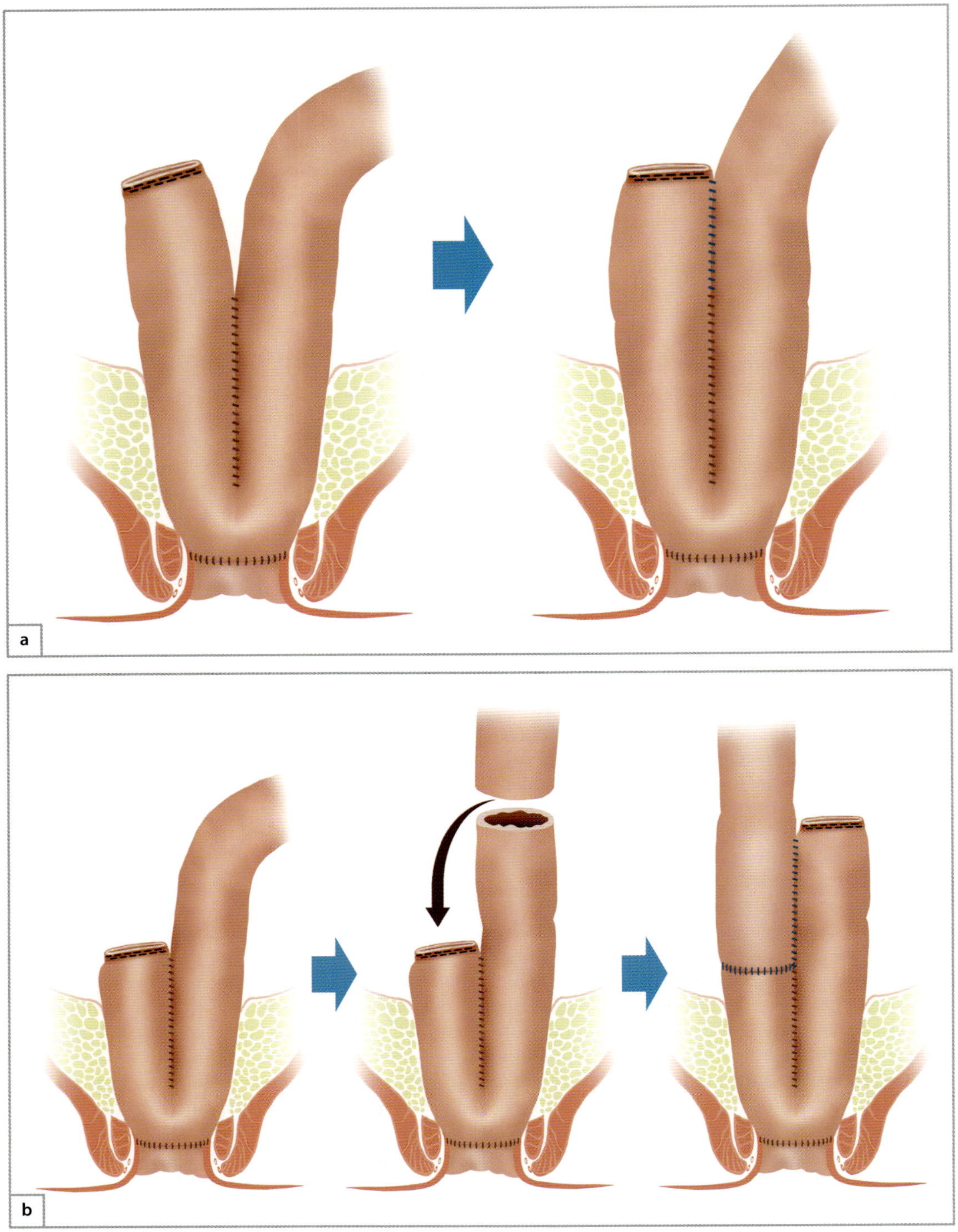

Figure 19.5 Continued

Pouch failure

Chronic pouchitis and development of Crohn's disease in the pouch are the most common causes of pouch failure nowadays, defined as the need for pouch excision and permanent diversion, followed by septic perineal complications (fistula-in-ano, pouch-vaginal fistula). A meta-analysis of 43 studies, published in 2005, reported a pooled pouch failure rate of 6.5% with a 3-year mean follow-up, increasing to 8.5% in patients followed up >60 months (Hueting et al. 2005).

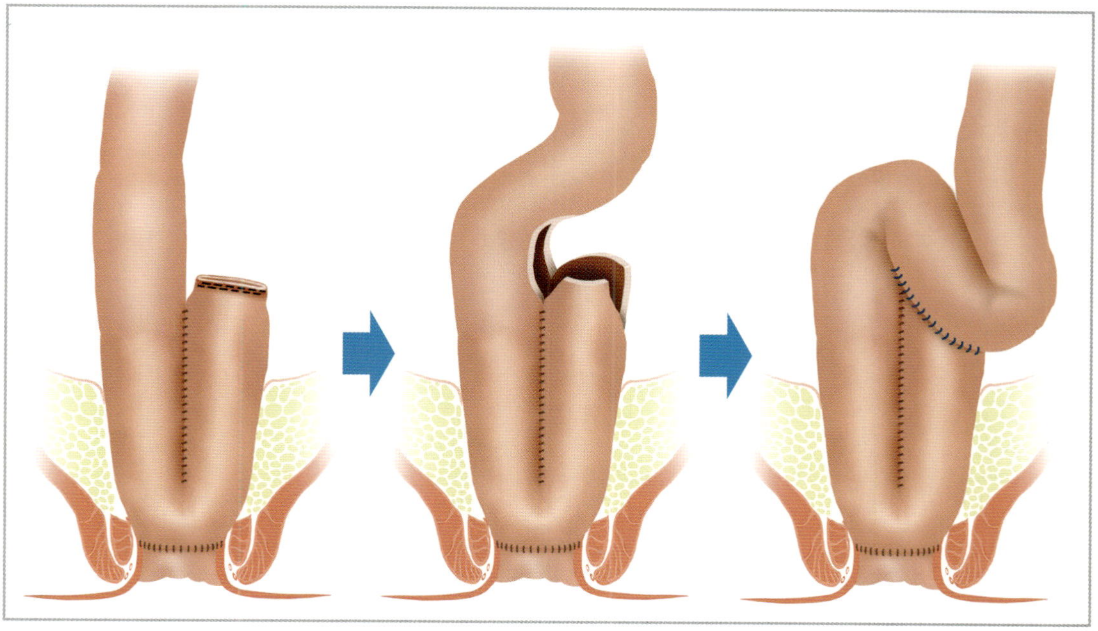

Figure 19.5 Ileal pouch enlargement techniques. (a) Type I, (b) type II, and (c) type III.

LATE POSTOPERATIVE COMPLICATIONS AFTER LESS COMMONLY PERFORMED SURGICAL PROCEDURES

Refractory proctitis or malignant transformation after abdominal colectomy with ileorectal anastomosis

Abdominal colectomy with ileorectal anastomosis is performed for ulcerative colitis in highly selected patients. The European guidelines (Travis et al. 2008) state that this procedure, more common in Europe than in the United States, can be proposed if the rectum has not lost its compliance and volume and there are no risk factors for ulcerative colitis-related rectal cancer (disease <10 years and no sign of colorectal adenoma or adenocarcinoma). The ileorectal procedure is associated with better functional outcomes and less impaired postoperative fertility than the IPAA procedure. Patients with ileorectal anastomosis require careful endoscopic follow-up.

In the event of an ulcerative colitis 'recurrence' in the rectum or in the presence of a neoplastic transformation, an IPAA can still subsequently be performed and result in comparable functional outcomes as a primary IPAA (Daude et al. 1993). A study from the Cleveland Clinic reported on the results of 86 ileorectal anastomosis for ulcerative colitis (da Luz Moreira et al. 2010). With a mean follow-up of >11 years, subsequent proctectomy was required in 53% of the patients, half of them because of refractory proctitis and the other half because of the occurrence of dysplasia or rectal cancer.

Ileostomy and perineal complications after proctocolectomy with permanent ileostomy

Stoma complications include ileostomy retraction, prolapse, stenosis, parastomal hernia, and, occasionally, varices. These complications usually require refashioning of the ileostomy. When a parastomal hernia is present, the new ileostomy should be resited to the contralateral side if at all possible.

Nonhealing of the perineal wound is a rare occurrence if the anal canal dissection is performed in the intersphincteric plane and the external anal sphincter is available for primary closure of the pelvic floor. It usually occurs after a perineal wound infection. In this case, drainage of the sepsis with extensive lavage and debridement is usually sufficient for secondary healing. Occasionally, myocutaneous flaps are necessary to fill the perineal space and provide cutaneous closure of the perineal wound (Michelassi et al. 2000).

REFERENCES

Aberra FN, Lewis JD, Hass D, et al. Corticosteroids and immunomodulators: postoperative infectious complication risk in inflammatory bowel disease patients. Gastroenterology 2003; 125:320–327.

Ahmed Ali U, Shen B, Remzi FH, Kiran RP. The management of anastomotic pouch sinus after IPAA. Dis Colon Rectum 2012; 55:541–548.

Akbari RP, Madoff RD, Parker SC, et al. Anastomotic sinuses after ileoanal pouch construction: incidence, management, and outcome. Dis Colon Rectum 2009; 52:452–455.

Bass EM, Del Pino A, Tan A, et al. Does preoperative stoma marking and education by the enterostomal therapist affect outcome? Dis Colon Rectum 1997; 40 440–442.

Belaiche E. Acute lower gastrointestinal bleeding in Crohn's disease: characteristics of a unique series of 34 patients. Am J Gastroenterol 1999; 94:2177–2181.

Bernell O, Lapidus A, Hellers G. Risk factors for surgery and postoperative recurrence in Crohn's disease. Ann Surg 2000; 231:38–45.

Brouquet A, Bretagnol F, Soprani A, et al. A laparoscopic approach to iterative ileocolonic resection for the recurrence of Crohn's disease. Surg Endosc 2010; 24:879–887.

Cattan P, Bonhomme N, Panis Y, et al. Fate of the rectum in patients undergoing total colectomy for Crohn's disease. Br J Surg 2002; 89:454–459.

Chardavoyne R, Flint GW, Pollack S, Wise L. Factors affecting recurrence following resection for Crohn's disease. Dis Colon Rectum 1986; 29:495–502.

Chaudhary B, Glancy D, Dixon AR. Laparoscopic surgery for recurrent ileocolic Crohn's disease is as safe and effective as primary resection. Colorectal Dis 2011; 13:1413–1416.

da Luz Moreira A, Kiran RP, Lavery I. Clinical outcomes of ileorectal anastomosis for ulcerative colitis. Br J Surg 2010; 97:65–69.

Daude F, Frileux P, Penna C, Tiret E, Parc R. [Transformations of ileo-rectal anastomosis into ileo-anal anastomosis in hemorrhagic rectocolitis. Indications and results]. Ann Chir 1993; 47:1014–1019.

Dehni N, Remacle G, Dozois RR, et al. Salvage reoperation for complications after ileal pouch-anal anastomosis. Br J Surg 2005; 92:748–753.

Dietz DW, Laureti S, Strong SA, et al. Safety and long-term efficacy of strictureplasty in 314 patients with obstructing small bowel Crohn's disease. J Am Coll Surg 2001; 192:330–338.

Dignass A, Van Assche G, Lindsay JO, et al. The second European evidence-based Consensus on the diagnosis and management of Crohn's disease: current management. J Crohns Colitis 2010; 4:28–62.

Fazio VW, Tjandra JJ. Pouch advancement and neoileoanal anastomosis for anastomotic stricture and anovaginal fistula complicating restorative proctocolectomy. Br J Surg 1992; 79:694–696.

Fazio VW, Wu JS, Lavery IC. Repeat ileal pouch-anal anastomosis to salvage septic complications of pelvic pouches: clinical outcome and quality of life assessment. Ann Surg 1998; 228:588–597.

Fazio VW, Ziv Y, Church JM, et al. Ileal pouch-anal anastomoses complications and function in 1005 patients. Ann Surg 1995; 222:120–127.

Fichera A, Silvestri MT, Hurst RD, Rubin MA, Michelassi F. Laparoscopic restorative proctocolectomy with ileal pouch anal anastomosis: a comparative observational study on long-term functional results. J Gastrointest Surg 2009; 13:526–532.

Gionchetti P, Rizzello F, Venturi A, et al. Oral bacteriotherapy as maintenance treatment in patients with chronic pouchitis: a double-blind, placebo-controlled trial. Gastroenterology 2000; 119:305–309.

Groom JS, Nicholls RJ, Hawley PR, Phillips RK. Pouch-vaginal fistula. Br J Surg 1993; 80:936–940.

Hahnloser D, Pemberton JH, Wolff BG, et al. Results at up to 20 years after ileal pouch-anal anastomosis for chronic ulcerative colitis. Br J Surg 2007; 94:333–340.

Hasegawa H, Watanabe M, Nishibori H, et al. Laparoscopic surgery for recurrent Crohn's disease. Br J Surg 2003; 90:970–973.

Heuschen UA, Allemeyer EH, Hinz U, et al. Outcome after septic complications in J pouch procedures. Br J Surg 2002; 89:194–200.

Heuschen UA, Hinz U, Allemeyer EH, et al. Risk factors for ileoanal J pouch-related septic complications in ulcerative colitis and familial adenomatous polyposis. Ann Surg 2002; 235:207–216.

Hueting WE, Buskens E, van der Tweel I, Gooszen HG, van Laarhoven CJ. Results and complications after ileal pouch anal anastomosis: a meta-analysis of 43 observational studies comprising 9,317 patients. Dig Surg 2005; 22:69–79.

Hurst RD, Molinari M, Chung TP, Rubin M, Michelassi F. Prospective study of the features, indications, and surgical treatment in 513 consecutive patients affected by Crohn's disease. Surgery 1997; 122:661–668.

Indar AA, Efron JE, Young-Fadok TM. Laparoscopic ileal pouch-anal anastomosis reduces abdominal and pelvic adhesions. Surg Endosc 2009; 23:174–177.

Jaskowiak NT, Michelassi F. Adenocarcinoma at a strictureplasty site in Crohn's disease: report of a case. Dis Colon Rectum 2001; 44:284–287.

Katariya RN, Sood S, Rao PG, Rao PL. Stricture-plasty for tubercular strictures of the gastro-intestinal tract. Br J Surg 1977; 64:496–498.

Kirat HT, Kiran RP, Oncel M, et al. Management of leak from the tip of the "J" in ileal pouch-anal anastomosis. Dis Colon Rectum 2011; 54:454–459.

Kumar S, Wong PF, Leaper DJ. Intra-peritoneal prophylactic agents for preventing adhesions and adhesive intestinal obstruction after non-gynaecological abdominal surgery. Cochrane Database Syst Rev 2009:CD005080.

Lee PY, Fazio VW, Church JM, et al. Vaginal fistula following restorative proctocolectomy. Dis Colon Rectum 1997; 40:752–759.

Lee EC, Papaioannou N. Minimal surgery for chronic obstruction in patients with extensive or universal Crohn's disease. Ann R Coll Surg Engl 1982; 64:229–233.

Lichtenstein GR, Hanauer SB, Sandborn WJ. Management of Crohn's disease in adults. Am J Gastroenterol 2009; 104:465–484.

Lolohea S, Lynch AC, Robertson GB, Frizelle FA. Ileal pouch-anal anastomosis-vaginal fistula: a review. Dis Colon Rectum 2005; 48:1802–1810.

Lovegrove RE, Heriot AG, Constantinides V, et al. Meta-analysis of short-term and long-term outcomes of J, W and S ileal reservoirs for restorative proctocolectomy. Colorectal Dis 2007; 9:310–320.

MacLean AR, Cohen Z, MacRae HM, et al. Risk of small bowel obstruction after the ileal pouch-anal anastomosis. Ann Surg 2002; 235:200–206.

Marchetti F, Fazio VW, Ozuner G. Adenocarcinoma arising from a strictureplasty site in Crohn's disease. Report of a case. Dis Colon Rectum 1996; 39:1315–1321.

Meagher AP, Farouk R, Dozois RR, Kelly KA, Pemberton JH. J ileal pouch-anal anastomosis for chronic ulcerative colitis: complications and long-term outcome in 1310 patients. Br J Surg 1998; 85:800–803.

Menon AM, Mirza AH, Moolla S, Morton DG. Adenocarcinoma of the small bowel arising from a previous strictureplasty for Crohn's disease: report of a case. Dis Colon Rectum 2007; 50:257–259.

Michelassi F. Side-to-side isoperistaltic strictureplasty for multiple Crohn's strictures. Dis Colon Rectum 1996; 39:345–349.

Michelassi F, Balestracci T, Chappell R, Block GE. Primary and recurrent Crohn's disease. Experience with 1379 patients. Ann Surg 1991; 214:230–240.

Michelassi F, Lee J, Rubin M, et al. Long-term functional results after ileal pouch anal restorative proctocolectomy for ulcerative colitis: a prospective observational study. Ann Surg 2003; 238:433–445.

Michelassi F, Melis M, Rubin M, Hurst RD. Surgical treatment of anorectal complications of Crohn's disease. Surgery 2000; 128:597–603.

Navaneethan U, Shen B. Diagnosis and management of pouchitis and ileoanal pouch dysfunction. Curr Gastroenterol Rep 2010; 12:485–494.

Oresland T, Fasth S, Nordgren S, Akervall S, Hulten L. Pouch size: the important functional determinant after restorative proctocolectomy. Br J Surg 1990; 77:265–269.

Parks AG, Nicholls RJ. Proctocolectomy without ileostomy for ulcerative colitis. Br Med J 1978; 2:85–88.

Partridge SK, Hodin RA. Small bowel adenocarcinoma at a strictureplasty site in a patient with Crohn's disease: report of a case. Dis Colon Rectum 2004; 47:778–781.

Post S, Herfarth C, Bohm E, et al. The impact of disease pattern, surgical management, and individual surgeons on the risk for relaparotomy for recurrent Crohn's disease. Ann Surg 1996; 223:253–260.

Raval MJ, Schnitzler M, O'Connor BI, Cohen Z, McLeod RS. Improved outcome due to increased experience and individualized management of leaks after ileal pouch-anal anastomosis. Ann Surg 2007; 246:763–770.

Rimola J, Rodriguez S, Garcia-Bosch O, et al. Magnetic resonance for assessment of disease activity and severity in ileocolonic Crohn's disease. Gut 2009; 58:1113–1120.

Roy P, Kumar D. Strictureplasty. Br J Surg 2004; 91:1428–1437.

Sagar PM, Pemberton JH. Intraoperative, postoperative and reoperative problems with ileoanal pouches. Br J Surg 2012; 99:454–468.

Sandborn WJ. Pouchitis following ileal pouch-anal anastomosis: definition, pathogenesis, and treatment. Gastroenterology 1994; 107:1856–1860.
Selvasekar CR, Cima RR, Larson DW, et al. Effect of infliximab on short-term complications in patients undergoing operation for chronic ulcerative colitis. J Am Coll Surg 2007; 204:956–963.
Tekkis PP, Heriot AG, Smith JJ, et al. Long-term results of abdominal salvage surgery following restorative proctocolectomy. Br J Surg 2006; 93:231–237.
Travis SP, Stange EF, Lemann M, et al. European evidence-based Consensus on the management of ulcerative colitis: Current management. J Crohns Colitis 2008; 2:24–62.
Tulchinsky H, Cohen CR, Nicholls RJ. Salvage surgery after restorative proctocolectomy. Br J Surg 2003; 90:909–921.
Wexner SD, Rothenberger DA, Jensen L, et al. Ileal pouch vaginal fistulas: incidence, etiology, and management. Dis Colon Rectum 1989; 32:460–465.
Wexner SD, Ruiz DE, Genua J, et al. Gracilis muscle interposition for the treatment of rectourethral, rectovaginal, and pouch-vaginal fistulas: results in 53 patients. Ann Surg 2008; 248:39–43.
Whitlow CB, Opelka FG, Gathright JB, Jr., Beck DE. Treatment of colorectal and ileoanal anastomotic sinuses. Dis Colon Rectum 1997; 40:760–763.
Yamamoto T, Bain IM, Allan RN, Keighley MR. Persistent perineal sinus after proctocolectomy for Crohn's disease. Dis Colon Rectum 1999; 42:96–101.
Yamamoto T, Fazio VW, Tekkis PP. Safety and efficacy of strictureplasty for Crohn's disease: a systematic review and meta-analysis. Dis Colon Rectum 2007; 50:1968–1986.
Yamamoto T, Keighley MR. Fate of the rectum and ileal recurrence rates after total colectomy for Crohn's disease. World J Surg 2000; 24:125–129.
Zappa M, Stefanescu C, Cazals-Hatem D, et al. Which magnetic resonance imaging findings accurately evaluate inflammation in small bowel Crohn's disease? A retrospective comparison with surgical pathologic analysis. Inflamm Bowel Dis 2011; 17:984–993.
Zmora O, Tulchinsky H, Gur E, et al. Gracilis muscle transposition for fistulas between the rectum and urethra or vagina. Dis Colon Rectum 2006; 49:1316–1321.

Chapter 20

Reoperative management of acute and chronic small and large bowel stoma complications

Susan Galandiuk

INTRODUCTION

Over 100,000 intestinal stomas are constructed in the United States alone every year, including ileostomies, colostomies, and ileal conduits. Complications of stomas occur early and late and can result due to technical error, patient disease, or body habitus. Reoperations, aside from closure, are not performed as often for temporary as compared with permanent stomas. This chapter will first describe complications that can occur with any stoma and then complications that are specific to different types of stoma. The chapter will describe reoperation for

- Acute stomal ischemia/necrosis
- Stomal stenosis/retraction
- Stoma prolapse
- Parastomal hernia
- The poorly sited stoma
- Caput medusae

The first two are typically technical complications related to ischemia of the distal bowel and the next two, stoma prolapse and hernia, can be technical issues but are most frequently related to stoma type (loop vs. end) and patient body habitus. Specific complications that tend to occur mainly with ileostomies include skin-related complications secondary to poor appliance fit as well as complications arising from recurrent Crohn's disease in or around an ileostomy or colostomy.

REOPERATION FOR ACUTE STOMAL ISCHEMIA/NECROSIS

Ischemia is a frequent reason for reoperation of stoma complications. Ischemia is either reversible or irreversible, which includes both necrosis and gangrene. This may require early reoperation within the first 24 hours postoperatively or result in a delayed stenosis and require later treatment. Necrosis with stomas usually occurs within 24 hours, but may be recognized as late as 3–5 days postoperatively. It is least frequent with loop stomas and may occur at different depths, i.e. above or below the fascia (**Figure 20.1**). Necrosis is usually caused by a disruption of blood supply with overly aggressive bowel mobilization or excessive mesentery tension, usually from insufficient mobilization of the bowel, or a higher amount of mesenteric adipose tissue or edema of the bowel wall. End sigmoid colostomy is the one at highest at risk of necrosis, and ischemia of colostomies is more generally frequent than with ileostomies (Leenen & Kuypers 1989).

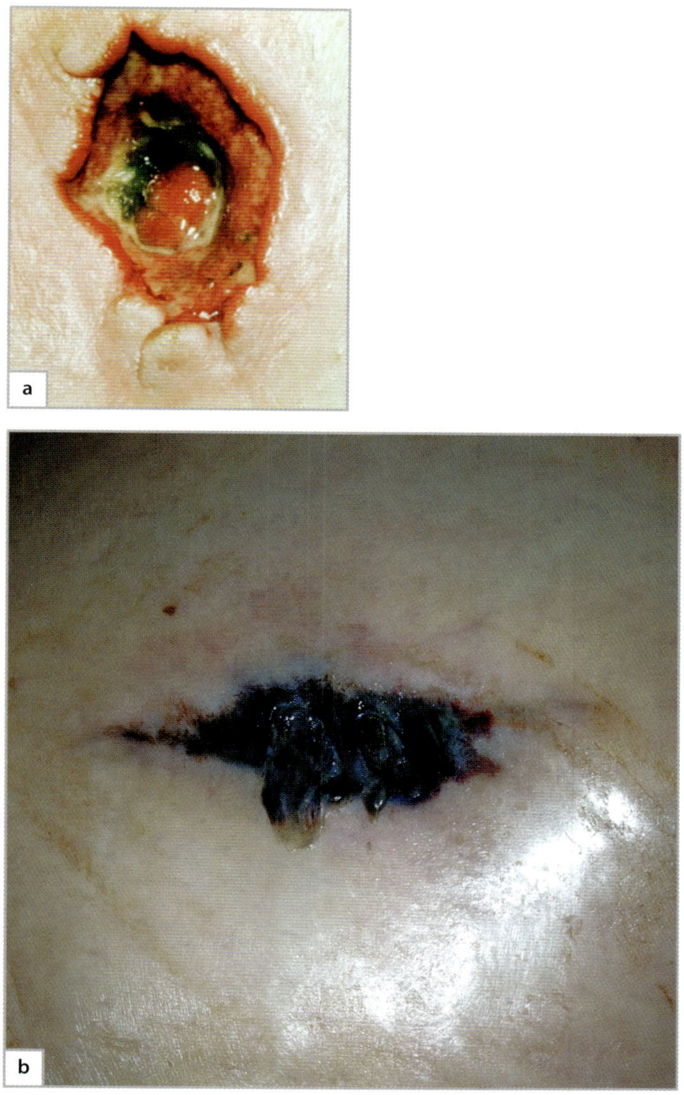

Figure 20.1 (a) Necrosis of a colostomy with sloughing of tissue, but viable bowel visible at level of fascia. (b) Full-thickness necrosis of an end ascending colon colostomy requiring reoperation.

In the acute postoperative setting, inserting a test tube test into the stoma is sometimes helpful at gauging whether or not there is viability below the fascial level by looking for perfused tissue. If there is no viability above the fascial level, this will often slough and result in a distal stricture that sometimes can be managed without reoperation. If full-thickness ischemia is restricted to *above* the fascial level, this can be treated conservatively, but followed closely (**Figure 20.1a**). The stoma site may require skin-level dilatation, and the patient may need to irrigate their stoma to ensure adequate emptying. If the ischemic area extends below the fascia, reoperation is mandatory; the sooner the better (**Figure 20.1b**). Skin-level stenosis leading to a need for reoperation is usually secondary to ischemia with or without tension. During reoperation, viability of the distal bowel can be assessed by looking for bleeding at the cut edge of the bowel or from cut epiploicae in the case of the colon, by using intravenously administered fluorescein dye and ultraviolet light illumination of the operative field, or more recently using indocyanine green arteriography (Horgan & Gorey 1992, Matsui et al. 2011).

It is often wise to check perfusion after the bowel has been passed through the stoma aperture in the abdominal wall. If perfusion is questionable intraoperatively, it will likely get worse postoperatively. It is imperative that a colostomy be constructed under no tension. In obese individuals, it may be necessary to mobilize the splenic flexure and ligate the inferior mesenteric artery at its origin as well as the inferior mesenteric vein, in order to obtain the necessary colonic mobility and length for an adequate left-sided colostomy. If there is tension, one can consider using a stoma rod in the case of a loop stoma, doing extracolonic mobilization as above, performing peritoneal windowing to obtain additional bowel length, or constructing a loop end stoma. It is also vital to perform an aperture large enough in the abdominal wall to avoid compression of the blood supply of the stoma. This is a particular judgment issue, since one always wishes to avoid a parastomal hernia.

REOPERATION FOR STOMAL STENOSIS

Stomal stenosis occurs in all stoma types and may interfere with output. It can be caused by improper sizing of either the fascia or skin aperture as the stoma is constructed or it can be due to scar formation due to necrosis, mucocutaneous separation, an inadequate amount of bowel mobilization during construction, recurrent disease processes, e.g. Crohn's disease or prior radiation. Stenosis can also be caused by excessive weight gain, pseudoverrucous lesions, a stoma that is not primarily matured, or chronic inflammation. Depending on the level of the stenosis, local surgical resection, fasciotomy, and stoma revision or major surgical revision, and reconstruction may be needed.

The normal 24-hour ileostomy output ranges from 500 to 800 mL. For several months following ileostomy creation, there is a decrease in stoma output secondary to ileal adaptation. An ileostomy that has over a 1000 mL output within a 24-hour period is designated as a high-output stoma. Very importantly, a sign of partial obstruction in the ileostomy patient is increased output with a very clear light green ileostomy affluent. Ileostomy stenosis can result in a functional outlet obstruction with such a dramatic increase in output that renal failure can occur (**Figure 20.2a**). Bowel obstruction can also be caused by a skin-level stenosis, a parastomal hernia, an impacted food bolus, or recurrent disease, as in Crohn's disease where facial level recurrence is common. Office follow-up of such patients should always include inserting an index finger into the stoma or, alternatively, a pediatric proctoscope or 10–12 French Hegar dilator in order to ensure that no distal stricture is present. If this is not possible, radiographic contrast studies performed retrograde through the stoma are helpful in documenting the degree and length of the stricture. It is best if the surgeon is present for such contrast studies. If there is concern regarding the presence of a stricture, the patient should be instructed to keep a diary of stoma output.

Colostomy stenosis has a very high rate of requiring surgical revision, whereas prolapse and hernia have a lesser rate of needing operation. Colostomy stenosis can be due to a too small skin aperture, ischemia, or serositis of the exposed bowel (**Figure 20.2b**). Stenosis is more likely to form if no solid stool is passing through, i.e. in patients who are doing irrigation or having diarrhea associated with chemotherapy. If the stenosis is not too fibrotic or rigid, it can be treated by dilatation. In some cases, this can be done by self-dilatation on part of the patient using a Hegar dilator. In some cases, if there is adequate mobility of the colon, one can excise the mucocutaneous junction, mobilize the bowel through a peristomal incision, and resuture (Allen-Mersh & Thomson 1988).

Early stoma retraction can occur due to prolonged ileus, abdominal distension, or an overly large abdominal wall aperture. Late stoma

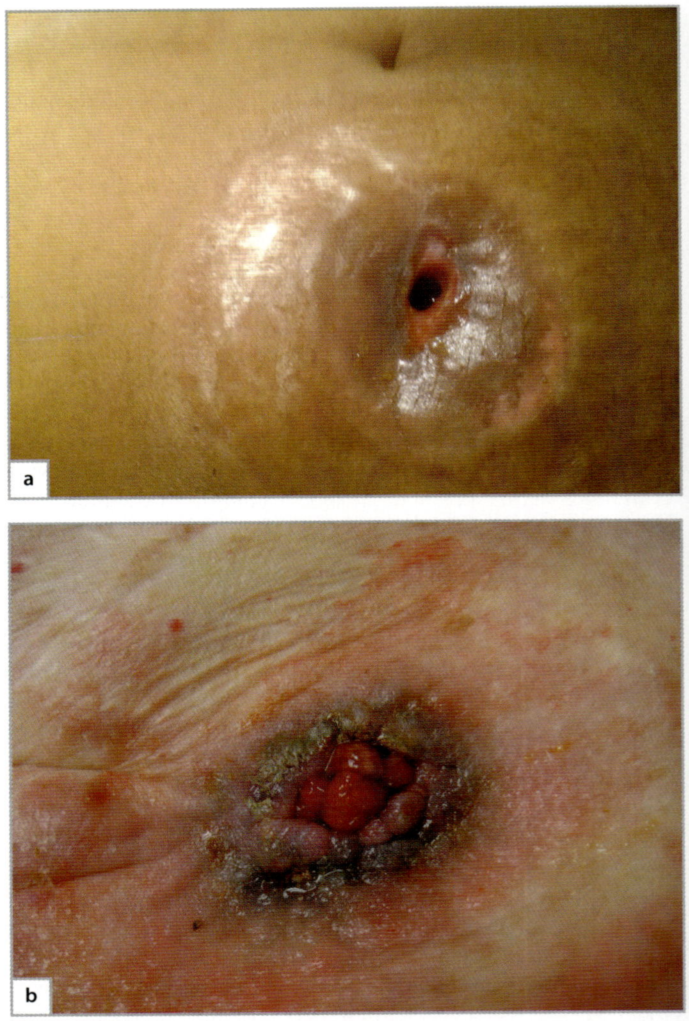

Figure 20.2 (a) Ileostomy stenosis. (b) Colostomy stenosis with surrounding pseudoepithelial hyperplasia.

retraction is often due to peristomal hernia or significant weight gain. This can be the usual American obesity or the gradual resumption of good health following surgery and after a chronic debilitating illness. Retraction of a stoma occurs in 10–15% of patients. This can lead to soiling, difficulty in keeping the appliance on, and is frequently due to weight gain. Since tension is the causative factor, this usually requires a major (as opposed to local) revision. As with ileostomies, colostomy retraction and stenosis can occur due to tension, ischemia, and infection. Colostomy stenosis can also prevent a patient from performing stoma irrigation.

REOPERATION FOR THE POORLY SITED OR RETRACTED STOMA

An improperly sited stoma is one of the most frequent reasons for reoperation. A well-sited, well-constructed stoma is less likely to cause skin or leakage problems, and will help the patient to cope with their altered body image and elimination. As with many things with surgery, the key to managing complications is to avoid them in the first place. One of the major points of reoperating for stoma complications is to select a good stoma site. Preoperative marking of stomas is essential. Preoperatively one needs to mark the patient in both a sitting and standing position. What looks flat on the operating table may not be when the patient is sitting upright. One should avoid proximity to the iliac crest, fat folds, the patient's beltline, old scars or other creases, as well as the patient's panniculus. Stoma appliances do not adhere well to scar tissue. It is also preferable to choose a stoma site that the patient can also see and reach without difficulty in order to be able to easily change the stoma appliance.

In order to minimize the risk of herniation, intestinal stoma sites should be placed within the rectus muscle sheath. The infraumbilical fat mound is the best stoma site in most patients. The abdominal wall aperture should be approximately 3.5 cm, which is approximately the size of two-fingerbreadths for the average surgeon. It is important to exteriorize enough bowel to have a stoma that is constructed without tension and therefore without ischemia. For an ileostomy, one should have 5–6 cm of ileum protruding above the level of the abdominal wall skin so that once the stoma is matured, the stoma will protrude 1.5–2.5 cm. For a colostomy, 3–4 cm of colon should protrude above the abdominal wall prior to maturation, leading to a 1 cm protrusion. This permits pouching of the stoma in the event that there is liquid stool, e.g. as when the patient receives chemotherapy. An easy way to assess viability of the stoma is to examine for bleeding at the cut edge after the bowel is pulled through the abdominal wall aperture. **Figures 20.3a and 20.3b** show some examples of remarkably poorly chosen stoma sites requiring reoperation.

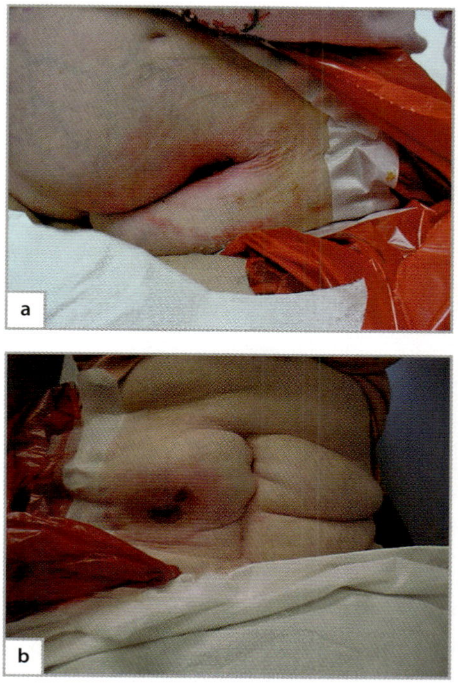

Figure 20.3 (a) Poorly sited colostomy underneath skin fold (pannus). (b) Poorly sited ileostomy; flush with skin and underneath abdominal fold.

REOPERATION FOR STOMA PROLAPSE

Intestinal stomas can be end, end-loop, or loop. By far, prolapse occurs most commonly following loop stomas, especially loop transverse colostomies. Prolapse of an end ileostomy can occur due to lack of mesenteric fixation or too big of an opening in the abdominal wall due to construction issues, or hernia (**Figure 20.4a and 20.4b**). Patients with stoma prolapse need a flexible pouching system. One-piece pouching systems tend to be most accommodating. Radial slitting of the stoma may help with stoma adhesion. The patient must be instructed so as to reduce the stoma prolapse. If necessary, the patient may need to be fit with a hernia belt. If the stoma prolapse is very large and interferes with appliance adherence, results in obstructive symptoms, or is cosmetically unacceptable, surgical correction is warranted (**Figure 20.4c**). In most cases, reducing the caliber of the stoma aperture and converting the loop stoma to an end stoma, if possible, is the best option. Occasionally, prolapsing loop colostomies have to be converted to end ileostomies due to recurrent prolapse problems.

REOPERATION FOR PARASTOMAL HERNIA

Acute peristomal evisceration or herniation of small bowel can occur if the stoma aperture is too wide and the patient develops an ileus or exerts a forceful Valsalva maneuver. Immediate surgical correction is mandatory, with downsizing of the aperture and reinforcement with some type of absorbable reinforcing prosthetic material, or stoma relocation (**Figure 20.5a**).

Peristomal hernia is a very common late complication. Operation is indicated if the hernia is symptomatic, as with abdominal pain or obstruction, or inability to keep an appliance on the stoma (**Figure 20.5b**). Different approaches for repair include relocation and repair, local direct repair, use of prosthetic material, or use of a stoma hernia belt (**Figure 20.5c and 20.5d**).

Peristomal hernias most frequently occur if the patient has had a stoma constructed lateral to the rectus sheath or due to patient weight gain. Several studies have, however, indicated that location within the rectus sheath may not be as important as previously thought (Carne et al. 2003, Leong et al. 1994). Diagnosis is often facilitated by inserting a finger through the stoma, both to assess the tortuosity of the bowel above fascial level and to gauge the size of the fascial opening. The patient should be assessed both supine and in the upright position (**Figure 20.6a and 20.6b**). Before reoperating, patients should first be managed conservatively with application of a stoma hernia belt and attempts at weight loss. These stoma hernia belts must be applied

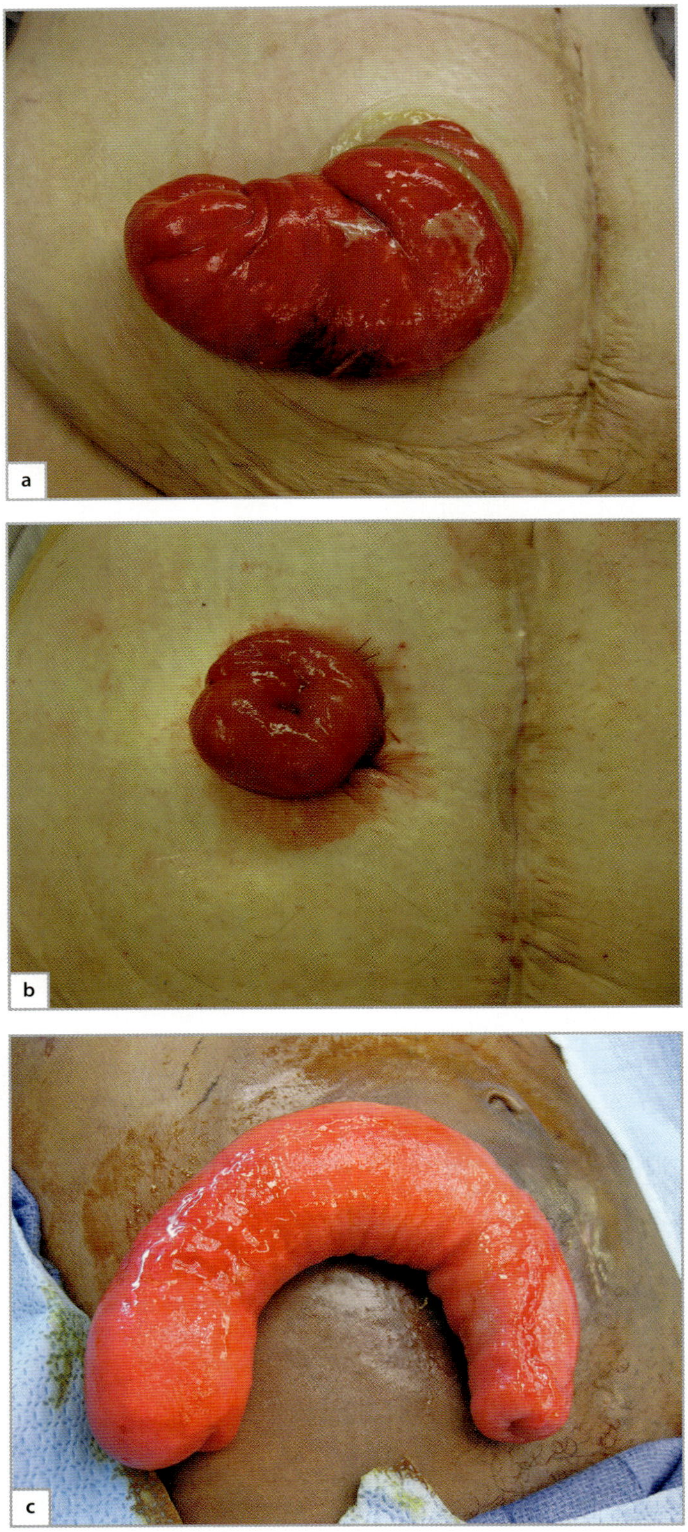

Figure 20.4 (a) Prolapse of end ileostomy, preoperative. (b) Prolapse of end ileostomy after local repair. (c) Prolapse of loop ileostomy causing symptoms of bowel obstruction.

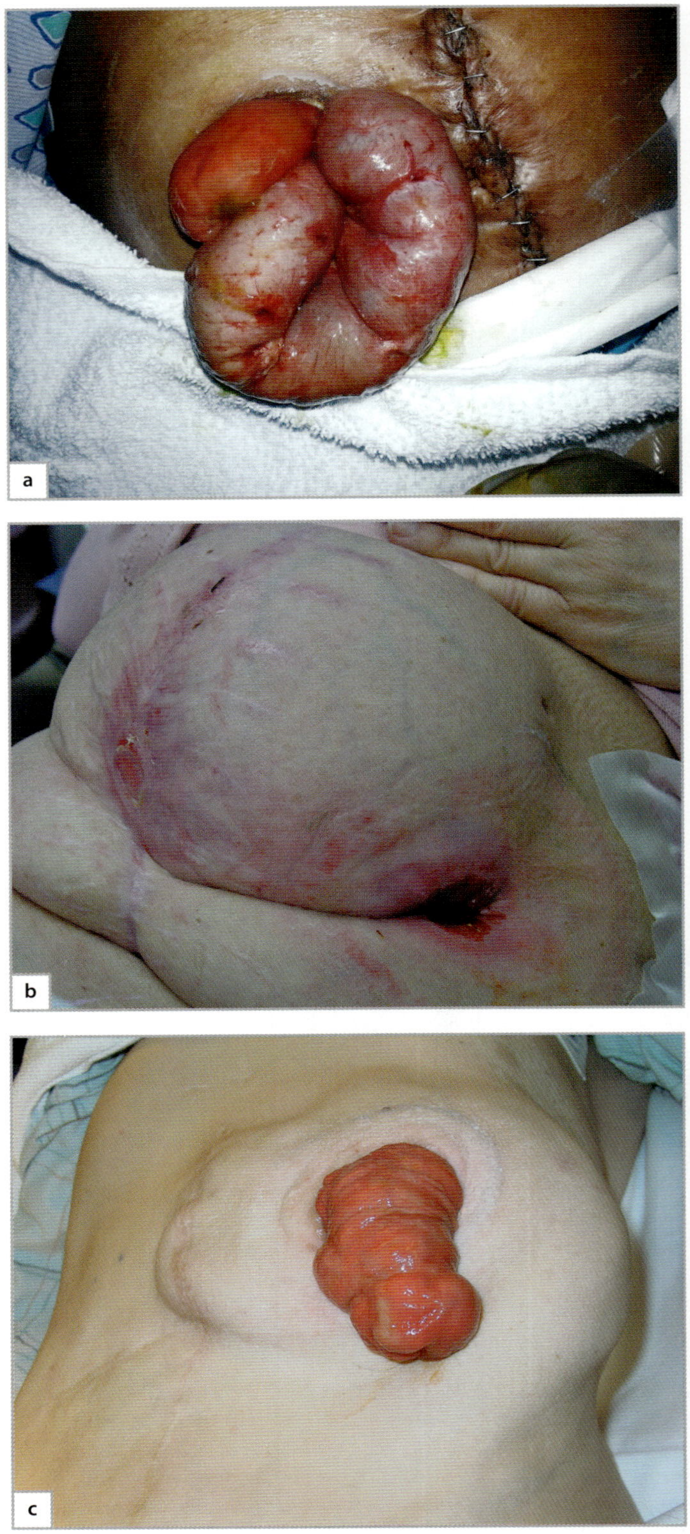

Figure 20.5 (a) Acute evisceration adjacent to ileostomy site. (b) Large parastomal hernia with poorly sited colostomy beneath skin fold. (c) Prolapsing colostomy with large parastomal hernia; preoperative. *Continued*

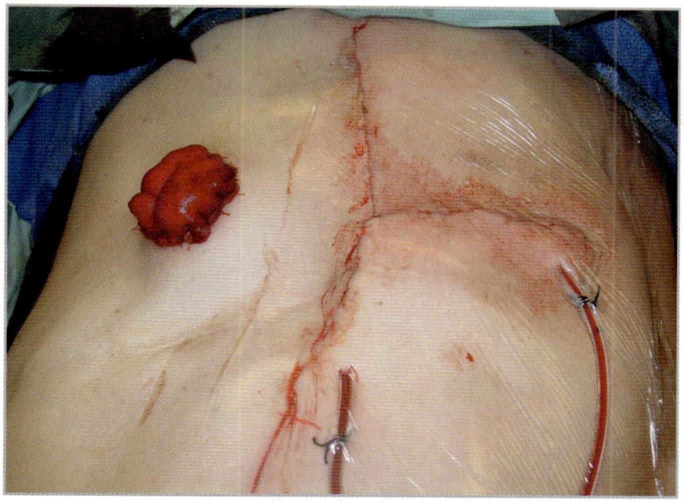

Figure 20.5 (d) Same patient as Figure 20.5c; postoperative view with relocation of colostomy and repair of parastomal hernia.

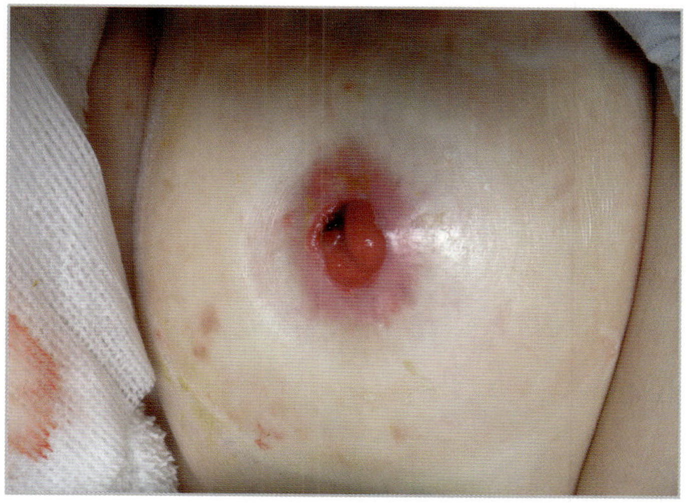

Figure 20.7 Caput medusae at ileostomy site.

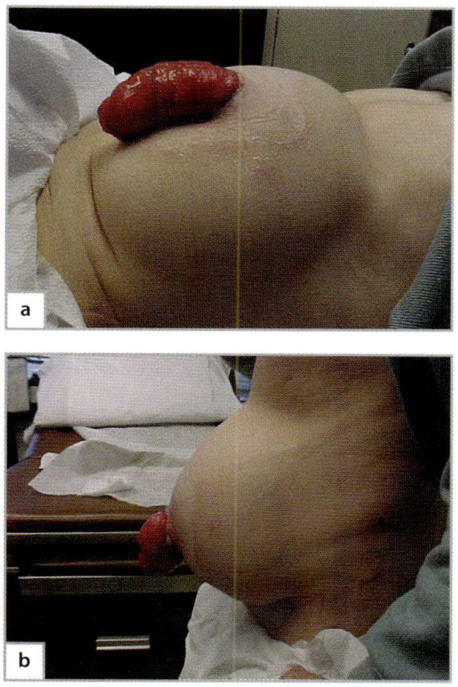

Figure 20.6 (a) Large paracolostomy hernia in recumbent patient. (b) Same patient as Figure 20.6a in standing position.

with the patient in the recumbent position. If the patient is symptomatic, i.e. the hernia is causing discomfort, obstructive symptoms, or is cosmetically disfiguring, surgical repair is warranted. There are numerous techniques to choose from, and as with surgery for rectal prolapse, where there are also numerous options, none are ideal, and hernia recurrence is common regardless of the approach used. The patient and family must be informed so.

Repair can be performed locally by an open or a laparoscopic approach. Alternatively, the stoma can be resited and the hernia repaired, again through either open or laparoscopic approaches. Several studies have shown that relocation is associated with a lower recurrence rate. Choice of a prosthetic material to reinforce the repair is problematic, particularly in the case of a colostomy, with higher risk of infection if this is nonresorbable. Different products are available, nonabsorbable, partially absorbable, and absorbable. Absorbable products are limited by their durability with respect to support for the abdominal wall. One prospective study using a partially resorbable product showed decreased hernia formation when this was used at the time of initial stoma creation (Serra-Aracil et al. 2009). Hansson et al. provide an excellent systematic review of surgical techniques for repair of parastomal hernias that is beyond the scope of this chapter (Hansson et al. 2012). They report that suture repair alone is associated with a higher recurrence rate than mesh repairs. Notwithstanding the controversy regarding the type of repair, this must be individualized to the patient, their comorbidities, the size of the hernia, and quality of the abdominal wall.

REOPERATION FOR CAPUT MEDUSAE

Peristomal varices are a late complication of ileostomies. This is frequently due to sclerosing cholangitis that has caused portal hypotension, but can occur secondary to portal hypertension of any etiology. This can be treated either with sclerotherapy or with mucocutaneous separation (Grundfest-Broniatowski & Fazio 1983). In the latter, a circumferential incision is made around the stoma with a 2-mL margin at the mucocutaneous junction down to the level of the fascia and the stoma then resutured to the same stoma site once the old mucocutaneous junction is trimmed away. This often results in a cessation of variceal bleeding for up 2 years. As an alternative, selective angioembolization or transjugular intrahepatic portosystemic shunt (TIPS) may also be helpful (Carrafiello et al. 2007, Pabon-Ramos et al. 2013).

COMPLICATIONS OFTEN TREATED NONOPERATIVELY

Many stomal problems can be treated with a good enterostomal therapist and minimize the need for reoperation. The in-office or direct participation of such a specialist is an enormous asset.

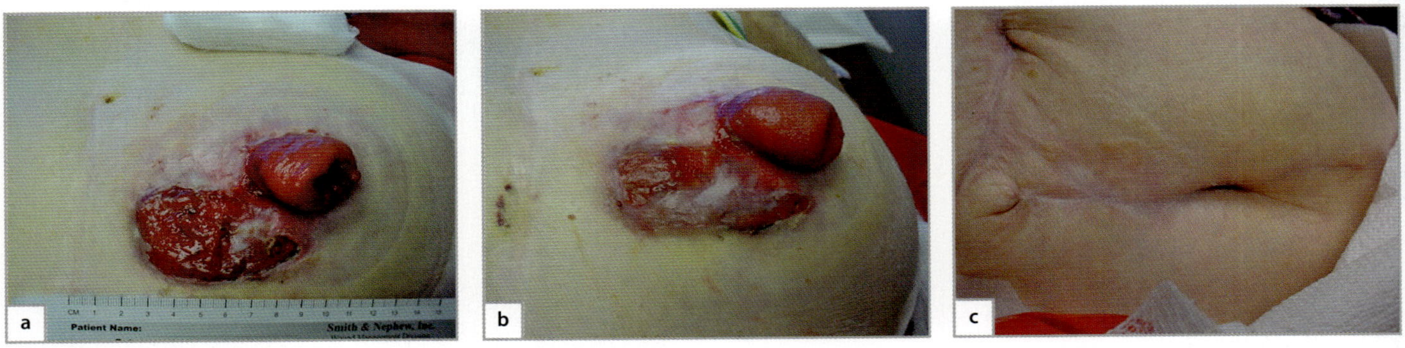

Figure 20.8 (a) Pyoderma gangrenosum adjacent to ileostomy overlying large parastomal hernia. (b) Slowly re-epithelializing pyoderma following intralesional steroid injection. (c) Same patient as Figures 20.8a and 20.8b after relocation of stoma and repair of parastomal hernia.

Enterostomal therapy aids that can minimize the need for reoperation include convex appliances, stoma belts, stoma adhesive paste, as well as hernia belts.

Mucocutaneous separations occur as commonly in patients who are malnourished, immunocompromised, or poorly perfused tissues. It can be circumferential or limited to a portion of the junction and can be superficial or deep. If it is deep, it needs to be filled in with an absorptive dressing, such as Aquacel or alginate. Mucocutaneous separation that occurs around an ileostomy can usually be treated with local measures, including application of stoma paste to the site, the use of sealing rings (Eakin seal) around the stoma, and a stoma belt. Mucocutaneous separation can occur superficially if the aperture is too large or the bowel too fibrotic to evert without tension, covering too bulky a mesentery or in the presence of superficial infection.

Fistulae can occur between the ileostomy and the skin if sutures are placed between the rigid fascia and bowel, and if the patient develops an ileus with abdominal distension and these sutures pull out.

Pyoderma is a frequent complication in patients with inflammatory bowel disease. Generally, this does not require surgery; therapy consists of intralesional steroid injections, biologic therapy with anti-tumor necrosis factor agents, or topical application of tacrolimus (Altieri et al. 2013, Kiran et al. 2005).

CONCLUSION

Reoperation for stoma problems is frequent and patient expectations must be addressed from the start. Careful assessment and preoperative planning are essential. Most acute stoma issues do not resolve without reoperation, but chronic ones can be managed as noted above.

REFERENCES

Allen-Mersh TG, Thomson JP. Surgical treatment of colostomy complications. Br J Surg 1988; 75:416–418.

AltieriM, Vaziri K, Orkin BA. Topical tacrolimus for parastomal pyoderma gangrenosum: a report of two cases. Ostomy Wound Manage 2010; 56:56–59.

Carne PW,Robertson GM, Frizelle FA. Parastomal hernia. Br J Surg 2003; 90:784–793.

Carrafiello G, Lagana D, Giorgianni A et al. Bleeding from peristomal varices in a cirrhotic patient with ileal conduit: treatment with transjugular intrahepatic portocaval shunt (TIPS). Emerg Radiol 2007; 13:341–343.

Grundfest-Broniatowski S, Fazio V. Conservative treatment of bleeding stomal varices. Arch Surg 1983; 118:981–985.

Hansson BM, Slater NJ, van der Velden AS et al. Surgical techniques for parastomal hernia repair: a systematic review of the literature. Ann Surg 2012; 255:685–695.

Horgan PG, Gorey TF. Operative assessment of intestinal viability. Surg Clin North Am 1992; 72:143–155.

Kiran RP, O'Brien-Ermlich B, Achkar JP, Fazio VW, Delaney CP. Management of peristomal pyoderma gangrenosum. Dis Colon Rectum 2005; 48:1397–1403.

Leenen LP, Kuypers JH. Some factors influencing the outcome of stoma surgery. Dis Colon Rectum 1989; 32:500–504.

Leong AP, Londono-Schimmer EE, Phillips RK. Life-table analysis of stomal complications following ileostomy. Br J Surg 1994; 81:727–729.

Matsui A, Winder JH, Laurence RG, Frangioni JV. Predicting the survival of experimental ischaemic small bowel using intraoperative near-infrared fluorescence angiography. Br J Surg 2011; 98:1725–1734.

Pabon-Ramos WM, Niemeyer MM, Dasika NL. Alternative treatment for bleeding peristomal varices: percutaneous parastomal embolization. Cardiovasc Intervent Radiol, 2013.

Serra-Aracil X, Bombardo-Junca J, Moreno-Matias J et al. Randomized, controlled, prospective trial of the use of a mesh to prevent parastomal hernia. Ann Surg 2009; 249:583–587.

Chapter 21 Surgical management of *Clostridium difficile* colitis

P. Ronan O'Connell, Olivier Gié

INTRODUCTION

Clostridium difficile

Clostridium difficile (from the Greek *kloster* (κλωστήρ): spindle) is a gram-positive anaerobic bacillus, which is widespread in nature, especially in the soil. Isolated in 1935 by Hall and O'Toole in the stool of healthy newborn (Hall & OToole 1935), at first its potential virulence was not realized and the association between antibiotics and colitis was identified only in 1973 by McNeill and Cohen (Cohen et al. 1973). One year later, in a prospective study involving patients treated with clindamycin, Tedesco et al. (1974) confirmed an incidence of diarrhea in 21% and pseudomembranous colitis in 10% of patients whose stool tested positively for *C. difficile*. Originally named 'bacillus difficilis' due to difficulty in isolation, this spore-forming bacteria was finally identified in 1978 by Bartlett et al. (1978) as the primary cause of pseudomembranous colitis in patients treated with antibiotics.

C. difficile most commonly exists in a vegetative form, is highly sensitive to oxygen, and can germinate in spores under stressful conditions. In this very resistant form, the spore can survive in extreme environments, such as gastric acid. This feature enables it to reach the small intestine and where it may develop into a vegetative form. The bacterium subsequently colonizes colonic mucosa and manifests virulence under specific circumstances. Several toxins are responsible for this. The most commonly described are TcdA and TcdB. Both are produced in response to environmental stimuli and enter the colonocyte through receptor-mediated endocytosis. This results in a severe inflammatory reaction in the colonic mucosa by inactivating the Ras superfamily of small GTPases via glycosylation (Voth & Ballard 2005).

TcdA is an enterotoxin, which stimulates cytokine production in human intestinal epithelial cells and monocytes. It generates inflammation with fluid accumulation in the bowel, infiltration of neutrophils, and activation of submucosal neurons with production of substance P. The role of toxin TcdB is cytotoxic and is not completely understood. It participates in the destruction of the actin cytoskeleton, which leads to cell death (Mitchell et al. 1987) and leakage of the tight junction between epithelial cells, which causes barrier loss. This effect may be determinant for the migration of neutrophils into the bowel lumen.

Epidemiology

C. difficile colonizes the gastrointestinal (GI) tract in 67% of newborns born in a hospital environment without causing particular symptoms (McFarland et al. 2000). The prevalence decreases to 3–5% among healthy adults and could be considered as a component of normal GI flora. *C. difficile* is transmitted in a fecal–oral mode and is widespread in hospital environment (McFarland et al. 1989). Despite increased emphasis on hygiene, there has been a sharp increase in *C. difficile* infection related to increasing use of antibiotics and the emergence of more resistant strains such that *C. difficile* is now the leading cause of hospital-acquired diarrhea in North American (Ricciardi et al. 2007) and Canadian (Loo et al. 2005) hospitals. The situation in Europe is similar. In the UK, two major outbreaks have been reported causing 38 deaths in <2 years (Smith 2005). These dramatic outbreaks were associated with a new hypervirulent bacterium characterized as BI by restriction endonuclease analysis, North America pulse-field type 1 (NAP1) by pulse-field gel electrophoresis and as ribotype 027 by PCR ribotyping. This particular strain of *C. difficile* showed a high production of TcdA and TcdB and combined a binary toxin named *C. difficile* toxin (CDT), which may potentiate enhancement of the action of toxins A and B. There are several theories to explain the recent increases in the incidence of *C. difficile*-related infection. First, improved detection methods have undoubtedly contributed to increased identification of the pathogen. Second, the broader use of antibiotics promotes the spread of *C. difficile* and contributes to its activation. There are currently an estimated 500,000 cases of clostridial infection annually within North American hospitals, with a healthcare cost of nearly US 1.1 billion dollars (Kyne et al. 2002).

Clinical manifestations

Symptoms of clostridial infection range from asymptomatic carriage to life-threatening toxic colitis. Exposure to *C. difficile* alone is probably not sufficient and disruption of the healthy colonic microbota secondary to antibiotic exposure is usually the first step in pathogenesis. This can occur after even a single dose of antibiotic has been administered. The most frequent manifestations of *C. difficile* infection are in order of increasing severity.

Asymptomatic

Widespread in hospital environment, *C. difficile* ingestion results, in the majority of cases, in an asymptomatic carriage without clinical evidence. McFarland et al. (1989) showed that 21% of patients admitted in hospital with negative cultures became infected with *C. difficile* during their stay; 63% of these patients remained asymptomatic. In long-term care facilities, the rate of carriage approaches 50% (Simor 2010). In health, the colonic microbiota limits clostridial growth and toxin production thus preventing toxic effects on the mucosa. Surprisingly, several studies have suggested that asymptomatic carriage of *C. difficile* actually protects against symptomatic disease (Giannasca & Warny 2004), as does an exaggerated immune response to the toxins with high production of antibodies (Kyne et al. 2000). Less symptomatic or asymptomatic subjects might be unwittingly responsible for the diffusion of the bacteria.

C. *difficile*-associated diarrhea (CDAD)

C. difficile is, by far, the leading cause of nosocomial diarrhea. Clindamycin, cephalosporins, fluoroquinolones, and penicillins are the antibiotics most frequently associated with CDAD (Owens et al. 2008). Watery diarrhea normally appears 48–72 hours after infection and is frequently accompanied by abdominal pain but symptoms can also arise several weeks later. In most, CDAD is self-limiting after stopping the antibiotic therapy; however, in some cases, an exacerbation of symptoms may be observed and spread of the contagion can lead to dramatic consequences if the infection is not promptly diagnosed and treated.

C. difficile-associated colitis (CDAC)

In the majority of cases *C. difficile* affects the colon without forming pseudomembranes. Clinical manifestations are more severe than with CDAD, with greater abdominal pain, watery diarrhea, leukocytosis, and fever. Colonoscopy reveals typical red patchy inflammation.

Pseudomembranous colitis

Pseudomembranous colitis is the most widely known infection due to *C. difficile*. The presence of yellow plaques scattered across the colorectal mucosa and sometimes the terminal ileum is the typical finding (**Figure 21.1**). These lesions are most commonly visible in the proximal colon and may be absent from the rectum. The histological examination shows a fibrinous exudate containing lymphocytes. The origin of the pseudomembrane is linked to cell destruction. The pseudomembrane is attached to mucosa and cannot easily be dislodged. Associated symptoms are severe abdominal pain and elevated white blood cells count. Patients suffering from pseudomembranous colitis need to be followed carefully because of a risk of toxic complications.

C. difficile fulminant colitis (CDFC)

Fulminant colitis occurs in 3–8% of patients infected with *C. difficile* (Olivas et al. 2010). There has recently been an increase in the incidence of CDFC due to the development of a new hypervirulent strain. The CDFC is frequently associated with organ failure and high mortality. Patients show a distended abdomen with severe pain and leukocytosis. Watery stools may be absent in the case of associated ileus. In such cases, medical therapy is often ineffective and patients may require salvage surgery. The reported operative mortality of CDFC is very high, reaching 80%, increasing with the patient's age.

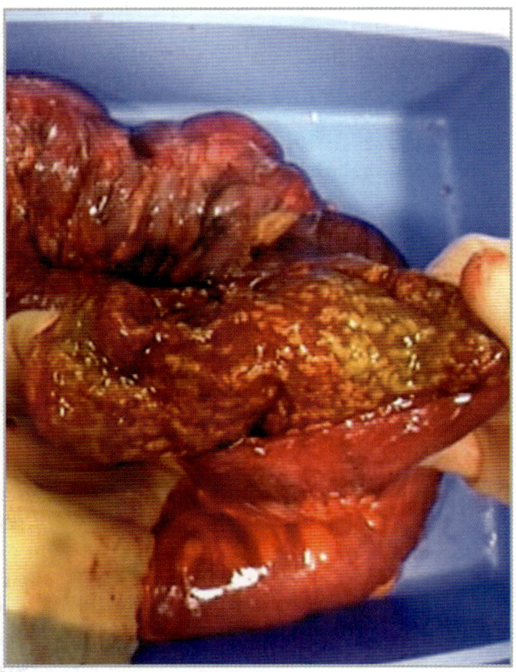

Figure 21.1 Macroscopic appearance of pseudomembranous colitis:
- The colonic wall is edematous
- Serosa is typically unaffected
- Pseudomembranes overlie an erythematous mucosa

C. difficile-associated enteritis

Enteritis is a rare complication of *C. difficile* infection but is increasingly recognized with emergence of a supervirulent strain. In the majority of cases, the enteritis occurs following recent GI surgery. Patients with pre-existing inflammatory bowel disease are particularly susceptible, especially after recent antibiotic therapy or a period of hospitalization (Kim & Muder 2011).

Imaging and laboratory tests

The diagnosis of a *C. difficile* infection is based on clinical symptoms, a recent intake of antibiotics even a single perioperative prophylactic dose, particularly of a cephalosporin, penicillin, or co-amoxiclav or the existence of other predisposing factors (see **Table 21.1**), as well as clinical investigations.

Laboratory tests

Identification of TcdA or TcdB in the stool is the easiest way to diagnose a clostridial infection. Toxin A can be directly observed in the stool using enzyme-linked immunosorbent assay (ELISA). This inexpensive procedure offers excellent specificity (95–100%) and results are available within 4 hours. However, this test has a low sensitivity (65–85%) and is therefore associated with high rate of false negative results (Turgeon et al. 2003).

The most sensitive technique (>90%), often considered as the 'gold standard' to detect *C. difficile*, is the stool culture and cytotoxin assay. This method is more sensitive but acquisition of results takes 4–5 days (Schmidt & Gilligan 2009).

Several molecular techniques provide detection of clostridial genome and allow its ribotyping. These methods include PCR ribotyping, pulsed field gel electrophoresis (PFGE), multilocus variable number tandem repeat analysis (MLVA), and multilocus sequence typing (MLST) (Kachrimanidou & Malisiovas 2011). Identification of a specific ribotype is fundamental to identify outbreaks.

CT scan

Computed tomography (CT) scanning can be useful in terms of diagnosis, often showing the typical 'thumb-printing' lesion of a distended colon (**Figures 21.2** and **21.3**). However, such images are not specific to clostridial infection. In severe clostridial disease, typical radiological findings show the 'accordion sign' produced by discontinuous edematous haustral folds interrupted by transverse mucosal ridges.

Table 21.1 Risk factors of *Clostridium difficile*-associated disease

Drug intake:
Antibiotics
Proton pump inhibitor
Valacyclovir
Comorbidities:
Inflammatory bowel diseases
Immunocompromised patients
Age
Surgical conditions:
History of previous gastrointestinal surgery
Post-transplantation patients
Peripartum
Others:
Prolonged stay in healthcare settings

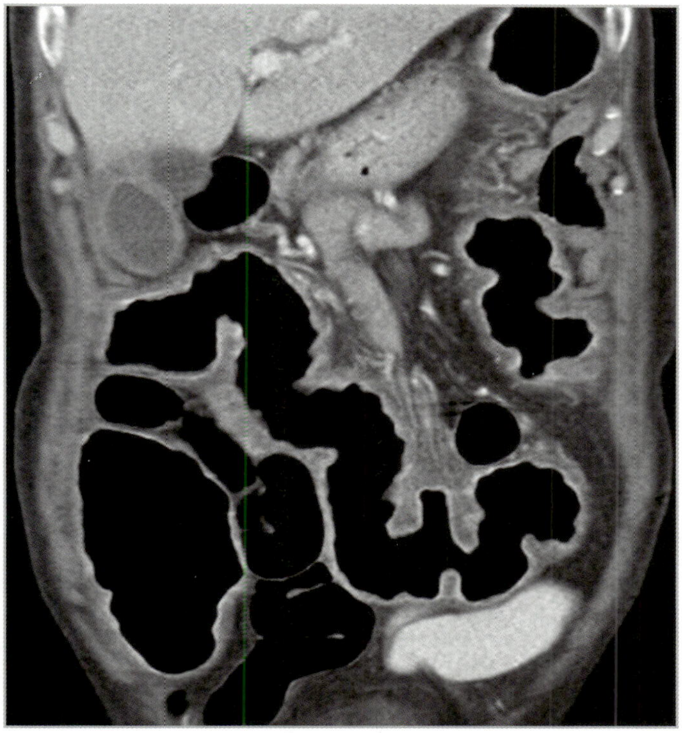

Figure 21.2 Computed tomography of patient with *Clostridium difficile* colitis (coronal). Colonic distension and wall thickening associated with submucosal edema.

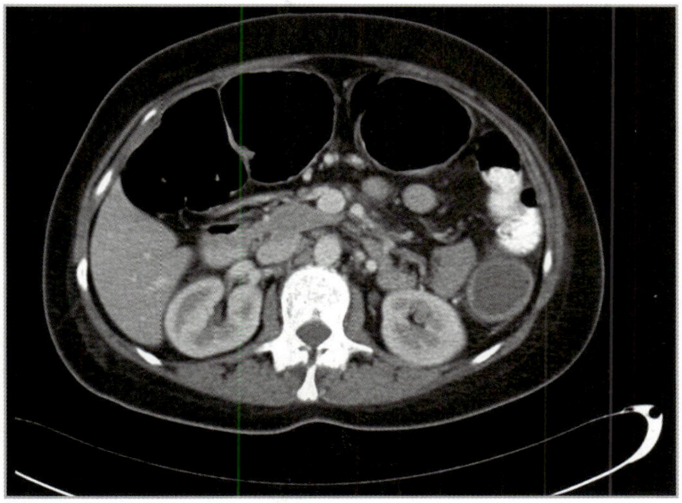

Figure 21.3 Computed tomography patient with *Clostridium difficile* colitis (axial).

Colonoscopy

Clostridial colitis is easily diagnosed in the presence of pseudomembranes (**Figure 21.4**) typically located proximally above the rectum. As reported by Hookman et al. there are four main indications for colonoscopy: (1) negative laboratory tests but high level of clinical suspicion, (2) prompt diagnosis is needed, (3) lack of response to antibiotic therapy, (4) atypical presentation (Hookman & Barkin 2009).

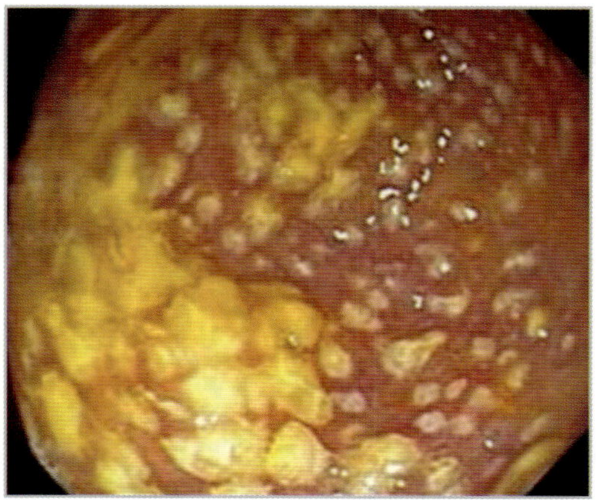

Figure 21.4 Endoscopic appearances of pseudomembranes.

Full colonoscopy is not indicated in the presence of a massively distended colon and in presence of fulminant colitis because of the risk of perforation; however, limited left-sided endoscopy may be diagnostic.

Medical management

The treatment of a clostridial infection is dependent on the seriousness of the symptoms. The diagnosis of the pathogen as well as the introduction of an efficient antibiotic therapy is crucial. It is absolutely necessary that this be continuously monitored. Constipating therapy must be avoided since one of the aims of the treatment is the elimination of toxins within the colonic lumen. Antibiotic treatment suspected as contributing to the development of the colitis must be cautiously suspended; if not, treatment success rate will be lower.

Antibiotics

Asymptomatic carriage of *C. difficile* is transient in most patients so that systematic screening followed by administration of metronidazole or vancomycin is ineffective (Johnson et al. 1992). Oral metronidazole (500 mg, tid) and vancomycin (125 mg, qid) are equally efficient in treatment of mild CDAD induced by ribotype 001. To avoid resistance and decrease the selection pressure for vancomycin-resistant enterococci, treatment should start with metronidazole. Vancomycin should be introduced only in refractory cases or in particular situations, such as (1) advanced age (>65 years), (2) immunocompromised patients, and (3) pre-existing inflammatory bowel disease. Both antibiotics should be administrated orally; vancomycin in particular, when given intravenously is poorly excreted into the bowel lumen and is less effective.

In severe CDAD, vancomycin is more effective compared with metronidazole (97% vs. 76%, $p = 0.02$) (Zar et al. 2007) and a higher dose (500 mg qid) is more appropriate. In presence of ileus, vancomycin can be administered per rectum (500 mg in 100 mL normal saline every 6 hours as a retention enema) in combination with intravenous metronidazole (500 mg, tid). Freeman et al. (2007) showed that new *C. difficile* ribotype 027 is more resistant to metronidazole in the intestinal lumen than ribotype 001.

Other antibiotics like nitazoxanide (Musher et al. 2007), fidaxomicin (Mullane et al. 2011), teicoplanin, and ramoplanin have efficacy in treatment of severe CDAD, but should be administered as second-line treatment only with the guidance of a microbiologist.

Table 21.2 summarizes recommendations for the treatment of a first episode of *C. difficile* infection according to the guidelines of the Society for Healthcare Epidemiology of America (SHEA) and the Infectious Diseases Society of America (IDSA) (Cohen et al. 2010).

Table 21.2 Recommendations for the treatment of a first episode of *Clostridium difficile* infection (CDI)

Clinical manifestation	Symptoms	Treatment
Mild CDI	Diarrhea, mild abdominal pain, leukocytosis <15,000 cells/μL	Metronidazole 500 mg orally tid for 10–14 days
Severe CDI	Diarrhea, abdominal pain, leukocytosis >15,000 cells/μL	Vancomycin 125 mg orally qid for 10–14 days
Severe, complicated CDI	Abdominal pain and distension, leukocytosis >15,000 cells/μL, +/– ileus.	Vancomycin 500 mg qid administered orally or nasogastric tube (and per rectum, if ileus is present, 500 mg in approximately 100 mL normal saline every 6 hours as a retention enema) with or without intravenously administered metronidazole (500 mg tid)

Intravenous immunoglobulin (IVIG)

Animal studies suggest that passive immunization with immunoglobulin protects against *C. difficile* infection and can prevent diarrhea (Lyerly et al. 1991). In humans, the rate of antitoxin A and B antibodies decreases with age (Aronsson et al. 1983, Bacon & Fekety 1994) and symptoms are less severe and of shorter duration in patients with a higher level of antitoxin A antibodies (Warny et al. 1994). On this basis, Leung et al. (1991) successfully treated children suffering from recurrent *C. difficile* colitis despite antibiotic use (Leung et al. 1991) with IVIG. Multiple studies have subsequently confirmed the efficiency of IVIG in relapsing and protracted *C. difficile* infection (Abougergi & Kwon 2011, Salcedo et al. 1997). In the absence of randomized trials, IVIG should be used only in adjunct with medical therapy.

Monoclonal antibodies

Thanks to encouraging results on an animal model (Babcock et al. 2006), Lowy et al. (2010) developed a fully human monoclonal antibody targeting TcdA and TcdB. In a randomized, double-blind, placebo-controlled study enrolling 200 patients, they showed a lower rate of recurrence of *C. difficile* infection among subjects treated with monoclonal antibodies for both conventional and epidemic BI/NAP1/027 strain and among patients with more than one previous episode of *C. difficile* infection. They concluded that the supplement of monoclonal antibodies with antibiotic significantly reduced the recurrence of *C. difficile* infection.

INDICATIONS FOR SURGERY

While there is a desire to avoid colectomy, inappropriate delay in a very ill patient can be fatal. Judgment on when to intervene is difficult and requires analysis of the factors that predict outcome with and without surgery. Greenstein et al. (2008) demonstrated in a multivariate logistic regression on a cohort of 35 patients that four factors are associated with progression to fulminant colitis:

- Leukocytosis >16,000/μL
- Surgery within the preceding 30 days
- History of inflammatory bowel disease
- History of past IVIG treatment

In the absence of colectomy, 95% of patients with a white blood cell count >50,000/μL or lactate >5 mmol/L died within 30 days. **Table 21.3** summarizes the factors linked with fulminant colitis, surgery, and high mortality.

Surgical management

The rate of surgery for fulminant colitis has risen (Dallal et al. 2002) and it is estimated that approximately 5% of clostridial-infected patients will undergo surgery for severe medically refractory *C. difficile* infection.

The decision to operate is largely based on clinical grounds and surgeon experience. Retrospective analysis has shown that, compared with medical treatment, colectomy seems to be advantageous in patients aged 65 years or older, with a leukocytosis ≥20 × 10^9/L or serum lactate between 2.9 and 4.9 mmol/L (Dallal et al. 2002). Then again surgery is mandatory in the cases where there are peritoneal signs or toxic megacolon associated with a need for vasopressor support.

Particular attention must be paid to patients suffering from inflammatory bowel disease since they have an increased risk of developing colitis requiring colectomy (Issa et al. 2007).

Although the laparoscopy has been reported, a vertical midline laparotomy is considered to be the best approach for *C. difficile*

Table 21.3 Factors linked with fulminant colitis, surgery, and high mortality

Factors predicting fulminant colitis	Factors predicting surgery	Factors predicting fatal outcomes
Leukocytosis >16,000	Leukocytosis >20,000	Leukocytosis >50,000
Surgery within 30 days	Lactate 2.9–4.9 mmol/L (Lamontagne et al. 2007)	Lactate >5 mmol/L
History of inflammatory bowel disease	Age >75	Hypoalbuminemia
History of past intravenous immunoglobulin treatment	Computed tomography results: Colon dilatation Colon thickening Free fluid Free air	Organ failure Vasopressors Steroid use ASA score >3 Apache II score >8
	Clinical findings: Abdominal distension Abdominal tenderness Peritonitis	

colitis. Once the abdomen is entered, it is not uncommon to find free ascitic fluid present surrounding distended, thickened loops of bowel. It is important to initially identify and control any perforation. Classically, the serosa is not affected and the extent of colonic involvement can be difficult to recognize. Serosal tears should be oversewn prior to commencing resection. Mobilization starts at the cecum, dividing the lateral peritoneal attachments and extending the dissection from right to left opening the lesser sac. Care must be exercised particularly when approaching the hepatic flexure. Colonic decompression should be considered if the bowel is distended and friable. Segmental resection is ineffective and is associated with an increased risk of further resection (Adams & Mercer 2007, Koss et al. 2006,) Therefore, the procedure of choice is a subtotal colectomy with preservation of the rectum and fashioning of an ileostomy. This approach has the best chance of restoring GI continuity after the acute insult has settled. Primary anastomosis is not recommended. An alternative to colectomy that may be considered in patients with intractable but not toxic colitis is irrigation of the colon with vancomycin (Apisarnthanarak et al. 2002) through a defunctioning ileostomy or a cecostomy. High volumes of saline solution containing polyethylene glycol followed by vancomycin flushes introduced through the efferent loop of the ileostomy may eradicate *C. difficile* bacteria and toxin from the colon (Castillo et al. 2012) with lower mortality and morbidity compared with colectomy (Neal et al. 2011).

Postoperative care

Most patients proceeding to colectomy are hemodynamically unstable. Fluid administration with concomitant use of vasopressors is often required. In the postoperative period, patients are often unstable and must be followed within an intensive care unit (ICU) where multiorgan support is available.

Sometimes, in spite of the surgical resection, clinical improvement is inadequate suggesting active disease in the rectal stump. Again intraluminal vancomycin therapy instilled through the anus is helpful to reduce the bacterial load inside the defunctioned rectum. Further surgery can be avoided by rinsing the stump with 500 mg of vancomycin in 100 mL normal saline every 6 hours.

Outcome of surgery

The mortality associated with colectomy for fulminant colitis ranges between 35% and 57% (Dallal et al. 2002, Issa et al. 2007). Retrospective multivariate analysis showed that medical treatment of >6 days with no improvement is associated with a higher mortality rate (Synnott et al. 1998) (**Table 21.4**). The survival rate is higher in patients without multiorgan failure (MOF) (87.5% vs. 33.3% in patient with MOF (Apisarnthanarak et al. 2002)). MOF is the most frequent cause of death in operated patients and therefore is imperative that such patients should be managed in an ICU setting postoperatively. In a cohort of 34 patients with fulminant colitis needing colectomy, the average ICU length of stay was 12 ± 14 days (Hall & Berger 2008) and the mean hospital stay exceeds 30 days in the majority of reported cases.

Special considerations

Rectal stump management

After colon mobilization and before colectomy, it is important to plan management of the rectal stump. Ideally this would minimize the risk

Table 21.4 Mortality following surgical intervention for *Clostridium difficile* colitis (n.s., not stated)

Investigator/Reference	Number of patients who underwent surgery/ Total number of patients with *Clostridium difficile* disease	Mortality (%)
Colectomy		
Al-Abed et al. (2010)	20/528 (3.7%)	40
Byrn et al. (2008)	73/5718 (1.3%)	34
Longo et al. (2004)	67/n.s.	48
Synnott et al. (1998)	5/138 (3.6%)	80
Koss et al. (2006)	14/3472 (0.4%)	35.7
Lamontagne et al. (2007)	38/165 (23%)	34
Trudel et al. (1995)	7/11 (64%)	71
Dallal et al. (2002)	44/2334 (1.9%)	57
Klipfel et al. (2000)	10/n.s.	80
Ali et al. (2008)	36/n.s.	47
Lipsett et al. (1994)	13/3300 (0.39%)	38
Greenstein et al. (2008)	35/6283 (0.56%)	40
Gash et al. (2010)	18/1398 (1.29%)	50
Dudukgian et al. (2010)	14/398 (3.52%)	28.6
Sailhamer et al. (2009)	50/4796 (1.04%)	24
Hall et al. (2008)	36/3237 (1.1%)	36.1
Pepin et al. (2009)	130/?	37
Diverting loop ileostomy		
Neal et al. (2011)	42/?	19

of rectal dehiscence, wound infection, pelvic sepsis, and facilitate restorative surgery.

Subcutaneous closure

The colon is divided at the level of the distal sigmoid to allow the distal limb to be brought into the laparotomy wound. No pelvic dissection takes place. The closed end is sutured above the fascia in the inferior edge of the laparotomy wound and the skin closed. The rectum should be drained using a wide bore transanal drainage tube. The disadvantages of this procedure are the need for a long stump with risk of persistent inflammation and a high risk of wound infection. In more than one-third of cases, the rectosigmoid stump opens spontaneously resulting in a mucous fistula. The advantages are reduced risk of rectal stump 'blow-out' with sometimes fatal peritonitis and easier later reconstruction.

Mucous fistula

The sigmoid colon is divided as above leaving sufficient length to allow a defunctioned colocutaneous anastomosis (mucus fistula) through the lower end of the laparotomy wound. This facilitates drainage of the remaining rectum and instillation of antibiotics. The advantages are those of the subcutaneous closure; however, the risk of wound infection is greater and a mucus fistula can be difficult for the patient to manage.

Intraperitoneal closure (Hartmann's closure)

For anatomical reasons or as a consequence of severe colonic inflammation, subcutaneous closure or a mucus fistula may not be possible. In these circumstances, the rectal stump is closed at the peritoneal reflection. Pelvic dissection should be avoided. The rectal stump must be drained with a transanal drain. The major risk is breakdown of the rectal closure resulting in stump 'blow out' that can occur in 12%. Rarely, closure of the rectal stump may be considered unsafe and a mucus fistula technically impossible. In such circumstances or when profuse rectal bleeding is present, proctectomy with either closure at the level of the pelvic floor or a completion proctectomy should be performed.

CONCLUSION

Clostridial-related complications are common in surgical patients. Patients who receive antibiotics, especially those undergoing GI surgery, are at increased risk. If active clostridial infection is suspected, samples should be sent for toxin levels and culture. Medical therapy should commence without delay. Despite medical treatment, fulminant colitis or toxic megacolon may ensue. Associated comorbidities often delay the decision to operate. Total abdominal colectomy preserving the rectum with end ileostomy is the procedure of choice. A primary anastomosis is not recommended. Care must be exercised in the management of the rectal stump.

REFERENCES

Abougergi MS, Kwon JH. Intravenous Immunoglobulin for the treatment of *Clostridium difficile* Infection: a review. Dig Dis Sci 2011; 56:19–23.

Adams SD, Mercer DW. Fulminant *Clostridium difficile* colitis. Curr Opin Crit Care 2007;13:450–455.

Al-Abed YA, Gray EA, Rothnie ND. Outcomes of emergency colectomy for fulminant *Clostridium difficile* colitis. The Surgeon 2010; 8:330–333.

Ali SO, Welch JP, Dring RJ. Early surgical intervention for fulminant pseudomembranous colitis. Am Surg 2008; 74:20–26.

Apisarnthanarak A, Khoury H, Reinus WR, Crippin JS, Mundy LM. Severe *Clostridium difficile* colitis: the role of intracolonic vancomycin? AM J Med 2002; 112:328–329.

Aronsson B, Granström M, Möllby R, Nord CE. Enzyme-linked immunosorbent assay (ELISA) for antibodies to *Clostridium difficile* toxins in patients with pseudomembranous colitis and antibiotic-associated diarrhoea J Immunol Methods 1983; 60:341–350.

Babcock GJ, Broering TJ, Hernandez HJ, et al. Human monoclonal antibodies directed against toxins A and B prevent *Clostridium difficile*-induced mortality in hamsters. Infect Immun 2006; 74:6339–6347.

Bacon AE III, Fekety R. Immunoglobulin G directed against toxin A and B of *Clostridium difficile* in the general population and patient with antibiotic-associated diarrhea. Diagn Microbiol Infect Dis 1994; 18:205–209.

Bartlett JG, Moon N, Chang TW, Taylor N, Onderdonk AB. Role of *Clostridium difficile* in antibiotic associated pseudomembranous colitis. Gastroenetrology 1978; 75:778–782.

Byrn JC, Maun DC, Gingold DS, et al. Predictors of mortality after colectomy for fulminant *Clostridium difficile* colitis. Arch Surg 2008; 143:150–154.

Castillo A, Lopez J, Panadero E, et al. Conservative surgical treatment for toxic megacolon due to *Clostridium difficile* infection in a transplanted pediatric patient. Transpl Infect Dis 2012; 14:E34–7.

Cohen SH, Gerding DN, Johnson S, et al. Clinical practice guidelines for *Clostridium difficile* infection in adult: 2010 update by the Society for Healthcare Epidemiology of America (SHEA) and the Infectious Diseases Society of America (IDSA). Infect Control Hosp Epidemiol 2010; 31:431–449.

Cohen LE, McNeill CJ, Wells RF. Clindamycin-associated colitis. JAMA 1973; 223:1379–1380.

Dallal RM, Harbrecht BG, Boujoukas AJ, et al. Fulminant *Clostridium difficile*: an underappreciated and increasing cause of death and complications. Ann Surg 2002; 235:363–372.

Dudukgian H, Sie E, Gonzalez-Ruiz C, Etzioni DA, Kaiser AM. C. difficile colitis – predictors of fatal outcome. J Gastrointest Surg 2010; 14:315–322.

Freeman J, Baines SD, Saxton K, Wilkox MH. Effect of metronidazole on growth and toxin production by epidemic *Clostridium difficile* PCR ribotype 001 and 027 in a human gut model. J Antimicrob Chemother 2007; 60:83–91.

Gash K, Brown E, Pullyblank A. Emergency subtotal colectomy for fulminant *Clostridium difficile* colitis -- is a surgical solution considered for all patients? Ann R Coll Surg Engl 2010; 92:56–60.

Giannasca PJ, Warny M. Active and passive immunization against *Clostridium difficile* diarrhea and colitis. Vaccine 2004; 22:848–856.

Greenstein AJ, Byrne JC, Zhang LP, et al. Risk factors for the development of fulminant *Clostridium difficile* colitis. Surgery 2008; 143:623–629.

Hall JF, Berger D. Outcome of colectomy for *Clostridium difficile* colitis: a plea for early surgical management. Am J Surg 2008; 196:384–388.

Hall IC, O'Toole E. Intestinal flora in newborn infants with a description of a new pathogenic anaerobe, Bacillus difficilis. Am J Dis Child 1935; 49:390–402.

Hookman P, Barkin JS. *Clostridium difficile* associated infection, diarrhea and colitis. World J Gastroenterol 2009; 15:1554–1580.

Issa M, Vijayapal A, Graham MB, et al. Impact of *Clostridium difficile* on inflammatory bowel disease. Clin Gastroeneterol Hepatol 2007; 5:345–351.

Johnson S, Homann SR, Bettin KM, et al. Treatment of asymptomatic *Clostridium difficile* carriers (fecal excretors) with vancomycin or metronidazole. A randomized, placebo-controlled trial. Ann Intern Med 1992; 117:297–302.

Kachrimanidou M, Malisiovas N. *Clostridium difficile* infection: a comprehensive review. Crit Rev Microbiol 2011; 37:178–187.

Kim JH, Muder RR. *Clostridium difficile* enteritis: a review and pole analysis of the cases. Anaerobe 2011; 17:52–55.

Klipfel AA, Schein M, Fahoum B, Wise L. Acute abdomen and *Clostridium difficile* colitis: still a lethal combination. Dig Surg 2000; 17:160–163.

Koss K, Clark MA, Sanders DS, et al. The outcome of surgery in fulminant *Clostridium difficile* colitis. Colorectal Dis 2006; 8:149–154.

Kyne L, Hamel MB, Polavaram R, Kelly PC. Health care costs and mortality associated diarrhea due to *Clostridium difficile*. Clin Infect Dis 2002; 34:346–353.

Kyne L, Warny M, Qamar A, Kelly CO. Asymptomatic carriage of *Clostridium difficile* and serum levels of IgG antibody against toxin A. N Engl J Med 2000; 342:390–397.

Lamontagne F, Labbé AC, Haeck O, et al. Impact of emergency colectomy on survival of patients with fulminant *Clostridium difficile* colitis during an epidemic caused by hypervirulent strain. Ann Surg 2007; 245:267–272.

Leung DY, Kelly CP, Boguniewicz M, et al. Treatment of intravenously administered gamma globulin of chronic relapsing colitis induced by *Clostridium difficile* toxin. J Pedriatr 1991; 118:633–637.

Lipsett PA, Samantaray DK, Tam ML, Bartlett JG, Lillemoe KD. Pseudomembranous colitis: a surgical disease? Surgery 1994; 116:491–496.

Longo WE, Mazuski JE, Virgo KS, et al. Outcome after colectomy for *Clostridium difficile* colitis. Dis Colon Rectum 2004; 47:1620–1626.

Loo VG, Poirier L, Miller MA, et al. A predominantly clonal multi-institutional outbreak of *Clostridium difficile*-associated diarrhea with high morbidity and mortality. N Engl J Med; 2005; 353:2442–2449.

Lowy I, Molrine DC, Leav BA, et al. Treatment with monoclonal antibodies against *Clostridium difficile* toxins. N Engl J Med 2010; 362:197–205.

Lyerly DM, Bostwick EF, Binion SB, Wilkins TD. Passive immunization of hamsters against disease caused by *Clostridium difficile* by use of bovine immunoglobulin G concentrate. Infect Immun 1991; 59:2215–2218.

McFarland LV, Brandmarker SA, Guandalini S. Pediatric *Clostridium difficile*: a phantom menace or clinical reality? J Pediatr Gastroenterol Nutr 2000; 31:220–231.

McFarland LV, Mulligan ME, Kwok RY, Stamm WE. Nosocomial acquisition of *Clostridium difficile* infection. N Engl J Med 1989; 320:204–210.

Mitchell MJ, Laughon BE, Lin S. Biochemical studies on the effect of *Clostridium difficile* toxin B on actin in vivo and in vitro. Infect Immun 1987; 55:1610–1615.

Mullane KM, Miller MA, Weiss K, et al. Efficacy of fidaxomicin versus vancomycin as therapy for *Clostridium difficile* infection in individuals taking concomitant antibiotics for other concurrent infections. Clin Infect Dis 2011; 53:440–447.

Musher D M, Logan N, Mehendiratta V, et al. *Clostridium difficile* colitis that fails conventional metronidazole therapy: response to nitazoxanide. J Antimicrob Chemother 2007; 59:705–710.

Neal MD, Alverdy JC, Hall DE, Simmons RL, Zuckerbraun BS. Diverting loop ileostomy and colonic lavage: an alternative to total abdominal colectomy for the treatment of severe, complicated *Clostridium difficile* associated disease. Ann Surg 2011; 254:423–427; discussion 427–429.

Olivas AD, Umanskiy K, Zuckerbraun B, Alverdy JC. Avoiding colectomy during surgical management of fulminant *Clostridium difficile* colitis. Surg Infect (Larchmt) 2010; 11:299–305.

Owens RC, Donskey CJ, Gaynes RP, Loo VG, Muto CA. Antimicrobial-associated risk factors for *Clostridium difficile* infection. Clin Infect Dis 2008; 46:S19–31.

Pepin J, Vo TT, Boutros M, et al. Risk factors for mortality following emergency colectomy for fulminant *Clostridium difficile* infection. Dis Colon Rectum 2009; 52:400–405.

Ricciardi R, Rothenberger DA, Madoff RD, Baxter NN. Increasing prevalence and severity of *Clostridium difficile* colitis in hospitalized patients in the United States. Arch Surg 2007; 142:624–631.

Sailhamer EA, Carson K, Chang Y, et al. Fulminant *Clostridium difficile* colitis: patterns of care and predictors of mortality. Arch Surg 2009; 144:433–439; discussion 439–440.

Salcedo J, Keates S, Pothoulakis C, et al. Intravenous immunoglobulin therapy for severe *Clostridium difficile* colitis. Gut 1997; 41:366–370.

Schmidt ML, Gilligan PH. *Clostridium difficile* testing algorithms: what is practical and feasible? Anaerobe 2009; 15:270–273.

Simor AE. Diagnosis, management, and prevention of *Clostridium difficile* infection in long-term care facilities: a review. J Am Geriatr Soc. 2010; 58:1556–1564.

Smith A. Outbreak of *Clostridium difficile* infection in an English Hospital linked to hypertoxin-producing strains in Canada and the US. Euro Surveill 2005; 10:(26):pii=2735.

Synnott K, Mealy K, Merry C, et al. Timing of surgery for fulminating pseudomembranous colitis. Br J Surg 1998; 85:229–231.

Tedesco FJ, Barton RW, Alpers DH. Clindamycin-associated colitis: a prospective study. Ann Intern Med 1974; 81:429–433.

Trudel JL, Deschenes M, Mayrand Ş, Barkun AN. Toxic megacolon complicating pseudomembranous enterocolitis. Dis Colon Rectum 1995; 38:1033–1038.

Turgeon DK, Novicki TJ, Quick J, et al. Six rapid tests for direct detection of *Clostridium difficile* and its toxin in fecal samples compared with the fibroblast cytotoxity assay. J Clin Microbiol 2003; 41:667–670.

Voth DE, Ballard JD. *Clostridium difficile* toxins: mechanism of action and role of disease. Clin Microbiol Rev 2005; 18:247–263.

Warny M, Vaerman JP, Avesani V, Delmee M. Human antibody response to *Clostridium difficile* toxin A in relation to clinical course of infection. Infect Immun 1994; 62:384–389.

Zar FA, Bakkanagari SR, Moorthi KM, Davis MB. A comparison of vancomycin and metronidazole for the treatment of *Clostridium difficile*-associated diarrhea, stratified by disease severity. Clin Infect Dis 2007; 5:302–307.

Chapter 22 Reoperative abdominal surgery for chronic vascular events

Peter Lamont

INTRODUCTION

Surgery of the abdominal aorta and visceral vessels within the abdomen, whether for aneurysmal or for occlusive disease, carries an excellent prospect of long-term cure once the immediate dangers of the surgery are overcome. Patients who have a successful abdominal aortic aneurysm (AAA) repair return to a normal life expectancy for their age and comorbidities. Graft patency rates of 95% 5 years after aortobiiliac/bifemoral bypass grafts can be expected. Long-term complications are rare, but when they do occur, can be challenging to deal with. In the case of open surgery, incisional herniation, intra-abdominal adhesions, and scarring around the vessels make access difficult. Contamination or infection of prosthetic graft materials offers a variety of problems with no clear-cut 'best' solution. The patients also often have significant comorbidities limiting the choice of intervention. The introduction of endovascular procedures within the abdominal vasculature has reduced the mortality risk from the initial procedure but is associated with a much higher risk of subsequent reintervention; should that reintervention involve open surgery, then the mortality risk may also be much higher than a primary open procedure.

Each patient needing reintervention presents different and often unique challenges. The decision of how best to tackle the problem mandates involvement of a multidisciplinary team involving vascular surgeons, interventional radiologists, vascular scientists, and vascular anesthetists. Input from microbiology, cardiology, renal medicine, and gastrointestinal (GI) surgery may be needed. These cases are never easy and should only be undertaken in a high-volume vascular center with full vascular imaging and critical care facilities.

THE NEED FOR VASCULAR REINTERVENTION

Graft-related complications after open AAA repair are rare and patients are more likely to need surgery for nonvascular complications, such as incisional hernia or adhesion-related small bowel obstruction (Kieffer et al. 2012). The risk of reintervention for graft-related complications seems to have improved, as surgical techniques, graft materials, and vascular sutures have evolved. In an early series of patients operated at the Mayo Clinic between 1957 and 1990, late graft complications were seen in 6.8% of patients (Hallett et al. 1997). More modern series from the past two or three decades show the risk of late vascular reintervention in the 2–3% range (Adam et al. 2006, Conrad et al. 2007, Kieffer et al. 2012). Graft-related complications include para-anastomotic aneurysms (true or false), graft infection, aortoenteric fistula, and graft thrombosis.

Graft-related complications after endovascular AAA repair (EVAR) are undoubtedly more common, although the majority can be managed by further endovascular means. Some 15–27% of patients require reintervention after EVAR, with some evidence that the risk of reintervention is higher in patients with earlier generation devices, which are now obsolete (Becquemin et al. 2004, Cao et al. 2004, Sampram et al. 2003). While only 2–3% of patients need open surgery for reintervention, the majority of these involve some form of extra-anatomic bypass, such as axillofemoral or femorofemoral bypass for graft limb thrombosis. The need for open abdominal surgery after EVAR is rare, under 1% of patients and usually for late rupture, endoleak or graft infection, but mortality risk is then high, of the order of 20% (**Figure 22.1**).

Aortoiliac or aortofemoral bypass for occlusive disease is now rarely performed in the modern era. The majority of patients can be managed either by percutaneous angioplasty, with or without stenting, by extra-anatomic bypass, or by a combination of angioplasty and extra-anatomic bypass. These latter strategies carry a much lower mortality risk than open aortic surgery and are now first choice of treatment. Just as with grafts for AAA repair, those patients who do undergo aortic bypass surgery may develop late graft-related complications such as graft infection, aortoenteric fistula, and graft thrombosis.

Late complications after visceral vessel reconstruction are rarely seen, perhaps because open visceral vessel reconstruction is itself rare. The majority of patients with mesenteric or renal artery stenosis requiring intervention are presently managed by angioplasty and stenting. Those patients who do undergo open surgical bypass are at risk of late graft complications requiring reintervention, predominantly graft stenosis, or thrombosis (**Figure 22.2**), although rare instances of graft infection have also been recorded.

Para-anastomotic and false aneurysms

Para-anastomotic aneurysms are the commonest graft-related complication and are twice as likely to occur after a ruptured AAA repair than after an elective repair (Cho et al. 1998). Imaging studies of patients who have survived >5 years after an elective AAA repair reveal new aneurysms developing in a large proportion, with up to 24% of patients developing a new aneurysm in the proximal aorta adjacent to the top end of the graft and 45% developing aneurysms in noncontiguous arterial segments, predominantly in the iliac arteries but also in the thoracic aorta (Conrad et al. 2007, Kalman et al. 1999). Few of these new, true aneurysms reach a size where intervention is needed but when they do, excluding them can be difficult. The proximal ones are often juxtarenal and the iliac ones may be very tortuous and so not suitable for endovascular repair (**Figure 22.3**).

False aneurysms at an anastomotic suture line are less common, occurring in around 5% of patients. Many vascular surgeons now try to avoid a distal anastomosis to the femoral artery in the groin as a high

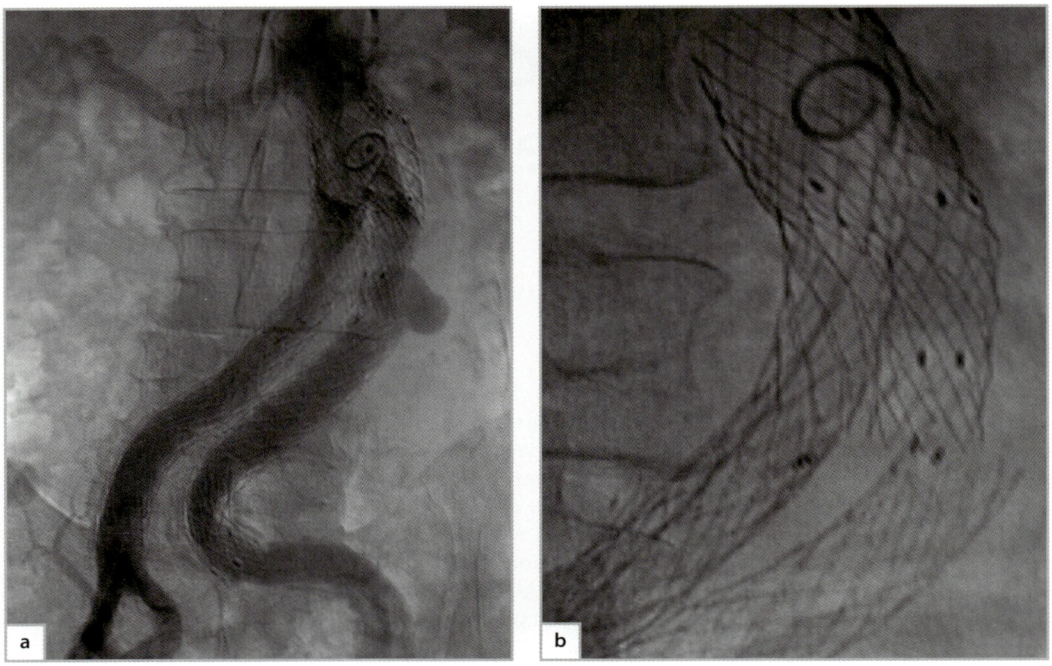

Figure 22.1 (a) A type III endoleak from an aortic stent graft due to migration of the left limb of the graft. (b) It proved impossible to pass a guidewire through the displaced, overlapping junction of the graft, and open repair was required.

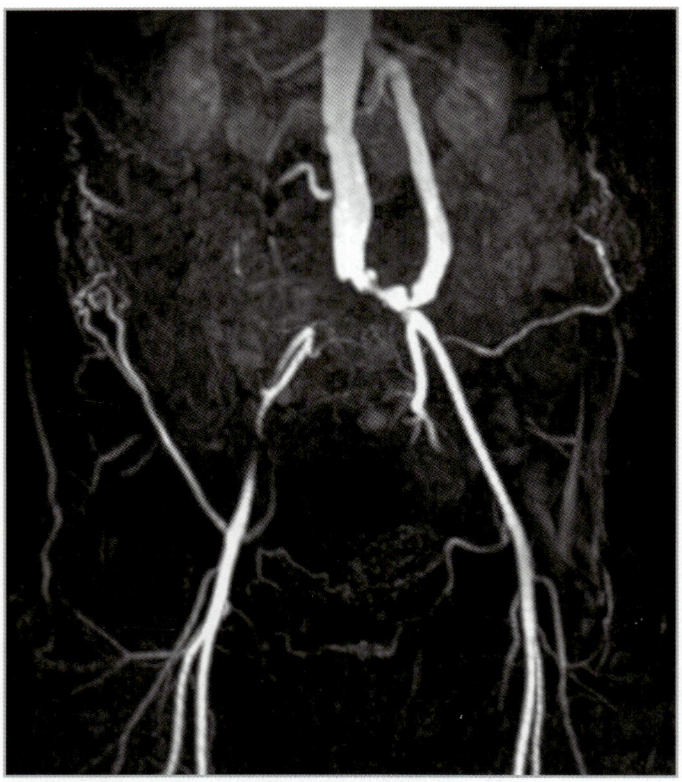

Figure 22.2 Progression of atherosclerosis and stenosis in the left common iliac artery threatens patency of a superior mesenteric bypass graft anastomosed to it. The patient complained of intestinal angina, and open surgery was required after balloon angioplasty of the stenosis failed.

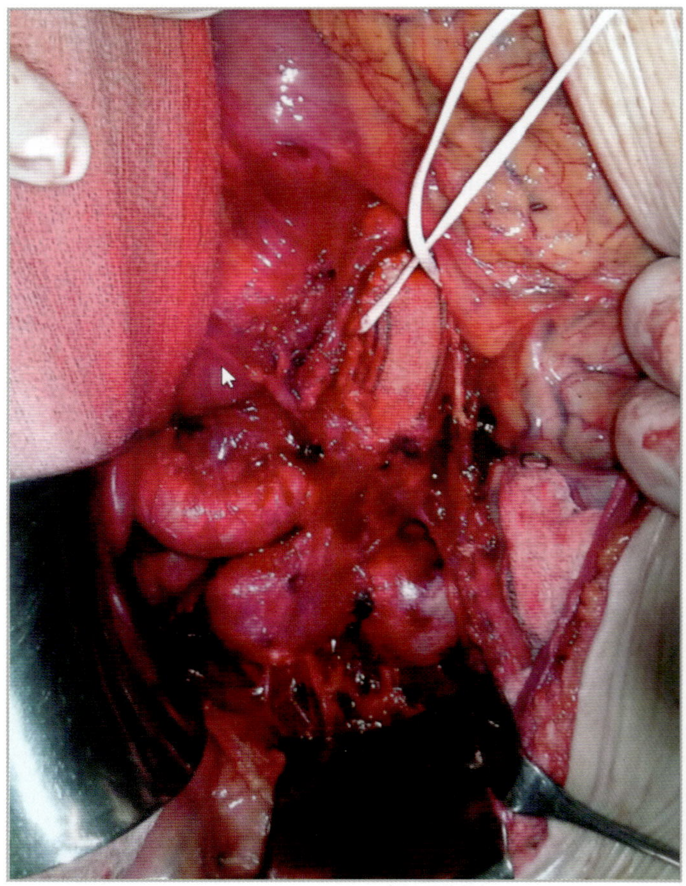

Figure 22.3 Extremely tortuous and aneurysmal iliac arteries below a previous tube graft repair of an abdominal aortic aneurysm.

proportion of late aortic graft infections occur in patients who suffered a groin wound infection after the initial AAA repair with a bifurcated graft. The majority of patients having a bifurcated graft for open AAA repair now have their distal anastomosis performed to the common iliac bifurcation or to the external iliac artery in preference to the femoral artery. While a false femoral aneurysm is clinically obvious, a false iliac aneurysm is unlikely to declare itself until complications supervene, such as rupture or thrombosis (**Figure 22.4**).

There is a 1% risk of late AAA rupture in patients who have been treated by EVAR, and many of these late ruptures are associated with endoleaks from the EVAR device. The aortic neck above the sac may continue to dilate over time, with a subsequent type I endoleak around the side of the device or slippage or migration of the graft out of the neck, which repressurizes the original aortic aneurysm sac and runs the risk of sac distension and late aneurysm rupture, necessitating open conversion of the AAA repair. The majority of EVAR devices are modular, with one of the limbs being inserted into the main body of the device from the contralateral side. Subsequent graft migration can occur, which may cause late separation of the contralateral limb, causing a late type III endoleak, The metallic struts on some of the earlier generation devices eroded through the Dacron stent covering, also leading to a late type III endoleak with a similar repressurization of the sac and risk of rupture, both these scenarios requiring an open conversion. Retrograde aortic aneurysm sac filling from collateral vessels such as the inferior mesenteric artery or lumbar arteries causes a type II endoleak, but these are often low pressure and are usually managed expectantly. Should the sac begin to expand in the presence of a type II endoleak, many units will attempt a percutaneous embolization of the feeding collateral vessel. Should this fail it might be possible to clip the collateral artery, especially the inferior mesenteric artery, via a laparoscope. Should this not be possible and the sac continues to expand, then open conversion may be required. Most units run a stent surveillance program with annual computed tomography (CT) or ultrasound scans to detect these late endoleaks, and the majority can be repaired by endovascular means, usually by relining the device with another stent. When this strategy fails, it may be necessary to undertake an open conversion and remove the device, repairing the aneurysm with a Dacron graft.

Graft infection and aortoenteric fistula

Late graft infection is uncommon, arising in 0.5–1.5% of patients after elective open AAA repair (Conrad et al. 1997, Hallett et al. 1997, Kieffer et al. 2012) and a similar incidence after EVAR (De Bruin et al. 2010, The United Kingdom EVAR Trial Investigators 2010). Late infection tends to occur with less virulent organisms, such as *Staphylococcus epidermidis*, which may curiously lie quiescent on the graft for many years before surfacing to cause a graft infection, often with no obvious precipitating factor. More virulent organisms may be deposited on the inner graft surface some years after AAA repair through hematogenous spread from a remote septic focus or something as innocuous as colonoscopy. Such infections may present in a myriad of ways; clinical features might include abdominal pain, weight loss, anorexia, anemia, the development of a false aneurysm or late wound sinus, septic emboli, and graft thrombosis. Any patient with unexplained malaise some years after AAA repair should certainly have aortic graft infection excluded by way of an abdominal CT scan, which may show an inflammatory phlegmon around the graft, fluid collections, or gas in the old AAA sac (**Figure 22.5**).

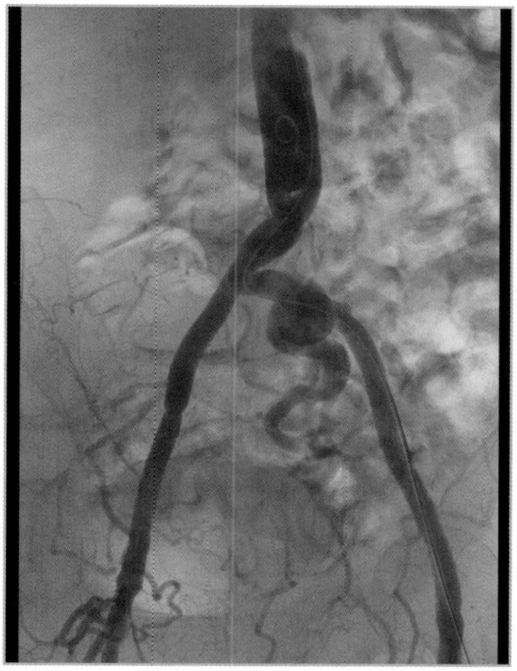

Figure 22.4 A false aneurysm at the distal anastomosis of a previous aortobiiliac graft to the left common iliac bifurcation. The patient presented with a leak from the false aneurysm, although on this occasion the aneurysm was successfully excluded with a wall stent rather than open surgery.

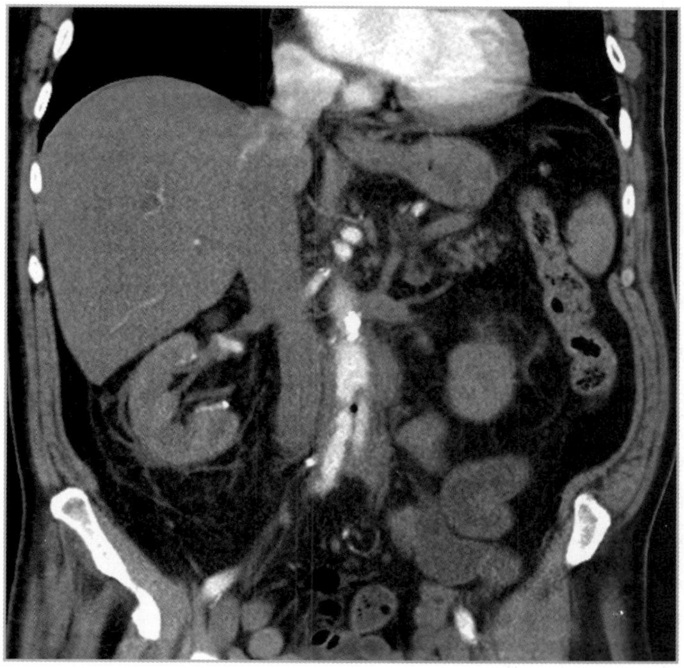

Figure 22.5 Abdominal computed tomography scan of a patient who presented 20 years after abdominal aortic aneurysm repair with unexplained sepsis. There is an inflammatory mass on the left side of the aorta together with a gas bubble overlying the aortic graft, indicating graft infection.

Strategies for managing aortic graft infection have gradually changed, as surgeons have realized that it is not an absolute prerequisite to perform graft explantation and extra-anatomic bypass; indeed mortality, amputation, graft patency, and graft reinfection rates may be better using graft explantation and in situ replacement (O'Connor et al. 2006, Oderich et al. 2006), perhaps supplemented with the use of local gentamicin-impregnated collagen fleeces or beads. In situ replacement has been performed with rifampicin-coated Dacron graft, cryopreserved aortic allograft, pericardial xenograft, or autogenous vein, and many surgeons now favor the latter conduit because it is autologous material and so more resistant to reinfection, although it can be time consuming to harvest the femoral vein and there is a risk of subsequent chronic venous insufficiency. Perhaps more controversially, some surgeons have advocated a conservative approach in high-risk patients, with drainage or debridement, antibiotic irrigation of the graft, and long-term antibiotic therapy. Given the mortality of over 20% with open surgical approaches, results have proved no worse with conservative measures.

Aortoenteric fistula complicating AAA repair is often thought to arise as a result of low-grade infection between the aortic graft and adjacent, adherent bowel, most commonly the duodenal–jejunal flexure. Adjacent collections of pus or overt signs of graft infection are not always present. It occurs after around 1% of open repairs and is rarely seen after EVAR (Cho et al. 1998). It is usually a late complication and presents with GI hemorrhage. There is often a sentinel bleed, giving warning of a more serious hemorrhage. Any patient presenting with a GI bleed who has had a previous AAA repair needs to have the diagnosis of aortoenteric fistula excluded and an extended gastroduodenoscopy all the way to the duodenojejunal flexure will often show the fistula at this point. While it might be tempting just to oversew the arterial side of the fistula, there is a risk of suture line breakdown in the presence of chronically infected aortic tissue and so it is better to partially or completely remove the graft, cut back the aorta to healthy tissue, and then consider either extra-anatomic bypass or in situ replacement as for aortic graft infection. It is usually possible to simply oversew the intestinal side of the fistula with an omental overlay rather than resecting the bowel.

Graft thrombosis

Graft thrombosis after open aortic aneurysm surgery is uncommon, occurring in 0.5–2% of patients (De Bruin et al. 2010, The United Kingdom EVAR Trial Investigators 2010). Aortoiliac anastomoses are usually of wide caliber with high flow rates and so late thrombosis is usually due to the progression of atherosclerotic disease distal to the graft, restricting outflow. Graft thrombosis is more commonly seen in the limbs of an EVAR device following endovascular AAA repair, where the risk is between 4% and 7% of patients. These grafts are more susceptible to kinking, to distortion of the graft outlet, and to graft migration that may restrict flow and lead to thrombosis. As it is much more common to thrombose one limb of a bifurcated graft or EVAR device rather than the main body, an extra-anatomic bypass such as a femorofemoral crossover graft is a much more likely strategy than redo aortic surgery, which carries a significantly higher mortality.

Visceral vessel grafts are of smaller caliber and are susceptible to intimal hyperplasia at the suture lines or to progression of atherosclerotic disease proximal or distal to the graft, causing medium-term or late thrombosis of the graft respectively. It is possible that many visceral vessel grafts thrombose without causing significant symptoms and so the surgery to redo such grafts is infrequent.

ANATOMICAL ISSUES

Intestinal adhesions

Intestinal adhesions are a hazard during any abdominal reoperation, but particularly during aortic surgery as the aorta is placed at the back of the abdominal cavity, and exposure of it through adhesions can require careful dissection to free the bowel and move it to the side. Such dissection can be very high stakes because any intestinal content spillage would make it hazardous to implant or expose a prosthetic graft because of the risk of subsequent graft infection. When a hostile abdomen is suspected, it may be better to consider a retroperitoneal approach to the aorta and iliac arteries. This approach is usually performed through a left subcostal incision, lifting the peritoneum off the posterior abdominal wall toward the midline to expose the aorta. This approach is also useful if access is needed to the left renal and superior mesenteric arteries, but the right renal artery can only be seen from inside the aorta and access to the right iliac artery may require a separate right iliac fossa incision. Care must be taken not to damage the spleen when mobilizing the peritoneum in the left upper quadrant.

Proximity to renal arteries

In many cases of redo abdominal aortic surgery, the renal arteries come into to play far more than during the primary procedure. A proximal abdominal aortic para-anastomotic or false aneurysm is likely to lie between the top end of the previous graft and the origins of the renal arteries (**Figure 22.6**), necessitating a suprarenal aortic clamp. Many current EVAR devices involve suprarenal stent graft fixation using barbed open metallic struts above the main, covered, body of the stent. Should the stent need to be removed for any reason, a suprarenal clamp may not therefore be high enough to get above the stent, and a period of supracoeliac clamping through the lesser sac may be required. This strategy still requires access to the suprarenal aorta so that the clamp can be moved down to the suprarenal area as soon as possible after explantation of the graft to minimize the splanchnic ischemic time.

Should a suprarenally fixated, hooked stent graft need to be removed during an open conversion, there is a significant risk of damage to the intima at the renal artery origins if the bare-metal struts above the main body of the device are pulled down without the proximal hooks being fully disengaged from the suprarenal aorta. In such cases, postoperative occlusion of the renal artery is possible from intimal flaps at their origin. Better then to simply divide the metal struts as they emerge from the main body of the device with wire cutters and leave the suprarenal component in situ, where it does little harm.

It has proved possible to repair para-anastomotic, juxtarenal aneurysms after previous open aneurysm repair using fenestrated and branched endovascular grafts, where side stents are used to reperfuse the renal arteries (Beck et al. 2009). Mortality and complication rates are low, although evidence is lacking as to whether the results are significantly better than open repair and the current extraordinary cost of such tailor-made devices can be difficult to justify. In such cases, it is better to use a bifurcated stent graft rather than a tube as there is a risk of fixation failure between the stent graft and the previous aortic graft.

One option for managing an infected aortic graft is graft excision and extra-anatomic bypass, and if the top end of the aortic graft is close to the renal artery origins, then two layer closure of the aortic stump may well compromise renal blood flow. It is often useful to have the option of a suprarenal clamp in these circumstances so that the renal origins can be clearly seen. If the infected graft is very

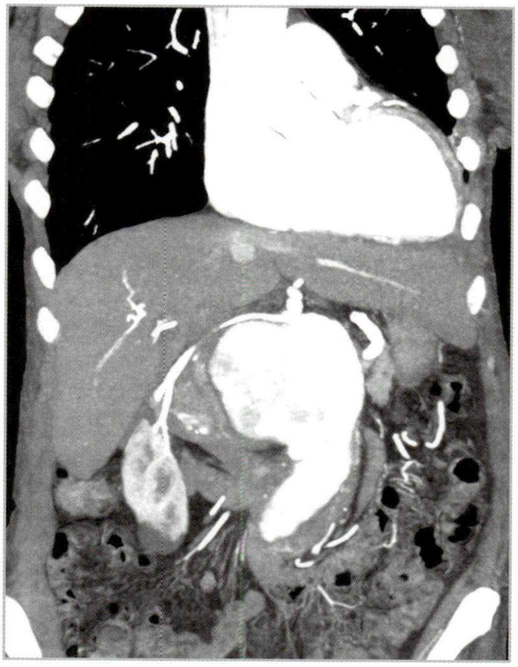

Figure 22.6 A ruptured para-anastomotic aneurysm lying between the top end of a previous abdominal aortic aneurysm graft repair and the renal arteries. The right renal artery is seen stretched around the top of the leaking aneurysm.

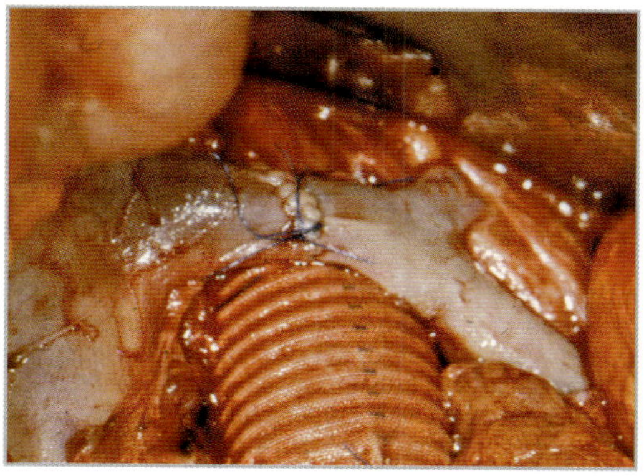

Figure 22.7 Reconstruction of a divided left renal vein with a continuous polypropylene suture. The vein was divided to allow access to the suprarenal aorta in a patient with an abdominal aortic aneurysm.

close to the renal arteries, then an in situ graft replacement strategy may be preferable.

Access to the suprarenal aorta is often restricted by the left renal vein, which usually lies across the front of the aorta just below the renal artery origins. There are two options to deal with this vein. It is easily mobilized by ligating and dividing the left gonadal vein and the left suprarenal vein (and sometimes a lumbar vein descending off the inferior surface of the left renal vein adjacent to the aortic wall). Once mobilized, the left renal vein can easily be slung out of the way. If this fails, then the left renal vein can be divided to provide access to the renal arteries, but it does provide some benefit in terms of postoperative renal function if the vein can be restored after the aorta has been dealt with. Thus, it is better to divide the left renal vein between arterial clamps and reconstruct it at the end of the procedure with a continuous polypropylene suture (**Figure 22.7**).

Proximity of the ureters

When it is necessary to expose the previous iliac limbs of an aortic bifurcation graft, usually for graft thrombosis but also for infected graft explantation, it is important to identify the course of the ureter as it crosses the graft. Normally the ureter is lifted forward off the common iliac artery during the course of the primary operation, and left to fall back onto the surface of the graft at the conclusion of the procedure, where it can become adherent to the graft exterior and difficult to identify because of surrounding scar tissue during re-exploration. When a decision is made to replace a kinked or thrombosed limb of an aortic bifurcation graft, a lower quadrant retroperitoneal approach can give a good exposure but the lower quadrant incision needs to be high enough to allow access to the aortic bifurcation and is ideally placed just below the level of the umbilicus. It is then possible to peel the ureter off the graft limb along with the peritoneum but it may be heavily scarred in place. Should the ureter is inadvertently divided, then immediate repair and ureteric stenting will be required on table, so it is vital to know both where the ureter is and that it is intact during the course of revisional aortoiliac surgery.

TIMING OF REOPERATION

A number of intra-abdominal vascular complications present as emergencies and need to be dealt with immediately to prevent life or limb loss. Rupture of a previously stented AAA, a para-anastomotic, or a false aneurysm leads to circulatory collapse requiring immediate resuscitation and surgery. Patients with an aortoenteric fistula may suffer a small sentinel bleed, remaining hemodynamically stable initially and giving rise to a false sense of security. It is impossible to predict how soon a major hemorrhage will occur after such a sentinel bleed and emergency surgery is mandated.

Graft infection requires urgent surgery once the patient's condition is stable. Given the length and complexity of surgery for graft infection, it is better scheduled for a daytime list with an experienced vascular team, including vascular anesthetists and scrub nurses. Should a strategy of graft excision and extra-anatomic bypass be used, there has been some debate around the timing of the bypass in relation to the graft excision. Since there is real risk of reinfection in the extra-anatomic bypass, the bypass should not be scheduled 2 or 3 days before graft excision, in case bacteremia from the graft excision seeds the new bypass graft. Most surgeons now excise and bypass at the same operation, but there is little evidence to suggest any difference in outcome whether the bypass is done before or after the graft has been excised. If the bypass is done before the graft excision, it does prevent any significant period of limb ischemia and so is preferred by some. Whichever order is used, it is important to completely exclude one operative field from the other and to use new instruments, re-prep and re-scrub in between the two phases of the operation to prevent cross-contamination, as the risk of reinfection of the new graft is around 10%.

The timing of surgery for false or para-anastomotic aneurysms that have not leaked will depend on the size of the aneurysm. Many will remain small and not need intervention during the lifetime of the patient. Intervention for contiguous aneurysms should be scheduled, once they reach the same size indications as for primary aneurysm, over 5.5 cm for an aortic aneurysm and over 3–3.5 cm for an iliac aneurysm. False aneurysms are more prone to complications and intervention may be timed at smaller diameters, particularly if they are expanding rapidly or causing symptoms.

While surgery can be scheduled electively for patients who present with sudden onset claudication or rest pain after thrombosis of one limb of a bifurcated graft or a stent, the chances of successful thrombectomy recede the longer the delay to operation and so an urgent approach is necessary. Should the patient presents with acute limb ischemia, then an emergency procedure will be required within 6 hours in order to avoid the risk of subsequent compartment syndrome on reperfusion of the limb. In such cases, it may be better to plan on table angiographic imaging rather than delay surgery while preoperative imaging is obtained. Planned fasciotomy prior to restoration of flow should be considered where ischemic time lasts beyond 6 hours.

PREOPERATIVE IMAGING

The majority of patients needing redo abdominal vascular surgery will undergo preoperative CT angiography (CTA). A modern CT workstation can produce excellent three-dimensional imaging of the aorta, the iliacs, and the visceral vessels (**Figure 22.8**). Multislice imaging means that there is no particular advantage for catheter angiography over CTA for arterial imaging. CT has the advantage over magnetic resonance angiography, in that it can give better anatomical detail, particularly for aneurysm disease, endoleaks, and the relationship of visceral arteries. Precise measurements and a clear evaluation of whether or not the patient is suitable for an endovascular or an open approach can be made. In cases of aneurysm rupture, CT is better than ultrasound at detecting retroperitoneal hematoma.

Graft infection is not always easy to diagnose. The typical feature of gas bubbles in the old aneurysm sac is not always present on CT and it can be a real dilemma when a patient with a previous graft presents with malaise and low-grade fever of no obvious origin. There may be some nonspecific soft tissue changes adjacent to the aortic sac or some para-aortic lymph node enlargement of uncertain aetiology. In such cases, the use of white blood cell labeled scanning has been superseded by the use of fluorodeoxyglucose positron emission tomography combined with CT (FDG-PET/CT). FDG is a radiopharmaceutical that accumulates in areas of infection, inflammation, and malignancy. Used in combination with CT, it allows accurate localization of inflammatory tissue adjacent to the graft and is superior to CT alone in detecting graft infection. Any suspicious areas can be sampled with CT-guided needle aspiration for microbial culture studies.

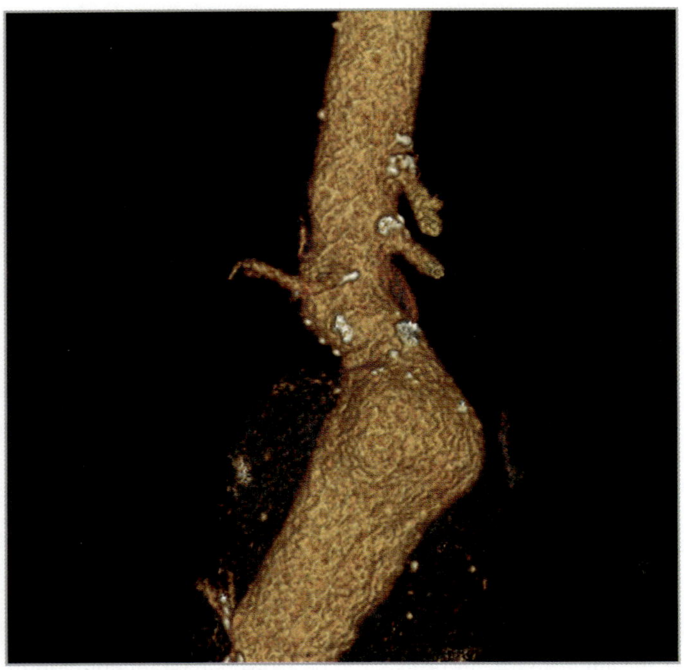

Figure 22.8 A three-dimensional reconstruction of the aorta from a computed tomography scan, with the surrounding soft tissues excluded, showing the origins of the coeliac axis, the superior mesenteric artery, and the right renal artery.

ANTICIPATED HEMORRHAGE

Any patient undergoing redo open abdominal vascular surgery is at risk of major intraoperative hemorrhage. The arteries are often difficult to identify within scar tissue and can be broached during dissection. False aneurysm walls or infected graft suture lines are friable and can disrupt easily during dissection, before proximal and distal control has been established. While local pressure may control the bleeding, dense scarring around the vessels may make it difficult to obtain good exposure of proximal and distal vessels, and significant blood loss can occur while such dissection takes place. It is therefore wise to plan ahead for this eventuality. In addition to cross-matched bank blood, a cell saver system should be used to salvage and transfuse as much of the anticipated blood loss as possible. It is also wise to obtain remote proximal control before tackling an infected proximal aortic suture line or false aneurysm or attempting to remove a suprarenally fixated stent graft. This can be done either by inserting a balloon catheter from the groin or iliac artery and positioning it above the renal arteries, where it can be inflated in the case of hemorrhage, or by dissecting out the supracoeliac aorta through the lesser sac where a clamp can be applied in case of need. Should these strategies be employed, it is important to keep the occlusion time above the splanchnic arteries to a minimum, preferably below 20 minutes, in order to avoid ischemic damage to the viscera or the kidneys.

The iliac veins and inferior vena cava are also at risk of injury during dissection, and consequent major venous bleeding is challenging to control. Proximal and distal compression should allow sight of the venous injury, and the walls of these major veins are usually quite robust, so it is possible often to grasp the injured vein wall with Allis tissue forceps so as to approximate the injured area and control the bleeding, while the vein wall is repaired with polypropylene sutures. Good vacuum suction is valuable here, preferably into a cell saver system and a good assistant can improve exposure; it is often helpful to operate with an experienced surgical colleague for these difficult cases.

Meticulous hemostasis is required as patients are susceptible to postoperative bleeding from suture lines or from extensive retroperitoneal dissection. Suture line bleeding can usually be controlled by the use of Teflon pledgets sutured across the bleeding point. More difficult is a generalized ooze from the operative field, which might occur as a result of massive blood loss and depletion of clotting factors or with the use of antiplatelet agents. Whenever possible, it is better to discontinue antiplatelet therapy at least a week before the surgery. Faced with generalized ooze, the patients clotting factors should be checked and any deficiencies reversed with fresh frozen plasma and platelet transfusions. Any systemic heparinization should be reversed with protamine sulfate. Antifibrinolytic agents may be given intravenously, such as epsilon-aminocaproic acid or tranexamic acid. Topical hemostatic agents and glues should be available. Warming of the patient is also helpful.

Following excision of an infected aortic graft, the proximal aorta should be carefully trimmed back to healthy tissue and closed in two layers of polypropylene sutures, then covered with an omental pedicle.

Any residual infection in the suture line can cause disruption, leading to an aortic stump blow out and fatal postoperative bleeding.

CONDUCT OF THE OPERATION

The majority of abdominal vascular reoperations can be conducted in the supine position. When a retroperitoneal approach is being considered, it can be useful to use a vacuum operating table beanbag under the patient to support the pelvis that is left supine, while the left shoulder is rotated 90° to the semiprone position to improve access. It also helps to strap the patient in position to allow the operating table to be rotated to the right, so bringing the left flank into a better view.

Para-anastomotic and false aneurysms

These aneurysms may be dealt with by either endovascular or open surgical means. A localized false aneurysm at a previous graft suture line can be excluded by deploying a covered stent across the neck of the aneurysm, provided there is an adequate landing zone to seal the stent above and below the aneurysm. A juxtarenal aneurysm may be considered for a fenestrated endograft (fEVAR). These grafts are both expensive and technically difficult to position, so should only be done in vascular centers with a large EVAR experience. The grafts are designed so that, when deployed in the correct position, fenestrations in the graft lie opposite the renal artery origins, which are sealed into the main body of the device with balloon expandable stents. Often a scallop on the top of the main body is positioned around the superior mesenteric artery origin to allow a good seal to the adjacent aorta above the renals.

If the aneurysm cannot be dealt with by endovascular means, either because access is difficult through tortuous or diseased iliac arteries or because a good seal cannot be obtained above or below the aneurysm, then open repair is performed. The principles of open surgery are the same as for primary repair of an aneurysm, with good proximal and distal control, opening of the aneurysm sac and inlay grafting with a prosthetic graft, taking account of all of the factors previously described. Care should be taken when closing the abdomen as the commonest reasons for redo surgery after aneurysm repair are incisional hernia and adhesive bowel obstruction.

Graft infection and aortoenteric fistula

Appropriate intraoperative antibiotic therapy, effective against the infecting organism, is preferable, although the infecting organism is not always identifiable before the operation; in such cases a suitable broad-spectrum antibiotic should be used on microbiology advice. Substantial doses and/or continuous infusion may be warranted. The main consideration when operating on graft infection or aortoenteric fistula is to have good proximal and distal control before entering the septic area. An infected suture line can fall apart with the application of minimal force and it is better to have control with a supracoeliac clamp or an intraluminal balloon catheter before this happens.

With the realization that mortality and morbidity can be less with a strategy of graft excision and in situ repair rather than extra-anatomic bypass, this has become the favored approach. Although the top end of the infected graft lies close to the renal arteries, aortic stump closure may be difficult without compromising renal blood flow and an in situ repair is less risky from this aspect, provided the aorta can be cut back to healthy tissue. The temptation to leave a cuff of the original graft to allow easier stump closure or anastomosis must be avoided; further surgery will almost certainly be required for recurrent infection. Thorough debridement of all purulent, infected, and necrotic material in the aortic bed back to healthy tissue is necessary and may be supplemented by antiseptic lavage. Segments of the graft and any pus or obviously infected tissue should be sent for microbial culture to try and identify the infecting organism and its antibiotic sensitivities.

The in situ approach requires that the newly implanted graft has some resistance to reinfection. Some gelatin-sealed Dacron grafts bind rifampicin and this may be especially suitable for staphylococcal graft infection. The rifampicin bonding can be done in theater by immersing a gelatin-sealed Dacron graft in rifampicin solution for 15–20 minutes. The development of tissue banks has increased interest in aortic allograft replacement of infected aortic grafts, and the early risk of aneurysmal degeneration and rupture has been reduced by the use of cryopreserved aortic allografts, although a significant risk of late graft occlusion remains. There have also been early promising reports of the use of pericardial xenografts, rolled into a suitable diameter, and sutured longitudinally to form a tube. The best results for in situ replacement, though, have come from the use of autogenous vein grafts, either long saphenous vein opened out into a ribbon and then sutured in a spiral fashion to form a larger diameter tube or femoral vein, harvested in a way that preserves the profunda femoral vein to reduce the risk of postoperative limb edema. Reported limb salvage, reinfection, and mortality rates have been lower than other techniques, but it does take a long time to complete the operation and there is a risk of subsequent deep venous insufficiency.

Once completed, the aortic reconstruction should be overlaid with omentum and consideration given to topical antibiotic delivery with gentamicin fleece or beads. The intestinal defect in patients with an aortoenteric fistula is usually quite small and can simply be closed in two layers without the need for bowel resection.

From a microbiologist point of view, typically indolent vascular graft infections are a curious breed per se. All measures should be on the menu, and few are more broadly applicable (but less frequently used) than transposition of healthy skeletal muscle into the operative bed. This has been common practice when radical groin dissection is required for some oncologic conditions; the sartorius muscle is easily transected at its origin and walled into and over the groin. This also applies to the psoas muscle in the upper abdomen and the sternocleidomastoidal muscle in the neck. Desperate measures for desperate circumstances!

Graft thrombosis

Unilateral aortic stent or graft thrombosis is more commonly seen than thrombosis of the entire graft; these are wide bore grafts with high blood flows and do not usually thrombose spontaneously. More often there is a kink or progression of distal atherosclerotic disease underlying the thrombosis and this needs to be corrected or recurrent thrombosis is likely. Often the patients do not present acutely but arrive complaining of sudden onset intermittent claudication starting a few weeks ago, by which stage it is too late for graft thrombectomy. Thrombectomy of the limb of a Dacron aortoiliac graft in any case often fails to re-establish good flow and it may be necessary to replace the blocked limb of the graft with a new segment. The thrombosed limb of the graft can usually be exposed by a lower quadrant Rutherford-Morrison incision with a retroperitoneal approach. When this proves difficult because of body habitus or previous surgery, an extra-anatomic approach might also be considered, with a femorofemoral crossover graft being the usual choice.

POSTOPERATIVE PRINCIPLES AND PRACTICES THAT MAXIMIZE RESULTS

Any patient undergoing major revisional aortic surgery requires high dependency care in the postoperative period so that their cardiovascular, respiratory, and renal function can be closely monitored. There is increasing evidence that units with low mortality have the same complication rates as those with higher mortalities, but are more successful at dealing with any complications that arise, aptly called rescue in North America. Timely intervention for complications is particularly important after revisional vascular surgery where mortality risk may be as high as 20% for open conversion of an endovascular stent graft or for removal of an infected aortic graft.

A low threshold for return to theater must be maintained if the patient's blood pressure and central venous pressure are proving difficult to maintain in the presence of an increasingly tense abdomen, which may signal postoperative bleeding. Likewise a sudden deterioration in renal or respiratory function and acidosis may be the only indication of colonic ischemia. It is also important to monitor the lower limb pulses and foot color so that should there be any postoperative graft thrombosis, it is detected early before irreversible ischemia develops. When there has been any period of renal ischemia during the surgery due to suprarenal clamping, postoperative renal function needs careful monitoring and if progressive deterioration sets in, an early threshold for hemofiltration should be maintained as the renal injury is often transient and will recover if kidney function is supported.

Whatever method is used to deal with an infected graft or aortoenteric fistula, prolonged antibiotic therapy will be required to try and prevent graft reinfection, preferably in line with the antibiotic sensitivities of the infecting organism. When an in situ technique has been used, a postoperative regime of 6 weeks intravenous antibiotic therapy may be used, followed by up to 6 months of oral antibiotics or longer if inflammatory markers fail to return to normal levels.

These patients are usually at high risk of postoperative deep vein thrombosis but often cannot wear compression stockings because of associated peripheral arterial disease. Venous thromboembolism prophylaxis with low molecular weight heparin should be prescribed and a policy of early mobilization is followed where possible. Long-term oral anticoagulation after clearing a thrombosed graft might be considered in order to prevent recurrent graft thrombosis, but only if no apparent reason for the initial graft thrombosis has been found and corrected.

REFERENCES

Adam DJ, Fitridge RA, Raptis S. Late reintervention for aortic graft-related events and new aortoiliac disease after open abdominal aortic aneurysm repair in an Australian population. J Vasc Surg 2006; 43:701–705.

Beck AW, Bos WT, Vourliotakis G, et al. Fenestrated and branched endograft repair of juxtarenal aneurysms after previous open aortic reconstruction. J Vasc Surg 2009; 49:1397–1394.

Becquemin JP, Kelley L, Zubilewicz T, et al. Outcomes of secondary interventions after abdominal aortic aneurysm endovascular repair. J Vasc Surg 2004; 39:298–305.

Cao P, Verzini F, Parlani G, et al. Clinical effect of abdominal aortic aneurysm endografting: 7-year concurrent comparison with open repair. J Vasc Surg 2004; 40:841–848.

Cho JS, Gloviczki P, Martelli E, et al. Long-term survival and late complications after repair of ruptured abdominal aortic aneurysms. J Vasc Surg 1998; 27:813–819.

Conrad MF, Crawford RS, Pedraza JD, et al. Long-term durability of open abdominal aortic aneurysm repair. J Vasc Surg 2007; 46:669–675.

De Bruin J, Baas AF, Buth J, Blankensteijn JD for the DREAM Study Group. Long-term outcome of open or endovascular repair of abdominal aortic aneurysm. N Engl J Med 2010; 362:1881–1889.

Hallett JW Jr, Marshall DM, Petterson TM, et al. Graft-related complications after abdominal aortic aneurysm repair: reassurance from a 36-year population-based experience. J Vasc Surg 1997; 25:277–284.

Kalman PG, Rappaport DC, Merchant N, Clarke K, Johnston KW. The value of late computed tomographic scanning in identification of vascular abnormalities after abdominal aortic aneurysm repair. J Vasc Surg 1999; 29:442–450.

Kieffer WKM, Sonnenberg S, Windhaber RA, Pal N, Pemberton RM. Complications and re-intervention following elective open abdominal aortic aneurysm repair: a 10-year retrospective analysis. Ann R Coll Surg Engl 2012; 94:177–180.

Oderich GS, Bower TC, Cherry KJ Jr, et al. Evolution from axillofemoral to in situ prosthetic reconstruction for the treatment of aortic graft infections at a single center. J Vasc Surg 2006; 43:1166–1174.

O'Connor S, Andrew P, Batt M, Becquemin JP. A systematic review and meta-analysis of treatments for aortic graft infection. J Vasc Surg 2006; 44:38–45.

Sampram ES, Karafa MT, Mascha EJ, et al. Nature, frequency and predictors of secondary procedures after endovascular repair of abdominal aortic aneurysm. J Vasc Surg 2003; 37:930–937.

The United Kingdom EVAR Trial Investigators. Endovascular versus open repair of abdominal aortic aneurysm. N Engl J Med 2010; 362:1863–1871.

Chapter 23 Surgery for recurrent small bowel obstruction

Herbert R. Freund

BACKGROUND

Intra-abdominal adhesions are bands of scar tissue that form between loops of bowel and the abdominal wall and other abdominal structures. Postoperative abdominal adhesions are considered by most surgeons 'inevitable' as >95% of abdominal operations will result in intra-abdominal adhesions (Menzies & Ellis 1990).

The issue of adhesions is of utmost importance as it carries the burden of recurrent operations, multiple repeat hospital readmissions, cost of operating room time, operative and postoperative complications, and lifelong impact on patients' welfare, infertility, and recurrent operations. So much so that in the forties of the previous century patients subjected to several laparotomies for recurrent intestinal obstruction were termed 'intestinal cripples' (Stanciu & Menzies 2007).

In recent years, the Surgical and Clinical Adhesions Research Group (SCAR) in the United Kingdom published a number of sentinel papers elucidating some of the issues and controversies of intra-abdominal adhesions.

In the first study of 29,790 patients undergoing open abdominal or pelvic surgery, 35%were readmitted at a mean of 2.1 times over 10 years for disorders directly or possibly related to adhesions, and for abdominal or pelvic surgery. About 5.7% of all readmissions were classified as directly related to adhesions with 3.8% managed operatively.

About 22.1% of all readmissions occurred in the first year postsurgery, but readmissions continued steadily over 10 years (Ellis et al. 1999). The many excellent publications by the UK group of researchers summarized all their experience by stating that adhesions are an integral part of everyday surgical practice and that the workload produced by them is enormous.

The impact of adhesions begins immediately after surgery but continues for the life of the patient. The costs of adhesions are cumulative and account for a significant proportion of the health service budget. Similar data were collected also in the United States from Medicare records. Within 2 years of small bowel surgery, 14.3% of patients suffered obstruction and 2.6% required adhesiolysis (Beck et al. 1999)

The three most common causes of small bowel obstruction (SBO) are adhesions, neoplasms, and hernias. Historically, hernias accounted for the majority of SBO, while currently postoperative adhesions are the leading cause of SBO. In the United States, 49–67% of SBO episodes are the result of adhesive SBO, followed by abdominal malignancies (13–16.2%) and incarcerated hernias (5–6%) (Carmichael & Mills 2006).

Among the most common abdominal procedures, appendectomy leads as the cause of adhesion ileus (23%), followed by colorectal surgery (21%), gynecological surgery (12%), foregut surgery (9%), and small bowel surgery (8%). Repeat laparotomies result in a 24% incidence of adhesion ileus.

Among patients with adhesion ileus, the episode of intestinal obstruction will occur within 1 month of surgery in 20% of patients, within 1 year of surgery in 30% of patients, within 1–5 years after surgery in 25% of patients, and after 5 years of surgery in 25% of patients.

Almost all patients develop adhesions following transperitoneal surgery. Adhesions occur between intraperitoneal organs, between intraperitoneal organ and the abdominal wall, as well as previous abdominal scars and omentum. The extent and severity of the adhesions depend on the extent of the original surgery, on the primary pathology requiring surgery, the type of incision, the number of previous laparotomies, damaged visceral or parietal peritoneum, intraperitoneal bleeding, leak of bowel content, and intra-abdominal or wound infection.

Obviously, children develop adhesions and their sequela as well. However, they suffer from obstructive symptoms and repeat surgeries for many more years. Grant et al. (2006) reported a cumulative 4 years readmission rate of 0.3–9.3% directly related to adhesions and a possibly related rate of 6.3–32.1% in children.

When operating for adhesion-related SBO, the use of various techniques, instruments, and energy sources is advocated. This should include sharp dissection with a blade or scissors, and various energy sources like coagulation, cutting, bipolar, harmonic scalpel, and others. Similar techniques and instruments are advocated for the release of adhesions between the bowel and various intra-abdominal structures. The surgeon entering such a 'hostile' abdomen should be experienced and familiar with as many techniques and technologies. Even so, one should tread very cautiously in this often hostile environment.

There are seven studies addressing time required to relieve adhesions in open surgery and one study addressing time required for laparoscopic release of adhesions. Previous surgery with adhesion formation extended operating time both to re-enter the abdomen as well as to dissect the site of pathology. Time necessary to explore an abdomen with adhesions ranged from 15 minutes to 4 hours (Beck et al. 2000, Fevang et al. 2004).

In a prospective study of 1701 patients undergoing colorectal surgery or surgery for SBO ($n = 90$), the mean time for lysis adhesions was 34 minutes (1–240 minutes) with the mean time required for lysis of adhesions being about 20% of the total mean operative time.

Bleeding, inadvertent enterotomies, damage to other intraperitoneal structures, and bowel ischemia are the most feared complications of intestinal obstruction–adhesion lysis surgery. It was reported that 20% of patients undergoing reoperation through a previous laparotomy scar for adhesion ileus suffer an inadvertent enterotomy. However, in another study accidental enterotomy requiring repair occurred in only 6% of patients operated for adhesive SBO (Van der Krabben et al. 2000).

Higher age and higher number of previous laparotomies predicted well the rate of inadvertent enterotomies. Patients with three or more previous laparotomies had a 10-fold increase in enterotomy rate compared with patients with only one or two previous laparotomies. Van Goor et al. (2007) claim that when SBO was the indication for surgery, 30% of patients sustained a bowel injury. Over 50% of enterotomies occurred with adhesions in the lower abdomen and pelvis.

It is important to remember that due to the extensive dissection and resultant raw surface, adhesiolysis is often also associated with considerable blood loss and injury to less-often reported organs like liver, spleen, and urinary bladder.

WHEN AND HOW TO MANAGE THE PATIENT WITH RECURRENT ADHESION ILEUS WHO HAS ALREADY BEEN OPERATED IN THE PAST

The classical patient with recurrent adhesion ileus would be hospitalized for at least a few days, often even 1–2 weeks for investigation, imaging, and a trial of conservative treatment in an attempt to avoid surgery. Obviously, during this period, he will have his gastrointestinal tract drained by a nasogastric tube and his oral intake discontinued. The ensuing protein-calorie malnutrition usually follows longer periods of inadequate oral intake due to abdominal pain, recurrent subileus, and progressive metabolic decline.

Also, during their pre-surgery hospital stay, these patients lose a considerable amount of fluids from the gastrointestinal tract and the abdominal cavity, making them even more susceptible to intraoperative and postoperative complications. It is thus of utmost importance to use the time in hospital not only for investigations and decision making but also for adequate hydration and intravenous nutrition therapy.

This brings one to the conclusion that no patient should reach the operating room with an albumin level lower than 21 mg. Furthermore, as the bowel of these patients is obstructed, there occurs not only intestinal bacterial overgrowth but also a change in flora representing the more resistant population of intestinal bacteria.

Also important is a hemodynamic stable state and the preoperative administration of broad-spectrum antibiotics, reflecting the flora of the specific hospital. Many of these patients are anemic as a reflection of their disadvantaged general condition. Preoperative blood transfusion should be considered and anyhow blood should be cross-matched for the operation as substantial blood loss during surgery might be encountered in such cases due to the extensive adhesiolysis-associated raw surface.

The technical challenges and the intraoperative decision making are so demanding that the recommendation is for two well-trained surgeons to join forces. Although not established as a routine procedure, it might prove beneficial to perform an ultrasound on the operating table as an adjunct to choose the more favorable site of the abdominal incision or site of the first laparoscopy trocar. A good preoperative CT scan might serve this purpose as well.

The surgeons will have to decide whether they prefer an open approach or laparoscopy. If the open approach is chosen, the decision should be whether to use the previous incision or to make a new one, more distant from previous ones, in the hope to gain easier and quicker access into the peritoneal cavity.

Entry through a previous laparotomy incision and dissection of adherent bowel loops off this dense scar tissue requires surgical skill, experience, patience, and the use of sharp dissection and all available surgical energy sources.

If possible the dissection should follow loops of bowel and other recognizable intra-abdominal organs and structures. If this seems impossible, parts of the abdominal wall can be sacrificed and reconstructed during closure of the abdomen. Inadvertent enterotomies should be avoided. If enterotomies occur, they should be repaired immediately. If immediate closure has to be deferred, the site of the enterotomy should be temporarily closed to avoid contamination and clearly marked for subsequent closure.

One should defer the decision about bowel resections until the entire bowel is freed and its integrity and viability inspected repeatedly and verified. Extensive resections should be avoided in an attempt not to cause a short bowel syndrome requiring long-term total parenteral nutrition therapy. The experienced surgeon should preserve the maximal length of small bowel, minimal number of suture lines, and perfectly viable bowel.

ANTIADHESION THERAPY

As many of these patients are operated repeatedly and there is a fair chance for some of them to need another surgical intervention for adhesion ileus, a brief discussion of available antiadhesion agents is expected. To reduce adhesion formation, a mechanical barrier composed of hyaluronic acid and carboxymethyl cellulose was developed.

The results of many uncontrolled studies of a hyaluronate-carboxymethylcellulose membrane (Seprafilm) for the prevention of abdominal adhesion led to no consensus. A meta-analysis of eight studies with a total of 4203 patients summarized that Seprafilm could not reduce postoperative intestinal obstruction. At the same time, Seprafilm did increase the incidence of abdominal abscesses and anastomotic leaks (Zeng et al. 2007).

With this conclusion it is impossible to recommend the routine use of Seprafilm unless dealing with patients who already underwent multiple sessions of adhesiolysis and in whom the odds for needing surgery again are high.

When discussing patients in whom intestinal obstructions occur frequently and regularly, the Mayo Clinic group published their experience with 40 patients operated repeatedly for relief of adhesions and presented with an abdomen encased and 'frozen' by chronic postoperative adhesions. The 40 reported patients had a mean of five previous operations and periods of total parenteral nutrition. The mean duration of the operation was 6.2 hours and 36 of 40 patients had small bowel resections.

The Mayo group concluded their experience in this extremely difficult group of recurrent patients stating that reoperation on the abdomen encased in dense abdominal adhesions can restore most patients to good health over the long term (Harris et al. 2002).

THE USE OF ORAL GASTROGRAFIN IN ADHESIVE SMALL BOWEL OBSTRUCTION

Many controversial reports on the possible beneficial effects of oral Gastrografin on adhesive SBO have been published and discussed. However, as all studies were lumped together with no consideration given to the severity of obstruction and the number of recurrent episodes of ileus no viable conclusions could be drawn. However, Gastrografin probably has a role in the treatment of adhesion ileus as concluded by the 2008 Cochrane collaboration report stating that:

1. Oral Gastrografin is a very accurate predictor of nonoperative resolution of adhesive SBO
2. Although Gastrografin does not reduce the need for surgery, it does reduce hospital stay in those patients who do not require surgery

These important conclusions lead us to recommend that unless signs of damaged bowel are present, a trial with Gastrografin should be attempted (Abbas et al. 2007).

TREATMENT OF MALIGNANT BOWEL OBSTRUCTION

Malignant bowel obstruction (MBO) occurs most commonly in patients with advanced ovarian or colorectal cancer. Several retrospective studies estimated MBO to occur in 25–50% of patients with ovarian cancer and conveyed a dismal prognosis. The goal of treatment in patients with MBO is clearly palliative attempting to improve the quality of life in a patient with a limited life expectancy due to a noncurable intra-abdominal malignancy. Obviously we are dealing with difficult, sometimes extensive, surgical procedures in sick and malnourished patients. Beyond the technical challenges and the issues of management, there are deep-rooted ethical and religious issues to be considered

A large study of 523 patients from the Ohio State University compared surgical versus nonsurgical treatment. The tumors in these patients were colorectal, gynecologic, genitourinary, neuroendocrine, and noncolorectal gastrointestinal. Nonsurgical therapy consisted of decompression, endoscopic procedures, stenting, and percutaneous ostomies.

Surgery included a variety of nonendoscopic procedures undertaken in the operating room for the relief of bowel obstruction and resuming gastrointestinal continuity. Survival for operated patients was 6.6 months versus 1.7 months in the nonoperated patients, indicating a better outcome when surgery is feasible.

The presence of ascites and carcinomatosis carried a worse prognosis and should probably indicate a nonoperative approach. Albumin level was also a predictor of survival, an observation made by other researchers as well.

MBO is a complex issue. However, every technical effort should be made in this difficult group of patients in an attempt to relieve bowel obstruction, achieve gastrointestinal continuity, resume oral intake, and enable the patient to eat and gain a few more months of life (Henry et al. 2012).

THE ROLE OF LAPAROSCOPY IN BOWEL OBSTRUCTION AND ADHESIOLYSIS

In recent years, laparoscopy became an accepted operative modality for the treatment of intestinal obstruction and for adhesiolysis. The rational is clear. As each additional laparotomy is associated with more adhesions, the use of laparoscopy might reduce the formation of some of these new adhesions. However, the blind, or even the open, introduction of trocars into a hostile abdomen with multiple adhesions and many dilated loops of bowel can be extremely dangerous, resulting in a high rate of bowel injury and bowel leaking.

Moreover, bowel injuries seem to go frequently undetected and their diagnosis and treatment are often delayed. A systemic review revealed that 67% of laparoscopy-associated, adhesiolysis-related bowel injuries were detected only within 24 hours postsurgery.

Another common cause of undiagnosed or late diagnosed enterotomy is electrocautery damage to the bowel during laparoscopic adhesiolysis (Van der Voort et al. 2004). Postoperative intra-abdominal hematomas, intra-abdominal abscess, fistula formation, and wound infection were found in 39% among 270 patients undergoing abdominal reoperations through a previous scar. The mortality in this group was 8%.

The mortality rate of patients with undetected bowel injuries is 20–50% and considerably higher than in patients with immediately recognized enterotomies (Perrone et al. 2005). Notwithstanding, a Cochrane database of 334 patients reported that laparoscopic adhesiolysis was associated with reduced overall and pulmonary complication rates compared with the open approach. Furthermore, no significant differences were noted for intraoperative injury to bowel, wound infection rates, and mortality rates (Li et al. 2012).

LAPAROSCOPY VERSUS LAPAROTOMY IN OBSTRUCTIVE ADHESIOLYSIS

Proponents of laparoscopic surgery claim that the reduced trauma to the peritoneum will minimize adhesions. Critics claim that the damage to the visceral peritoneum is even more severe during laparoscopy. Moreover, they cite the additional morbidity and mortality associated with trocar injuries and inadvertent enterotomies.

Several studies compared laparotomy with laparoscopy in the induction and treatment of abdominal adhesions. The designs of these studies were different and the results nonconclusive. In a Swedish study of 105 women operated for tubal pregnancy by either laparotomy or laparoscopy, laparotomy resulted in significantly more adhesions than laparoscopy as observed at a second-look laparoscopy (Lundorf et al. 1991).

An additional gynecological multicenter study assessed the frequency and severity of adhesions in 68 women undergoing operative laparoscopic procedures including adhesiolysis, followed by a second operative procedure within 90 days. The total adhesion score decreased by 52% at the second-look procedure. Adhesion reformation occurred in 66 of 68 women. However, de novo adhesion reformation occurred in only 8 of 68 women (12%) (Operative Laparoscopy Study Group 1991).

The controversy as to the advantage of laparoscopy versus laparotomy for the treatment of recurrent adhesive SBO is certainly not settled yet. However, with the accumulation of more and more experience with a wide range of advanced laparoscopic procedures and advances in techniques and technology, laparoscopy seems to gain more popularity in the treatment of adhesive bowel obstruction and should certainly be attempted in most cases.

REFERENCES

Abbas S, Bisse IP, Parry BR. Oral water soluble contrast for the management of adhesive small bowel obstruction. Cochrane Database Syst Rev 2007; (3):CDOO4651.

Beck DE, FergusonMA, Opelka FG, et al. Effect of previous surgery on operating time. Dis Colon Rectum 2000; 43:1749–1753.

Beck DE, Opelka FG, Bailey R, et al. Incidence of small bowel obstruction after open colorectal and grneral surgery. Dis Colon Rectum 1999; 42:241–248.

Carmichael JC, Mills S. Reoperation for small bowel obstruction: how critical is the timing. Clin Colon Rectal Surg 2006; 19:181–187.

Ellis H, Morgan BJ, Thompson NJ, et al. Adhesion related hospital admissions after abdominal and pelvic surgery: a retrospective study. Lancet 1999; 353:1476–1480.

Fevang BT, Fevang J, Lie A, et al. Long term prognosis after operation for adhesive small bowel obstruction. Ann Surg 2004; 240:193–201.

Grant HW, Parker MC, Wilson MS, et al. Population based analysis adhesion related readmissions after abdominal surgery in children. J Ped Surgery 2006; 41:1453–1456.

Harris EA, Kelly AW, Pockaj BA, et al. Reoperation on the abdomen encased in adhesions. Am J Surg 2002; 184:499–504.

Henry JC, Severin P, Sullivan R, et al. A scoring system for prognosis and treatment of malignant bowel obstruction. Surgery 2012; 152:747–756.

Li MZ, Lian L, Xiao LB, et al. Laparoscopic versus open adhesiolysis in patients with adhesive small bowel obstruction: a systematic review and meta-analysis. Am J Surg 2012; 204:779–786.

Lundorff P, Hahiin, Kallfelte B, et al. Adhesion formation after laparoscopic surgery in tubal pregnancy: a randomized trial versus laparotomy. Fertil Steril 1991; 55:911–915.

Menzies D, Ellis H. Intestinal obstruction from adhesions: How big is the problem. Ann R Coll Surg Engl 1990; 72:60–63.

Operative Laparoscopy Study Group. Postoperative adhesion development after laparoscopy: evaluation at second-look procedure. Fertil Steril 1991; 55:700–704.

Perrone JM, Soper NJ, Eagon JC, et al. Perioperative outcome and complications of laparoscopic ventral hernia repair. Surgery 2005; 138:708–716.

Stanciu D, Menzies D. The magnitude of adhesion related problems. Colorectal Dis 2007; 9:35–38.

Van der Krabben AA, Dijkstra FR, Nieuwehuizen M, et al. Morbidity and mortality of inadvertent enterotomy during adhesiolysis. Br J Surg 2000; 87:467–471.

Van Goor H. Consequences and complications of peritoneal adhesions. Colorectal Dis 2007; 9:25–32.

Van der Voort M, Heijnsdijk EA, Gouma DJ, et al. Bowel injury as a complication of laparoscopy. Br J Surg 2004; 91:1253–1258.

Zeng Q, Yu Z, You J, Zhang Q. Efficacy and safety of Seprafilm for preventing postoperative abdominal adhesions. World J Surg 2007; 11:2125–2131.

Chapter 24 The surgical approach to acute and chronic complications of radiation injury and chemotherapy

Sandra L. Wong, Khaled S. Hafez

INTRODUCTION

Historically, surgical resection was considered the only curative treatment for many solid tumors. Even if an operation could be performed, recurrent disease was often a harbinger of poor prognosis. However, modern cancer care includes multimodality treatments with radiation and chemotherapy (or both). These advances have improved outcomes for many solid organ tumors but their effect on surgical management has occasionally been to complicate it. With increased use of radiation and chemotherapy, acute and chronic complications are sometimes related to cancer-directed treatments, but occasionally are not.

There have been expanding indications for radiation and chemotherapy in the neoadjuvant, adjuvant, and palliative settings. Concomitant with this is the noted expansion of indications for surgical management, and it is in this context that the effects of multimodality treatment on the surgical approach will be discussed in this chapter. Contemporary administration of radiation, chemotherapy, or chemoradiation employs generally safer and better tolerated techniques and relies on a cadre of supportive adjuncts such as effective antiemetics and bone marrow support. This allows for an improved ability to tolerate a complete course of treatment. However, different patterns of side effects and complications are also seen because improved therapeutic windows allow for more dose-dense and immunosuppressive chemotherapy and higher doses of radiation.

BACKGROUND

Radiation therapy

Known impediments to wound healing include tissue hypoperfusion and active neoplasm. In many patients, both of these factors are present and may have additive effects. Tissue hypoperfusion is commonly associated with operations conducted on patients in shock (hypotension and acidosis), but it can certainly be seen more insidiously with irradiated tissue due to microangiopathy. In these patients, an abnormal inflammatory response is seen in tissues with reduced capillary blood supply and increased fibrosis. Radiation affects soft tissue on a macroscopic and microscopic level. The same biologic effects of radiation that make it so effective for cell kill also lead to adverse effects for surrounding normal tissue. Modern techniques such as accelerated or hyperfractionated radiation schemes are used to maximize treatment effects while keeping normal tissue toxicity at a minimum, but the therapeutic index remains narrow. Tissue and cellular responses can be classified into acute, subacute, and delayed phases of injury. Dose-limiting toxicity is usually based on end-organ damage from late effects, but all phases of injury must be considered when caring for patients who have undergone radiation.

Fascinatingly, Spratt and Heinbecker examined radiation injury to the canine small bowel nearly 50 years ago (Spratt et al. 1961). They concluded that by reducing intraluminal bacteria (as with a sulfa bowel prep) facilitated healing of the acute injury. Interestingly, the concept has not been studied clinically despite hundreds of papers on antimicrobial bowel prep for large bowel surgery (Polk, 1987).

The acute response of tissues to radiation includes effects that are seen immediately – hours to days – after treatment. Early-responding tissues include skin, mucosa (including bowel), bone marrow, and tumor cells. These tissues exhibit rapid cell turnover, and the extent of toxicity is a function of cell regeneration from surviving stem cells. Prolonging overall treatment time decreases the severity of acute toxicity, but severe acute toxicity can progress to chronic tissue injury. Subacute injury occurs a few months after exposure and delayed injuries are seen 6 months to years later. Acute effects are typically managed expectantly and with supportive treatments aimed at minimizing symptoms. For instance, acute injury to the intestines can result in cramping, diarrhea, nausea, and vomiting that can be treated with antidiarrheal agents, antiemetics, and low-residue diets (**Figure 24.1**). Radiation can contribute to problems with fistulae, which typically close on their own with appropriate management but can be a particularly vexing chronic problem when they are related multifactorial causes (including prior surgery, chemotherapy, and/or active cancer).

Tissues that have a later response to treatment include spinal cord, central and peripheral nerve tissues, heart myocytes, and kidney nephrons. These tissues are characterized by terminally differentiated cells with slow cellular turnover and low levels of repopulation. The extent of late injury is not dependent on the length of treatment, but rather total radiation dose. Late effects lead to irreversible end-organ damage. In addition to known damage to small vessel vascular damage (endarteritis), the 'fibroatrophic effect' from radiation-induced release of bioactive cytokines and stem cell depletion is associated with parenchymal cell damage and progressive fibrosis and long-term tissue injury (Delanian & Lefaix 2004). The molecular mechanisms of this injury involve induction of a cascade of cytokines that result in collagen deposition and vascular injury (Anscher & Vujaskovic 2005) This sublethal radiation damage causes progressive endarteritis that leads to hypoxic and hypovascular tissue. Tissue breakdown then occurs because of the inability to replace collagen and cellular loss. Toxicity can manifest as stricture, mucosal ulceration, and chronic inflammation.

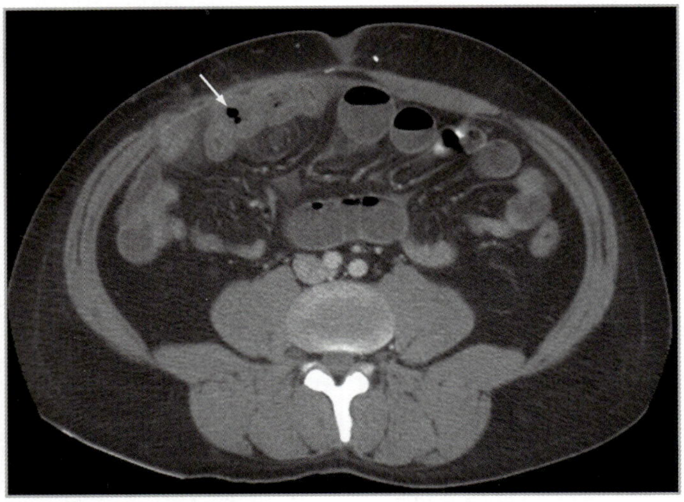

Figure 24.1 A 32-year-old man s/p resection of high-grade extraosseous Ewing sarcoma of the right anterior abdominal wall who was undergoing adjuvant radiation therapy when he presented with abdominal pain. Computed tomography scan demonstrates a severely thickened loop of bowel underlying the area of radiation (note the postoperative appearance of the right rectus sheath). The thickening represented acute radiation changes to the underlying bowel, causing pain and abdominal cramping.

Regardless of timing of radiation toxicity, tissue damage can be manifest as obvious necrosis, thickening, and fibrosis of the epidermal layer of skin, though there may be no obvious macroscopic changes. Importantly, all radiated tissue is accompanied by a varying degree of decreased compliance and decreased vascularity, both of which must be noted if operating in or around previously irradiated tissues because of limited vascular ingrowth following irradiation.

Chemotherapy

The use of systemic chemotherapy in solid organ tumors is largely relegated to the adjuvant setting or the palliative setting. There are well-described, though uncommon, toxicities of systemic therapy that require operative management and these are usually seen in the emergent setting. When bulky disease is treated, the risk of tumor complications must be considered and include perforation, bleeding, fistulae, obstruction, and neutropenic enterocolitis. Operative management for perforation and complete bowel obstruction is mandatory unless the patient's overall prognosis is extremely poor. For cases of gastrointestinal bleeding (either associated with an in situ tumor or from peptic ulcers or thrombocytopenia) and entercolitis associated with chemotherapy-induced neutropenia, nonoperative approaches are usually successful. The myelosuppressive and immunosuppressive effects of chemotherapy are typically short-lived and improve with time after treatments are completed. However, patients who have received multiple lines of systemic treatment may have ongoing problems with myelosuppression that can limit a patient's ability to tolerate major operative procedures.

A poorly understood phenomenon is that of radiation recall, an acute inflammatory reaction ranging from a mild rash and swelling to necrosis and ulceration at the site of prior irradiation that is triggered by certain chemotherapy agents when administered after radiation (Burris & Hurtig 2010). Diagnosis is made clinically and biopsies of the site are usually not required. Management is usually symptom-based and operations should be avoided. Upfront or neoadjuvant chemotherapy, administered before a planned surgical resection, can often make a tumor more amenable to resection with tumor shrinkage. However, systemic treatments can affect the tumor adversely, aside from the potential for in situ tumor growth while on treatment.

ANATOMIC CONSIDERATIONS

Cancer type and site, as well as treatment intent, are the main determinants of complications from radiation and/or chemotherapy.

Abdomen/pelvis/retroperitoneum

Gastrointestinal cancers

Neoadjuvant chemotherapy and/or radiation therapy are used in selected cases of esophageal, gastric, hepatopancreaticobiliary, colon, and rectal cancers. The main rationale for a neoadjuvant approach includes allowing for an in situ treatment response to allow for better resectability or to treat the lethal effects of systemic disease when the risk of metastatic disease is high. Upfront chemotherapy also importantly informs the effectiveness of any given chemotherapy regimen and has the benefit of administering treatment in advance of a major operation when a patient is thought to be better able to tolerate treatment. Further, postoperative complications or a prolonged recovery may affect a patient's ability to tolerate systemic treatment in a timely manner.

However, adverse effects of chemotherapy can be serious and include progression of disease despite treatment (occasionally enough to render the tumor unresectable) and physiologic effects such as immunosuppression, myelosuppression, cardiotoxicity, or renal insufficiency (possibly making an operation more difficult). With the increasing use of combination chemotherapy and molecularly targeted agents for the treatment of liver metastases from colon and rectal cancers, the potential for treatment-associated liver injury must be considered prior to metastasectomy. Treatment regimens containing irinotecan or oxaliplatin are associated with steatosis/steatohepatitis (termed chemotherapy-associated steatohepatitis) and sinusoidal obstruction syndrome, either of which leads to increased morbidity and mortality associated with liver injury and hepatic insufficiency following resection (Kneuertz et al. 2011).

Preoperative radiation is also increasingly used in gastrointestinal cancers with the main focus on treating the local fields when anatomic constraints may preclude wide resection margins. Because of the physiologic effects of radiation, timing of the operation following radiation must be planned well in advance to allow for adequate recovery from the acute effects of radiation but not let so much time elapse as to allow for tissue fibrosis and associated problems with intraoperative dissection. For many gastrointestinal cancers, local recurrences are a harbinger of more advanced disease. There are, however, highly selected cases in which the local recurrence may be the only site of disease. There is a paucity of reports of surgical outcomes in the contemporary literature, but small series demonstrate acceptable results with limited experiences in reoperative surgery [e.g. pancreatectomy (Lavu et al. 2011) and adrenalectomy (Tan et al. 2009)]. Reoperation in previously radiated fields is associated with the additive difficulties of adhesions from the prior resection and fibrosis from radiation.

Pelvic surgery

Radiation is instrumental in the prevention of potentially morbid local recurrences in the pelvis from advanced rectal cancer. Rectal cancers serve as important examples of benefit from preoperative radiation in terms of an improved toxicity profile compared with postoperative administration (Sauer et al. 2004). Because postoperative anastomotic leak is associated with pelvic sepsis, routine use of a temporary diverting loop ileostomy is commonly used when low anastomoses following rectal cancer resection are performed in a radiated field. Importantly, diversion does not prevent the leak but acts to mitigate the adverse effects if one occurs. Loop ileostomies are not without their own set of problems (dehydration from high stoma output and need for an additional operation to restore intestinal continuity), but the risk–benefit ratio for radiation appears to be supported because of the vastly improved oncologic outcomes.

In the past, whole abdominal radiation was used for high-risk uterine cancers, but results of a randomized controlled trial demonstrated an advantage for systemic chemotherapy. Currently, tumor-directed radiation [either external beam radiation therapy (EBRT) or brachytherapy] is typically used in high-risk cases of cervical cancer or endometrial cancers with extrauterine extension. The radiation fields encompass the pelvic structures and can encompass extended pelvic fields, along lymph node basins up to the level of the renal vessels (Randall et al. 2006). Complications of radiation include vaginal stenosis, fistulae, cystitis, proctitis, and intestinal obstruction.

Reoperation for rectal cancer or gynecologic cancer recurrences in the setting of prior radiation can be daunting and associated with major complications in over 20% of cases even in highly selected patients (Verrees et al. 1996). When operating for recurrent disease, the use of autologous tissue flaps can be a useful adjunct in complex pelvic operations, especially in the setting of highly invasive tumors necessitating extensive resection or additional radiation. Muscle or myocutaneous flaps can be used to fill large anatomic defects and provide well-vascularized tissue in the area. This is particularly helpful when dealing with fistulizing complications such as vesicovaginal fistula or rectovaginal fistula (Galandiuk 2005).

Soft tissue sarcoma

Use of radiation in soft tissue sarcoma was instrumental in the advent of limb-sparing procedures, with a randomized controlled trial compared pre- and postoperative radiation for extremity sarcomas and demonstrated that the use of radiation following a local resection had similar results to more morbid amputations (Rosenberg et al. 1982). Local control and overall survival rates were similar, but wound-complication rates were significantly higher in the neoadjuvant group (35% vs. 17%) and this was worse with lower extremity tumors compared with upper extremity tumors (43% vs. 6%). Early limb function was worse in the neoadjuvant group due to fibrosis, stiffness, and edema, but longer term limb function was fairly similar (Davis et al. 2005, O'Sullivan et al. 2002). While radiation is standardly applied to extremity and truncal sarcomas, retroperitoneal sarcomas are more complicated because of intra-abdominal anatomic considerations. Postoperative radiation is particularly problematic because of the typically wide fields with overlying bowel and other visceral structures that reach therapeutic toxicity at doses lower than what is thought to be needed for sarcoma treatment that can lead to adverse long-term effects related to radiation fibrosis (**Figure 24.2**). Attempts at using mesh slings or temporary tissue expanders to 'protect' surrounding structures have been uniformly unsuccessful. This has led to consideration of neoadjuvant approaches so that the tumor is treated in situ while sparing surrounding structures from directed radiation toxicity because of a 'placeholder' effect, but strong evidence of treatment benefit is sparse and treatment is therefore selectively used.

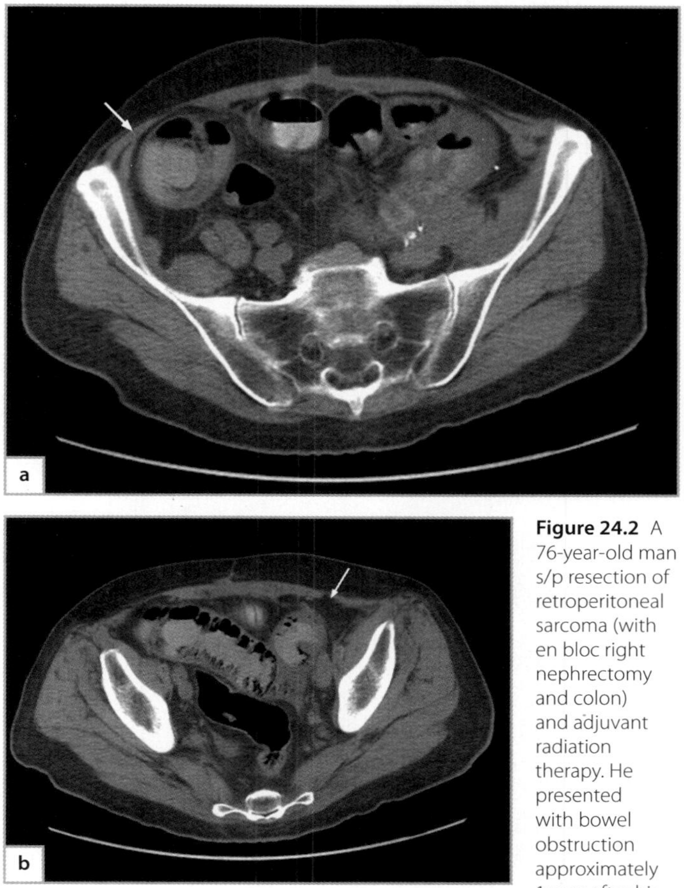

Figure 24.2 A 76-year-old man s/p resection of retroperitoneal sarcoma (with en bloc right nephrectomy and colon) and adjuvant radiation therapy. He presented with bowel obstruction approximately 1 year after his index operation. Computed tomography scan demonstrates (a) appearance of intussusception and bowel obstruction with (b) pneumatosis from compromised bowel. Intraoperative findings included massive intra-abdominal adhesions with a 'Gordian knot' of bowel in the right abdomen from radiation-associated fibrosis.

Testes cancer

The success of cisplatin-based chemotherapy in the management of testicular cancer has rendered a large number of patients with high-stage disease candidates for postchemotherapy retroperitoneal lymph node dissection (RPLND), and the high cure rate of this combined modality approach has been well established. Still, the significant morbidity of this major procedure relative to primary RPLND continues to be a challenge for the genitourinary oncological surgeon. Series have reported complication rates of 20.7–35% (Baniel et al. 1995, Baniel & Sella 1999). Contemporary experiences demonstrate lower rates of major complications with primary RPLND, especially when performed at tertiary care centers by experienced surgeons (Steyerberg et al. 1995). The rates of renovascular injury have decreased with use of bilateral infrahilar surgical templates and the rates of small bowel obstruction have remained low over time. The most common major complications encountered with postchemotherapy RPLND include chylous ascites, pulmonary complications, renovascular injury, and mechanical small bowel obstruction. Chylous ascites occurs in 2–7% of patients and usually resolves with conservative management, including low-fat diet, diuretics, total parenteral nutrition, or paracentesis (**Figure 24.3**). In a minority of cases, rapid or refractory ascites may

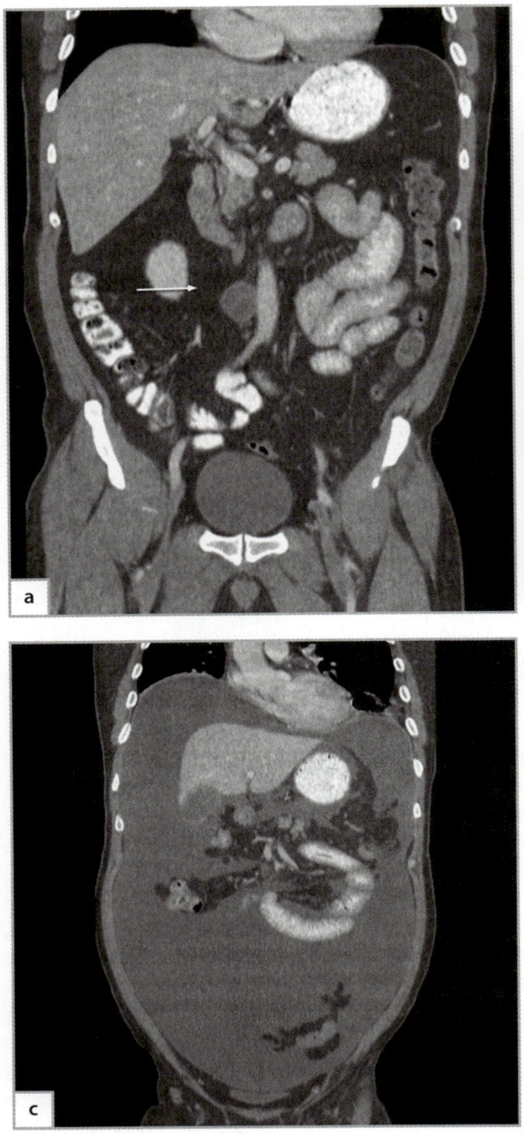

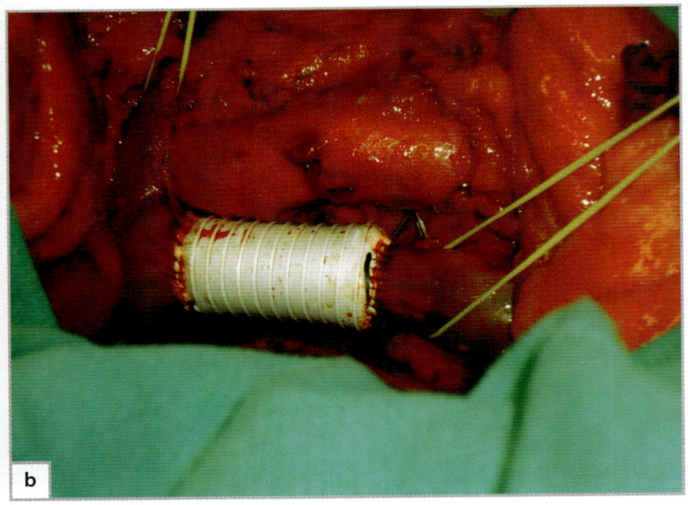

Figure 24.3 A 48-year-old man with stage II mixed germ cell tumor who received primary chemotherapy followed by retroperitoneal lymph node dissection. He later presented with recurrent tumor (a, arrow) and was treated with salvage chemotherapy followed by extensive repeat lymph node dissection necessitating en bloc resection of the inferior vena cava, reconstructed with a GoreTex interposition graft (b). Postoperatively he developed chylous ascites (c) as demonstrated on the computed tomography scan. He was managed nonoperatively, and the process resolved.

require peritoneovenous shunting (Baniel & Sella 1999, Evans et al. 2006).

Major pulmonary complications can occur in patients who have received bleomycin and require general anesthesia. Patients who received bleomycin should undergo preoperative pulmonary function testing and if a diffusion defect is identified, should be managed by an experienced anesthesia team using judicious fluid management and the lowest fraction of inspired oxygen possible to maintain oxygenation. Postoperative fluid management should continue to be carefully managed and should preferentially use colloid over crystalloid (Baniel & Sella 1999).

Prostate cancer

If a patient decides to undergo radiation treatment of prostate cancer, there is a dizzying array of options including conventional EBRT, three-dimensional conformal radiation, intensity-modulated radiotherapy (IMRT), or brachytherapy with or without an external beam boost and all of these therapies are delivered at vastly different doses with different numbers of fractions. The accuracy in the delivery of brachytherapy transperineally has been dramatically improved with the integration of ultrasound and CT scans. Variability in dosimetry due to placement of a source slightly closer to the urethra or rectum than planned can substantially increase the dose to those structures (Wallner et al. 1995). There is a clear dose response to radiation, and more radiation translates into better recurrence-free survival (Kuban et al. 2008). Unfortunately, dose escalation and increasing toxicity are correlated, especially with rectal and bladder complications (Garg et al. 2006).

The bladder and bladder neck, the rectum, and the femoral heads are all within close proximity of the prostate and their tolerance of radiation exposure is what limits the delivery of higher doses. In the lower urinary tract, these effects translate into chronic cystitis with mucosal ulceration with bleeding and bladder contracture (Lopez-Beltran et al. 2002). Unfortunately, even with more sophisticated dose distribution most methods of delivery of radiation cannot limit the dose delivered to the urethra since it traverses the prostate (Roach 2004). Urethral strictures are an uncommon but troublesome complication after radiation therapy to the prostate. The rectum is especially sensitive to radiation and radiation exposure can lead to proctitis symptoms (Garg et al. 2006). Management of complications is guided by the principles that a radiation-induced damage occurs in poorly vascularized tissue and is difficult to treat (**Figure 24.4**).

Rectourethral fistulas (RUF) are one of the most devastating complications that can occur after radiation to the pelvis. Unfortunately, spontaneous closure of this kind of fistula is rare and surgical repair with flaps or urinary and bowel diversion is necessary (Nyam & Pemberton 1999). The rate of fistulas after radiation is difficult to estimate. RUF typically present 1–3 years after the radiation therapy, but have been reported as early as 4.4 months or as late as 20 years after the radiotherapy (Lane et al. 2006). After brachytherapy monotherapy, 0.2% of men develop RUF, but after brachytherapy combined with EBRT, the incidence is 2.9% and salvage brachytherapy after EBRT has a 8.8–14% rate of fistulization (Nguyen et al. 2007, Theodorescu et al. 2000). They most commonly present as urine leaking from the rectum, pain, fecaluria, intractable urinary tract infections, hematuria, or significant rectal bleeding that can be life threatening (Lane et al. 2006, Theodorescu et al. 2000). A significant risk factor for RUF is rectal biopsy, usually done for rectal symptoms so due caution is warranted during evaluation of these patients.

Special cases

Repeat operations for peritoneal surface malignancy (primary or secondary) are complex procedures that are frequently performed in the setting of prior cytoreduction and hyperthermic intraperitoneal chemotherapy (HIPEC) and should only be managed at expert centers.

Other sites

Breast cancer

Radiation therapy is a commonly used modality of adjuvant treatment following either lumpectomy or mastectomy for breast cancer. Consideration must be given to the effect of radiation on breast reconstruction options. With an irradiated chest wall, reconstruction with autogenous tissue is preferred. Transposition of previously nonirradiated tissue into a radiated site can replace damaged native tissue but such procedures are typically associated with more extensive operations and longer recovery time. Reconstruction with artificial prostheses is more straightforward but relies on a certain degree of malleability and durability of the radiated soft tissue covering the implant. Complications from this type of reconstruction can be related to the infection, seroma, hematoma, wound dehiscence, failure of tissue expansion, or implant failure related to the device itself (e.g. rupture) or its surrounding tissue (e.g. device rotation or displacement, capsular contraction) (Lin et al. 2012). Radiation will be increasingly applied to the axillary nodal basin as the role of completion axillary lymph node dissection in early breast cancers (Giuliano et al. 2011) begins to decline. However, we are now approaching 40 years of regular screening mammography and there is a gaining consensus that this radiation exposure needs to be part of the clinician's calculus. Results of repeat operation for regional recurrences is poorly defined at the current time, but concerns of increased complications with superficial and deep infection, seroma, lymphocele, and lymphedema may be valid.

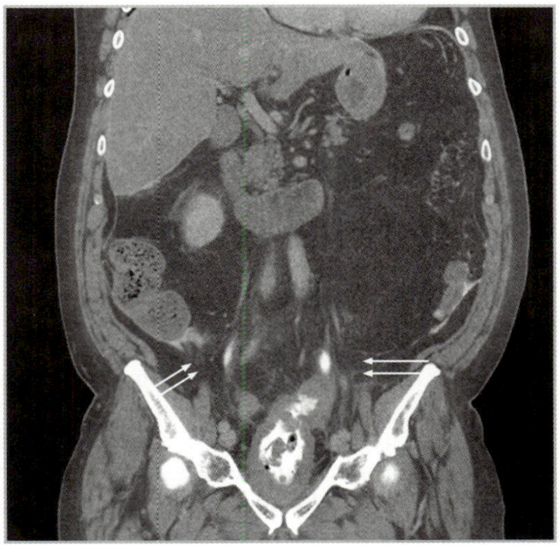

Figure 24.4 A 61-year-old man treated with external beam radiation therapy for high-risk prostate cancer, complicated by severe radiation cystitis. He developed intraperitoneal bladder perforation during cystoscopy for clot evacuation. He underwent urgent cystectomy with a colon conduit because the ileum had sustained radiation enteritis. The computed tomography cystogram demonstrates contrast extravasation from a thickened bladder (arrow) and bilateral ureteral reflux (double arrows).

Head and neck cancers

Multimodality treatment for head and neck cancers has evolved to include combination therapy (resection with radiation and/or chemotherapy) and functional organ preservation approaches (definitive radiation as primary therapy). Most treatment decisions are based on location and histology and must take potential major complications into consideration. Difficult decisions must be made in cases of local or regional recurrence or secondary cancers since salvage operations are often indicated if the disease is technically resectable. Operating in previously irradiated aerodigestive fields poses unique challenges because of consequences to postoperative function, inability to clear all microscopic disease, and increased operative risks of nerve injury and organ dysfunction. Toxicity from radiation can be severe and aside from general mucosal atrophy and soft tissue fibrosis, includes carotid artery stenosis, organ dysfunction (xerostomia, odynophagia, dysphagia, mucositis), hypothyroidism, and transverse myelitis. If repeat radiation is planned, wound closure or reconstruction should include the incorporation of well-vascularized tissue into the field. In addition, chemotherapy may not significantly increase the difficulty of an operation, but does add to morbidity because of downstream consequences of neck and mucosal edema with cervical lymphadenectomy (Gokhale 2001).

PREOPERATIVE PLANNING

Emergent cases requiring surgical intervention should not be delayed because of prior or concomitant radiation or chemotherapy. In many cases, acute complications from treatment may be the root cause of the problem. For example, perforation, obstruction, and bleeding could be directly or indirectly related to treatment and not always directly related to the site of the tumor being treated. Preoperative planning should include a thorough review of treatment records, including any prior operations or use of adjunctive therapies, to help anticipate intraoperative obstacles to the conduct of the operation.

Similarly, even in the longer term, emergency returns to the operating room can be directly or indirectly related to prior treatment. If time allows, directed preparation for an operation should include thorough review of the medical records with a focus on treatment history and details of prior operations. In elective cases, some known risk factors for perioperative complications may be able to be optimized prior to the procedure. While it is difficult to mitigate the effects of prior radiation, these patients should be encouraged to decrease the effects of malnutrition, smoking, and poorly controlled diabetes. In all cases, preoperative planning should include thorough review of treatment records and anticipation of potential intraoperative findings.

For cases that may employ pelvic or retroperitoneal dissection, consideration should be given to arranging a multidisciplinary approach to operative management. For instance, a urologist could provide assistance with ureteral stent placements, allowing for ease of ureteral identification in a highly scarred retroperitoneum or pelvis. While stents aid in identification of the ureter, they do not specifically prevent injury to that particular structure and a surgeon must be prepared to repair or reconstruct if necessary. Similarly, a well-versed plastic and reconstructive surgeon may need to be available for help with soft tissue coverage depending on the extent of resection. For example, skin grafts have a high failure rate if the site is irradiated and more durable soft tissue coverage should be used if radiation is an important part of treatment. Furthermore, different subspecialists may be able to provide specific help depending on the extent of the procedure (e.g. if there is tumor involvement with vessels, a vascular surgeon should be available if exposure is complicated or if reconstruction is needed).

Need for an operation may be unrelated to the primary tumor. Chronic treatment-related complications include nonhealing or poorly healing wounds, fistulae, and bowel obstruction. Specific issues should be dealt with according to the complication itself, but demand consideration of treatment nuances because of prior radiation or chemotherapy. For example, approach to bowel obstruction in the setting of prior abdominal surgery and irradiation is different than if radiation were not previously used because of the likelihood of problems beyond simple adhesions is much higher. Preoperative discussions with the patient should include these possible scenarios since the outcome of the operation is unpredictable.

CONDUCT OF THE OPERATION

Practical and pragmatic operative judgment is informed by a few key considerations in the setting of prior radiation or chemotherapy treatment. Preoperatively, attention should be given to upfront preparation for a lengthy and tedious adhesiolysis or anticipation for access to the deep pelvis or perineum to allow for proper patient positioning. If a long case is planned, proper preoperative discussion with the anesthesiology team and operative assistants is mandatory.

Anticipation of increased blood loss associated with dissection through severely inflamed tissues resultant from recent chemotherapy or radiation can help with on demand repletion, though transfusions should otherwise be used conservatively. Other complications may not occur immediately, but intraoperative care should be taken to minimize complications of fistulae, poor wound healing, and anastomotic leak since these patients are at high risk. For example, meticulous fascial closure should follow well-established principles: wide tissue bites, short stitch intervals, and nonstrangulating suture tension. There is little evidence regarding the efficacy of internal retention sutures in avoiding dehiscence or incisional hernia, but most surgeons avoid the use of external retention sutures because of their high rates of associated tissue trauma and ischemia. While there are no specific surgical techniques to prevent all complications, steps can be taken to minimize devastating effects of the complication should they occur. For example, diverting ileostomies can minimize the effects of an anastomotic leak. In cases requiring extensive reconstruction, planning for a staged procedure may be the most oncologically safe approach if clearance of margins is in question. Use of a temporary covering (biologic implant or standard wet-to-dry dressing) to the defect will allow final pathologic evaluation of all margins prior to definitive closure of a large soft tissue defect. This short delay often allows for granulation of the local site, which may ultimately help in healing if invasive infection is avoided.

Patients with complicated fistulae may initially present with sepsis or severe bleeding; so they must first be medically stabilized and any life-threatening complications treated. These patients are also most likely deconditioned with low albumin and chronic anemia. Cross-sectional imaging can help rule out intra-abdominal abscess. Once a patient has been resuscitated, further workup can be performed. With rectal or ureteral/urethral/bladder involvement, a sigmoidoscopy and cystoscopy are performed. Fecal diversion is often considered (Chrouser et al. 2005, Lane et al. 2006), but many factors must be considered before this is undertaken. Fistula size and location must be documented, as well as the condition or degree of necrosis in adjacent tissue. Preservation of physiologic bowel and urinary function may be possible with a fistula repair. The competence of the anal sphincters must be assessed, since the patient will be incontinent of stool despite repair of the fistula if they are compromised. Similarly, urinary continence, any associated urethral strictures, as well as bladder capacity must be documented during cystoscopy. If there is severe anal sphincter injury or the patient cannot tolerate or does not want downstream reconstruction, a permanent fecal diversion (e.g. end colostomy) would be preferred over a temporary fecal diversion (e.g. ileostomy or loop colostomy).

If the bladder is unsalvageable because of radiation cystitis, severe urethral strictures, or severe urinary incontinence, an ileal conduit should be performed simultaneously with the fecal diversion and a simple cystectomy should be performed. The bladder should not be left in situ, if at all possible, since it is at high risk of complications such as hemorrhage, abscess formation (Chrouser et al. 2005), and pyocystis, the accumulation of mucosal debris and fluid with secondary infection. Management of severe RUF illustrates the complexity of decision making in these cases. In the event that both the bladder and rectum are deemed salvageable, after the suprapubic catheter and an ileostomy/loop colostomy at least 3–6 months should be allowed for healing while diverted before undertaking any reconstruction. Regardless of the approach employed recurrences are common and a healthy tissue flap is necessary to protect the repair. Hyperbaric oxygen therapy has been attempted to heal RUF after a catheter has been placed, but the results have been disappointing (Moreira et al. 2004, Theodorescu et al. 2000).

POSTOPERATIVE MANAGEMENT/ SURVEILLANCE

The general principles of postoperative care apply. In immunosuppressed or neutropenic patients, awareness of specific problems can pre-empt downstream complications of delayed wound healing. For example, vigilance and prompt attention to early wound infections may avoid the development of more severe surgical site infections. The concomitant use of corticosteroids with some chemotherapy regimens may lead to signs of adrenal insufficiency such as hypotension, myalgia/arthralgia, fever, electrolyte abnormalities, and eosinophilia, but current evidence does not support the routine use of prophylactic 'stress dose' steroids (Bromberg et al. 1995).

Short-term morbidity may be related to longer term outcomes, particularly if complications lead to delays in planned adjuvant therapy. Surveillance for delayed complications or disease recurrence can result in the earlier detection and management of problems.

Specific secondary cancers deserve special mention since awareness of the risk of radiation-associated cancers may facilitate earlier diagnosis (and subsequent earlier and appropriately aggressive surgical management). Radiation-associated solid organ cancers typically appear several years after exposure, ranging from 8 to 20 or more years later (Little 1993). Cervical and mediastinal radiation for head and neck cancers, medulloblastoma, or hematogenous malignancies can predispose to secondary thyroid malignancies, skin cancers, or sarcomas. The increasing use of breast conservation therapy, which includes breast radiation, is associated with soft tissue sarcomas, often aggressive angiosarcomas (Abbott & Palmieri 2008). Prior chemotherapy is not causally associated with secondary solid tumors.

SUMMARY

There are expanding indications for the use of radiation and chemotherapy in modern cancer care. The effects of multimodality treatment can complicate the role of surgical management, and due consideration to these effects must be made based on acuity and anatomic location in the context of careful preoperative planning and meticulous surgical technique and judgment.

REFERENCES

Abbott R, Palmieri C. Angiosarcoma of the breast following surgery and radiotherapy for breast cancer. Nat Clin Pract Oncol 2008; 5:727–736.

Anscher MS, Vujaskovic Z. Mechanisms and potential targets for prevention and treatment of normal tissue injury after radiation therapy. Semin Oncol 2005; 32:S86–S91.

Baniel J, Foster RS, Rowland RG, et al. Complications of post-chemotherapy retroperitoneal lymph node dissection. J Urol 1995; 153:976–980.

Baniel J, Sella A. Complications of retroperitoneal lymph node dissection in testicular cancer: primary and postchemotherapy. Semin Surg Oncol 1999; 17:263–267.

Bromberg JS, Baliga P, Cofer JB, et al. Stress steroids are not required for patients receiving a renal allograft and undergoing operation. J Am Coll Surg 1995; 180:532–536.

Burris HA, Hurtig J. Radiation recall with anticancer agents. Oncologist 2010; 15:1227–1237.

Chrouser KL, Leibovich BC, Sweat SD, et al. Urinary fistulas following external radiation or permanent brachytherapy for the treatment of prostate cancer. J Urol 2005; 173(6):1953–1957.

Davis AM, O'Sullivan B, Turcotte R, et al. Late radiation morbidity following randomization to preoperative versus postoperative radiotherapy in extremity soft tissue sarcoma. Radiother Oncol 2005; 75: 48–53.

Delanian S, Lefaix JL. The radiation-induced fibroatrophic process: therapeutic perspective via the antioxidant pathway. Radiother Oncol 2004; 73:119–131.

Evans JG, Spiess PE, Kamat AM, et al. Chylous ascites after post-chemotherapy retroperitoneal lymph node dissection: review of the M. D. Anderson experience. J Urol 2006; 176:1463–1467.

Galandiuk S, Jorden J, Mahid S, et al. The use of tissue flaps as an adjunct to pelvic surgery. Am J Surg 2005; 190:186–190.

Garg AK, Mai WY, McGary JE, et al. Radiation proctopathy in the treatment of prostate cancer. Int J Radiat Oncol Biol Phys 2006; 66:1294–1305.

Gokhale AS, Lavertu P. Surgical salvage after chemoradiation of head and neck cancer: complications and outcomes. Curr Oncol Rep 2001; 3:72–76.

Giuliano AE, Hunt KK, Ballman KV, et al. Axillary dissection vs no axillary dissection in women with invasive breast cancer and sentinel node metastasis: a randomized clinical trial. JAMA 2011; 305:569–575.

Kneuertz PJ, Maithel SK, Staley CA, Kooby DA. Chemotherapy-associated liver injury: impact on surgical management of colorectal cancer liver metastases. Ann Surg Oncol 2011; 18:181–190.

Kuban DA, Tucker SL, Dong L, et al. Long-term results of the M.D. Anderson randomized dose-escalation trial for prostate cancer. Int J Radiat Oncol Biol Phys 2008; 70:67–74.

Lane BR, Stein DE, Remzi FH, et al. Management of radiotherapy induced rectourethral fistula. J Urol 2006; 175:1382–1387.

Lavu H, Nowcid LJ, Klinge MJ, et al. Reoperative completion pancreatectomy for suspected malignant disease of the pancreas. J Surg Res 2011; 170:89–95.

Lin KY, Blechman AB, Brenin DR. Implant-based, two-stage breast reconstruction in the setting of radiation injury: an outcome study. Plas Recons Surg 2012; 129:817–823.

Little JB. Cellular, molecular, carcinogenic effects of radiation. Hematol Oncol Clin North Am 1993; 7:337–352.

Lopez-Beltran A, Luque RJ, Mazzucchelli R, et al. Changes produced in the urothelium by traditional and newer therapeutic procedures for bladder cancer. J Clin Pathol 2002; 55:641–647.

Moreira SG,Jr, Seigne JD, Ordorica RC, et al. Devastating complications after brachytherapy in the treatment of prostate adenocarcinoma. BJU Int 2004; 93:31–35.

Nguyen PL, Chen MH, D'Amico AV, et al. Magnetic resonance image-guided salvage brachytherapy after radiation in select men who initially presented with favorable-risk prostate cancer: a prospective phase 2 study. Cancer 2007; 110:1485–1492.

Nyam DC, Pemberton JH. Management of iatrogenic rectourethral fistula. Dis Colon Rectum 1999; 42:994–997.

O'Sullivan B, Davis AM, Turcotte R, et al. Preoperative versus postoperative radiotherapy in soft-tissue sarcoma of the limbs: a randomised trial. Lancet 2002; 359:2235–2241.

Polk HC Jr. Contributions of alimentary tract surgery to modern infection control. Am J Surg 1987; 153:2–8.

Randall ME, Filiaci VL, Muss H, et al. Randomized phase III trial of whole-abdominal irradiation versus doxorubicin and cisplatin chemotherapy in advanced endometrial carcinoma: a Gynecologic Oncology Group Study. J Clin Oncol 2006; 24:36–44.

Roach M. Reducing the toxicity associated with the use of radiotherapy in men with localized prostate cancer. Urol Clin North Am 2004; 31:353–366.

Rosenberg SA, Tepper J, Glatstein E, et al. The treatment of soft-tissue sarcomas of the extremities: prospective randomized evaluations of (1) limb-sparing surgery plus radiation therapy compared with amputation and (2) the role of adjuvant chemotherapy. Ann Surg 1982; 196:305–315.

Sauer R, Becker H, Hohenberger W, et al. Preoperative versus postoperative chemoradiotherapy for rectal cancer. N Engl J Med 2004; 351:1731–1740.

Spratt JS. Heinbecker P, Saltzstein SL. The influence of succinylsulfathiasole (sulfasuxidine) upon the response of canine small intestine to irradiation. Cancer 1961; 14:862–874.

Steyerberg EW, Keizer HJ, Fossa SD, et al. Prediction of residual retroperitoneal mass histology after chemotherapy for metastatic nonseminomatous germ cell tumor: multivariate analysis of individual patient data from six study groups. J Clin Oncol 1995; 13:1177–1187.

Tan CT, Meyer-Rochow GY, Sywak MS, et al. Reoperative adrenal surgery: lessons learnt. ANZ J Surg 2009; 79:371–377.

Theodorescu D, Gillenwater JY, Koutrouvelis PG. Prostatourethral-rectal fistula after prostate brachytherapy. Cancer 2000; 89:2085–2091.

Verrees JF, Fernandez-Trigo V, Sugarbaker PH. Rectal cancer recurrence after prior resection and radiotherapy: palliation following additional surgery. Int J Colorectal Dis 1996; 11:211–216.

Wallner K, Roy J, Harrison L. Dosimetry guidelines to minimize urethral and rectal morbidity following transperineal I-125 prostate brachytherapy. Int J Radiat Oncol Biol Phys 1995; 32:465–471.

Chapter 25 The approach to reoperations in the geriatric population

Paul J. Speicher, Sandhya A. Lagoo-Deenadayalan

INTRODUCTION

As our society continues to age, the incidence of elderly patients presenting with surgical diseases will continue increasing. Advances in surgical techniques and understanding of perioperative physiology have led to the conclusion that age alone is no longer a contraindication to most operative interventions. Because of this, the number of geriatric patients requiring abdominal operations, and consequently reoperations, is expected to continue to rise. While the natural tendency is often to frame the geriatric patient as simply an older adult, it is becoming more apparent that this subset of patients represents a unique population with specific requirements regarding diagnosis and management of surgical disease.

As patients age there is a functional decline in most organ systems, and comorbidities such as cardiovascular disease and chronic pulmonary disease are more common (Schwandner et al. 1999). Many important factors must be factored into the preoperative workup, intraoperative management, and postoperative care of the geriatric patient, particularly in the setting of prior abdominal surgeries. The goal of this chapter is to address the approach to the geriatric patient undergoing reoperative abdominal surgery, including an overview of common elective and emergent presentations, technical considerations, and appropriate perioperative management.

INCIDENCE

The past century has been witness to a progressive ageing of the population, with average life expectancy in the United States now estimated at 77.9 years according to recent reports (Arias 2001). It is predicted that this ongoing aging will lead to a disproportionately large increase in surgical disease burden, particularly for the general surgeon. As individuals age, the likelihood of developing cancers, diverticular disease, hernia, and other abdominal pathology increases. Somewhere between 36% and 60% of all general surgical procedures are currently performed on patients over the age of 65 (Etzioni et al. 2003, Lawrence et al. 2004). Similarly, as age increases so does the likelihood of need for emergency operations. Studies have demonstrated emergent operations are more common with advanced age, with >15% of all operations in the elderly being done on an emergent basis (Barlow et al. 1989, Keller et al. 1987).

PREOPERATIVE WORKUP

The preoperative approach to the geriatric surgical patient is of utmost importance, as it allows the surgeon to minimize risk while optimizing perioperative planning. A thorough history and physical examination is essential, particularly with respect to comorbid medical conditions and functional status. A detailed past surgical history must be obtained, focusing not only on the nature of past operations but also on the timing and indications. Similarly, the physical examination should not only focus on the standard neurologic, cardiopulmonary, and abdominal findings, but should also include a detailed examination of abdominal scars indicative of previous surgical procedures and/or trauma. If timing allows, such as in the case of scheduled procedures, obtaining past medical records is extremely important for operative planning. Prior operative reports are a critical component of the preoperative workup, as they can be used to guide not only surgical approach but also to anticipate findings in the operating room.

Two important factors that should always be assessed in the geriatric surgical patient are nutritional status and frailty index. Advanced age is associated with poor nutritional standing, with undernutrition being a largely unrecognized yet prevalent problem in the elderly (Forster & Gariballa 2005). Serum albumin, an important marker of nutritional status, has been shown to be protective against perioperative mortality (Huang et al. 2010). Additionally, a history of preoperative weight loss and weight extremes (BMI >30 or <18.5) is associated with increased postoperative complications (Collins et al. 1999, Hickman et al. 1980). Similarly, the concept of frailty, defined as 'a state of reduced physiologic reserve associated with increased susceptibility to disability' is important when assessing perioperative risk in the elderly (Buchner & Wagner 1992). While calculating an actual frailty index [such as the Canadian Study of Health and Aging Frailty Index (Farhat et al. 2012)] is generally not necessary, the surgeon must be conscious of the patient's overall physiologic reserve and tailor surgical planning appropriately.

Part of the perioperative workup should always include taking the time to fully understand patient wishes and attempting to manage expectations. Medical decision makers, including patients, their families, and their physicians, should be counseled preoperatively and be made aware of the specific risks involved for a patient's age, functional status, and previous operations. Even in the setting of emergency surgery, it is essential that adequate time be taken during the initial consultation and preoperative consent process to discuss these risks and to fully understand the patient's wishes.

Often overlooked risk factors include (Galandiuk and Polk (2009)):

- serum albumin <2 mg/dL
- white cell count >11,000mg/dL
- medications interfering with coagulation (patients may forget to disclose their use)
- impaired mobility, e.g. necessitating use of a wheelchair

Unfortunately, elderly patients often present with clinical presentations necessitating urgent operative intervention. While preoperative resuscitation is important in almost all situations, it is particularly important in the geriatric population. Aging is associated with declining physiologic reserves, and in situations of surgical stress or acute illness, these reserves may become inadequate. Studies have demonstrated that elderly patients undergoing emergent operations have significantly worse outcomes (Basili et al. 2008, Ong et al. 2008, Tan et al. 2006). As such, preoperative optimization by way of early and aggressive resuscitation, particularly in the case of reoperations, is essential. In most cases, timing of emergent surgical interventions in the elderly should be deferred long enough to establish a degree of resuscitation and adequate workup, but should not be delayed with unnecessary studies. As a general rule, early intervention is often favored over both immediate and delayed action.

Another common concern, often related to the urgency of an operation, is the degree to which preoperative imaging studies are warranted. In cases of frank peritonitis, obviously incarcerated and/or strangulated hernia, or other ominous physical findings, preoperative imaging may not be indicated. When the diagnosis is less clear, or in cases where the information gained from imaging studies will help guide operative decision making, particular concerns must be addressed in the elderly population. As patients age, renal function tends to diminish, and concern for nephrotoxicity from intravenous contrast is of great importance. In such situations, fluid resuscitation in an attempt to optimize volume status can help reduce the risk of contrast-induced nephropathy. Ultimately, the decision regarding whether to order preoperative imaging relies on a combination of surgeon experience, clinical severity, and patient presentation.

COMMON SITUATIONS FOR ELDERLY REOPERATIONS

While reoperations in the geriatric population can be related to nearly any clinical scenario, in our experience there are a number of situations that most commonly lead to repeat abdominal operations in older patients. These can be divided into the general categories of elective procedures in patients who have previously undergone multiple abdominal procedures, early bowel obstructions after abdominal surgery, planned second looks, emergent re-exploration, and staged approach to multiple surgical issues.

Early postoperative bowel obstruction can be a challenging situation for the general surgeon to manage. Distinguishing bowel obstruction from postoperative ileus can be difficult, but often presents as persistent nausea and vomiting with classic symptomatology of mechanical obstruction. The geriatric patient is no exception, although the clinical picture may be confounded by additional comorbidities. Furthermore, preoperative malnourishment is more likely to be a concern in this population, and may make a conservative 'watchful waiting' approach less desirable. In patients who are seriously malnourished, prolonged waiting may necessitate the use of total parenteral nutrition (TPN) for nutritional support. Unfortunately, this is not without risk. The surgeon must weigh the potential immediate risks of surgical intervention against the risks of TPN, including infections, hepatic dysfunction, and central venous catheter complications.

The value of diagnostic laparoscopy in these situations is often understated, as this often not only identifies the problem but can also be therapeutic. It is not uncommon for a small loop or knuckle of bowel to become adherent to a port site or mesh in the early postoperative period, leading to symptoms of mechanical obstruction. In our experience, this is most often seen following laparoscopic colorectal procedures and hernia repairs. By utilizing a minimally invasive laparoscopic approach, it is often possible to mobilize the adherent bowel, freeing the obstruction and speeding recovery. If no correctable pathology is identified, the morbidity of a negative diagnostic laparoscopy is generally small enough even in the elderly to justify its routine use in these situations (**Figure 25.1**).

A more urgent situation requiring repeat intervention is the presence of postoperative bleeding. While younger individuals can often be managed with close hemodynamic monitoring and resuscitation with fluids and blood products, the geriatric patient may be better served by early take back for surgical control of the bleeding. The significantly higher burden of cardiopulmonary comorbidities in the older patient population may make these patients less tolerant of hemorrhagic blood loss and large volume resuscitations. Rather than attempting lengthy supportive care with multiple transfusions, we often endorse early take back to the operating room for definitive control. That said, elderly patients are frequently on therapeutic anticoagulation for a number of reasons, including coronary stents, atrial fibrillation, and peripheral vascular disease, and therefore the importance of correcting coagulopathies cannot be overemphasized.

As mentioned earlier, advanced age is associated with a higher proportion of emergent surgical procedures. During the course of an exploratory laparotomy for urgent or emergent indications, concern for the viability of a portion of bowel may arise. While obviously necrotic or damaged portions of bowel should be managed at the time of the initial procedure, there are often segments of bowel that appear mottled, dusky, or otherwise ischemic. For these areas that are not frankly necrotic, it can be very helpful to defer definitive management until a subsequent early return to the operating room. By temporizing the problem with a 'damage control' approach, the initial procedure duration can be reduced, and the patient can be resuscitated sooner and often more effectively, usually in the intensive care setting. In the geriatric patient, it can be particularly difficult to predict the viability of compromised-appearing bowel, and returning for a second look in 24–48 hours allows for definitive management and appropriate resuscitation while potentially eliminating unnecessary or redundant procedures.

Whether emergent or planned, multiple surgical problems are often encountered in the course of an operation, particularly in the elderly population. When this is the case, proper preparation with respect to anticipated return for reoperation is essential. One such situation most commonly seen in our experience is the identification hernia in patients undergoing operations for other intra-abdominal processes. In such cases, it is often wise to defer definitive management of the hernia until a later date. The clean-contaminated nature of most of these cases would require the use of an absorbable mesh for hernia

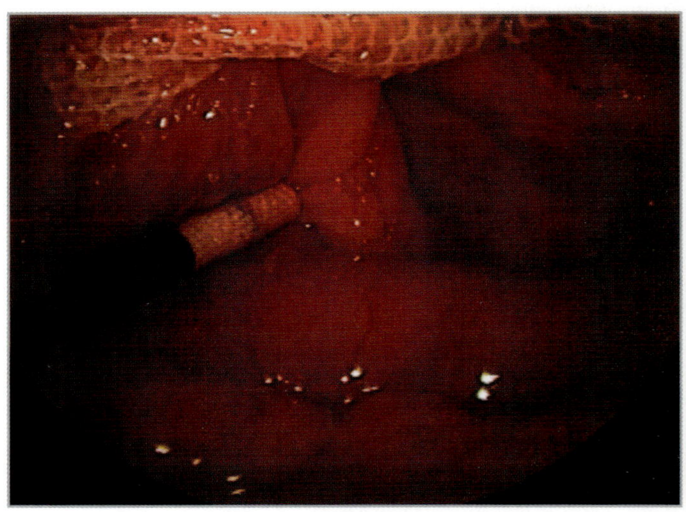

Figure 25.1 Examples of early postoperative adhesions. Note that a single knuckle of adherent bowel can often be the cause of early postoperative mechanical obstruction. In these cases, gentle laparoscopic mobilization of the adherent section of bowel can alleviate the obstruction with minimal morbidity.

repair at the time of the initial operation, as the risk of mesh infection and subsequent morbidity is too significant for permanent mesh repair. By addressing the primary issue and returning for a subsequent elective procedure, the surgeon gains the advantage of performing a more durable and permanent hernia repair using nonabsorbable mesh.

In contrast, there are times when the elderly patient has multiple surgical concerns that are identified preoperatively. This is commonly seen in patients undergoing gallbladder, upper GI, or colon surgery, and who also have a concomitant large ventral hernia in need of repair. The decision to do a staged operation is based on a number of factors. In such cases, it is often wise to take an approach similar to if the hernia was discovered incidentally in the operating room. This is particularly true if the surgeon prefers a laparoscopic approach for hernia repair, utilizing nonabsorbable mesh. In such situations, a staged approach is favored, and repair of the hernia should be deferred until a later date, allowing for the use of permanent mesh with significantly less concern for infection. In cases of smaller hernia, or if the repair is amenable to a bilateral separation of components, a primary repair or one utilizing only absorbable mesh can be considered.

Another rare but important situation is the elderly patient diagnosed with both colorectal cancer and an abdominal aortic aneurysm (AAA). If both colorectal resection and aneurysm repair are surgically indicated, the question arises as to the order in which to address these issues. If the colorectal cancer is managed first, there is a small but significant risk of life-threatening aneurysm rupture postoperatively (Baxter et al. 2002). If the aneurysm is addressed first, there can be a significant delay in treatment of the patient's colorectal cancer. There have been a few small studies focusing on patients in this situation, and it appears that in properly selected patients, it may be prudent and safe to attempt both procedures concomitantly (Baxter et al. 2002, Matsumoto et al. 2002). In all situations, the risk of repeat anesthesia in an older individual must be balanced against the risks of attempting multiple procedures during the same operation.

INTRAOPERATIVE CARE

In the elderly patient undergoing repeat surgery, two of the most important goals of intraoperative care are minimizing surgical stress and using the patient's past surgical history to assist in formulating a plan. Laparoscopic surgery has gained significant favor in the past decade as a means of limiting operative trauma; however, this comes at the expense of generally longer operative times (Panis 2000). While some studies have supported a laparoscopic approach in the elderly, the data are limited and no current guidelines exist (Grailey et al. 2012, Tan et al. 2010). The role of laparoscopy remains even less clear in the setting of prior related operations. Reoperative cases, by nature, involve the risk of significant adhesions and altered anatomy, which makes a laparoscopic approach potentially more challenging.

The approach to surgical access in an elderly patient undergoing redo operations depends on a number of factors, including prior surgeries, medical comorbidities, and the nature of the operation being undertaken. For patients undergoing redo abdominal operations, a thorough review of past operative records as well as abdominal scars is mandatory. If a laparoscopic approach is to be attempted, we recommend using the Veress needle technique. This can usually be done safely; however, feeding gastrostomy and jejunostomy tubes are not uncommon in the elderly population, and the presence of these can limit the traditional access approach in the left upper quadrant. In these situations, or in any situation where anticipated abnormalities or adhesions might interfere with needle placement, many surgeons find it safer instead of using the more direct Hasson technique. Ultimately, surgeon experience and comfort is probably the most important factor in deciding on a means of laparoscopically gaining entry to the redo geriatric abdomen. It cannot be overemphasized, however, that conversion to an open procedure should not be viewed as a failure, but rather as a natural progression of particular operations in order to achieve the best possible outcome for the patient.

Along similar lines, in patients with a history of multiple redo abdominal operations, it may be best to forgo any attempt at laparoscopic access and simply proceed with an exploratory laparotomy incision. The presence of significant adhesions or a so-called 'hostile' abdomen can render a laparoscopic approach too risky, particularly in older patients who might not tolerate the long operative times required for a laparoscopic lysis of adhesions. In such individuals, careful entry into the abdominal cavity via an open approach may allow for better visualization, shorter operative times, and less potential for undetected intraoperative injuries. This may be particularly true in patients who have previously undergone repair of large ventral hernia, and who might have a layer of incorporated mesh in their abdominal wall. In such cases, an open approach is typically favored, and the mesh should be transected along the surgical plane and then simply reapproximated normally upon closure of the abdomen, as the mesh has already been incorporated into its surrounding tissues.

Once surgical access is established and the problem of interest is solved, the surgeon should always evaluate for other coexisting problems. In patients who have had previous abdominal operations, it is important that other more rare problems be entertained, including obturator and femoral hernia, adhesive bands, and internal hernia. This is particularly relevant in older patients taken to the operating room without a specific diagnosis, such as the case with urgent or emergent exploratory operations, or in cases of small bowel obstruction.

SPECIFIC SITUATIONS

Hernia is a common problem in the elderly, likely a result of the reduced strength of the abdominal wall with age (Gianetta et al. 1997). As mentioned previously, in the case of redo ventral hernia repairs, the patient's past surgical history is of utmost importance. The approach should be guided by the location, size, and prior operative technique. If a separation of components has been previously attempted, a laparoscopic approach utilizing mesh should be entertained. In cases of inguinal hernia, there has been much debate regarding the proper approach to reoperations. Traditional teaching has generally recommended utilizing a surgical approach that avoids the scar-tissue plane from the previous operation. A number of randomized trials have examined the various techniques for reoperation of recurrent inguinal hernia, and a recent meta-analysis failed to demonstrate any significant difference among techniques in rates of re-recurrence or pain (Karthikesalingam et al. 2010). Despite this, our recommendation is to take an alternate approach as compared with the original repair technique: if the repair was originally done laparoscopically, we favor an open technique; if the original repair was done open, then laparoscopic approach should be considered. In the rare case of multiple failures, where both open and laparoscopic techniques have been utilized, an open preperitoneal approach may also be attempted.

In the setting of paraesophageal hernia repair, approximately 2–10% of patients will suffer from recurrent reflux symptoms, dysphagia, or discomfort (Ellis et al. 1996, Hatch et al. 2004). In the presence of such symptoms, redo repair may be indicated.

Recent studies have demonstrated that while reoperation for paraesophageal hernia recurrence is more expensive, challenging, and morbid as compared with primary repair, long-term results are good and usually lead to a significantly improved quality of life (Cowgill et al. 2007, Vignal et al. 2012). The major preoperative consideration in such cases is the determination of whether a repeat operation is likely to lead to improved quality of life and reduced symptom severity or frequency.

Similarly, in the elderly patient requiring repeat colorectal surgery, a number of important considerations must be addressed. In patients with a history of previous partial colectomy for any reason, it is often necessary to convert this to a total colectomy in recurrent cases requiring further resection. Additionally, particularly in elderly individuals undergoing emergent colon operations, the surgeon is faced with the decision on whether or not to create a proximal diverting ostomy. While there are certainly cases were this is mandated, and many where the indication is less strong, the nuances of this decision making are complex and a subject of much debate. In situations where there is concern for marginal bowel viability or frank ischemia, it can be prudent to fashion an end ileostomy for diversion, though this is often postponed until a second-look operation 24–48 hours later. It should also be noted that ostomy takedown is not without morbidity in and of itself, and appropriate planning must also be made for this type of procedure. Another important consideration when dealing with the elderly patient is baseline continence. That is, if the patient is known to be incontinent of stool at baseline, a diverting ostomy may be preferred. In all cases, because of the inevitable scar tissue that forms after initial pelvic surgery, ureteral stents should always be considered in repeat colorectal operations, as this can reduce operating times in a safe and reliable manner (Pokala et al. 2007).

POSTOPERATIVE MANAGEMENT

While a full discussion of postoperative management is well beyond the scope of this chapter, certain issues are particularly relevant to the geriatric population. Every reasonable attempt should be made to promote wound healing and prevent postoperative infections. Advanced age has been shown to be associated with higher rates of hospital-acquired infections, and a significant increase in associated mortality (Avci et al. 2012). Wounds should be assessed daily, as well as the need for all lines and urinary catheters.

Another important consideration in the geriatric patient is postoperative delirium, which affects somewhere between 37% and 74% of elderly patients (Dyer et al. 1995, Francis et al. 1990, Levkoff et al. 1992). A more recent study demonstrated that for elderly patients who are undergoing major abdominal surgery and are identified as high risk, the rate of postoperative delirium was 60%, with a mortality rate of 20% (Ganai et al. 2007). Care should be taken to minimize the likelihood of postoperative delirium in at-risk geriatric patients, defined as those with severe illness, visual impairment, cognitive impairment, or elevated BUN to creatinine ratio (Inouye et al. 1993). Some of the drugs that cause confusion are (Galandiuk and Polk 2009):

- Alcohol
- Alprazolam
- Diazepam
- Dilaudid
- Hydrocodone
- Meperidine
- Oxycodone
- Drugs associated with withdrawal symptoms

CONCLUSION

Improvements in medical practice and healthcare delivery have led to continued increases in life expectancy over the past half century, and individuals over the age of 65 remain the fastest growing section of our society. As our population continues to age, more and more patients will present with surgical disease, and an increasing number will have had previous operations. While the general attitude toward surgery in the elderly has changed in recent years with a shift toward more aggressive intervention, the approach to the geriatric patient undergoing repeat operation is somewhat unique. There must be strong emphasis placed both on preoperative resuscitation and optimization, as well as on a detailed surgical history and physical. With a better understanding of geriatric physiology and disease processes, surgeons will be able to optimize perioperative management and allow patients to make the most informed decisions possible.

REFERENCES

Arias E. United States life tables, 2007. Natl Vital Stat Rep 2011; 59:1–60.

Avci M, Ozgenc O, Coskuner SA, Olut AI. Hospital acquired infections (HAI) in the elderly: comparison with the younger patients. Arch Gerontol Geriatr 2012; 54:247–250, doi:10.1016/j.archger.2011.03.014.

Barlow AP, Zarifa Z, Shillito RG, et al. Surgery in a geriatric population. Ann R Coll Surg Engl 1989; 71:110–114.

Basili G, Lorenzetti L, Biondi G et al. Colorectal cancer in the elderly. Is there a role for safe and curative surgery? ANZ J Surg 2008; 78:466–470, doi:10.1111/j.1445-2197.2008.04536.x (2008).

Baxter NN, Noel AA, Cherry K, Wolff BG. Management of patients with colorectal cancer and concomitant abdominal aortic aneurysm. Dis Colon Rectum 2002; 45:165–170.

Buchner DM, Wagner EH. Preventing frail health. Clin Geriatr Med 1992; 8:1–17.

Collins TC, Daley J, Henderson WH, Khuri SF. Risk factors for prolonged length of stay after major elective surgery. Ann Surg 1999; 230:251–259.

Cowgill SM, Arnaoutakis D, Villadolid D, Rosemurgy AS. "Redo" fundoplications: satisfactory symptomatic outcomes with higher cost of care. J Surg Res 2007; 143:183–188, doi:10.1016/j.jss.2007.03.078.

Dyer CB, Ashton CM, Teasdale TA. Postoperative delirium. A review of 80 primary data-collection studies. Arch Intern Med 1995; 155:461–465.

Ellis FH, Jr., Gibb SP, Heatley GJ. Reoperation after failed antireflex surgery. Review of 101 cases. Eur J Cardiothorac Surg 1996; 10:225–231; discussion 222–231.

Etzioni DA, Liu JH, Maggard MA, Ko CY. The aging population and its impact on the surgery workforce. Ann Surg 2003; 238:170–177, doi:10.1097/01.SLA.0000081085.98792.3d.

Farhat JS, Velanovich V, Falvo AJ et al. Are the frail destined to fail? Frailty index as predictor of surgical morbidity and mortality in the elderly. J Trauma Acute Care Surg 2012; 72:1526–1530; discussion 1530-1521, doi:10.1097/TA.0b013e3182542fab.

Forster S, Gariballa S. Age as a determinant of nutritional status: a cross sectional study. Nutr J 2005; 4:28, doi:10.1186/1475-2891-4-28.

Francis J, Martin D, Kapoor WN. A prospective study of delirium in hospitalized elderly. JAMA 1990; 263:1097–1101.

Galandiuk S, Polk HC Jr. Surgical principles in the aged. In: Arenson C, et al. (eds), Reichel's care of the elderly: clinical aspects of aging, 6th edn. Cambridge: Cambridge University Press, 2009:442–446

Ganai S, Lee KF, Merrill A et al. Adverse outcomes of geriatric patients undergoing abdominal surgery who are at high risk for delirium. Arch Surg (Chicago, Ill:1960) 2007; 142:1072–1078, doi:10.1001/archsurg.142.11.1072.

Gianetta E, de Cian F, Cuneo S et al. Hernia repair in elderly patients. Br J Surg 1997; 84:983–985.

Grailey K, et al. Laparoscopic versus open colorectal resection in the elderly population. Surg Endosc 2012, doi:10.1007/s00464-012-2414-1.

Hatch KF, Daily MF, Christensen BJ, Glasgow RE. Failed fundoplications. Am J Surg 2004; 188:786–791, doi:10.1016/j.amjsurg.2004.08.062.

Hickman DM, Miller RA, Rombeau J L, Twomey P L, Frey CF. Serum albumin and body weight as predictors of postoperative course in colorectal cancer. JPEN. J Parenter Enteral Nutr 1980; 4:314–316.

Huang TS, Hu FC, Fan CW et al. A simple novel model to predict hospital mortality, surgical site infection, and pneumonia in elderly patients undergoing operation. Dig Surg 2010; 27:224–231, doi:10.1159/000274485.

Inouye SK, Viscoli CM, Horwitz RI, Hurst LD, Tinetti ME. A predictive model for delirium in hospitalized elderly medical patients based on admission characteristics. Ann Intern Med 1993; 119:474–481.

Keller SM, Markovitz LJ, Wilcer JR, Aufses AH, Jr. Emergency surgery in patients aged over 70 years. Mt Sinai J Med 1987; 54:25–28.

Levkoff SE, Evans DA, Liptzin B et al. Delirium. The occurrence and persistence of symptoms among elderly hospitalized patients. Arch Intern Med 1992; 152:334–340.

Lawrence VA, et al. Functional independence after major abdominal surgery in the elderly. J Am Coll Surg 2004; 199:762–772, doi:10.1016/j.jamcollsurg.2004.05.280.

Karthikesalingam A, Markar SR, Holt PJ, Praseedom RK. Meta-analysis of randomized controlled trials comparing laparoscopic with open mesh repair of recurrent inguinal hernia. Br J Surg 2010; 97:4–11, doi:10.1002/bjs.6902.

Matsumoto K, Murayama T, Nagasaki K, et al. One-stage surgical management of concomitant abdominal aortic aneurysm and gastric or colorectal cancer. World J Surg 2002; 26:434–437, doi:10.1007/s00268-001-0244-8.

Ong ES, Alassas M, Dunn KB, Rajput A. Colorectal cancer surgery in the elderly: acceptable morbidity? Am J Surg 2008; 195:344–348; discussion 348, doi:10.1016/j.amjsurg.2007.12.022.

Panis, Y. [Laparoscopic surgery for benign colorectal diseases]. J Chir (Paris) 2000; 137:261–267.

Pokala N, et al. A randomized controlled trial comparing simultaneous intra-operative vs sequential prophylactic ureteric catheter insertion in re-operative and complicated colorectal surgery. Int J Colorectal Dis 2004; 22:683–687, doi:10.1007/s00384-006-0219-1.

Schwandner O, Schiedeck TH, Bruch HP. Advanced age – indication or contraindication for laparoscopic colorectal surgery? Dis Colon Rectum 1999; 42:356–362.

Tan KY, Chen CM, Ng C, Tan SM, Tay KH. Which octogenarians do poorly after major open abdominal surgery in our Asian population? World J Surg 2006; 30:547–552, doi:10.1007/s00268-005-0224-5.

Tan KY, Konishi F, Tan L et al. Optimizing the management of elderly colorectal surgery patients. Surg Today 2010; 40:999–1010, doi:10.1007/s00595-010-4354-5.

Vignal JC, Luc G, Wagner T, Cunha AS, Collet D. Re-operation for failed gastro-esophageal fundoplication. What results to expect? J Visc Surg 2012; 149:e61–65, doi:10.1016/j.jviscsurg.2011.12.004.

Index

Note: Page numbers in **bold** or *italic* refer to tables or figures respectively.

A

AAA *see* Abdominal aortic aneurysm (AAA)
Abdomen
  burst 12–13
  open (*see* Open abdomen)
Abdominal abscess, postoperative 30–31, **31**, *31*, *32* *see also* Abdominal wall infection/intra-abdominal abscess
Abdominal aortic aneurysm (AAA) 185 *see also* Vascular surgery, reoperative
  endovascular repair of 85
    graft maldeployment **85**, *85*, 85–86
    graft thrombosis 86
    hemorrhage after 85
    infection after 86
  open surgical repair of 83
    anastomotic aneurysms after 83–84, *84*
    graft thrombosis after 84–85
    hemorrhage and 83
    infection and aortoenteric fistula 83, *84*
    ischemic colitis after 83
    reintervention for laparotomy-related complications 85
Abdominal colectomy with ileorectal anastomosis, for ulcerative colitis 167
Abdominal compartment syndrome (ACS) 37 *see also* Open abdomen
  damage control laparotomy and 37
  intra-abdominal hypertension and 38–39
  and reoperative surgery 11
Abdominal organ transplants 149 *see also* Transplantation, reoperations in
Abdominal wall infection/intra-abdominal abscess 29
  algorithm for selecting percutaneous *versus* reoperative drainage *32*
  infection, diagnosis of 30–32, **31**, *31*, 32
  intraoperative management 34–35
    antiseptic solution, use of 34
    culture material, collection of 34–35
    entering and draining abscess away from intestine 34
    patient positioning 34
    preoperative imaging studies, use of 34
    re-entry into abdomen through prior incision 34
    suture line leaks, management of 34
    temporary closure 35
  pathogenesis of 29–30, **30**, *30*
  postrelaparotomy management 35
    antibiotic management 35
    fever and leukocytosis 35
    mobilization of patient 35
    nutritional support 35
    open abdomen, management of 35
  preoperative preparation for relaparotomy 33–34
    antibiotics use 33
    central venous pressure (CVP) monitoring 33
    hemoglobin concentration 33
    intraoperative blood loss and 33
    intraoperative hypothermia and 34
    volume resuscitation 33
  recurrence after drainage of abscess 31, *32*
  timing of reoperation 32–33, **33**
Abdominal wall reconstruction, delayed *42*, 42–43
Acetaminophen, for postoperative pain 24
Achalasia, recurrent 55–56
Acidemia, in trauma patients 72
Acidosis after hemorrhagic shock 69
ACS *see* Abdominal compartment syndrome (ACS)
Activated clotting time (ACT) 67
Acute respiratory distress syndrome (ARDS) 62
Adhesion formation *see also* Intestinal/intra-abdominal adhesions
  abdominal surgery and 9, 51, 188
  antiadhesion agents 194
  clinical implications of 9
  and infertility in female patients 9, 10
  pathophysiology of 9–10, *10*
  prevention of 10–11
  time course of 10
Adhesion ileus 193
  recurrent 194
Adrenalectomy, cortical sparing 52
Adrenal mass, laparoscopic reoperation of 51–53, *52*, *53*
American Association for the Surgery of Trauma (AAST) 74
  colon injury scale 74, **74**
  liver injury scale 76, **76**
  pancreatic injury scale 75, **75**
  renal injury scale 80, **80**
  ureteral injury scale 78, **78**
Anastomotic aneurysms 83–84, *84*
Anastomotic leakage, and reoperative surgery 11, 12
Anesthetic management 19
  intraoperative
    anesthesia, type of 21
    fluid management 23
    glucose management 24
    normothermia 21–23, **22**, *23*
    supplemental oxygen 23–24
  postoperative
    nausea and vomiting, management of 25
    pain, management of 24
    respiratory management 25
  preoperative
    antibiotic prophylaxis 19–20
    antiplatelet therapy and stents 20, *20*
    beta-blockers and cardiac medications 19
    cardiovascular assessment 19
    obstructive sleep apnea 20–21
    respiratory assessment 20, **20**
    smoking cessation 21
    statin therapy 19
Angiography-based endovascular technique, for hemorrhage control 64
Antibiotic prophylaxis, in reoperative surgery 14, 19–20
Antiplatelet therapy, in perioperative period 20
Antireflux procedure, laparoscopic, reoperation after 55
Antireflux surgery, reoperative 55
Arctic Sun system 69
Argon beam coagulation, for diffuse capsular and parenchymal bleeding 66

B

Bair Hugger 69
Baori flap 78–79, *79*
Bariatric procedures, reoperative 109
  indications and types of **109**, 109–110
  LAGB related 113–114, **114**
    band erosion 115
    band prolapse *114*, 114–115
  management
    postoperative 117
    preoperative 116
  non-LAGB-related reoperations 110, **110**
    gastrogastric fistula *111*, 111–112
    internal herniation and small bowel obstruction 113, *113*
    leaks *112*, 112–113
    marginal ulceration 111, *111*
    reversal and conversion 110
    revisional 110–111
    stricture formation *111*, 111–112
  port-related 115
    megaesophagus 115–116, *116*
  preoperative considerations 116
  preoperative imaging 116
  procedure for 117
  prolonged surgery and consults 116
Barker's vacuum pack 41
Basal/bolus insulin (BBI) approach 24
Beta-blockers, in perioperative period 19
Bile peritonitis 139
Biliary strictures (BS) 125, 142

cause of 125
treatment of 126, *126*
Biliary tract surgery complications, reoperation for 137
bile duct injuries and 138–141, *140, 141*
biliary strictures and 142, *143*
cholecystectomy 137
gallbladder carcinoma and 142–143
postcholecystectomy syndrome and 144, *144*
postoperative care 142
and postoperative hemorrhage 142
preoperative imaging 138, *138*
preventive operative techniques 137–138
Biliopancreatic diversion and duodenal switch (BPD-DS) 109
Bioprosthetic meshes 42
Bleeding, postoperative 11, 56 *see also* Hemorrhage, postoperative
liver transplantation and 153
reasons for 11
reoperative surgery for 11, 63–64
Blood loss, intraoperative, in relaparotomy patient 33
Bogota bag 37
Bowel leakage and enterocutaneous fistula, postoperative 91
management of *92*, 92–93
presentation and diagnosis 91–92
Bowel leakage, reoperative surgery for 11–12
Bowel obstruction, small *see also* Small bowel obstruction (SBO)
acute 56–57
reoperative surgery for 51
Bowel perforations, and reoperative surgery 11
Bowel stoma *see* Intestinal stomas, reoperation for
Burr closure device 41
Burst abdomen, reoperative surgery for 12–13

C
Calot's triangle 137
Caput medusae, reoperation for 175
Carbapenem antibiotics 15
Cardiac arrhythmias, in trauma patients 72
Cardiac conditions, active 19
Cardiac medications, in perioperative period 19
Cardiovascular assessment, preoperative 19
Carotid artery stenting (CAS) 87
hemorrhage after 87
maldeployment 87
restenosis after 87–88
stroke after 87
Carotid endarterectomy (CEA) 86
hemorrhage after 86
infection after 87
restenosis following *86*, 87
stroke after 86–87
CAS *see* Carotid artery stenting (CAS)
CEA *see* Carotid endarterectomy (CEA)
Cellulose-based matrices 64
Central venous catheters 60–61
Chemotherapy-associated liver injury 130–131
Child–Pugh class 130
Chlorhexidine 34
Cholecystectomy *see* Biliary tract surgery complications, reoperation for
Choledocholithiasis 144–146, *145*
Cholelithiasis 137 *see also* Biliary tract surgery complications, reoperation for
Chylous ascites 199, *200*
Cirrhotic patients, reoperative liver resection in 130
Clostridium difficile infection 177
diagnosis of
colonoscopy 179, *179*
CT scan 178, *179*
laboratory tests 178
epidemiology 177
manifestations of 177
asymptomatic 177
C. difficile-associated diarrhea (CDAD) 177–178
C. difficile-associated enteritis 178
C. difficile-colitis (CDAC) 178
C. difficile fulminant colitis (CDFC) 178
pseudomembranous colitis 178, *178*
medical management 179
antibiotics 179, **180**
intravenous immunoglobulin (IVIG) 180
monoclonal antibodies 180
rectal stump management 181–182
intraperitoneal closure 182
mucous fistula 182
subcutaneous closure 182
risk factors **178**
surgical management 180–181
indications for 180, **180**
outcome of 181, **181**
postoperative care 181
Coagulopathy, in trauma patients 72
Colon and rectal cancer, recurrent, reoperative laparoscopy in 49–50
Colonoscopy 48
in clostridial colitis 179, *179*
Colon repair, in trauma patients 74–75
Colorectal cancer, metastatic, repeat hepatectomy for 129, 133, *133* *see also* Liver surgery, reoperative
Colostomy stenosis *172*, 172–173
Common bile duct (CBD) injuries 137 *see also* Biliary tract surgery complications, reoperation for
Components separation technique 42–43, 104–105
Computed tomography (CT)
abdominal abscess and 31, *31*
Clostridium difficile infection 178, *179*
for Crohn's disease 159
enterocutaneous fistula and 92
in liver transplantation 154
for recurrent hernia 96, *97*, 102
in redo abdominal vascular surgery 190
Convective air warming system 13
Corkscrew stomach 112
Crohn's disease, reoperation in 48–49, *49*, 58, 159
postoperative complications and
hemorrhage 160, 162
recurrence 162
septic complications 162
small bowel obstruction 162
preoperative evaluation and planning 159–160
strictureplasty techniques and 160
Finney strictureplasty *161*
Heineke–Mikulicz strictureplasty *160*
side-to-side isoperistaltic strictureplasty *161*

D
Damage control laparotomy 37
Damage control resuscitation 62
Damage control surgery 65–66
Decompressive laparotomy 39
Deep venous thrombophlebitis (DVT) 33
Dysphagia, after antireflux surgery 55

E
EAF *see* Enteroatmospheric fistula (EAF)
Elderly patients, reoperation in 205
colorectal surgery, considerations in 208
hernia repair, approach for 207
intraoperative care 207
paraesophageal hernia repair, considerations in 207–208
postoperative management 208
preoperative approach for 205–206
consultation and consent process 205
frailty index 205
history and physical examination 205
nutritional status 205
preoperative imaging studies 206
risk factors 205–206
situations for *206*, 206–207
Embolization, for hemorrhage control 64–65
Endograft, infection of 86
Endoleaks **85,** 85–86
Endoscopic nasopancreatic drainage (ENPD) 123
Endoscopic retrograde cholangiography (ERC) 154
Endoscopic retrograde cholangiopancreatography (ERCP) 76, 137
for biliary system 138, 139, *139*
in management of bile leak 139, *140*, 144
Endoscopic ultrasound (EUS) 53
Endovascular aneurysm repair (EVAR) 85 *see also* Abdominal aortic aneurysm (AAA)
End sigmoid colostomy 171
Enteroatmospheric fistula (EAF) 41, 91, 92–93
and catabolic black hole 43
deep 43
management of 43
and nutritional support 43
prevention of 43
superficial 43, 44
Enterocutaneous fistula 91
after appendectomy *49*
anastomotic leakage and 91 (*see also* Bowel leakage and enterocutaneous fistula, postoperative)
Enterostomal therapy 176
Enzyme-linked immunosorbent assay (ELISA) 178
Esophageal dilation 115
Esophagogastroduodenoscopy (EGD) 116
Euro-Collins solution (ECS) 152
EVAR *see* Endovascular aneurysm repair (EVAR)

F
False aneurysms 185–187, *187*, 191
Fibrin gel matrix 10
Finger adhesiolysis 47
Fistula-in-ano 165
Fistulography 92
FlowTrac 68
Fluid management, in perioperative period 23
Fluorodeoxyglucose positron emission tomography ((FDG-PET) 190
Fresh frozen plasma (FFP), in surgical/traumatic bleeding 61, **61**
Frozen abdomen 9, 41, 43, 64, 93

G
Gabapentin, for postoperative pain 24
Gallbladder carcinoma 142–143
Gallstones 137 *see also* Biliary tract surgery complications, reoperation for

Gastric repair, in trauma patients 74
Gastroduodenal artery 142
Gastroduodenal artery stump from pancreatic leakage and fistula, protection of 123, *124*
Gastrogastric fistula *111,* 111–112
Gastrografin, oral, in adhesive SBO 194
Gastrointestinal bleeding 67
Gastrointestinal (GI) endoscopy 63
Gelfoam 64
Gerota's fascia 79
Glucose management, in perioperative period 24
Graft thrombosis
  after EVAR 86
  after open AAA repair 84–85, 188
Graft-to-body weight ratio (GBWR) 151
Greater omentum graft 123, *124*
Groin hernia, reoperation for 95
  anatomical issues in 95–96, *96*
  hernia repair approach, historical perspective on 95, *95*
  history and physical examination in 95
  inguinodynia and 98, *98, 99*
  operation
    open and laparoscopic previous recurrences and 97–98
    previous laparoscopic recurrence and 97
    previous open inguinal hernia recurrence and 97
  postoperative care 98
  preoperative considerations, other 97
  preoperative imaging 96–97, *97*
  surgical considerations 97
  timing of 96

H
Hand-assisted laparoscopic surgery technique 47–48
  Crohn's disease and 49
Hartmann's procedure 50
  laparoscopic reversal of 50–51
Heaney technique 77
Hematoma, after carotid endarterectomy 86
Hemobezoars 113
Hemodynamic instability, and laparoscopy 57
Hemorrhage, postoperative 59
  carotid artery stenting and 87
  carotid endarterectomy and 86
  diagnostic evaluation and resuscitation
    initial evaluation and therapy 60–61, **61**
  diagnostic imaging in 63
  endovascular treatment of lower extremity occlusive disease and 88
  EVAR and 85
  initial diagnosis of
    clinical signs 60, **60**
    hypovolemia and 60, **60**
    patient's history in **59,** 59–60
  intervention for 63
    angiography and endovascular embolization 64–65
    reoperative surgery 63–64
  lower extremity bypass and 88
  open AAA repair and 83
  organ/disease-specific considerations
    elective procedures, damage control for 68
    gastrointestinal bleeding 67
    liver 66
    pancreas/duodenum 66–67
    pelvis 67
    spleen 66
    trauma/damage control surgery *65,* 65–66
    vascular procedures 67–68
  postintervention resuscitation and care 68–69
  resuscitation for hemorrhagic shock **61,** 61–63, *62*
Hepatectomy, repeat 132–133 *see also* Liver surgery, reoperative
Hepatic artery embolization 65, 66
Hepatic bleeding after surgery 66
Hepatic vascular isolation, total 132
Hepatobiliary iminodiacetic acid scan (HIDA) 144
Hepatobiliary scintigraphy 138
Hepatocellular carcinoma (HCC), repeat hepatectomy for 129, *132,* 132–133 *see also* Liver surgery, reoperative
HepaVision 154, *155*
Hiatal hernia, recurrent 55
Hippel–Lindau syndrome, recurrent pancreatic NET in 53–55, *54*
Histidine – tryptophan – ketoglutarate solution (HTK) 152
Human acellular dermal matrix (HADM) 102
Hypothermia
  in perioperative period **22,** 22–23, *23*
  in trauma patients 72
  treatment of 69
Hypovolemic shock 60, **60**

I
Ileal pouch advancement technique 163, *164*
Ileal pouch-anal anastomosis (IPAA) 159, 162 *see also* Ulcerative colitis, reoperation in
Ileal pouch enlargement techniques 165, *166–167*
Ileoanal pouch, creation of 48
Ileostomy stenosis 172, *172*
Incisional hernias
  abdominal CT scan 13, *13*
  in abdominal surgery 9
Inferior vena cava (IVC) 52
Inflammatory bowel disease, reoperation in 159
  considerations in
    intraoperative 160
    preoperative 159–160
  Crohn's disease 48–49, *49,* 159, 160–162
  postoperative complications after
    abdominal colectomy with ileorectal anastomosis 167
    proctocolectomy with permanent ileostomy 167
  small bowel adenocarcinoma and 162
  ulcerative colitis 48, 159, 162–166
Inguinodynia 98, *98, 99*
Inlay mesh, for defect reconstruction *14,* 14–15
Internal herniation (IH), gastric bypass procedure and 113
Intestinal/intra-abdominal adhesions 51, 193
  aortic surgery and 188
  laparoscopic management of 51
  and small bowel obstruction 193
Intestinal stomas, nonoperative treatment 175–176
Intestinal stomas, reoperation for 171
  acute stomal ischemia/necrosis *171,* 171–172
  caput medusae 175
  parastomal hernia 173, *174,* 175
  poorly sited/retracted stoma 173, *173*
  stomal stenosis *172,* 172–173
  stoma prolapse 173, *174*
Intra-abdominal hypertension (IAH) 38–39
Intra-abdominal pressure (IAP) 38, 57
Intraoperative cholangiography (IOC) 137–138
Intravenous immunoglobulin (IVIG) 180
Ioban, sheets of 65
Ischemia, and stoma complications 171

K
Ketamine, for postoperative pain 24
Kidney, repair of, in trauma patients 79–80, **80**
Kidney transplants, reoperations in 151 *see also* Transplantation, reoperations in
Kocher maneuver 80

L
Lactated ringers solution 60
Laparoscopic adhesiolysis 51, 56, 195
Laparoscopic adjustable gastric banding (LAGB) 109 *see also* Bariatric procedures, reoperative
Laparoscopic adrenalectomy, primary adrenal tumors 51
Laparoscopic argon beam coagulator 53
Laparoscopic foregut surgery, reoperative 55
Laparoscopic sleeve gastrectomy (LSG) 109 *see also* Bariatric procedures, reoperative
Laparoscopic sleeve gastrectomy leak 112, *112*
Laparoscopic ultrasound, in laparoscopic ultrasound 53–54
Laparotomy, trauma 71–72
Lesser sac 34
LiDCO 68
LigaSure device 66
Limb thrombosis 86
Live donation 156
Liver injuries, repair of, in trauma patients **76,** 76–77
Liver surgery, reoperative 129
  anatomical challenges in *129*
  anesthesia 131
  bleeding in, limiting of 131–132
  indications for 130
  laparoscopic repeat hepatic resection 133, *134*
  operative planning 130
    chemotherapy-associated liver injury 130–131
    extent of resection 130
    liver cirrhosis 130
    preoperative portal vein embolization 130
  patient positioning and incisions 131, *131*
  preoperative imaging 131
  repeat hepatectomy 132
    for metastatic colorectal cancer 133, *133*
    for recurrent hepatocellular carcinoma *132,* 132–133
  segmental liver anatomy and *129*
Liver transplantation 149–151 *see also* Transplantation, reoperations in
Loop stoma 40
Lower extremity occlusive disease 88
  lower extremity bypass
    and graft infection 88
    graft occlusion and restenosis 88, **88**
    hemorrhage after 88
  percutaneous endovascular intervention
    arterial embolization and occlusion 88–89
    hemorrhage 88
    restenosis after 89

M
Magnetic resonance imaging (MRI) 13, 52, 96, 159
Maldeployment, endograft 85
Malignant bowel obstruction (MBO) 195

Massive transfusion protocol (MTP) 62
Megaesophagus 115–116, *116*
Mesh, 39
biologic 102
composite 102
heavyweight polypropylene 102
infection 101
lightweight 102
multifiber 102
preperitoneal placement of 104, *105*
for recurrent hernia repair 101–102
synthetic 102
synthetic *versus* biologic 102
Methicillin-resistant *Staphylococcus aureus* (MRSA) 33
Methylene blue 74
Microembolization 89
Minigastric bypass procedures 110
MR cholangiopancreatography, abdominal 138
MR enterography (MRE), for Crohn's disease 159
Mucocutaneous separations 176
Myocutaneous flaps, for perineal space 167

N
Nasogastric tube, postoperative 15
Necrosis of colostomy 171, *171*
Negative pressure sponge technique 41
Neuroendocrine tumor (NET), pancreatic 53–55, *54*
Noninvasive positive pressure ventilation 25
Nonsteroidal antiinflammatory drugs (NSAIDs), for postoperative pain 24
Normothermia, in perioperative period 21–23, **22,** *23*

O
Obstructive sleep apnea (OSA), perioperative management 20–21, 25
Omentum 9
Open abdomen 37
abdominal compartment syndrome and 38–39
in abdominal infection 38
care of *39,* 39–40
closure of 41–42
delayed abdominal wall reconstruction, options for *42,* 42–43
and enteroatmospheric fistula 43–44
healing process of 40
indications for 37–38
planned ventral hernia approach *40,* 40–41
Opiate therapy, for postoperative pain 24

P
Packed red blood cells (pRBC), in surgical/traumatic bleeding 61, **61**
Packs, removal of 73
Pain, postoperative, management of 24
Pancreas/duodenum operations, and postoperative bleeding 66–67
Pancreas transplants, reoperations in 151 *see also* Transplantation, reoperations in
Pancreatic fistula, postoperative 55
Pancreatic injuries, repair of, in trauma patients **75,** 75–76
Pancreatic surgery complications, reoperations for 121
biliary stricture 125–126 (*see also* Biliary strictures (BS))
case example 126–127
postpancreatectomy hemorrhage 121–125 (*see also* Postpancreatectomy hemorrhage (PPH))
Pancreatic tumors, laparoscopic reoperation of 53–55, *54*
Pancreatitis, and reoperative surgery 11
Pancreatoduodenectomy (PD), two-stage 123, *124*
Panniculectomy, with ventral hernia repair 106
Para-anastomotic aneurysms 185–187, *186,* 191
Parastomal hernia, reoperation for 173, *174,* 175
Parkland/Harborview 'vac-pack' closure 65, *65*
Pelvic sinus 162
Pelvic surgery/fracture, and hemorrhage 67
Percutaneous coronary intervention (PCI), prior 20, *20*
Percutaneous transhepatic cholangiography (PTC) 138, *138*
Perifascial space 29, *30* *see also* Abdominal wall infection/intra-abdominal abscess
Perineal wound, nonhealing of 167
Peristomal hernias 173
Piggyback technique 150, *150*
Pinch test 41
Pneumatic compression devices 69
Portal hypertension 130
Portal vein embolization (PVE) 129, 130
Portocaval plane 130
Positron emission tomography (PET), in resection for metastatic liver tumors 131
Postoperative nausea and vomiting (PONV), management of 25
Postpancreatectomy hemorrhage (PPH) 121
cause of 121
continuous irrigation methods 124–125, *125*
definition of 121–122
delayed *123*
early 122, *122*
preoperative imaging 122
prevention of 123–125
sites of 121, *122*
timing of reoperation 122–123
type of operation for 123
Pouch-cutaneous fistula 163
Pouchitis 165
Pouch-vaginal fistula 165
PPH *see* Postpancreatectomy hemorrhage (PPH)
Pregabalin, for postoperative pain 24
Primary graft failure (PGF) 152
Pringle maneuver 66, 76, 132
Prolapse of end ileostomy 173, *174*
Pseudomembranous colitis 178, *178*
Psoas hitch 79, *79*
Pulmonary artery catheters (PACs) 68–69
Pulmonary embolism (PE) 33
Pyoderma 176

R
Radiation and chemotherapy complications, and surgical management 197
breast cancer and 201
chemotherapy 198
conduct of operation 202
gastrointestinal cancers and 198
head and neck cancers and 201
pelvic surgery and 198–199
postoperative care 202–203
preoperative planning 201–202
prostate cancer and 200–201, *201*
radiation therapy, toxicity from 197–198, *198*
soft tissue sarcoma and 199, *199*
testes cancer and 199–200, *200*
Recombinant factor VII (rVIIa) 62
Rectal injuries, repair of, in trauma patients 75
Rectourethral fistulas (RUF) 201, 202
Regional anesthesia, cancer recurrence rates and 21
Renal vein, left 189, *189*
Reoperative laparoscopy 47
achalasia and 55–56
adhesive acute small bowel obstruction 56–57
adrenal tumors, recurrent 51–53, *52, 53*
antireflux procedure and 55
contraindications to 57
Crohn's disease and 48–49, *49*
emergency 56
general principles 47
hand port, use of 47–48
history examination 47
patient positioning and room setup 47
port placement 47
previous operations, information about 47
Hartmann's procedure, laparoscopic reversal of 50–51
hiatal hernia, recurrent 55
pancreatic neuroendocrine tumors, recurrent 53–55, *54*
for recurrent colon cancer 49–50
results of 57–58
small bowel obstruction and abdominal adhesions, recurrent 51
ulcerative colitis and 48
Reoperative surgery 1–2, 9
acute 3
adhesion formation 9
pathophysiology 9–10, *10*
prophylaxis 10
time course 10–11
anatomical issues in 9
clinical judgment in, importance of 3
complication rates from 3
conduct of operation 14–15
abdominal wall closure 14
adhesiolysis 14
antibiotic prophylaxis 14
choice of incision 14
defect reconstruction *14,* 14–15
drain placement 14
emergency 11–13
anastomotic leakage 12, *12*
bile duct anastomosis leakage 12
bowel leakage 11–12
burst abdomen 12–13
colon/small bowel leaks 12
pancreatic leakage and fistula 12
postoperative bleeding 11
indications for 11
and informed consent 4
defenses to informed consent claim 6–7
requirements 4
standards 4–6, **5–6**
long operation time and blood loss 13
medical ethics in, principles of 4
patient positioning 14
planned secondary reconstruction 13
postoperative principles 15
antibiotic therapy 15
laparostoma care 15, *15*
nutrition 15
wound management 15
preoperative imaging 13, *13*
remote occurrence 3
timing of 11
Respiratory assessment, preoperative 20, **20**
Resuscitation, for hemorrhagic shock 61–63, *62*

Retransplantation 153
Retroperitoneal lymph node dissection (RPLND), postchemotherapy 199
The Rives-Stoppa technique, for open ventral hernia repair 104
Round ligament of liver 130
Roux-en-Y gastric bypass (RYGB) 109 *see also* Bariatric procedures, reoperative
Roux-en-Y gastric bypass leak 112, *112*
Roux-en-Y hepaticojejunostomy 139, *141*

S
Seprafilm 163, 194
Sequential compression devices 33
Seromas, postoperative, prevention of 106
Sleeve pouchectomy 165
Small bowel obstruction (SBO)
  in Crohn's disease 162
  gastric bypass procedure and 113
  recurrent adhesive SBO 193
    laparoscopy, role of 195
    laparoscopy *versus* laparotomy in 195
    malignant bowel obstruction 195
    recurrent adhesion ileus, reoperation in 194
Small bowel repair, in trauma patients 74
Smoking, cessation of 21
Somatostatin analog 53
Splenectomy, and hemorrhage 66
Splenic artery embolization 66
Staged laparotomy, for trauma 71
Staphylococcus epidermidis 187
Statins, in perioperative period 19
Stoma, bowel *see* Intestinal stomas, reoperation for
Strasberg classification, of bile duct injuries 138
Stricture formation, after bariatric surgery 112
Strictureplasties, for Crohn's disease 160
  Finney strictureplasty *161*
  Heineke–Mikulicz strictureplasty *160*
  side-to-side isoperistaltic strictureplasty *161*
Stroke, after carotid artery stenting 87
Supplemental oxygen, perioperative 23–24
Surgical and Clinical Adhesions Research Group (SCAR), on intra-abdominal adhesions 193
Surgical site infections (SSI)
  antibiotic prophylaxis and 20
  in hernia patients 106
  hypothermia and 22

T
Talc (magnesium silicate hydroxide) 106
TcdA 177
TcdB 177
Thromboelastography (TEG) 62, *62*
Tissue expanders 43
Tissue hypoperfusion 197
Total parenteral nutrition (TPN) 15, 91, 92
Tranexamic acid (TXA) 62
Trans-femoral balloon catheter, IVC 52, *52*
Transplantation, reoperations in 149
  anatomical and physiological issues in 149
  causes for 149
  conduct of 155
  donor reoperations 154
  indication for 153
  kidney and pancreas 151
  liver 149
    arterial revascularization 150
    partial liver grafts *150,* 150–151, **151**
    portal venous revascularization 149
    venous outflow 149–150, *150*
  long case and need for consultants 154–155
  preoperative imaging 154, *155*
  recipient reoperations 154
  timing of 151
    bleeding 151–152
    drainage and leakage 152
    graft loss and retransplantation 153
    infections 153
    initial graft dysfunction 152
    intestinal obstructions 153
    persistent graft dysfunction 152
    primary graft failure 152
    vascular stenosis occlusion 152
Transuretero-ureterostomy 78
Trauma, reoperative surgery in 71
  acidemia in 72
  coagulopathy in 72
  gastrointestinal injuries and
    colonic repair **74**, 74–75
    gastric repair 74
    rectal repair 75
    small bowel repair 74
  hypothermia in 72
  laparotomy 71–72
  liver injuries and 76–77
  pancreatic injuries and **75,** 75–76
  physiological resuscitation in ICU 72–73
  preoperative check list 73
  reconstructive work 73–74
  re-exploration 73
  reoperation, planned 73
  staged surgery 71
  urinary reconstruction
    kidney repair 79–80, *80*
    ureter repair **78**, *78,* 78–79, *79*
'Triad of death' 71, 72

U
Ulcerative colitis, reoperation in 48, 159, 162
  postoperative complications and
    abdominal colectomy with ileostomy and closure of rectal stump and 163
    anastomotic dehiscence and pelvic sepsis 163
    anastomotic stenosis 163, *164*
    bowel obstruction 162, 163
    chronic pouchitis 165
    Crohn's features in pouches 165
    fistula-in-ano 165
    pouch-cutaneous fistula 163
    pouch failure 166
    pouch-vaginal fistula 165
    pouch with insufficient capacity 165, *166–167*
    pouch with large capacity 165
  recurrence and 167
Ureteral injuries, repair of, in trauma patients **78,** *78,* 78–79, *79*
Ureteral stents 50
Uretero-uretostomy 78, **78,** *78*

V
Vacuum-assisted laparostoma treatment 15, *15*
Vacuum-assisted wound management 41
Vacuum pack dressing 39, *39*
Vancomycin 33, 179, *180*
Vascular procedures, postoperative bleeding after 67–68
Vascular surgery, reoperative 83, 185
  abdominal aortic aneurysm 83–86
  anatomical issues in
    intestinal adhesions 188
    renal arteries, proximity to 188–189, *189*
    ureters, proximity of 189
  carotid artery stenosis 86–88 (*see also* Carotid artery stenting (CAS); Carotid endarterectomy (CEA))
  conduct of
    aortic stent/graft thrombosis and 191
    infection and 191
    para-anastomotic and false aneurysms 191
    patient positioning 191
  intraoperative hemorrhage, risk of 190–191
  lower extremity occlusive disease 88–89
  need for 185, *186*
    false aneurysms 185, 187, *187*
    graft infection and aortoenteric fistula *187,* 187–188
    graft thrombosis 188
    late AAA rupture risk 187
    para-anastomotic aneurysms 185, *186*
  postoperative care 192
  preoperative imaging 190, *190*
  timing of 189–190
Vasopressin 162
Vasopressive agents 69
Vena cava filter, prior to relaparotomy 33
Venous thromboembolism (VTE) 69
Ventral hernia, planned *40,* 40–41
Ventral hernias, recurrent 101
  components separation 104, 106
  drains, placement of 106
  hernia recurrence, reasons for 101
  laparoscopic repair 103, *103*
  mesh for repair of 101–102, **102**
  open repair 104, *105*
  panniculectomy 106
  postoperative complications and treatment 106
  preoperative care and imaging 102–103
  seroma formation, prevention of 106
Ventral Hernia Working Group (VHWG), grading system for ventral incisional hernias 102, **102**
Visceral vessel grafts 188
Vitamin K 33

W
Water-based thermo-wrap system 13
Wound management 15